DECISION MAKING IN
Pediatric Ophthalmology

Clinical Decision Making™ Series

Berman:
Pediatric Decision Making
Bready, Smith:
Decision Making in Anesthesiology
Bucholz, Lippert, Wenger, Ezaki:
Orthopaedic Decision Making
Callaham, Barton, Schumaker:
Decision Making in Emergency Medicine
Cibis, Tongue, Stass-Isern:
Decision Making in Pediatric Ophthalmology
Cohn, Doty, McElvein:
Decision Making in Cardiothoracic Surgery
DeCherney, Polan, Lee, Boyers:
Decision Making in Infertility
Greene, Johnson, Maricic:
Decision Making in Medicine
Karlinsky, Lau, Goldstein:
Decision Making in Pulmonary Medicine
Korones, Bada-Ellzey:
Neonatal Decision Making
Levine:
Decision Making in Gastroenterology
Marsh:
Decision Making in Plastic Surgery
Nichols, Hyslop, Bartlett:
Decision Making in Surgical Sepsis
Ramamurthy, Rogers:
Decision Making in Pain Management
Resnick, Caldamone, Spirnak:
Decision Making in Urology
Schein:
Decision Making in Oncology
van Heuven, Zwaan:
Decision Making in Ophthalmology
Weisberg, Strub, Garcia:
Decision Making in Adult Neurology

DECISION MAKING IN

Pediatric Ophthalmology

Gerhard W. Cibis, M.D.

Associate Clinical Professor of Ophthalmology
University of Missouri—Kansas City School of Medicine
Chief of Ophthalmology
The Children's Mercy Hospital
Kansas City, Missouri

Andrea Cibis Tongue, M.D.

Clinical Associate Professor of Ophthalmology
Oregon Health Sciences University School of Medicine
Portland, Oregon

Merrill L. Stass-Isern, M.D.

Clinical Assistant Professor of Ophthalmology
University of Missouri—Kansas City School of Medicine
Clinical Assistant Professor of Medicine
Department of Ophthalmology
The Children's Mercy Hospital
Kansas City, Missouri

B. C. Decker
An imprint of Mosby–Year Book

Mosby
Dedicated to Publishing Excellence

BC Decker

Publisher: George Stamathis
Editor: Susan M. Gay
Editorial Assistant: Cecelia H. Bayruns
Project Manager: Victoria Hoenigke

Printed in the United States of America.

Mosby–Year Book, Inc.
11830 Westline Industrial Drive
St. Louis, Missouri 63146

NOTICE
The authors and publisher have made every effort to ensure that the patient care recommended herein, including choice of drugs and drug dosages, is in accord with the accepted standards and practice at the time of publication. However, since research and regulation constantly change clinical standards, the reader is urged to check the product information sheet included in the package of each drug, which includes recommended doses, warnings, and contraindications. This is particularly important with new or infrequently used drugs.

ISBN 1-5566-4296-2

92 93 94 95 96 CL/MY 9 8 7 6 5 4 3 2 1

CONTRIBUTORS

JOHN D. BAKER, M.D.

Clinical Associate Professor of Ophthalmology, Wayne State University School of Medicine; Co-Chief, Department of Ophthalmology, Children's Hospital of Michigan, Detroit, Michigan

HOLLY L. BARBOUR, M.D.

Clinical Fellow, Oculoplastic, Orbital and Lacrimal Surgery, Ophthalmic Oncology, Duke University Eye Center, Durham, North Carolina

CRISTIE BECKER, M.D.

Instructor, Department of Radiology, Wayne State University School of Medicine; Director, Pediatric Neuroradiology, Children's Hospital of Michigan, Detroit, Michigan

MICHAEL L. BEGLEITER, M.S.

Instructor in Medicine, University of Missouri—Kansas City School of Medicine; Genetic Counselor, The Children's Mercy Hospital, Kansas City, Missouri

FREDERICK C. BLODI, M.D.

Professor (Emeritus) of Ophthalmology, University of Iowa College of Medicine, Iowa City, Iowa

ROY D. BROD, M.D.

Assistant Professor of Ophthalmology, Jefferson Medical College of Thomas Jefferson University, Philadelphia, Pennsylvania; Clinical Assistant Professor of Ophthalmology, Pennsylvania State University School of Medicine, Hershey, Pennsylvania

DAVID M. BROWN, M.D.

Associate Ophthalmologist, Department of Ophthalmology, University of Iowa Hospitals and Clinics, Iowa City, Iowa

YVONNE J. BRYSON, M.D.

Professor of Pediatrics, Division of Infectious Diseases, Department of Pediatrics, University of California, Los Angeles, UCLA School of Medicine, Los Angeles, California

EDWARD G. BUCKLEY, M.D.

Associate Professor of Ophthalmology, and Assistant Professor of Pediatrics, Duke University Eye Center, Durham, North Carolina

J. RAYMOND BUNCIC, M.D., FRCS (C)

Associate Professor of Ophthalmology, University of Toronto Faculty of Medicine; Ophthalmologist-in-Chief, The Hospital for Sick Children, Toronto, Ontario, Canada

JOHN P. BURKE, M.D., FRCS

Senior Registrar, Department of Ophthalmology, University of Sheffield, England

DONNA BURROWS, M.D.

Resident in Ophthalmology, University of Texas Health Science Center, Houston, Texas

JOSEPH H. CALHOUN, M.D.

Clinical Professor of Ophthalmology, Jefferson Medical College of Thomas Jefferson University; Director, Pediatric Ophthalmology and Strabismus, Wills Eye Hospital, Philadelphia, Pennsylvania

TIMOTHY B. CAVANAUGH, M.D.

Clinical Instructor, Department of Ophthalmology, University of Kansas School of Medicine, Kansas City, Kansas

HONG-MING CHENG, O.D., PH.D.

Associate Professor of Ophthalmology, Harvard Medical School, Boston, Massachusetts

COLLEEN J. CHRISTIAN, M.D.

Clinical Associate, Department of Ophthalmology, Jefferson Medical College of Thomas Jefferson University; Instructor, Department of Pediatric Ophthalmology, Wills Eye Hospital; Associate Surgeon, Children's Hospital of Philadelphia, Philadelphia, Pennsylvania

GERHARD W. CIBIS, M.D.

Associate Clinical Professor of Ophthalmology, University of Missouri–Kansas City School of Medicine; Chief of Ophthalmology, The Children's Mercy Hospital, Eye Foundation, Kansas City, Missouri

THOMAS B. CONNOR, JR., M.D.

Assistant Chief of Service, Wilmer Ophthalmological Institute, The Johns Hopkins Hospital, Baltimore, Maryland

DONNELL J. CREEL, PH.D.

Research Professor, Department of Ophthalmology, University of Utah School of Medicine; Research Career Scientist, Veterans Administration Medical Center, Salt Lake City, Utah

EARL R. CROUCH, JR., M.D.

Professor of Ophthalmology, Chairman, Department of Ophthalmology, and Associate Professor of Pediatrics, Eastern Virginia Medical School of the Medical College of Hampton Roads; Surgical Director, Department of Ophthalmology, Children's Hospital of the King's Daughter, Norfolk, Virginia

OSCAR A. CRUZ, M.D.

Assistant Professor of Ophthalmology, Bethesda Eye Institute, Saint Louis University School of Medicine, Saint Louis, Missouri

SUSAN H. DAY, M.D.

Consultant in Pediatric Ophthalmology and Strabismus, California Pacific Medical Center, San Francisco, California

LUIS C. F. DE SA, M.D.

Consultant, Department of Ophthalmology, University of São Paulo, São Paulo, Brazil

MONTE A. Del MONTE, M.D.

Skillman Professor of Pediatric Ophthalmology, University of Michigan Medical School; Director of Pediatric Ophthalmology and Strabismus, C. S. Mott Children's Hospital and W. K. Kellogg Eye Center, University of Michigan Medical Center, Ann Arbor, Michigan

ARLENE V. DRACK, M.D.

Associate Pediatric Ophthalmology Service, University of Iowa Hospitals and Clinics, Iowa City, Iowa

DANIEL S. DURRIE, M.D.

Clinical Associate Professor, Department of Ophthalmology, University of Nebraska Medical Center, Omaha, Nebraska; Director, Refractive Service, Hunkeler Eye Clinic, Kansas City, Missouri

JONATHAN J. DUTTON, M.D., Ph.D.

Associate Professor, Oculoplastic, Orbital and Lacrimal Surgery, Ophthalmic Oncology, Duke University Eye Center, Durham, North Carolina

FORREST D. ELLIS, M.D.

Professor Ophthalmology, Indiana University School of Medicine, Indianapolis, Indiana

KATHLEEN FITZGERALD, R EP T

Technical Director, Vision Sciences Laboratory, Section of Ophthalmology, University of Missouri–Kansas City, Kansas City, Missouri

DONALD C. FLETCHER, M.D.

Assistant Professor, and Medical Director, Low Vision Rehabilitation Program, Department of Ophthalmology, University of Missouri–Kansas City School of Medicine, Kansas City, Missouri

HARRY W. FLYNN, Jr., M.D.

Associate Professor of Ophthalmology, Bascom Palmer Eye Institute, University of Miami School of Medicine, Miami, Florida

JOHN T. FLYNN, M.D.

Professor of Ophthalmology, Bascom Palmer Eye Institute, University of Miami School of Medicine, Miami, Florida

BENJAMIN M. FRISHBERG, M.D.

Clinical Instructor in Neurology, George Washington University School of Medicine and Health Sciences, Washington, District of Columbia

CONRAD L. GILES, M.D.

Clinical Professor of Ophthalmology, Kresge Eye Institute, Wayne State University School of Medicine, Detroit, Michigan

WILLIAM A. GODFREY, M.D.

Professor of Ophthalmology, University of Kansas School of Medicine, Kansas City, Kansas

WILLIAM V. GOOD, M.D.

Assistant Professor of Ophthalmology, and Director of Residency and Medical Student Education, University of California, San Francisco, School of Medicine, San Francisco, California

MARK J. GREENWALD, M.D.

Associate Professor of Clinical Ophthalmology, Northwestern University Medical School; Head, Division of Ophthalmology, Children's Memorial Hospital, Chicago, Illinois

TRUDI R. GRIN, M.D.

Clinical Assistant Professor of Ophthalmology, University of Missouri–Kansas City School of Medicine; Clinical Assistant Professor of Medicine, The Children's Mercy Hospital, Kansas City, Missouri

BARRETT G. HAIK, M.D.

Professor of Ophthalmology, and Clinical Professor of Pediatrics, Tulane University School of Medicine; Director, Tulane University Medical Center Ophthalmic Oncology and Orbital Disease Service, New Orleans, Louisiana

DAVID J. HARRIS, M.D.

Professor of Pediatrics and Biological Science, University of Missouri–Kansas City School of Medicine; Chief, Section of Genetics, The Children's Mercy Hospital, Kansas City, Missouri

BARBARA K. HECHT, Ph.D.

Jacksonville, Florida.

FREDERICK HECHT, M.D.

President, Hecht Associates, Inc., Jacksonville, Florida; Visiting Professor, Department of Cytogenetics and Molecular Genetics, Adelaide Children's Hospital, Adelaide, South Australia; Professor of Medicine, Faculté de Medecine, Nice, France

JOHN R. HECKENLIVELY, M.D.

Professor of Ophthalmology, University of California, Los Angeles, UCLA School of Medicine, Los Angeles, California

EUGENE M. HELVESTON, M.D.

Professor of Ophthalmology, and Chief, Section of Pediatric Ophthalmology, Indiana University School of Medicine, Indianapolis, Indiana

RICHARD W. HERTLE, M.D.

Assistant Professor of Ophthalmology, Division of Pediatric Ophthalmology, Scheie Eye Institute, University of Pennsylvania School of Medicine; Children's Hospital of Philadelphia, Philadelphia, Pennsylvania

JONATHAN M. HOLMES, B.M., B.Ch.

Assistant Professor of Pediatric Ophthalmology, Loyola University of Chicago Stritch School of Medicine, Maywood, Illinois

CREIG S. HOYT, M.D.
Professor of Ophthalmology and Pediatrics, and Vice-Chairman, Department of Ophthalmology, University of California, San Francisco, School of Medicine, San Francisco, California

SHERWIN J. ISENBERG, M.D.
Professor of Ophthalmology, and Vice-Chairman, Department of Ophthalmology, University of California, Los Angeles, UCLA School of Medicine, Los Angeles, California; Chief of Ophthalmology, Harbor/UCLA Medical Center, Torrance, California; Jules Stein Eye Institute, Los Angeles, California

JOHN B. JEFFERS, D.V.M., M.D.
Associate Professor of Ophthalmology, Jefferson Medical College of Thomas Jefferson University; Senior Assistant Surgeon, Wills Eye Hospital, Philadelphia, Pennsylvania

ZEYNEL A. KARCIOGLU, M.D.
Professor of Ophthalmology and Pathology, Tulane University School of Medicine, New Orleans, Louisiana

RANDY H. KARDON, M.D., Ph.D.
Assistant Professor of Ophthalmology, University of Iowa College of Medicine; Neuro-ophthalmology Division, Department of Ophthalmology, Veterans Affairs Medical Center, Iowa City, Iowa

JAMES A. KATOWITZ, M.D.
Associate Professor of Ophthalmology, University of Pennsylvania School of Medicine; Director of Oculoplastic and Orbital Surgery, Division of Ophthalmology, Children's Hospital of Philadelphia; Chief, Section of Ophthalmology, Center for Human Appearance, University of Pennsylvania Medical Center, Philadelphia, Pennsylvania

RONALD V. KEECH, M.D.
Associate Professor of Ophthalmology, University of Iowa College of Medicine; Department of Ophthalmology, University of Iowa Hospitals and Clinics, Iowa City, Iowa

ROSS A. KENNEDY, M.D., C.M., FRCS(C)
Assistant Professor of Ophthalmology, University of British Columbia Faculty of Medicine, Vancouver, Canada

PETER C. KOHLER, M.D.
Ophthalmologist, Private Practice, Eastern Maine Medical Center, Bangor, Maine

SUSMITHA P. KOLLI, B.A.
Student, The University of Chicago Pritzker School of Medicine, Chicago, Illinois

SCOTT R. LAMBERT, M.D.
Assistant Professor of Ophthalmology and Pediatrics, Emory University School of Medicine, Atlanta, Georgia

KAMERAN LASHKARI, M.D.
Chief Resident, Department of Ophthalmology, University of Missouri—Kansas City School of Medicine, Eye Foundation of Kansas City, Kansas City, Missouri

ANDREW W. LAWTON, M.D.
Assistant Professor of Ophthalmology and Neurology, Louisiana State University School of Medicine; Director, Neuro-ophthalmology Service, Louisiana State University Medical Center, New Orleans, Louisiana

BRIAN L. LEE, B.S.
Senior Medical Student, University of California, Los Angeles, UCLA School of Medicine, Los Angeles, California

KING Y. LEE, M.D.
Professor of Ophthalmology, University of Missouri—Kansas City School of Medicine, Kansas City, Missouri

JUNPING LI, M.D.
Research Assistant, Visual Sciences Center, The University of Chicago Pritzker School of Medicine, Chicago, Illinois

ROBERT W. LINGUA, M.D.
Associate Clinical Professor of Ophthalmology, Loma Linda University School of Medicine, Loma Linda, California

DON LIU, M.D.
Associate Professor of Ophthalmology, University of Southern California School of Medicine, Doheny Eye Institute, Los Angeles, California

THOMAS LUKE, B.S.
Lee's Summit, Missouri

MAX S. MANCILLAS, O.D.
Staff Optometrist, Humana Health Care Plans, Mission, Kansas

CURTIS E. MARGO, M.D.
Professor of Ophthalmology and Pathology, University of South Florida College of Medicine; Chief, Section of Ophthalmology, James A. Haley Veterans Administration Hospital, Tampa, Florida

LOIS J. MARTYN, M.D.
Associate Professor of Ophthalmology, and Associate Professor in Pediatrics, Temple University School of Medicine; Pediatric Ophthalmologist, St. Christopher's Hospital for Children, Philadelphia, Pennsylvania

WILLIAM D. MATHERS, M.D.
Associate Professor of Ophthalmology, University of Iowa College of Medicine; Director, Corneal Service, University of Iowa Hospitals and Clinics, Iowa City, Iowa

MALCOLM L. MAZOW, M.D., F.A.C.S
Professor of Ophthalmology and Pediatrics, University of Texas Medical School at Houston, Houston, Texas

JOHN C. MERRIAM, M.D.
Assistant Clinical Professor of Ophthalmology, Columbia University College of Physicians and Surgeons; Assistant Attending in Ophthalmology, Columbia-Presbyterian Medical Center, New York, New York

PETER H. MESTAD, M.D.

Associate Professor of Pediatrics and Anesthesiology, University of Missouri—Kansas City School of Medicine, Kansas City, Missouri

MARILYN NEWMAN METZL, Ph.D.

Associate Clinical Professor of Psychology, University of Kansas School of Medicine, Kansas City, Kansas; Clinical Director, Psychological-Educational Associates, Kansas City, Missouri

KEVIN M. MILLER, M.D.

Assistant Professor of Clinical Ophthalmology, University of California, Los Angeles, UCLA School of Medicine, Los Angeles, California

MARILYN T. MILLER, M.D.

Professor of Ophthalmology, and Director of Pediatric Ophthalmology and Strabismus, University of Illinois College of Medicine at Chicago, Chicago, Illinois

A. LINN MURPHREE, M.D.

Professor of Ophthalmology and Pediatrics, University of Southern California School of Medicine; Head, Division of Ophthalmology, Children's Hospital of Los Angeles, Los Angeles, California

MARVA K. NEWBERRY, M.S.

Educational Diagnostician, Psychological-Educational Associates, Kansas City, Missouri

PHILLIP L. PEARL, M.D.

Clinical Assistant Professor of Pediatrics and Neurology, University of Maryland School of Medicine, Baltimore, Maryland; Clinical Assistant Professor of Pediatrics and Neurology, George Washington University School of Medicine and Health Sciences; Clinical Instructor in Pediatrics, Georgetown University School of Medicine, Washington, District of Columbia

STEFAN-MATTHIAS PULST, M.D., Dr. med.

Warschaw Chair of Neurology, and Associate Professor of Medicine, University of California, Los Angeles, UCLA School of Medicine; Division of Neurology, Cedars-Sinai Medical Center, Los Angeles, California

MICHAEL X. REPKA, M.D.

Associate Professor of Ophthalmology, and Associate Professor of Pediatrics, The Johns Hopkins University School of Medicine; Department of Ophthalmology, The Wilmer Ophthalmological Institute, The Johns Hopkins Hospital, Baltimore, Maryland

SHAWN M. RIEDEL, B.S.

Senior Medical Student, Kansas City, Missouri

JILL CELLARS ROGERS, M.S.

Instructor in Medicine, University of Missouri—Kansas City School of Medicine; Genetic Counselor, The Children's Mercy Hospital, Kansas City, Missouri

PAUL E. ROMANO, M.D., M.S.O.

Former Professor of Ophthalmology, University of Florida College of Medicine, Gainesville, Florida

HAMID SAJJADI, M.D.

Associate Professor of Ophthalmology, University of Kansas School of Medicine; Director, Cornea and External Disease, Department of Ophthalmology, University of Kansas Medical Center; Medical Director, Kansas Eye Bank, Kansas City, Kansas

JOHN R. SAMPLES, M.D.

Associate Professor of Ophthalmology, Oregon Health Sciences University School of Medicine; Glaucoma Service, Casey Eye Institute, Portland, Oregon

ANDREA M. SCALISE-GORDY, D.O.

Active Staff, Pediatric Ophthalmology, Mary Immaculate Hospital; Active Staff, Pediatric Ophthalmology, Riverside Regional Medical Center, Newport News, Virginia; Active Staff, Pediatric Ophthalmology, Sentera Hampton General Hospital, Hampton, Virginia

WILLIAM E. SCOTT, M.D.

Professor of Ophthalmology, University of Iowa College of Medicine; Director of Pediatric Ophthalmology, University of Iowa Hospitals and Clinics, Iowa City, Iowa

KAREN S. SHIMSHAK, M.D.

Clinical Assistant Professor of Ophthalmology, University of Missouri—Kansas City School of Medicine, Kansas City, Missouri; Clinical Instructor, Department of Ophthalmology, University of Kansas School of Medicine, Kansas City, Kansas; Attending Staff, Eye Department, The Children's Mercy Hospital, Kansas City, Missouri

THOMAS L. SLOVIS, M.D.

Professor of Radiology, Wayne State University School of Medicine; Chief of Pediatric Radiology, Children's Hospital of Michigan, Detroit, Michigan

MICHAEL E. SOMERS, M.D.

Midwest Eye Institute, North Kansas City, Missouri

ANDREA R. SPERDUTO, M.D.

Clinical Instructor, Division of Infectious Diseases, Department of Pediatrics, Center for the Health Sciences, University of California, Los Angeles, UCLA School of Medicine, UCLA Medical Center, Los Angeles, California

MERRILL L. STASS-ISERN, M.D.

Clinical Assistant Professor of Ophthalmology, University of Missouri—Kansas City School of Medicine; Clinical Assistant Professor of Medicine, Department of Ophthalmology, The Children's Mercy Hospital, Kansas City, Missouri

ROSA ANA TANG, M.D.

Clinical Professor of Ophthalmology, University of Texas Medical Branch, University of Texas Medical School at Galveston, Galveston, Texas; Clinical Associate Professor of Ophthalmology, University of Texas Medical School at Houston, Houston, Texas

H. STANLEY THOMPSON, M.D.

Professor of Ophthalmology, University of Iowa College of Medicine, Iowa City, Iowa

ANDREA CIBIS TONGUE, M.D.

Clinical Associate Professor of Ophthalmology, Oregon Health Sciences University School of Medicine, Portland, Oregon; Child Eye Care Associates, Lake Oswego, Oregon

ELIAS I. TRABOULSI, M.D.

Assistant Professor of Ophthalmology and Pediatrics, The Johns Hopkins School of Medicine, Baltimore, Maryland

BRENDA J. TRIPATHI, PH.D.

Research Associate (Professor) of Ophthalmology and Visual Science, and Senior Lecturer, Department of Organismal Biology and Anatomy, The University of Chicago Pritzker School of Medicine, Chicago, Illinois

RAMESH C. TRIPATHI, M.D., PH.D., F.A.C.S.

Professor of Ophthalmology and Visual Science, The University of Chicago Pritzker School of Medicine; Attending Ophthalmologist, University of Chicago Hospitals, Chicago, Illinois; Attending Ophthalmologist, Oak Forest Hospital, Oak Forest, Illinois

JOANNE WAELTERMANN, M.D.

Clinical Assistant Professor of Ophthalmology, University of Maryland School of Medicine; Head of Pediatric Ophthalmology, St. Agnes Hospital; Instructor, Greater Baltimore Medical Center Eye Clinic, Baltimore, Maryland

METTE WARBURG, M.D., PH.D.

Adjunct Professor, Department of Ophthalmology, University of Arhus, Denmark; Consultant Ophthalmologist, Gentofte Hospital, Copenhagen, Denmark

MARY WARREN, M.S., OTR

Coordinator, Occupational Therapy Service, Low Vision Rehabilitation Program, Department of Ophthalmology, University of Missouri—Kansas City School of Medicine, Kansas City, Missouri

THOMAS A. WEINGEIST, M.D., PH.D.

Professor of Ophthalmology, and Head, Department of Ophthalmology, University of Iowa College of Medicine; Director, Vitreoretinal Service, Department of Ophthalmology, University of Iowa Hospitals and Clinics, Iowa City, Iowa

AVERY H. WEISS, M.D.

Associate Professor of Ophthalmology, University of Washington School of Medicine; Chief, Division of Ophthalmology, Department of Surgery, The Children's Hospital and Medical Center, Seattle, Washington

DAVID L. ZWICK, M.D.

Associate Professor of Pathology and Pediatrics, University of Missouri—Kansas City School of Medicine, Kansas City, Missouri; Associate Clinical Professor, Department of Pathology, University of Kansas School of Medicine, Kansas City, Kansas; Pathologist-in-Chief, and Medical Director, Blood Bank, The Children's Mercy Hospital, Kansas City, Missouri

To Drs. Paul and Lisa Cibis and all who knew them

PREFACE

Pediatric ophthalmology, as other subspecialties within ophthalmology, requires complicated decision-making processes based on interlocking information. *Decision Making in Pediatric Ophthalmology* is an effort to provide "expert" algorithms for solving common clinical problems. The book is organized both by the symptoms and the chronologic age of the child. With the help of numerous authors chosen for their expertise in each field, many common presenting complaints are expertly dissected; these range from "Can my child see?," "He holds his head funny" (torticollis), or "My child sees lights and spots," to the more standard exotropia, headaches, or unequal pupils. Genetics and molecular biology, as they apply to routine care, are also emphasized.

Pediatricians, family practitioners, optometrists, and nurses, as well as ophthalmologists and pediatric eye care specialists will benefit from this book. Where possible, the practical details of "how to" and "how much" are spelled out. References allow for more detailed reading, but the practical aspects of each chapter should be sufficient to guide the readers into their next course of action. The book can also be used in coordination with the new CPT-4 problem-solving and decision-making complexity level format. Each chapter is documentation of the decision-making complexity for a particular problem presentation.

We are grateful to all of the contributing authors; Children's Mercy Hospital for its uplifting pediatric care environment; and our residents, students, fellows, and patients, who constantly hone our skills. Special thanks go to Carol Jenks, whose patience, care, and insight into the clarity and sequence of the subject matter were invaluable.

Gerhard W. Cibis, M.D.
Andrea Cibis Tongue, M.D.
Merrill L. Stass-Isern, M.D.

CONTENTS

THE PRESCHOOL AND SCHOOL-AGE CHILD

Acquired Periorbital Anomalies

Acquired Media Opacities or Anomalies

Visual Problems

Systemic Diseases

Acquired Strabismus

Eye and Head Pain

Ocular Infections

Glaucoma

DECISION MAKING IN

Pediatric Ophthalmology

MEDICAL AND GENETIC HISTORY TAKING AND COUNSELING

MEDICAL AND GENETIC HISTORY TAKING AND COUNSELING

Andrea Cibis Tongue, M.D.
Barbara K. Hecht, Ph.D.,
Frederick Hecht, M.D.

A. The most important part of history taking is eliciting details of why the patient is being seen. Is the patient here because of noted eye or vision problems, because the child is at risk for eye problems, or just for a routine eye examination? Genetic counseling also depends upon the collection and analysis of critical data before the diagnosis, prognosis, and treatment can be accurately communicated and implemented.

B. All relevant information needs to be taken into account. This includes review of the medical records and photos (see C below), genetic family history (p 114), results of the general history and physical examination, the anomaly checklist (p 112), and relevant laboratory data such as cytogenetics (p 124), biochemical genetics (e.g., enzyme assays), and molecular genetics (p 126).

C. It is important to detail the age of onset, the duration and frequency, whether the signs or symptoms appear to be getting better or worse, if there are associated or concomitant problems not related to the eye, who first noted the abnormality, and who suggested that the patient be seen by an ophthalmologist. In the case of strabismus, parents should be asked to point to the eye in question. Often what they call left is the patient's right eye, or vice versa. Vague terms (e.g., wandering eye, lazy eye) need to be clarified, as do generalized symptoms (e.g., headaches or eye pain). Compile a clear picture of the parent's or patient's perceived concerns. It takes time but it is often vital to obtain and review medical records of the patient and pertinent family members. With visible stigmata as in Marfan syndrome, neurofibromatosis, and many other genetic disorders, family photographs are extraordinarily informative. Most families are delighted that a physician is interested and bring whatever family records and photographs they have available.

D. Medical history should identify age, sex, and a brief prenatal and perinatal history, including birth weight, gestational age at the time of birth, and, if any time was spent in a neonatal nursery, the infant's medical problems. General growth and development need to be addressed as well as a complete review of systems. Parents often view an eye examination as nonmedical and fail to mention medical problems unless specifically questioned. Have parents fill out a basic history questionnaire (see Figure on p 4 for prototype). Inquire about allergies, especially to medications, medications currently being taken, and medical problems that might impact the examination or put the patient at risk for certain eye diseases or vision disorders. *Question specifically* about seizure disorders, developmental delay, skin abnormalities, heart murmurs, asthma, anatomic anomalies, and hearing problems.

E. Establish whether the patient is an adopted, foster, or biologic child or other relation to the person giving the history. Accuracy of the history may be significantly impacted by who is giving it. A more detailed history is tailored to elicit more specific information, and the extent of the history taking depends primarily on the chief complaint; for example, if a child is brought in because of possible strabismus, parents need to be asked if any family member has crossed or wandering eyes, a lazy eye, unexplained poor vision or glasses since a young age, and so forth.

F. If an asymptomatic patient is seen for a consultation because of risk of an eye condition, specific questions regarding signs or symptoms of that condition need to be addressed. An asymptomatic patient referred because of juvenile rheumatoid arthritis needs to be questioned concerning any history of red eyes, pain, photophobia, and so forth. History taking is an evolutionary process that changes direction with the findings. If an ocular abnormality is noted which may be associated with systemic disease or anomalies, questions specifically addressing signs or symptoms of the associated disease need to be asked. The history is an important clinical tool that, in conjunction with the examination findings, dictates treatment.

G. Extensive genetic history is imperative with the presence or risk of genetic eye disease, particularly if there is a question as to the mode of inheritance or the risk for disease in the patient or other family members. See pp 112 and 114 for outlines of methods for obtaining a family pedigree and genetic history. If the child has signs or symptoms of an eye disease that is X-linked, dominantly inherited, or has carrier manifestations, biologic family members accompanying the child should be examined. Negative or positive findings in immediate family members may impact further clinical investigation.

H. A process of differential diagnosis strives toward an accurate and precise diagnosis, essential before doing genetic counseling because many genetic disorders are heterogeneous and need to be differentiated from each other. It determines prognosis, natural history, treatment, and recurrence risks. In the absence of a solid diagnosis, you may choose to defer genetic counseling.

(Continued on p. 4.)

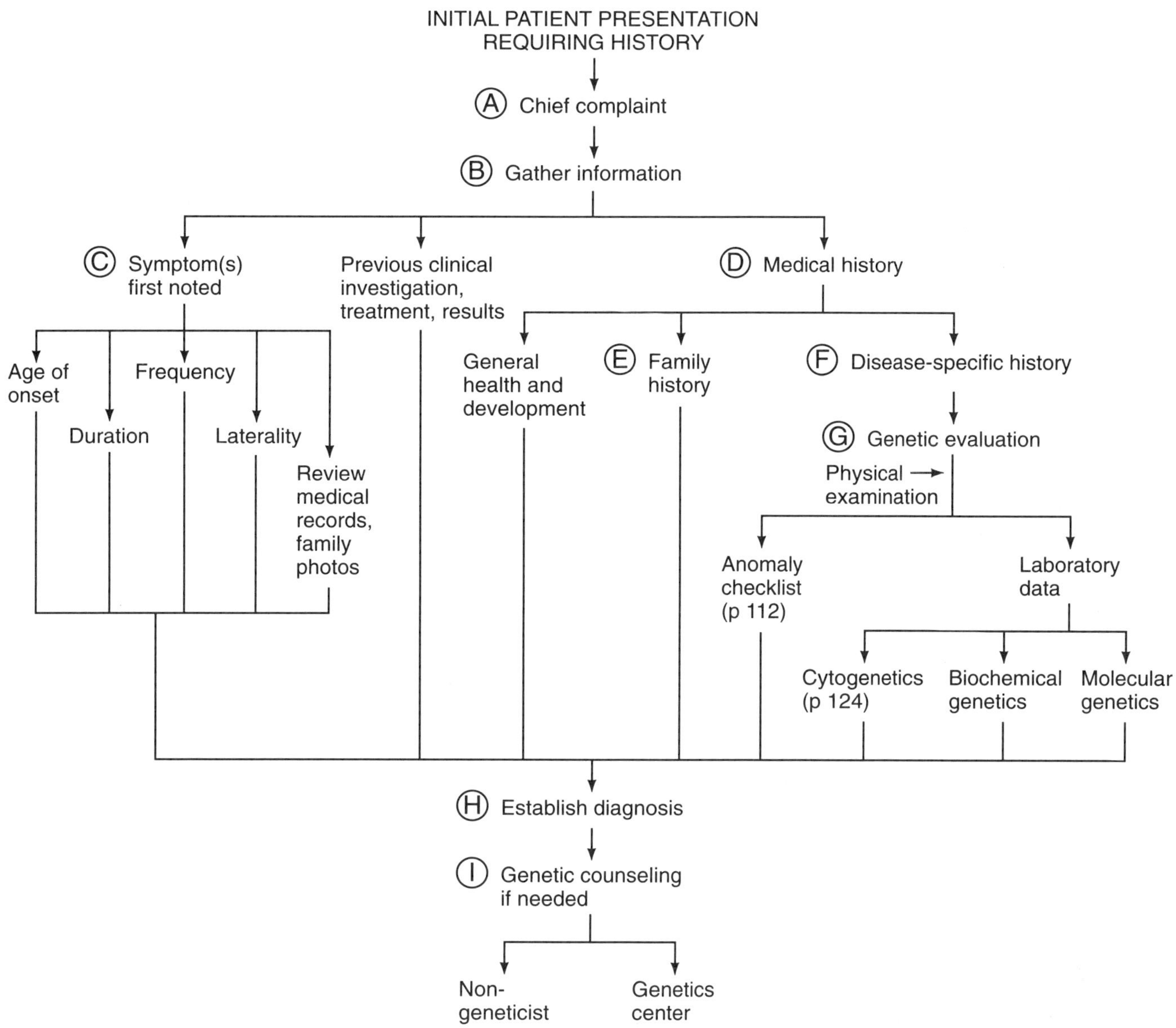
INITIAL PATIENT PRESENTATION REQUIRING HISTORY
(A) Chief complaint
(B) Gather information
(C) Symptom(s) first noted
Previous clinical investigation, treatment, results
(D) Medical history
Age of onset
Frequency
Duration
Laterality
Review medical records, family photos
General health and development
(E) Family history
(F) Disease-specific history
(G) Genetic evaluation
Physical examination
Anomaly checklist (p 112)
Laboratory data
Cytogenetics (p 124)
Biochemical genetics
Molecular genetics
(H) Establish diagnosis
(I) Genetic counseling if needed
Non-geneticist
Genetics center

MEDICAL HISTORY QUESTIONNAIRE

Name ______________________ Birth Date __________ Sex ___ Race__________

Allergies to medications ______________________
Prior hospitalizations and surgeries ______________________
Current medications (dose and reason for taking medication) ______________________
____
Birth weight __________ Premature or full-term? __________
Prenatal problems ______________________
Birth or neonatal problems ______________________
____
Pediatrician or family doctor ______________________ Last physical exam __________
Are immunizations up to date? ______________________

System Review:
Does your child have or has your child had any of the following?
Diabetes mellitus __________ Cancer or leukemia __________
Juvenile rheumatoid arthritis __________ Bleeding disorder __________
Hepatitis __________ HIV virus __________
Chromosome abnormality ______________________
Syndrome or identified genetic disease ______________________
Other disease ______________________
Serious injury ______________________
Skin problems or abnormalities ______________________
Neurologic problems ______________________
Cerebral palsy ______ Seizure disorder ______ Developmental delay ______
Learning disability ______ ADD ______ Hypdrocephalus ______
Other ______________________
Heart murmur __________ Cardiac abnormality ______________________
Asthma __________ Other lung problems ______________________
Hearing problems ______________________
Bone, joint, or limb abnormalities ______________________
Kidney or urinary tract problems ______________________
Bleeding disorder ______________________
Has your child had an abnormal reaction to eye medication? ______________________
Previous eye care ______________________

Family History:
Is your child adopted or foster child? ______________________
Please list patient's relation to any biologic family members who have or had the following:
Eye muscle problem ______________________
Amblyopia or "lazy eye" ______________________
Glasses as young child or infant ______________________
Cataracts (diagnosed under age 40) ______________________
Glaucoma ______________________
Poor eyesight not corrected with glasses or contacts ______________________
Tear duct problems ______________________
Poor color vision ______________________
Other ______________________

Date __________ Signed ______________________ Relation to patient __________

I. Decide who should explain the genetics. If you can do it effectively, do it. Otherwise, refer the patient and family to a genetics center for counseling. Genetic counseling can be directive or nondirective. In directive counseling the patient is directed as to the course of action, whereas in nondirective counseling the facts and options are discussed with the patient or family so they can make their own informed decisons. Genetic counseling may be need to:
   1. Explain diagnosis, causation, treament, prognosis.
   2. Clarify recurrence risks for sibs and offspring.
   3. Review options for patient/family.
   4. Help with adjustment to diagnosis and to decison making.
   5. Communicate with other care providers.
   6. Refer patient/family appropriately.

References

McKusick VA. Mendelian inheritance in man. Catalog of autosomal dominant, autosomal recessive and X-linked phenotypes. 9th ed. Baltimore: John Hopkins University Press, 1990.

Thompson MW, McInnes RR, Willard HF. Thompson and Thompson's genetics in medicine. 5th ed. Philadelphia: WB Saunders Company, 1991.

University of Colorado Health Sciences Center. Genetic Applications: A Health Perspective. Lawrence, Kansas: Learner Managed Designs, 1988.

THE NEONATE

CONGENITAL LID AND SKIN ANOMALIES

John C. Merriam, M.D.
Merrill L. Stass-Isern, M.D.

Most congenital anomalies of the eyelids occur during the second month of gestation as a result of either a failure of fusion or an arrest of development. Others occur without a known cause. These can anatomically obscure the visual axis or be irritating to the ocular structures and therefore have possible amblyogenic effects. Skin anomalies, however, may be an isolated finding not representing a structural abnormality or have association with systemic disease.

A. Congenital ectropion, entropion, coloboma, and microblepharon are developmental lid anomalies often misdiagnosed as "conjunctivitis" and treated with topical antibiotics. A thorough ocular examination is necessary to determine if there are associated ocular anomalies (e.g., corneal dysgenesis, congenital cataract, colobomata of the retina and iris, optic nerve hypoplasia, or microphthalmia). Prenatal teratogen exposure should be investigated. Severe lid anomalies are generally associated with facial or ocular anomalies. Coloboma and microblepharon, more rare than entropion and ectropion, are manifestations of a clefting disorder and are more likely to be associated with other anomalies.

B. Exposure (ectropion, coloboma, microblepharon) or lashes rubbing the eye (entropion, trichiasis, distichiasis) may cause irritation.

C. Lid margins and lashes must be examined to determine if trichiasis (aberrant direction of lashes) or distichiasis (accessory row of posterior lashes) is the cause. Small numbers of irritating lashes may be removed by electrolysis. Distichiasis is managed by excision of abnormal lashes. Trichiasis may be associated with microblepharon, entropion, or coloboma.

D. With entropion, the bulbar conjunctiva and cornea may be abraded by lashes, but most infants have surprisingly few symptoms.

E. With true ectropion, the exposed conjunctiva may become irritated.

F. True congenital ectropion is due to a deficiency of skin and may be treated, if necessary, as acquired cicatricial ectropion. Apparent eversion of the lid margin may be associated with hypoplasia of all layers of the lid and occasionally anomalous development of the orbit, as in Treacher-Collins syndrome. Rarely, a newborn may have a lid that is floppy and everts spontaneously. Surgery usually is not necessary.

G. Entropion and ectropion may improve with growth, so observation is appropriate. Lubricating agents and topical antibiotics may help. Parents may be taught lid massage to try to return it to a normal position. Persistent abrasion or ulceration of the cornea may require surgery.

H. True cicatricial ectropion may be repaired with a full-thickness skin graft from another lid, if possible, or from the retroauricular area. Complex lid anomalies, such as microblepharon or various craniofaical syndromes, which may also have lid eversion, generally require evaluation by a plastic surgeon and geneticist.

I. Surgery for congenital entropion may involve resection of an ellipse of skin and tarsal orbicularis muscle, tightening of the lower lid retractors, or tarsal repositioning (Wies procedure).

J. Coloboma typically affects the nasal third of the upper lid but may involve any portion of the lids or canthi. Multiple colobomata may be found in a single lid. The defect may range from a subtle notch at the lid margin to hypoplasia of the tarsus to a full-thickness defect that may be associated with a shallow or absent fornix in the area of the defect.

K. Microblepharon, a deficiency of all layers of the lid, may range from subtle lagophthalmos to severe exposure. Generally more than one lid is affected. Colobomata may be associated.

L. Coloboma and microblepharon, manifestations of a clefting disorder, require evaluation for associated ocular, craniofacial, and other anomalies.

M. Corneal exposure due to a full-thickness lid defect or lagophthalmos may lead to neovascularization, ulceration, or perforation. Severity of exposure and visual potential of the eye must be assessed to plan therapy. With a healthy cornea, conservative topical wetting agents are sufficient.

N. Corneal ulceration requires surgery. If the child has other surgical problems, surgeries should be coordinated to minimize anesthesia time.

O. Repair of lid coloboma generally involves excision of the margins of the coloboma, restoration of the fornix, and direct side-to-side closure. The lateral canthal tendon may be released. A rotation flap from the opposite lid should be avoided because of greater risk of occlusion amblyopia.

P. Microblepharon is repaired with large, full-thickness skin grafts to the affected lid. Lateral and/or nasal tarsorrhaphy may help prevent contracture of the grafts and protect the cornea postoperatively.

Q. Any lid abnormality may cause corneal irregularity or astigmatism. Surgery of the lid may lead to occlusion of the eye. Evaluate carefully for amblyopia.

R. In the nonirritated eye, blepharophimosis, an autosomal dominant syndrome, includes telecanthus, epicanthus inversus, and severe ptosis. Lower eyelid entropion, a poorly developed nasal bridge, hypoplasia of the superior orbital rims, and hypertelorism may also be found. Reconstruction is usually in multiple phases. The epicanthus is corrected with V-Y and Z plasties with transnasal wiring of the elongated medial canthal tendons. Then the ptosis is addressed. Euryblepharon, an unusual condition, results in horizontal elongation of the palpebral fissure, unilateral or bilateral. Impaired blinking, poor closure, and lagophthalmos may lead to exposure keratitis. Treatment, if necessary, consists of full-thickness resection of excess

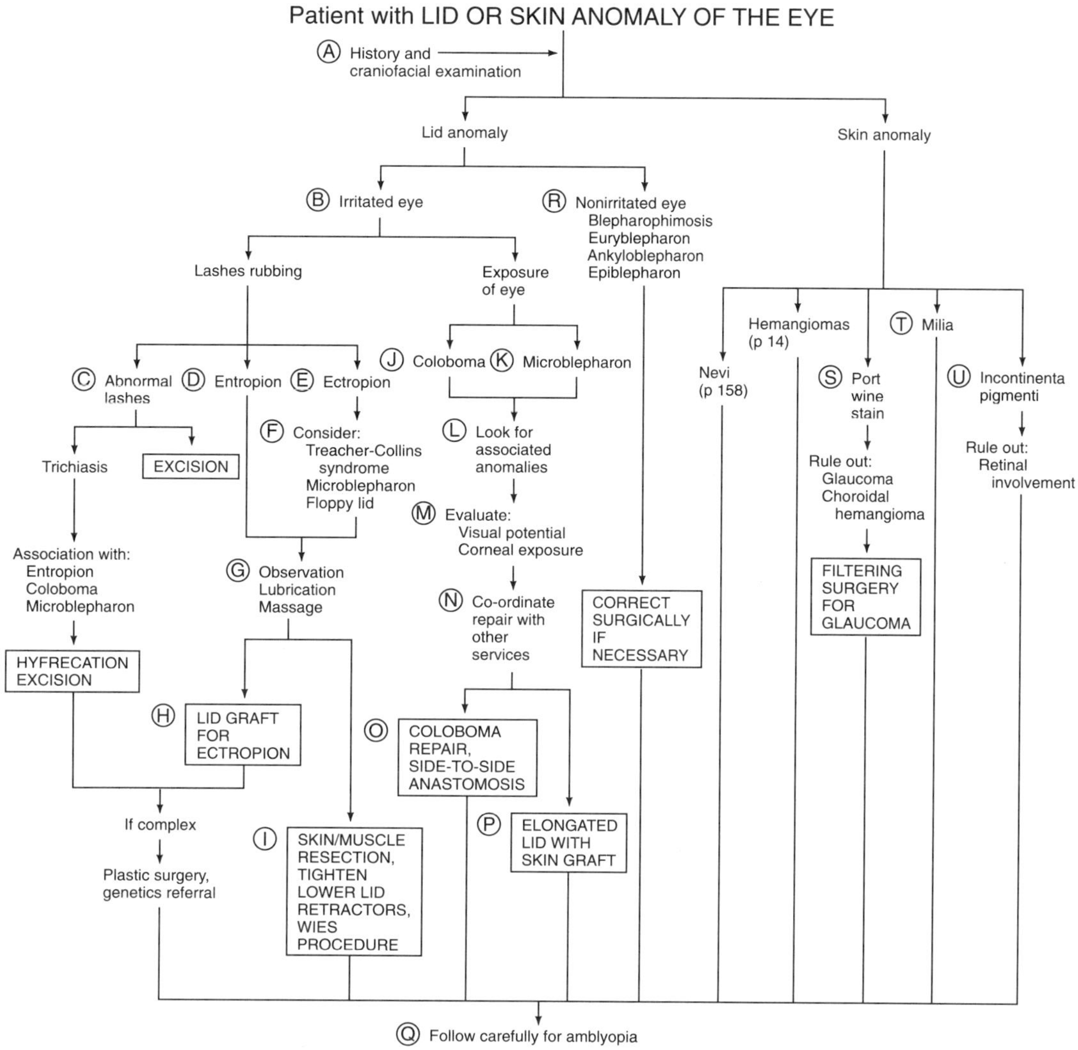

eyelid length and canthoplasty. Ankyloblepharon results in partial fusion of the eyelids by webs of skin. Correction consists of clamping the web and then cutting. With epiblepharon the pretarsal orbicularis muscle and skin ride above the lid margin, forming a horizontal fold and allowing the lashes to assume a vertical position. The lid margin is in a normal position with respect to the globe. Most often the lashes do not contact the globe. This tends to disappear with maturation of the face and does not require treatment.

S. Nevus flammeus (cutaneous) angioma (port wine stain) may be associated with the Sturge-Weber syndrome. It involves the area of distribution of the first and second divisions of the trigeminal nerve. Thirty percent of patients with Sturge-Weber syndrome have glaucoma. The glaucoma involves the side with the facial angioma and is more common if the upper eyelid is involved. Onset of the glaucoma may occur from infancy to adulthood.

T. Milia neonatorum, white pinhead-sized papules, occur on the eyelids or anywhere on the face in about 40% of newborns. They resolve spontaneously and need no treatment.

U. Incontinentia pigmenti is a disease of abnormal skin pigmentation rarely limited to the eyelids. The presenting skin lesion is a bulla that evolves to whorl-like or linear patches of pigmentation. About one-third of these patients have ocular abnormalities consisting of retinal dysplasia or an exudative chorioretinitis. There is no effective ocular treatment.

Other diseases involve the eyelids in neonates, but their appearance is usually not limited to the eyelid and they are not addressed here.

References

Bartley GB, Nerad JA, Kersten RC, Maguire LJ. Congenital entropion with intact lower eyelid retractor insertion. Am J Ophthalmol 1991; 112:437.

Collin JRO. A manual of systematic eyelid surgery. 2nd ed. New York: Churchill Livingstone, 1989.

Merriam JC, Stalnecker MC, Merriam GR Jr. Reconstruction of the lids of a child with microblepharon and multiple congenital anomalies. Trans Am Ophthalmol Soc 1988; 86:55.

EPICANTHUS

Trudi R. Grin, M.D.

Epicanthus or epicanthal fold is a crescent-shaped fold of skin running vertically from the upper and/or lower lid and partially covering the inner canthus. Most commonly it is bilateral, but it may be unilateral or asymmetric, giving the appearance of esotropia (see p).

A. Four types of epicanthal folds have been described. In *epicanthus tarsalis* the fold is most prominent in the upper lid. It arises from the tarsal fold and terminates in the inner canthus. Epicanthus tarsalis is most frequently associated with the Asian and the Eskimo eye. In *epicanthus inversus* the fold is most prominent in the lower lid. It is seen almost exclusively as a part of the blepharophimosis syndrome. *Epicanthus palpebralis* is a fold equally distributed in the upper and lower lids. It arises from the upper lid above the tarsal region and extends to the lower margin of the orbit. *Epicanthus supraciliaris* is a more prominent fold, arising from the brow region and running toward the nasolacrimal sac area.

B. Epiblepharon is a congenital anomaly in which an extra horizontal skin fold exists, located adjacent to the upper or lower lid margin. Epiblepharon of the upper eyelids is considered to be an exaggeration of epicanthus tarsalis. Epiblepharon is relatively common in infants and is a frequent finding in the Asian eye. It tends to regress spontaneously during the first 2 years of life. On occasion the skin fold may overlap the lid margin and turn the lashes of the medial half of the lid against the cornea. The cornea usually tolerates this quite well, but occasionally corneal irritation occurs and ophthalmic ointment may be necessary to control the symptoms. If epithelial erosion develops, surgical management consisting of simple excision of the skin fold may be necessary. In general, surgical correction should be delayed because epiblepharon spontaneously resolves in most cases.

C. Epicanthus is a frequent finding among normal infants. It is rare to see epicanthus at birth (3%), but it may be seen in as many as 30% of children under 2 years of age. Epicanthus as an isolated feature can also be transmitted as an autosomal dominant trait. In the majority of infants, the folds gradually decrease with maturation of the facial bones, especially as the bridge of the nose develops. In the Asian eye, epicanthus tarsalis tends to persist into adult life. Treatment for isolated epicanthus is usually for cosmetic reasons. In general, surgical correction should be delayed until the teen years when facial maturity has occurred. Cases requiring treatment can be successfully repaired with linear revisions such as a Z- plasty or Y-V plasty.

D. Epicanthus inversus is often part of a dominantly inherited congenital syndrome in conjunction with blepharophimosis, ptosis, and telecanthus (Kohn-Romano syndrome). The palpebral fissures are shortened horizontally and vertically (blepharophimosis), the ptosis is severe, and the lid folds are absent. Associated ocular abnormalities may occur and include lower lid ectropion, hypoplasia of the superior orbital rims, poorly developed nasal bridge, lacrimal system abnormalities, strabismus, micropthalmos, and nystagmus. Systemic manifestations are uncommon but include amenorrhea due to primary hypogonadism, low-set and cupped ears, generalized myopathy, dwarfism, and heart disease. Surgical treatment is often performed at an early age to correct the severe ptosis, but correction of the epicanthal deformity is usually delayed until the preschool years when the clinical features stabilize.

E. Because epicanthus is such a common finding in normal children, this lid configuration has little diagnostic value by itself. When present in combination with other features, it contributes to typical facies of many syndromes and genetic abnormalities, such as fetal alcohol syndrome and trisomy 21 (Table 1).

TABLE 1 Genetic Abnormalities Associated with Epicanthus

Trisomy: 13, 21
Duplication: 2p, 3q, 11p, 12p
Deletion: 4p, 5p, 10p, 13q, 22q
Ring: 22
45,X, 48,XXXX

From Punnet HH, Harley RD. Genetics in pediatric ophthalmology. In: Harley RD. Pediatric ophthalmology. 2nd ed. Philadelphia: WB Saunders, 1983:40; with permission.

References

Crawford JS. Congenital eyelid anomalies in children. J Pediatr Ophthalmol 1984; 21:140.

Crawford JS, Pashby RC, Apt RK. Embryology and congenital anomalies. In: Stewart WB, ed. Ophthalmic plastic and reconstructive surgery. American Academy of Ophthalmology, 1984:101.

Johnson CC: Epicanthus and epiblepharon. Arch Ophthalmol 1978; 96:1030.

Nelson LB, Brown GC, Arentsen JJ. Recognizing patterns of ocular childhood diseases. Thorofare, NJ: Slack, 1985:142.

Palmer EA. Teratogenic agents. In: Isenberg SJ. The eye in infancy. Chicago: Year Book, 1989:110.

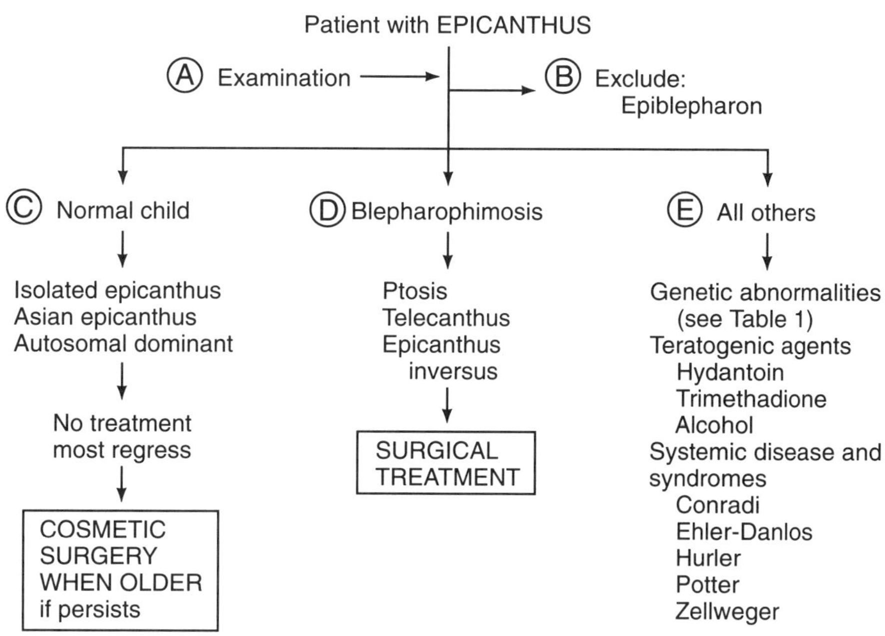
Patient with EPICANTHUS
(A) Examination
(B) Exclude:
Epiblepharon
(C) Normal child
Isolated epicanthus
Asian epicanthus
Autosomal dominant
No treatment
most regress
COSMETIC
SURGERY
WHEN OLDER
if persists
(D) Blepharophimosis
Ptosis
Telecanthus
Epicanthus
inversus
SURGICAL
TREATMENT
(E) All others
Genetic abnormalities
(see Table 1)
Teratogenic agents
Hydantoin
Trimethadione
Alcohol
Systemic disease and
syndromes
Conradi
Ehler-Danlos
Hurler
Potter
Zellweger

ORBITAL ANOMALY

Richard W. Hertle, M.D.
James A. Katowitz M.D.

A. The first step in evaluation is the history, and trauma is initially ruled out. Important considerations include when and who first noticed the anomaly and how long it has been present. The presence of associated systemic abnormalities and familial similarities help in the initial differential diagnosis.

B. In most cases traumatic anomalies are diagnosed historically. After a thorough ocular and adnexal examination, radiographic examination is carried out. The main purpose is to characterize the clinical deformity in terms of disrupted bony and soft tissue architecture. Delineation of fractures is important for surgical reconstruction.

C. The differential diagnosis of orbital anomalies is cumbersome when one is confronted with all the inherited metabolic and inflammatory developmental conditions and tumors that are potential causes. A quick way to narrow the differential diagnosis is first to determine whether the condition is unilateral or bilateral. Certain conditions are more commonly unilateral.

D. One must determine whether the condition is congenital or acquired. Some conditions can be present only from birth (e.g., Crouzon syndrome) whereas other anomalies are most often acquired (e.g., osteopetrosis). Similar malformations can be distinguished in this way (e.g., microphthalmos versus radiation-induced hypoplasia).

E. It is almost always necessary to obtain radiographic evaluation of orbital anomalies. A CT scan is preferred for the evaluation of bony structures and is excellent for detecting intracranial and intraorbital abnormalities. If further soft tissue characterization is needed, an MR scan is obtained.

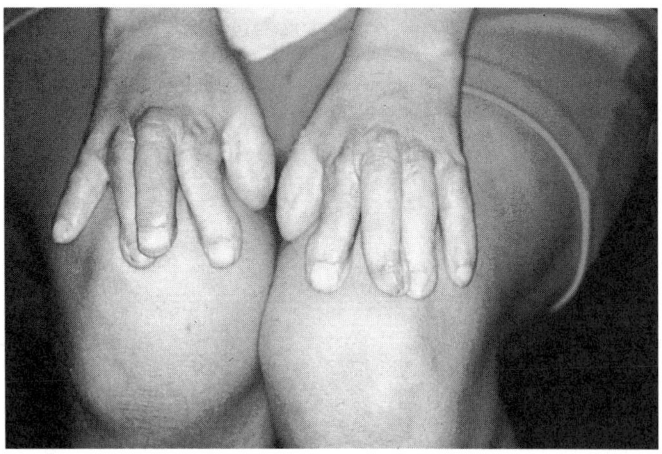

Figure 1 Syndactyly in Apert syndrome (acrocephalosyndactyly).

F. The anomaly can be placed in one of two categories based on the radiographic and clinical evaluation. The anomaly is either (1) part of a syndrome or (2) a tumor. Included in the syndrome diagnosis is every orbital process except tumors, e.g., hereditary (Apert, Crouzon), developmental (clefts, encephalocele, microphthalmos, anophthalmos), inflammatory (pseudotumor, cellulitis), metabolic (osteopetrosis, hyperthyroidism), and degenerative (enucleation, radiation). Once the diagnosis of tumor is made, other radiographic and clinical signs help in differentiating benign from malignant processes.

G. A team evaluation is needed for the complete diagnosis and management of orbital syndromes. Support from specialists including pediatricians, geneticists, plastic surgeons, neurosurgeons, social workers, speech and hearing therapists, growth and development specialists, and psychiatrists is necessary. The ophthalmic treatment is part of this team approach. Visual, adnexal, and orbital consequences of these diagnoses are treated in standard fashion, coordinated with the other specialists caring for the patient.

H. When a tumor is diagnosed, the ophthalmic surgeon's role continues as an integral part of the diagnosis and therapy. The first step is the exact tissue diagnosis, and this often requires biopsy and/or removal of the tumor. Benign lesions are then either removed or followed. Malignant lesions are treated by further excision, radiation, chemotherapy, or a combination of the three. This requires that the ophthalmologist work with other surgical subspecialists and oncologists. Finally, secondary visual, adnexal, and orbital consequences of the tumor or the treatment must be continually evaluated.

References

Fries PD, Katowitz JA. Congenital craniofacial anomalies of ophthalmic importance. Surv Ophthalmol 1990; 35:87.

Kennerdell JS, Dresner SC. The non-specific orbital inflammatory syndromes. Surv Ophthalmol 1984; 29:93.

Shields JA, Bakewell B, Augsburger JJ, et al. Space occupying orbital masses in children. A review of 250 consecutive biopsies. Ophthalmology 1986; 93:379.

Weiss A, Friendly D, Eglin K, et al. Bacterial periorbital and orbital cellulitis in childhood. Ophthalmology 1983; 90:195.

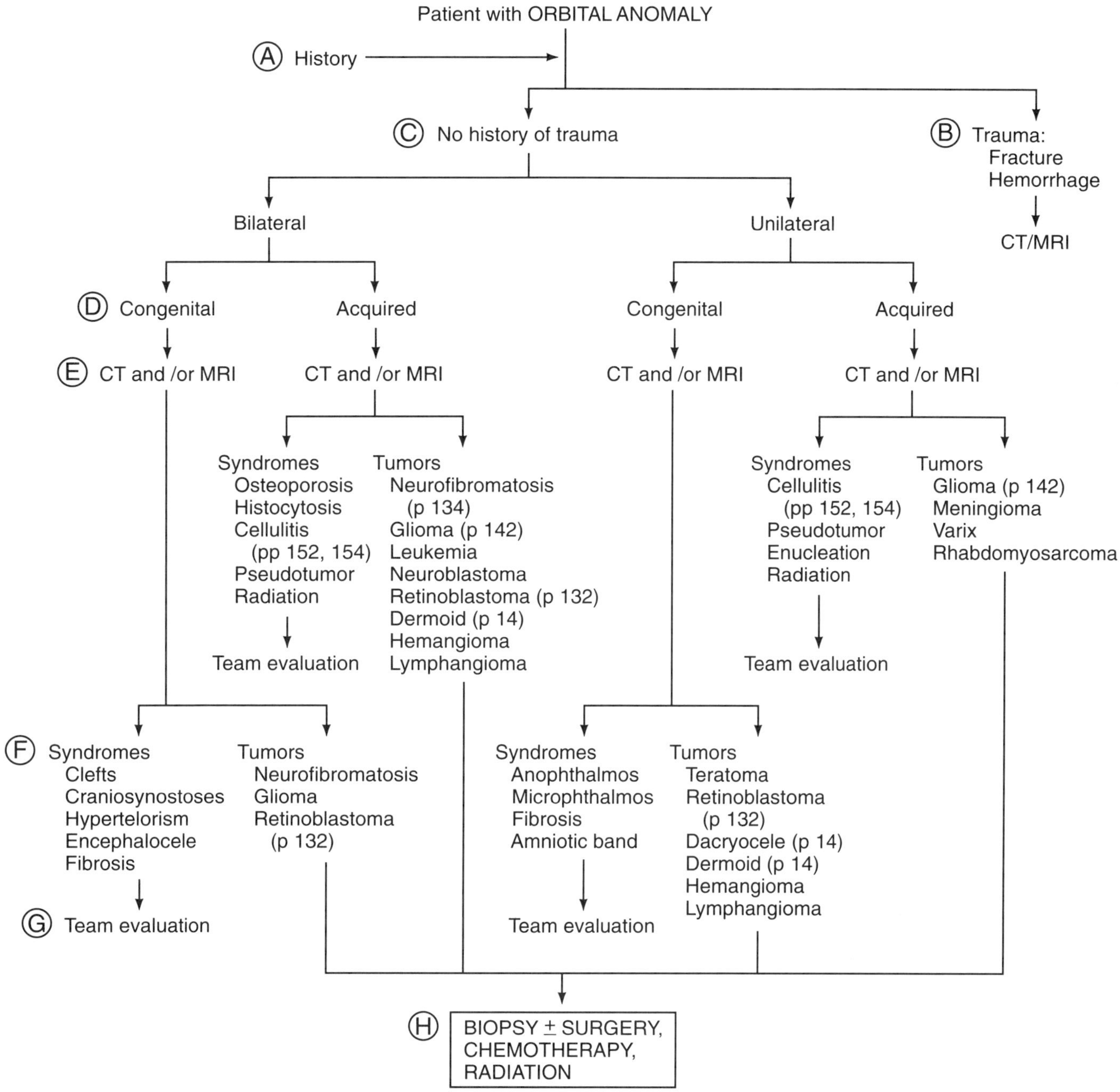
Patient with ORBITAL ANOMALY
(A) History
(C) No history of trauma
(B) Trauma:
Fracture
Hemorrhage
CT/MRI
Bilateral
Unilateral
(D) Congenital
Acquired
Congenital
Acquired
(E) CT and /or MRI
CT and /or MRI
CT and /or MRI
CT and /or MRI
Syndromes
Osteoporosis
Histocytosis
Cellulitis
(pp 152, 154)
Pseudotumor
Radiation
Team evaluation
Tumors
Neurofibromatosis
(p 134)
Glioma (p 142)
Leukemia
Neuroblastoma
Retinoblastoma (p 132)
Dermoid (p 14)
Hemangioma
Lymphangioma
Syndromes
Cellulitis
(pp 152, 154)
Pseudotumor
Enucleation
Radiation
Team evaluation
Tumors
Glioma (p 142)
Meningioma
Varix
Rhabdomyosarcoma
(F) Syndromes
Clefts
Craniosynostoses
Hypertelorism
Encephalocele
Fibrosis
(G) Team evaluation
Tumors
Neurofibromatosis
Glioma
Retinoblastoma
(p 132)
Syndromes
Anophthalmos
Microphthalmos
Fibrosis
Amniotic band
Team evaluation
Tumors
Teratoma
Retinoblastoma
(p 132)
Dacryocele (p 14)
Dermoid (p 14)
Hemangioma
Lymphangioma
(H) BIOPSY ± SURGERY,
CHEMOTHERAPY,
RADIATION

LID AND ADNEXAL MASSES IN THE NEONATE

Trudi R. Grin, M.D.

A. When evaluating the neonate with a lid or adnexal mass, a careful history is important to rule out any associated systemic disease, such as plexiform neurofibroma seen with neurofibromatosis. A complete ophthalmic evaluation is essential to determine if any associated ocular abnormalities are present.

B. Nevi are common benign, congenital tumors that may be flat or slightly elevated. Pigmentation may be present at birth, but nevi may darken or enlarge at puberty. The lid margin is a common location. Surgical excision (except for cosmesis) is not necessary unless the nevus increases in size or pigmentation.

C. Dermoid cysts are choristomas that are thought to form as a result of developmental invagination of ectodermal tissue. Typically this cyst is firm, nontender, rubbery, and well circumscribed. Dermoid cysts are usually attached to the periosteum, limiting movement to some degree on palpation. Approximately one-half are located in the upper temporal quadrant (lateral brow region) and one-fourth in the upper nasal quadrant. Twenty-five percent are present at birth, and the natural history is one of gradual enlargement of the cyst. Rarely, bony defects may be seen underlying the cyst, and a CT scan may be helpful, especially with nasal dermoids (Fig. 1). Complete surgical excision is generally recommended because the cyst may occasionally rupture and cause a severe inflammatory reaction. Incompletely excised dermoids may recur.

D. Lid involvement in neurofibromatosis is rare in the first year of life. Neurofibromas or plexiform neuromas tend to involve the upper lid in a diffuse fashion. These masses may cause ptosis or a severe cosmetic defect. Surgical removal of these tumors is difficult owing to the diffuse involvement of the lid.

E. Capillary hemangiomas (strawberry nevi) are nonheritable, benign tumors composed of proliferating endothelial cells and anastomosing, blood-filled channels. These tumors range in size from a small strawberry mark to a large cauliflower-shaped mass. Capillary hemangiomas are quite common, occurring in 1% of all infants. Twenty percent are present at birth, and most are visible within the first 3 months of life. The usual presentation is a small red spot or mass that enlarges during the first 6 months of life. More than 80% regress spontaneously, beginning by age 2 years, and regression is generally complete by age 7 years. When the tumor involves the lid or orbit, ocular complications may ensue such as amblyopia (either from lid occlusion or induced astigmatism from compression of the globe by tumor), strabismus, proptosis, or optic nerve compression. If anisometropia and or amblyopia develops, the refractive error should be corrected promptly and occlusion therapy instituted. If vision is threatened by lid occlusion from the tumor or globe distortion, intervention with intralesional corticosteroid injection should be considered. Use a 25-gauge needle with 1 ml of 50:50 mixture of triamcinolone acetonide (40 mg/ml) and betamethasone (6 mg/ml). Complications include formation of crystalline deposits, fat atrophy, eyelid necrosis, and adrenal suppression.

F. Lymphangiomas are uncommon lesions consisting of endothelium-lined vascular spaces filled with lymph. When they occur in the lid, associated facial or conjunctival involvement is often present. About one-third are present at birth, and most are manifest by 5 years of age. Clinically, a lymphangioma appears as a bluish, noncompressible mass. In contrast to capillary hemangiomas, they tend to increase gradually in size and do not regress. A common feature is enlargement with upper respiratory tract infection. Spontaneous hemorrhage or hemorrhage with minor trauma is also more common with lymphangiomas. Surgical excision is generally not advised unless the lesion causes a significant functional or cosmetic problem. Bleeding within the lesion (chocolate cysts) may be associated with acute onset of proptosis or ptosis. Complete surgical excision is difficult owing to the diffuse nature of lymphangiomas and may be complicated by damage to the normal lid structures. Recent work with the CO_2 laser shows promise in dealing with these lesions.

G. Nevus flammeus (port wine stain) usually involves the facial distribution of the trigeminal nerve. Clinically the lesion is dark pink to purple in color, nonelevated, and, in contrast to capillary hemangiomas, does not blanch with pressure. Nevus flammeus is present at birth and does not regress over time. Two percent of all patients with nevus flammeus have leptomeningeal

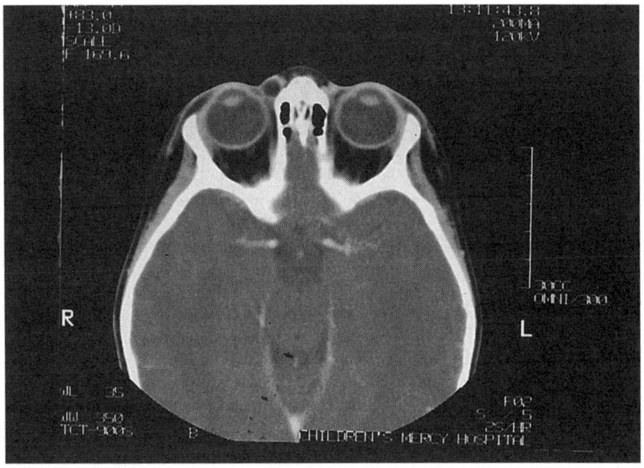

Figure 1 CT of nasal dermoid.

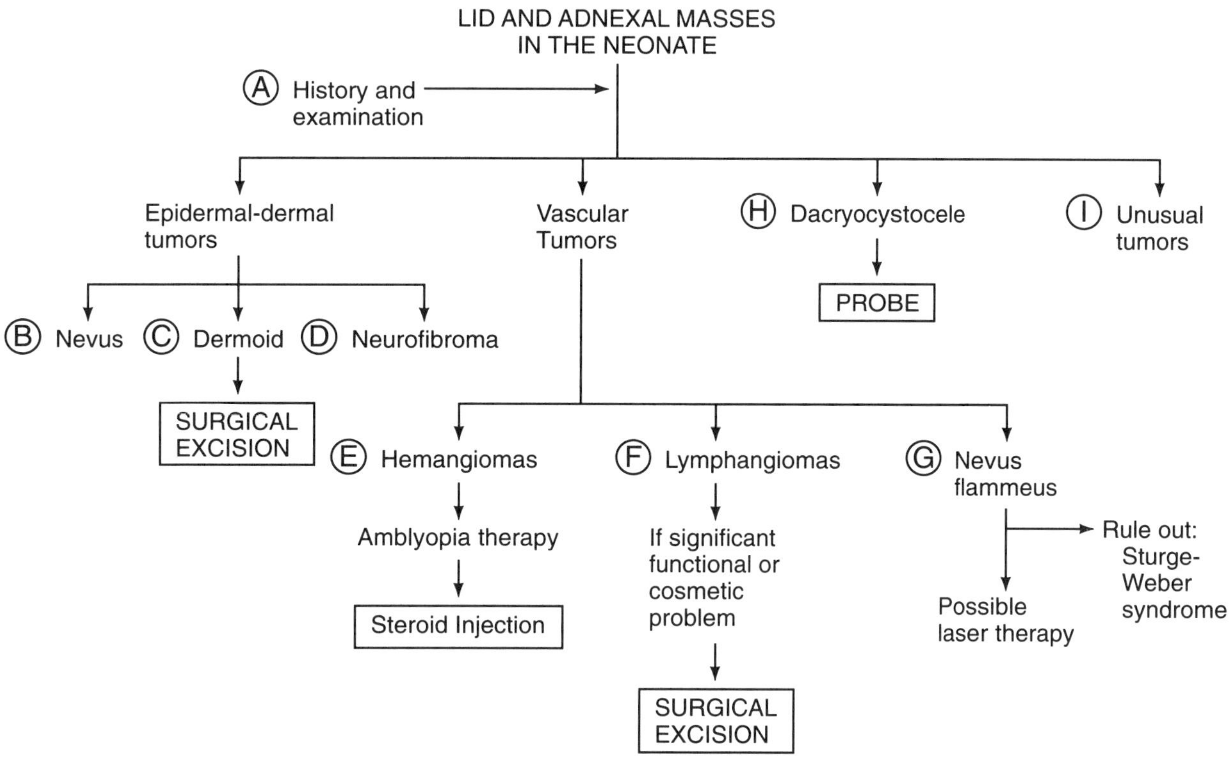

angiomas (Sturge-Weber syndrome; see p 134) and, of these, 30% have glaucoma. Recently, laser therapy has been shown to be extremely effective in the treatment of the port wine stain.

H. Congenital dacryocystocele (mucocele, amniotocele) is an uncommon variant of congenital nasolacrimal duct obstruction. This condition is characterized by unilateral or bilateral distention of the nasolacrimal sac, with a grey-blue cystic mass just below the medial canthus. The findings are typically seen at birth or develop within the first few weeks of life. A secondary dacryocystitis frequently develops. The lesion is sometimes mistaken for an hemangioma and must be differentiated from a midline encephalocele. Nasolacrimal duct cysts resulting from distention of the distal nasolacrimal duct have recently been reported in association with dacryocystocele and when bilateral may cause nasal obstruction and respiratory distress. A CT or MR scan may be helpful if the diagnosis is unclear. Treatment consists of decompression of the sac with massage and antibiotics if dacryocystitis is present. Nasolacrimal duct probing with nasal examination is recommended for patients who do not respond to conservative treatment.

I. Rhabdomyosarcoma may arise in the lid from the lid muscles but more frequently involves the orbit. This tumor is rare in the first year of life. The lids may be involved in metastatic neuroblastoma and should be considered in the differential diagnosis of a lid mass in an infant, especially if ecchymosis of the lid is a prominent feature.

References

Ashinoff R, Geronemus R. Flash lamp pumped pulse dye laser for port wine stains in infancy: Earlier vs. later treatment. J Am Acad Dermatol 1991; 24:467.

Grin TR, Mertz JM, Stass-Isern M. Congenital nasolacrimal duct cysts in dacryocystocele. Ophthalmology 1991; 98:1238.

Kushner BJ. Intralesional corticosteroid injection for infantile adnexal hemangioma. Am J Ophthalmol 1982; 93:496.

Pollard ZF, Harley RD, Calhoun J. Dermoid cysts in children. Pediatrics 1976; 57:379.

Stigmar G, Crawford JS, Ward CM, Thomson HG. Ophthalmic sequelae of infantile hemangiomas of the eyelids and orbit. Am J Ophthalmol 1978; 85:806.

Weiss AH. Adrenal suppression after corticosteroid injection of peri-ocular hemangiomas. Am J Ophthalmol 1989; 107:518.

NEONATAL CONJUNCTIVAL DISCHARGE

Sherwin J. Isenberg, M.D.

A. If within 30 days of birth the discharge from a red eye in an infant is colored, the diagnosis is either toxic or infectious conjunctivitis. One should seek a history of venereal disease or discharge from the parents and find out which agent was used for ophthalmic prophylaxis. The time of onset of conjunctivitis and the type and intensity of discharge are helpful in the diagnosis (Table 1).

B. Following a cesarean section within 3 hours of rupture of membranes, the conjunctiva has been shown either to be sterile or to bear a few aerobic cutaneous-type bacteria.

C. If the infection began within 3 days of birth and the laboratory tests prove negative, the probable diagnosis is toxic conjunctivitis, particularly if silver nitrate was used as the prophylactic agent. If laboratory tests are positive for a venereal organism, the parents should be worked up and parents and child treated appropriately.

D. Conjunctival epithelial cells should be obtained with a spatula. Most other techniques do not gather enough cells for analysis.

E. On Giemsa stain, chlamydial infection can be diagnosed if one sees paranuclear cytoplasmic inclusion bodies in a field of mixed inflammatory cells, especially polymorphonuclear leukocytes. A finding of intranuclear inclusions and multinucleate giant cells suggests the presence of herpes simplex virus.

F. To obtain a specimen of conjunctival exudate, place a moistened cotton-tipped applicator deeply into the inferior conjunctival fornix. Avoid contact with the eyelid speculum or bent paper clip used to evert or widen the eyelids.

G. A clear discharge suggests a noninfectious cause. Family history may indicate infantile glaucoma or familial lacrimal hypersecretion. Ocular examination may demonstrate the enlarged and cloudy cornea of glaucoma, swelling in the area of the nasolacrimal sac of dacryocystocele or nasolacrimal duct obstruction, or increased lacrimation on feeding indicative of the gustatory-lacrimal reflex. The initial clear discharge resulting from nasolacrimal duct obstruction may later become colored as infection ensues.

TABLE 1 Differential Diagnosis of Colored Discharge

Cause	*Discharge*		
	Onset after birth	*Type*	*Intensity*
Toxic	2–72 hr	Mucopurulent	Mild to moderate
Gonococcus	1–21 days	Purulent	Severe
Chlamydia	4–30 days	Mucopurulent	Mild to moderate
Other bacteria	2–30 days	Mucopurulent	Mild to moderate

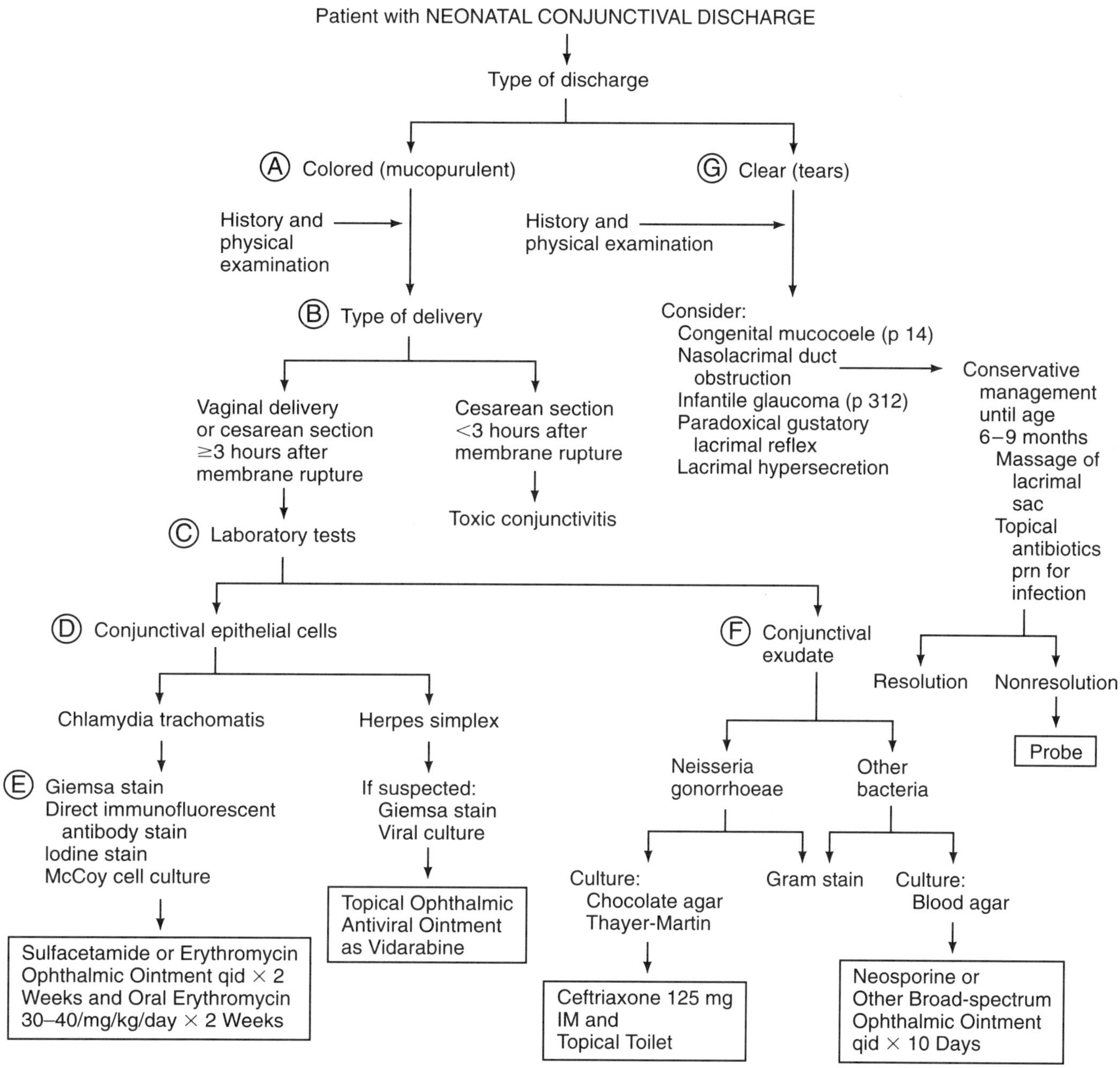

References

Holland GN. Infectious diseases. In: Isenberg SJ, ed. The eye in infancy. Chicago: Year Book, 1989:387.

Isenberg SJ, Apt L, Yoshimori R, et al. The source of the conjunctival flora at birth and implications for ophthalmia neonatorum prophylaxis. Am J Ophthalmol 1988; 106:458.

Rapoza PA, Quinn TC, Kiessling LA, et al. Epidemiology of neonatal conjunctivitis. Ophthalmology 1986; 93:456.

Sandstrom I. Treatment of neonatal conjunctivitis. Arch Ophthalmol 1987; 105:925.

ABNORMALITIES OF CORNEAL SIZE

Colleen J. Christian, M.D.

The normal newborn cornea measures approximately 10 mm in diameter and reaches the average adult measurement of 11.75 mm by 2 years of age. Corneal diameter >12 mm or <10 mm at birth is abnormal and must be thoroughly evaluated. Anterior and posterior segments are inspected for associated anomalies. Intraocular pressure is measured. This can be done in the office with a Tonopen (Biorad) or a Perkins hand-held tonometer. A-scan ultrasonography and retinoscopy can be used to evaluate axial length. Precise diagnosis is necessary to predict the natural history of the disorder, to begin appropriate medical or surgical therapy, and to aid in detection of any associated systemic abnormalities. Embryologically, neural crest–derived mesenchymal cells differentiate into the cornea (except the epithelium), the angle structures, and the iris stroma. These structures are subject to common influences during development, and abnormalities often occur in more than one.

A. Megalocornea refers to a cornea measuring 13 mm or more in horizontal diameter. It is glaucoma until proven otherwise (p 312). Diagnosis of megalocornea can be made in a child with an enlarged cornea only when no evidence of glaucoma is found.

B. Megalocornea has two forms: simple megalocornea and anterior megalophthalmos. It is often clinically difficult to distinguish these two disorders in the infant, and long-term follow-up may be necessary to separate them. Simple megalocornea is a nonprogressive, bilateral condition in which the cornea is enlarged without other associated ocular abnormalities. All patterns of inheritance have been reported. Some patients are myopic owing to increased corneal curvature, although the curvature may also be normal. Once the diagnosis is clearly made, follow-up is necessary only for refractive correction.

C. Anterior megalopthalmos is an X-linked recessive, bilateral disorder including megalocornea, iris abnormalities, and an enlarged ciliary ring. Abnormal spatial relationships in the anterior segment may result in high astigmatism and lens subluxation. Transillumination defects and an ectopic pupil can be seen due to iris abnormalities. Although simple megalocornea requires no special long-term follow-up, anterior megalophthalmos is associated with three complications that occur later in life: ectopia lentis, glaucoma due to angle anomalies, and premature cataracts. These patients require lifelong annual examinations and surgical intervention when appropriate.

D. Microcornea refers to a cornea with horizontal diameter <10 mm. It may be an isolated abnormality in an otherwise normal eye or may accompany abnormalities of the iris, angle, or lens. It may be a component of microphthalmos, in which the whole eye is small. Microcornea is also found in sclerocornea, anterior segment dysgenesis (a developmental abnormality involving various anterior segment structures), and congenital cataracts; axial length is normal in these disorders. Ultrasonography-documented axial length helps to separate these two categories.

E. Microphthalmos is a developmental abnormality of ocular size. It is suspected on the basis of microcornea, high hyperopia, or a small palpebral fissure. Diagnosis is established by an axial length measurement at least two standard deviations below the age-adjusted normal value. Microphthalmos can be divided into two types: complex, in which the eye is malformed, and simple, in which the eye is anatomically intact.

F. In complex microphthalmos, because either the anterior or posterior segment may be abnormal, the appearance of the globe varies considerably. Colobomatous and noncolobomatous forms have been described (p 48). When malformation severely limits visual potential, cosmesis becomes a priority. Tissue expanders of increasing size are placed in the eye to stimulate normal fissure and orbit growth. This allows placement of an appropriately sized prosthesis as the child grows.

G. Uveal colobomata are frequently associated with microphthalmos (p 122).

H. In noncolobomatous complex microphthalmos, the eye is small and malformed. Reported malformations include anterior segment dysgenesis, cataract, persistent hyperplastic primary vitreous (PHPV), and retinal dysplasia. All inheritance patterns have been reported. Treatment varies according the underlying pathology. When possible, surgery is done to maintain a clear visual axis. This is followed by correction of refractive errors and patching for amblyopia when the malformation is asymmetric or unilateral. When malformation severely limits visual potential, tissue expanders are used.

I. Simple microphthalmos is characterized by microcornea, high hyperopia, and a shortened axial length. The posterior segment is disproportionately reduced in size. Simple microphthalmos has been called *nanophthalmos.* It can be associated with such systemic disorders as fetal alcohol syndrome, myotonic dystrophy, and the mucopolysaccharidosis and mucolipidosis syndromes. Retinal detachment, glaucoma, and premature cataracts often develop between the third and fifth decades of life. Any ocular surgery may be complicated by severe uveal effusion and should be attempted with this in mind. In children, a careful refraction should be done and any amblyogenic asymmetry treated.

J. Anterior segment dysgenesis (neurocristopathies; p 140).

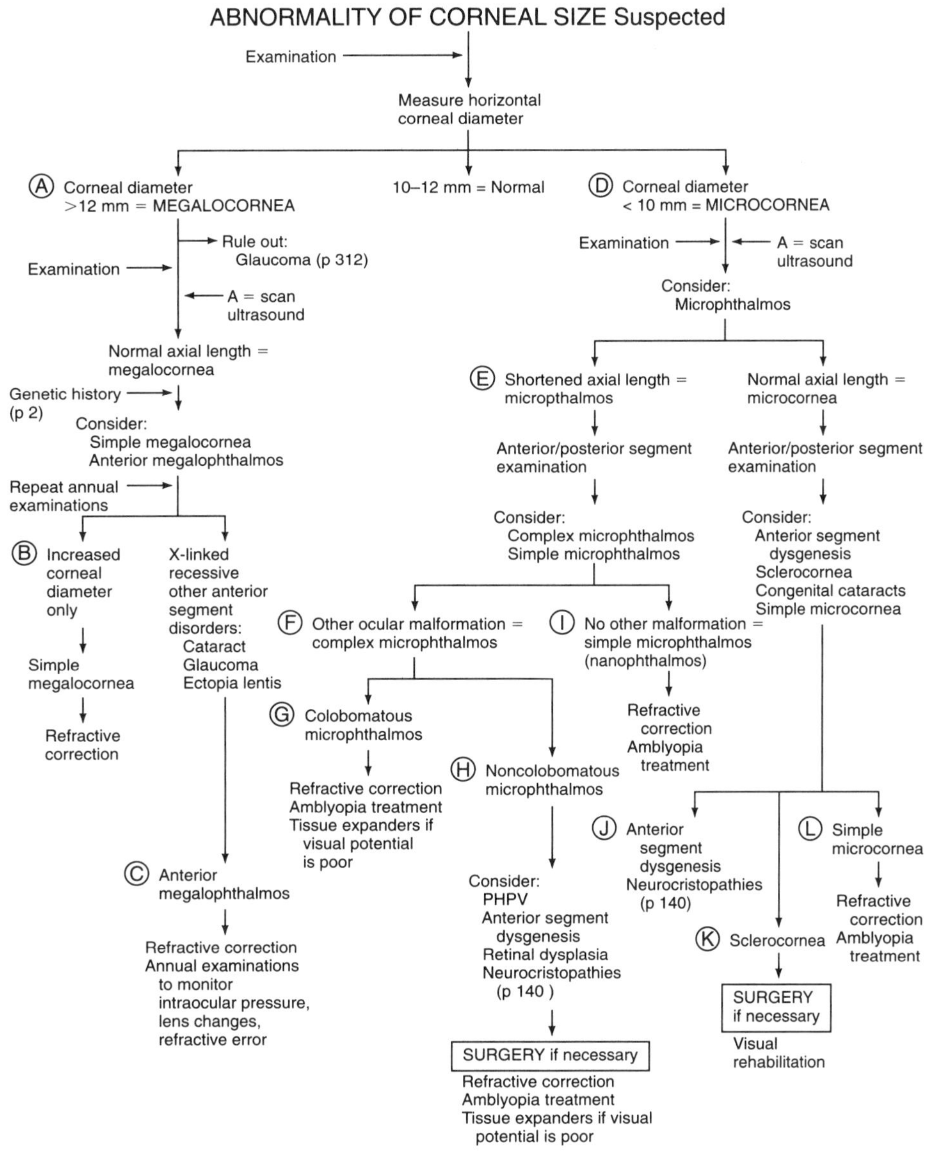

K. Sclerocornea is a congenital, bilateral, often asymmetric peripheral corneal opacification with vascularization. The limbus is usually ill-defined, and superficial vessels that are extensions of normal scleral, episcleral, and conjunctival vessels cross the cornea. Scleralization may be only peripheral but usually involves the entire cornea. Even when opacification is complete, the central cornea is often slightly less opaque than the periphery. When only the periphery is involved, the corneal diameter appears small. Sclerocornea is a nonprogressive disorder. Flattened cornea (cornea plana), shallowing of the anterior chamber, iris abnormalities, glaucoma, and microphthalmos have been described in association with sclerocornea. Ninety percent of cases are bilateral, and no pattern of inheritance has been identified. Glaucoma should be excluded and careful refraction done, as these patients are often hyperopic.

L. Microcornea may be an isolated abnormality in an otherwise normal eye. All inheritance patterns have been reported. Hyperopia is common owing to decreased corneal curvature, but the curvature may also be normal. Lifelong annual examinations are necessary to monitor the intraocular pressure, which is more commonly elevated in eyes with microcornea.

References

Good W, Hoyt C. Corneal abnormalities in childhood. In: Taylor D, ed. Pediatric ophthalmology. London: Blackwell, 1990:178.

Laibson PR, Waring GO. Diseases of the cornea. In: Nelson LB, Calhoun JH, Harley RD, eds. Pediatric ophthalmology. 3rd ed. Philadelphia: WB Saunders, 1991:191.

Weiss AH, Kousseff BG, Ross EA, Longbottom J. Complex microphthalmos. Arch Ophthalmol 1989; 107:1619.

Weiss AH, Kousseff BG, Ross EA, Longbottom J. Simple microphthalmos. Arch Ophthalmol 1989; 107:1625.

Wilson FM. Congenital anomalies. In: Smoling G, Thoft RA, eds. The cornea. 2nd ed. Boston: Little, Brown & Co, 1987:457.

CONGENITAL CORNEAL CLOUDING

Gerhard W. Cibis, M.D.

A. Evaluating a newborn for corneal clouding should include taking a history for possible forceps injury, familial diseases or dystrophies, intrauterine infections, and any drugs taken during pregnancy. Proper blood titers should be ordered when indicated. Gross examination in the nursery may be adequate. An evaluation under anesthesia (EUA), when the infant is able to tolerate it, is appropriate where needed and should not be delayed because of age. Gross inspection includes an examination for systemic findings that may indicate the ocular cause of clouding. This includes cataracts in TORCH (toxoplasmosis, rubella, cytomegalovirus, and herpes simplex) preaurical tags associated with corneal dermoids, dysmorphisms or anomalies of the extremities in cases of chromosomal disorders, and the presence of photophobia and tearing which would support the diagnosis of glaucoma (see pp 120, 312, 314).

B. Infectious keratitis is usually not present at birth. With most TORCH infections, especially rubella, keratitis manifests later. Glaucoma can be superimposed on the anterior chamber disruption and must be differentiated. TORCH and syphilis titers, as well as metabolic work-up, are indicated. EUA may be needed. Look for other associated systemic and ocular findings for the suspected diagnosis such as cataracts, chorioretinitis, and skeletal anomalies.

C. Microphthalmos is covered on page 18. An opacified cornea of small diameter may be seen in association with rubella, trisomy 13, sclerocornea, and glaucoma in the presence of microphthalmos. Colobomatous microphthalmos occurs when the embryonic cleft of the optic vesicle fails to close. Sclerocornea and microcornea (see p 18) can be present in a normal-sized globe. Both are often associated with systemic findings such as chromosomal anomalies and may be part of other syndromes. When they are bilateral, a chromosomal work-up is indicated.

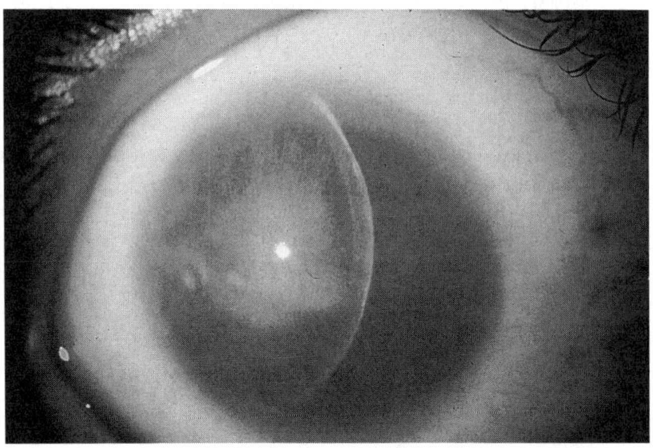

Figure 1 Congenital hereditary endothelial dystrophy (CHED).

D. *Neurocristopathies* (p 140) is the current term for what was previously called "mesodermal dysgenesis" or "anterior chamber cleavage anomalies," now known to be defects in migration, differentiation, or regression of neural crest cells. Associated systemic findings should be looked for. EUA for gonioscopy may be needed. Posterior embryotoxon is a prominent Schwalbe's line found in up to 15% of normal individuals and may therefore be totally benign. Axenfeld anomaly, prominent iris processes to Schwalbe's line without other iris or pupillary anomalies, is usually benign but can be associated with glaucoma. Rieger syndrome is associated with iris hypoplasia and corectopia. Glaucoma, infantile or late onset, is common. This is often autosomal dominant. Examination of family members is indicated in all neurocristopathies. Peters anomaly includes central corneal clouding due to adhesion of lens to cornea in anterior chamber formation. It can be familial but is also seen in association with other systemic findings, as in fetal alcohol syndrome or chromosomal anomalies. It occurs with Walker-Warburg syndrome associated with developmental brain abnormalities (lissencephaly), retinal dysgenesis, and Fukuyama congenital muscular dystrophy. Brain imaging studies are appropriate.

E. Forceps injuries are usually unilateral, are associated with facial lesions from the forceps on the side of injury, and have a clear history of forceps being used. One should also look for conjunctival hemorrhages. The resultant corneal edema from Descemet's rupture (Haab striae) clears within a few weeks as endothelium covers the defect. Steroid eye drops enhance healing by reducing anterior chamber inflammation. Patching for amblyopia and glasses for induced astigmatism and anisometropia are often indicated.

F. Buphthalmos at birth is rare. Most congenital glaucomas manifest in the first year of life (see p 312). An EUA for gonioscopy, intraocular pressure, axial length, optic nerve inspection, and possible surgery is mandatory (see p 310 on congenital glaucoma management). Buphthalmos may be confused with simple megalocornea.

G. Congenital hereditary endothelial dystrophy (CHED), posterior polymorphous dystrophy (PPMD), and congenital stromal dystrophy can manifest at birth. They are differentiated from glaucoma by normal intraocular tension and corneal size, preponderance of deep stromal and less epithelial edema, and characteristic corneal and iris findings. CHED and PPMD can be associated with glaucoma, congenital or late onset. EUA is not mandatory if clinical signs are clear and glaucoma is not present.

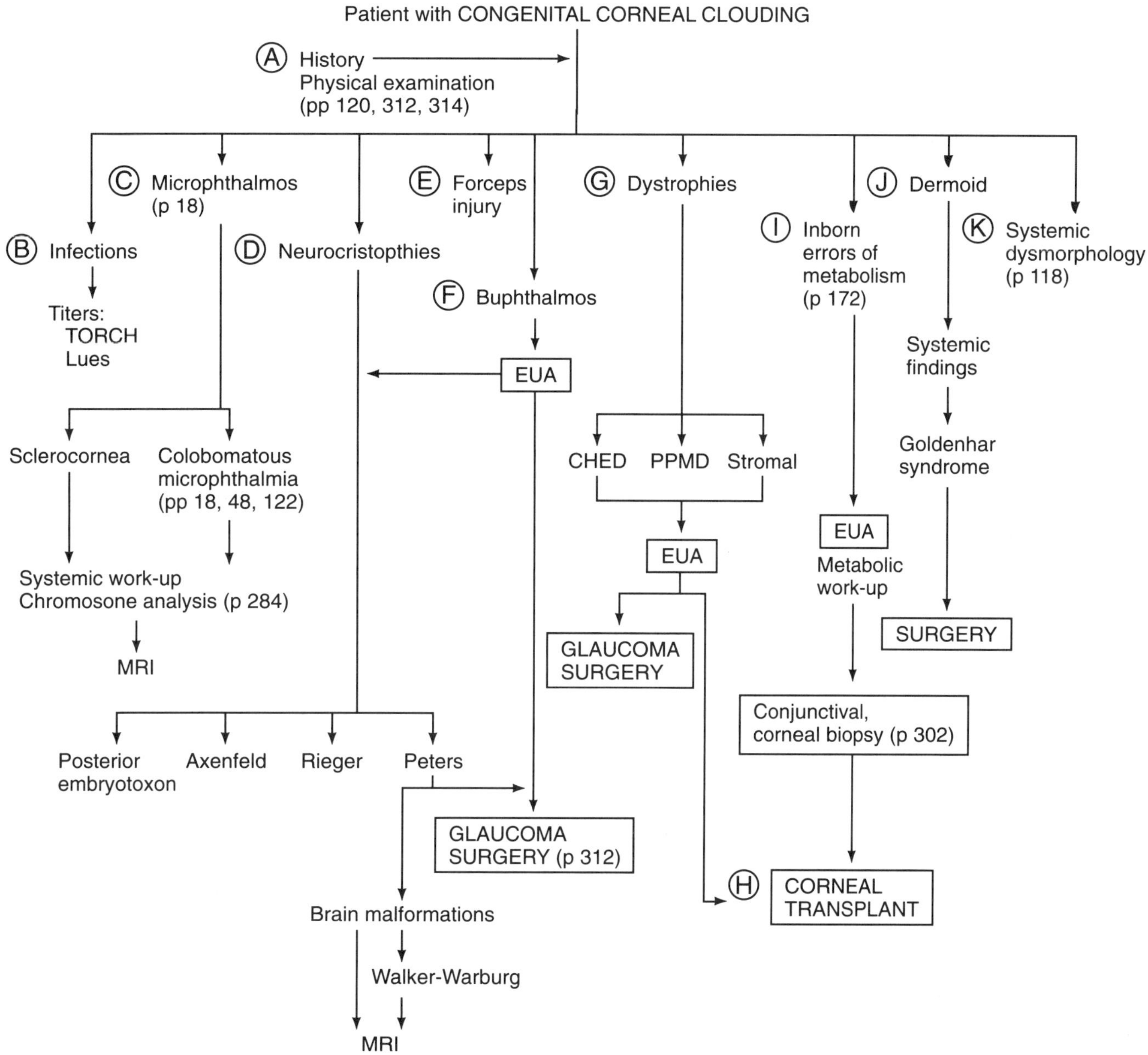

H. Any cause of corneal clouding in infancy, when sufficiently severe and prolonged to be amblyogenic, raises the question of therapy including corneal transplantation as part of management (see p 184, Amblyopia Management, and p 26, Corneal Transplantation in Children).

I. Many inborn errors of metabolism cause corneal clouding. Usually the corneal clouding is not present at birth (see p 172).

J. Corneal dermoids are choristomas, i.e., normal tissue at an inappropriate location. They are commonly associated with preaurical tags in Goldenhar syndrome, as well as other skull, limb, facial, and skeletal anomalies.

K. Any cloudy cornea with dysmorphology should be worked up as on p 118.

References

Cibis GW. Congenital glaucoma. J Am Optom Assoc 1987; 58:728.

Cibis GW, Krachmer JH, Phelps CD, Weingeist TA. The clinical spectrum of posterior polymorphous dystrophy. Arch Ophthalmol 1977; 95:1529.

Elston J. Developmental abnormalities of the cornea and iris. In: Taylor D, ed. Pediatric ophthalmology. Boston: Blackwell Scientific, 1990:168.

Good W, Hoyt C. Corneal abnormalities in childhood. In: Taylor D, ed. Pediatric ophthalmology. Boston: Blackwell Scientific, 1990:178.

CORNEAL TRANSPLANTS IN CHILDREN

Daniel S. Durrie, M.D.
Timothy B. Cavanaugh, M.D.
Shawn M. Riedel, B.S.

Potential benefits for pediatric corneal transplant must outweigh the risk.

A. First evaluate the cause of the corneal opacity. Trauma is established by history. Child abuse must be ruled out. Corneal infections such as congenital herpes, rubella, and syphilis are ruled out by maternal history. Treatment and counseling may be initiated. Congenital glaucoma causes corneal opacities and may be associated with opacities from congenital anomalies (p 24). Recent advances in filtering surgery, goniopIasty, and glaucoma shunts have advanced glaucoma treatment in eyes with congenital anomalies. Corneal transplantation is more successful than in the past. Parent co-operation is paramount in surgical follow-up. Unless parents are willing to undertake intense patching programs, comply with follow-up visits, and control the child's behavior to prevent eye rubbing or injury postoperatively, surgical intervention should not be undertaken.

B. Is the corneal opacity bilateral and obstructing development of vision in both eyes? If neither eye has the ability to see owing to the opacity, surgery is usually indicated.

C. With unilateral corneal opacities, if there is good functional vision in the contralateral eye, corneal transplantation is indicated only under ideal conditions, in which the visual potential in the eye is very high.

D. Positive results from visual function tests are useful. Clinical testing showing good visual function favors transplantation. Tests include observation of good fixation and following movements, optic nerve function by potential acuity measurements, color perception, entoptic phenomenon, pupillary responses, two-point discrimination, and direct examination. Electrophysiology testing is indicated when clinical tests are questionable. Visual evoked response (VER) is abnormal both with organic causes and with amblyopia. A flat or highly abnormal electroretinogram (ERG) is a poor prognostic sign (see pp 294, 298).

E. Amblyopia is a major obstacle in the success of unilateral surgery. Factors to consider prior to surgery include age of the child, density of the opacity, and the ability of patient and family to patch intensively. *One should proceed with surgery only if there is a high likelihood that amblyopia therapy will be successful.*

F. Retinal pathology can preclude the success of a corneal transplant. Strabismus necessitates preoperative and postoperative evaluation and appropriate management. Pre-existing lens opacities or the possibility of inducing further lens changes needs to be considered prior to surgery. An aphakic child with a transplant who becomes contact lens intolerant is extremely difficult to manage. Despite a clear cornea, amblyopia can easily develop.

G. If the cataract is incompatible with good acuity, lens extraction should be performed with corneal surgery. Small anterior polar cataracts are compatible with good acuity. Especially in bilateral cases, they frequently can be left for future surgical intervention.

H. Lens implants (triple procedures): Advances in surgery make posterior chamber intraocular lenses in children a viable alternative. Parents need to be advised that posterior chamber intraocular lenses have not been used in children until recently. Although the long-term prognosis of implants in children is untested, the risk may be worth taking. Aphakic contact lens fitting and wear in transplanted children are difficult and can interfere with amblyopia therapy.

I. If the corneal opacity is limited to the anterior one-half of the cornea, lamellar keratoplasty is ideal. Avoidance of intraocular infection, rejection reaction, and surgical trauma make lamellar keratoplasty the first choice for superficial opacities. Penetrating keratoplasty (PK) is needed if the corneal opacity is deep in the stroma.

J. Transplant tissue for PK should reflect the recipient's age. Younger corneas have greater endothelial cell density (approaching 3500 cells/mm^2) and are less likely to contain abnormalities such as guttata. Even in newborn recipients, corneas less than 2 years of age are not recommended. Such tissue is floppy and difficult to handle. The corneal curvature is very steep, yielding excessive myopia after keratoplasty. Use of steep infant donor tissue is indicated in aphakic grafts, in which the high corneal curvature serves to reduce the refractive error.

K. Pediatric transplants must be done under general anesthesia in a hospital setting involving the pediatrician. Scleral rigidity is unpredictable in children. Even in phakic grafts, ocular collapse can occur owing to excessively thin sclera. Because it is somewhat unpredictable, we tend to use a Flieringa ring. A Honan balloon is recommended to soften the globe preoperatively. We have not found it necessary to use osmotic agents. We use the same surgical techniques as with adult transplants. Trephine size depends on corneal diameter and ranges from 7 to 8.5 mm. We generally oversize the donor tissue by 0.25 mm unless dealing with an extremely flat cornea preoperatively. With sclerocornea or cornea plana, an 0.50 mm oversized donor button should be used. A Hessburg Barron vacuum trephine is recommended because it provides the most controlled entry in phakic transplants, in

CONSIDERATIONS FOR CORNEAL TRANSPLANTS IN CHILDREN

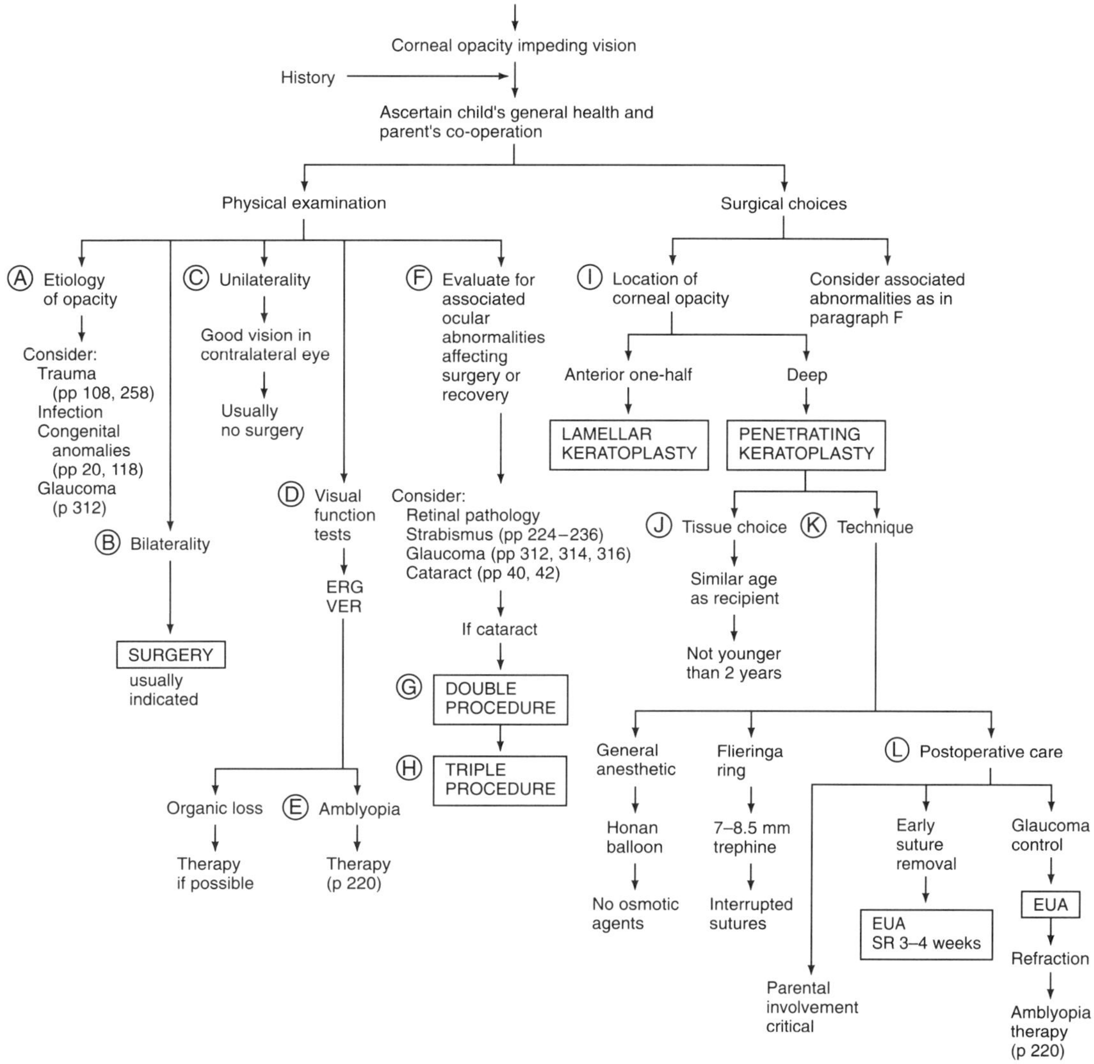

which lens protection is vital. Invariably there is a great deal of posterior pressure. Expect a flat anterior chamber upon removal of host tissue. This flattening does not respond to manipulation of the lid speculum, drapes, or other conventional methods. It does not represent impending expulsive hemorrhage and is dealt with by injecting viscoelastic into the chamber angle over the iris and lens. This protects the lens from trauma and provides a barrier between the donor endothelium and underlying structures during graft suturing. One must be very careful not to sew iris to the wound. Once the first eight sutures are placed, the chamber usually deepens. Placement of the remaining sutures is simpler. Sixteen to 20 interrupted 10-0 nylon sutures are recommended. Pediatric patients heal quickly. Sutures vascularize rapidly, which precludes the use of running suture. In children over 10 years, running suture is possible. For lamellar keratoplasties, 24-bite 10-0 nylon sutures are recommended to prevent graft edge lift between sutures.

L. Success depends on diligent efforts by both the surgeon and the patient's parents. Uncomplicated opacities have a good prognosis. Success diminishes with concurrent conditions such as congenital glaucoma. Early suture removal is vital. The graft wounds heal quickly with rapid scarring. Vascularization, if left unattended, can lead to severe allograft rejection and failure. In patients less than 6 months old we recommend examination under anesthesia (EUA) with removal of any loose or vascularized sutures at 1 week. Remaining sutures should be removed at 3 to 4 weeks. In children age 6 months to 4 years, we perform partial suture removal at 2 weeks and strive to have all sutures out by 4 to 8 weeks. Risk of graft dehiscence is minimal even with suture removal within the first week. Parents must be educated to monitor the child closely for the warning signs of graft rejection. The importance of early diagnosis and treatment of rejections cannot be overemphasized. Postoperative astigmatism control is an ongoing problem. Treatment includes eyeglass or contact lens correction. Refractive surgical procedures are playing an increasingly important role in the treatment of postkeratoplasty astigmatism in pediatric transplants.

IRREGULAR PUPILS

Joanne Waeltermann, M.D.

A. Aniridia is the congenital absence of iris tissue, causing the appearance of fully dilated pupils. Variable expression is the rule, ranging from mild hypoplasia of the iris to total lack of all but the most rudimentary iris tissue beneath the corneoscleral junction. The cause is a defect in neuroectodermal or mesodermal elements. There are two modes of inheritance for aniridia: the autosomal dominant and the sporadic, which is associated with a chromosome 11 defect, Wilms' tumor, and mental retardation. Ocular findings include macular hypoplasia, glaucoma, and corneal opacity.

B. Iris colobomata give the pupils a keyhole shape caused by a segmental lack of iris tissue. Typical inferonasal colobomata result from failure of the embryonic fissure to close and are associated with chorioretinal and disc colobomata. Notching or iris defects elsewhere are "atypical" and not associated with retinal findings. Iris colobomata may be confined to the stroma or pigment epithelial layers. Colobomata often have persistent pupillary membranes and, where the iris strands bridge the opening, may simulate polycoria. When colobomata are found in patients with multiple malformations, syndromes to be considered include; CHARGE, Aicardi, trisomy 13, and Goldenhar. When isolated, they are inherited as an autosomal dominant trait. Anisometropic amblyopia, obscuration of the visual axis, and retinal complications may also occur (see p 62).

C. Persistent pupillary membranes are common findings and consist of fine pigmented strands of anterior iris stroma bridging the pupil. They may be thick and distort the pupil but only rarely cause visual impairment. The strands may also attach to the anterior lens capsule, creating anterior polar type of cataract, or leave star-shaped pigment deposits. They are caused by the incomplete involution of the iris' anterior vascular arcades.

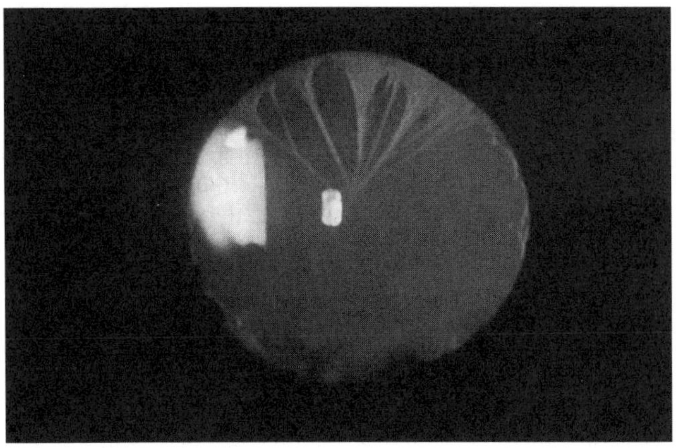

Figure 1 Persistent pupillary membrane seen in retroillumination.

D. Primary iris cysts of the pigment epithelium may appear at the pupillary margin (iris flocculi) and cause an irregular pupil. These cysts are dark brown pigmented, globular structures that ring the pupil. When unilateral, they are not heritable and may be single or multiple. The bilateral cases are familial and multiple. The cause is unclear but may be due to faulty closure of the optic cup layers. These have a benign course.

E. Congenital ectropion uveae (CEU) is a rare unilateral stable condition in which hyperplasia of the iris pigment epithelium extends onto the anterior surface of the iris. The pupil may appear larger or may be oval. This is differentiated from bilateral pupillary ruffs, in which a double layer of pigment epithelium forms a crenated pupillary border. Glaucoma is very common in CEU and is usually diagnosed in childhood. CEU is most commonly associated with neurofibromatosis, although Rieger anomaly (p 134), Prader-Willi syndrome, and chromosomal abnormalities have also been found. CEU is best thought of as a neurocristopathy (see p 140).

F. Congenital miosis and congenital mydriasis are extremely rare conditions. Microcoria is due to an absence of the iris dilator muscle. It is bilateral, frequently autosomal dominant, and associated with good vision. The pupils are 1 to 1.5 mm and poorly reactive. The diagnosis of congenital mydriasis should not be made until neurologic disease and loss of parasympathetic input have been excluded (see p 30). The congenitally dilated pupils are fixed to light and pharmacologics. Because this is autosomal dominant, examination of other family members may avoid a neurologic work-up. The lack of iris musculature has been suggested as a cause.

G. Ectopia, or displacement of the pupil, may be congenital and may be associated with ectopia lentis. Ectopia lentis et pupillae is occasionally missed because the pupillary displacement may be minimal. This condition is rare and autosomal recessive. Additional findings include persistent pupillary membranes, iridodonesis, and iris transillumination. Neuroectodermal defects are the cause of this disorder.

H. Polycoria is rare and must be differentiated from the more common pseudopolycoria caused by iris atro-

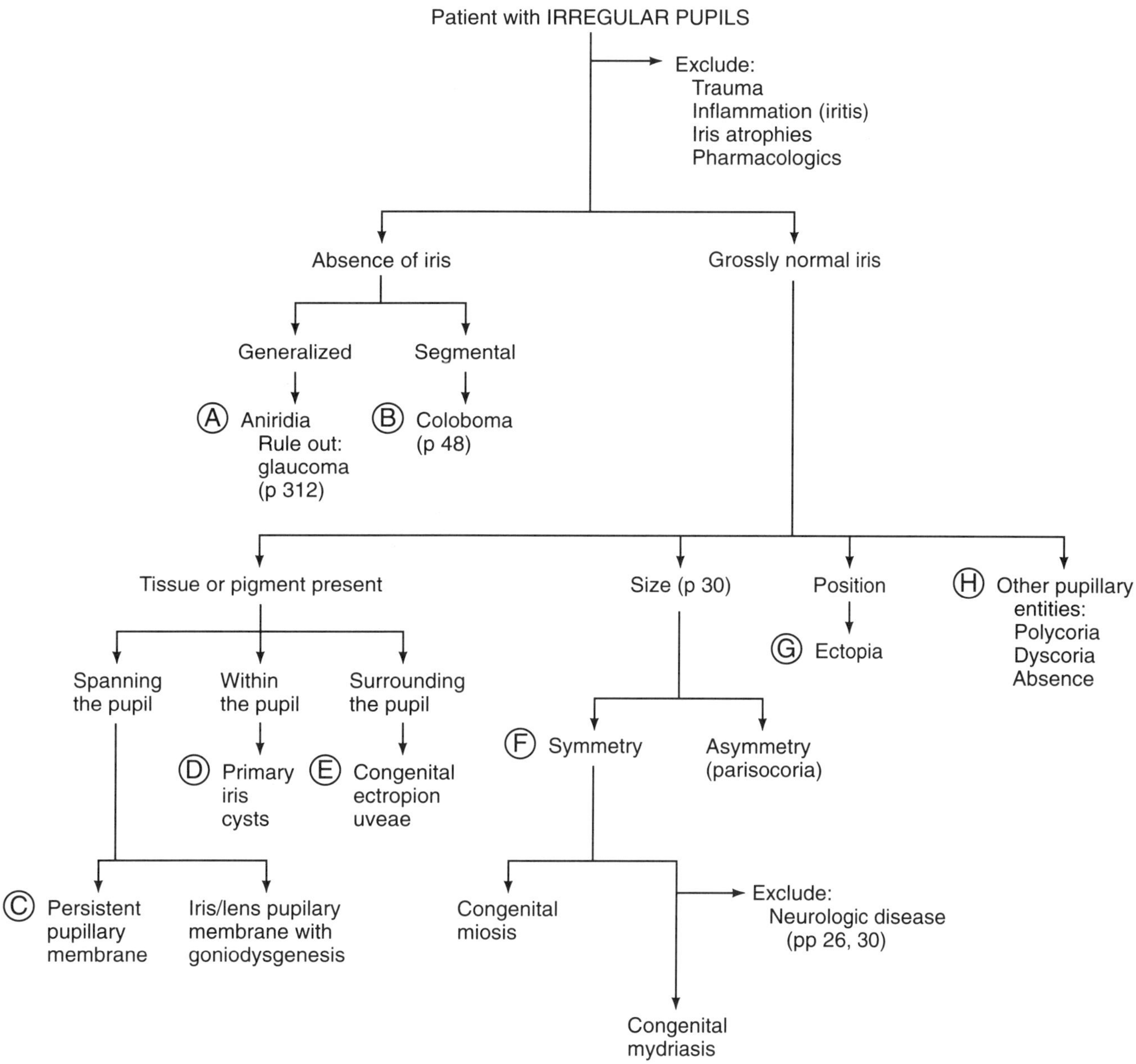

phies (iris defects), trauma, or colobomata (see B). True polycoria has more than one iris aperture with each opening surrounded by a sphincter. Dyscoria, or an abnormally shaped pupil, may be congenital or acquired. Congenital forms are slitlike and usually bilateral. Absence of the pupillary openings has also been reported.

References

Cibis GW, Waeltermann JM, Hurst E, et al. Congenital pupillary-iris-lens membrane with goniodysgenesis (a new entity). Ophthalmology 1986; 93:847.

Goldberg MF. Clinical manifestations of ectopia lentis et pupillae in 16 patients. Ophthalmology 1988; 95:1080.

Ritch R, Forbes M, Hetherington J Jr, et al. Congenital ectropion uveae with glaucoma. Ophthalmology 1984; 91:326.

Shields JA. Primary cysts of the iris. Trans Am Ophthalmol Soc 1981; 79:771.

Waeltermann JM, Hettinger ME, Cibis GW. Congenital cysts of the iris stroma. Am J Ophthalmol 1985; 100:549.

CONGENITAL AND ACQUIRED ANISOCORIA IN CHILDREN

Randy H. Kardon, M.D., Ph.D.
H. Stanley Thompson, M.D.

Pupil inequality, or anisocoria, is usually noticed in room light. Poorly understood, its causality may be asymmetric central inhibitory input to the Edinger-Westphal (parasympathetic) nucleus. Simple anisocoria may fluctuate over minutes, hours, or days, or may always be the same in a given individual. Horner's syndrome (p 30) may be confused with simple anisocoria. Ptosis and anhidrosis differentiate this oculosympathetic deficit. Both conditions show maximal pupil inequality in the dark.

Most other common causes of anisocoria result from sphincter muscle effects. These include (1) trauma, (2) denervation (e.g., post-varicella, Adie's tonic pupil, or third cranial nerve palsy), (3) accidental anticholinergic pharmacologic (e.g., plants, household medicines), (4) inflammatory scarring of the iris to the lens (e.g., uveitis).

A. Careful examination of family photos can be helpful in establishing how the anisocoria was noted, giving clues to etiology. Ptosis and strabismus can be discerned. Birth trauma, head or neck trauma and cardiac trauma (surgery) may help explain the anisocoria. Imaging studies should be reviewed with radiology.

B. The first step in the examination of anisocoria is to decide which is the abnormal pupil, the larger or the smaller. Observe whether the anisocoria increases or decreases in bright light. A weak sphincter cannot constrict well and bright light enhances the anisocoria. If the problem is in the smaller pupil (e.g., simple anisocoria or oculosympathetic defect), the pupillary inequality decreases in bright light. The larger pupil "catches up" with the smaller pupil, which has reached its mechanical limit to constriction sooner.

C. The differential diagnosis when anisocoria decreases is Horner's syndrome, simple anisocoria, mechanical restriction, and aberrant reinnervation from third nerve palsy or long-standing tonic pupil.

D. Horner's syndrome (oculosympathetic deficit) is covered on p 30.

E. If bright light increases anisocoria, the larger pupil is the abnormal one. Causes include parasympathetic nerve damage without reinnervation (e.g., acute Adie's syndrome), or direct sphincter damage (e.g., trauma, ischemia from acute angle closure glaucoma), synechiae, or pharmacologic plegia (anticholinergics inhibiting the sphincter or adrenergic drugs stimulating the dilator) are the differential.

Central inhibition of the pupillomotor center in crying infants may prevent pupil constriction even in bright light. In such a case, try having the mother give the baby its feeding and let it go to sleep. This disinhibits the Edinger-Westphal nucleus and drives a normal pupil down to a very small size, even in low illumination, but not the pupil with a weak sphincter or scarring. Gently lifting the lids of a sleeping infant to observe the pupils in dim light is clearly preferable to struggling with a terrified child in bright illumination.

F. If anisocoria increases in bright light, look for unequal accommodation. Cholinergic drug blockade or denervation as with Adie's tonic pupil or third nerve palsy may be the underlying cause. If accommodation causes anisocoria to diminish or reverse (light-near dissociation), reinnervation from an Adie's pupil or third nerve palsy should be suspected. With equal accommodation and no reduction in anisocoria at near, direct sphincter muscle damage or synechiae to the lens should be considered. Anisocoria from adrenergic drugs acting on the dilator is usually partially overcome by bright light or the near response owing to the more powerful iris sphincter.

G. Segmental sphincter palsy with asymmetric bunching or streaming in areas responding to light or accommodation is usually Adie's pupil or less commonly third nerve palsy. Sphincter tears are a clue to previous orbital trauma, and child abuse needs to be kept in mind when no history of trauma can be elicited. Evidence of uveitis suggests juvenile rheumatoid arthritis.

H. One percent pilocarpine differentiates between sphincter damage, pharmacologic blockage, scarring, and denervation. If both pupils become smaller in the dark 30 minutes after 1% pilocarpine is administered, the bigger pupil was either denervated (in which case it may constrict even more owing to supersensitivity) or dilated with a weak adrenergic drug (which is easily overcome by sphincter cholinergic stimulation). The most common cause of a denervated sphincter without a motility problem or ptosis is a tonic pupil, which in children often occurs following chickenpox.

I. If the larger pupil is associated with a motility abnormality such as poor adduction and infraduction and decreased accommodation, but normal supraduction and no ptosis, then the inferior division of the third nerve has been damaged. Imaging studies are warranted when there is suspicion of third nerve involvement. If normal, follow for resolution. If the condition resolves within 1 to 3 weeks and headache was present (or a family history of migraine exists), a diagnosis of ophthalmoplegic migraine should be considered. If the palsy fails to resolve or is accompanied by signs of aberrant reinnervation or other cranial nerve involvement, reimaging is warranted.

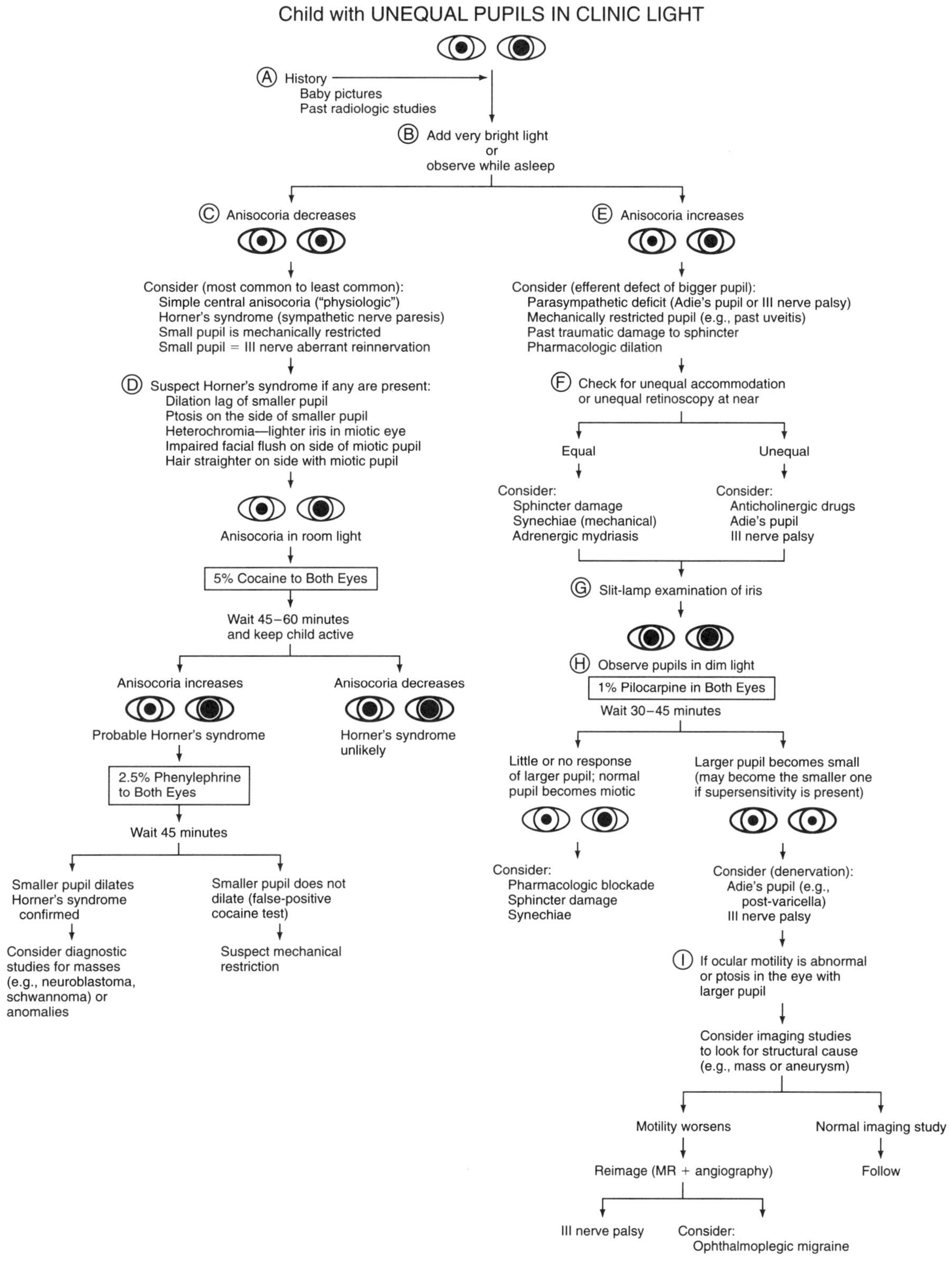

References

Durkan GP, Troost BT, Slamovitz TL, et al. Recurrent painless oculomotor palsy in children. A variant of ophthalmoplegic migraine? Headache 1981; 21:58.

Lam B, Thompson HS. The prevalence of simple anisocoria. Am J Ophthalmol 1987; 104:69.

Loewenfeld IE. "Simple central" anisocoria: A common condition, seldom recognized. Trans Am Acad Ophthalmol Otolaryngol 1977; 83:832.

Thompson HS. Segmental palsy of the iris sphincter in Adie's syndrome. Arch Ophthalmol 1978; 96:1615.

Thompson HS, Pilley FJ. Unequal pupils. A flow chart for sorting out anisocorias. Surv Ophthalmol 1976; 21:45.

LEUKOKORIA

Frederick C. Blodi, M.D.

A. The term *leukokoria* was introduced in 1950 and literally means "white pupil." By definition, cataract is not included. For practical purposes, therefore, leukokoria is any white tissue mass behind a clear lens obscuring the pupil and occurring in infants or young children. The most important cause of leukokoria is retinoblastoma, a highly malignant tumor of infancy. This tumor must always be considered, whether the condition is unilateral or bilateral and regardless of the age of the child at the time of diagnosis. Because of the possible lethal outcome and because of the need to treat early, retinoblastoma always remains number one in the differential diagnosis of leukokoria. Because of its importance, this tumor is discussed in a separate chapter.

B. Only one eye is affected; the other eye is absolutely normal.

C. The condition is diagnosed before the age of 1 year.

D. Persistence and hyperplasia of the primary vitreous (PHPV) is a congenital lesion characterized by a persistence of primary mesenchymal vitreous. With it remnants of the hyaloid arterial system may be present. This is a case of arrested development as the connective tissue of the primary vitreous does not absorb and may proliferate. The affected eye is usually smaller than normal. A grey-white tissue lies behind the lens. Blood vessels are seen in the center of the mass radiating toward the periphery. Ciliary processes often adhere to the mass and are elongated because the central tissue contracts. This contracture eventually breaks the lens capsule, leading somewhat later in life to cataract. The posterior segment of the eye is usually normal, and therefore early surgical intervention may be indicated. (This condition may rarely occur in both eyes.)

E. Retinal dysplasia occurs usually in a small eye (microphthalmos). Characteristic is the malformation of the retina with rosettes, folds, and detachment. Other associated anomalies usually reflect arrested development (e.g., colobomata, persistence of primary vitreous, formation of cartilage). The eye does not usually perceive light.

F. Trauma may certainly produce a white tissue mass behind the lens. This may be an organizing vitreous hemorrhage, an extensive retinal detachment, or gliosis of the retina when large retinal lesions (hemorrhage, exudation) are replaced by glial overgrowth. In cases with equivocal history, consider child abuse!

G. The condition is diagnosed after the age of one.

H. Coats disease is a congenital anomaly of retinal vessels, which show aneurysms, tortuousity, and newly formed vascular structures. These abnormal vessels bleed easily and therefore lead to extensive retinal hemorrhages and hemophthalmos. Characteristic are large yellow retinal exudates and cholesterol deposits. These retinal changes sooner or later lead to a complete detachment, causing a yellowish white mass behind the lens. Characteristic are abnormal newly formed blood vessels on its surface. The condition occurs more often in boys than in girls and usually occurs in the first decade.

I. During septicemia, infected emboli may occlude retinal vessels. The resulting ischemic infarcts may cause extensive retinal necrosis, detachment, and organization of inflammatory cells in the vitreous. Often the history reveals a period of diffuse and intensive inflammatory signs within and around the globe. The cause of the septicemia may be an acute exanthematous disease, herpes simplex, herpes zoster, endocarditis, or drug abuse.

J. *Toxocara canis* infection is a special kind of endophthalmitis caused by the larva of the dog ascarid (visceral larva migrans). The infestation is usually transmitted through the excrement of puppies. Children, when eating dirt or sand, may become infected. The dying nematode produces an eosinophilic granuloma in the vitreous which becomes organized and can detach the retina by traction. A cataract may follow. Enzyme-linked immunosorbent assay (ELISA) of the aqueous may be a helpful diagnostic test. MRI can be helpful in differentiating retinoblastoma from Coats disease and *Toxocara canis* infection.

K. Both eyes are involved.

L. Norrie disease is a sex-linked recessive disease affecting only males. The patients not only have eye disease, but also become deaf owing to a sensorineural hearing loss. The changes in the eye are characterized by anomalies of the retinal vessels, hemorrhages, organization, traction retinal detachment, and formation of a white tissue mass behind the lens.

M. Incontinentia pigmenti is a sex-linked dominant trait that is lethal to males and can therefore be seen only in girls. There is a generalized pigmentary disorder, which may involve the retinal pigment epithelium. The skin changes are characteristic but may be transient. Bullae and papules develop into flat blotches of pigment, often arranged in whorls. The teeth and the central nervous system (seizures, mental retardation) may be affected. In about one third of the children, the eyes are involved. Changes in the retinal vascular system cause retinal detachment, uveitis, proliferation of retinal pigment epithelium, and a retrolental mass.

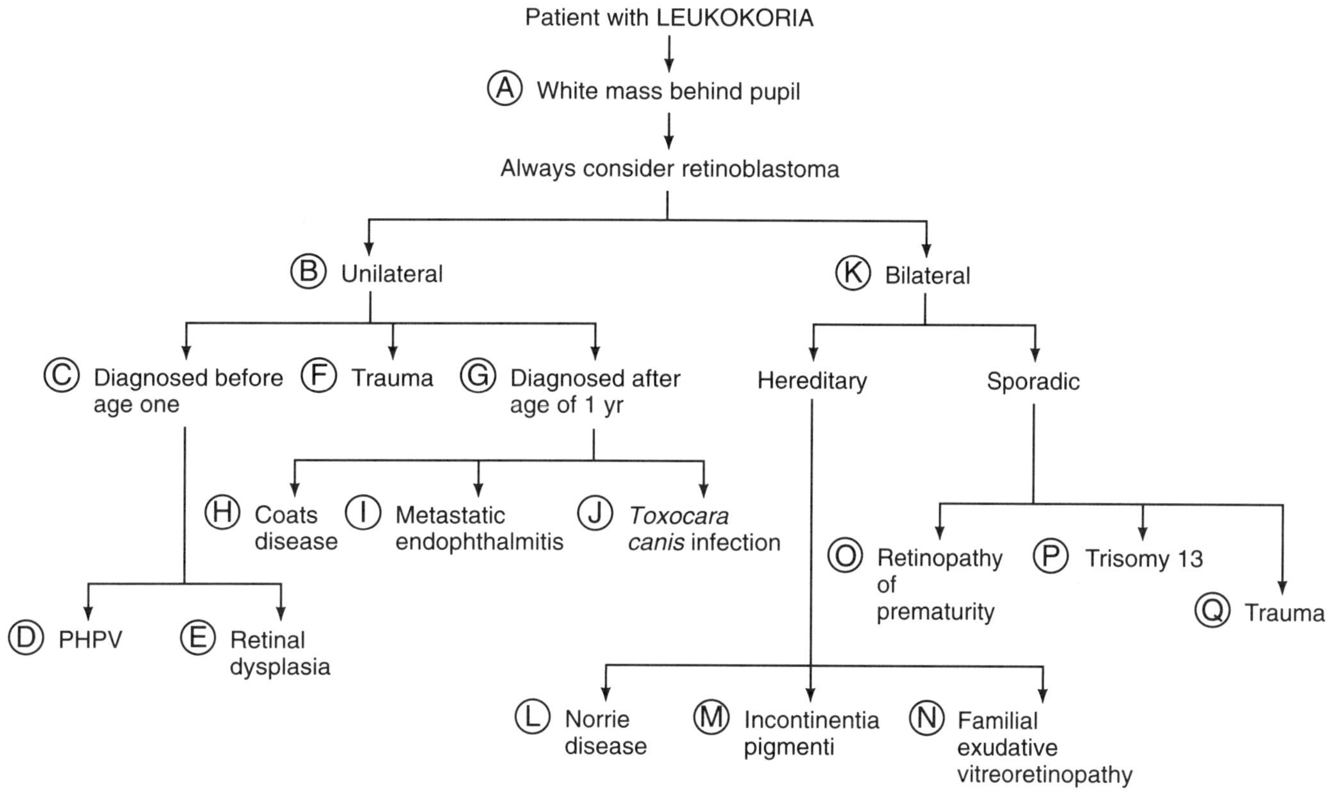

N. Familial exudative vitreoretinopathy is an autosomal dominant disease. The course resembles that of retinopathy of prematurity. See O.

O. Retinopathy of prematurity is usually associated with low birth weight and exposure to supplemental oxygen. When premature infants are exposed to a high oxygen concentration, the retinal vessels occlude and stop growing. Secondarily, there is proliferation of newly formed blood vessels in and on the retina. These thin-walled vessels may sprout into the vitreous. Hemorrhages, organization, and retinal detachment follow. *Note:* The process need not be symmetric. One eye may even appear normal when the disease regresses completely.

P. Trisomy 13 (Patau syndrome) is usually lethal because of severe involvement of the central nervous system. Many organs are affected (e.g., face, skeleton). The eye lesions constitute a complete dysembryogenesis, resembling retinal dysplasia (see E) but affecting both eyes.

Q. The various manifestations (see F) may occur in both eyes.

References

Apple DJ, Puklin JE. Leukokoria. In: Peyman GA, Sanders DR, Goldberg M, eds. Principles and practice of ophthalmology. Philadelphia: WB Saunders, 1980.

Gold DH, Weingeist TA. The eye in systemic disease. Philadelphia: JB Lippincott, 1990.

Reese AB, Blodi FC. Retinal dysplasia. Am J Ophthalmol 1950; 33:23.

THE HORNER SYNDROME

Gerhard W. Cibis, M.D.

A. In children, the causes of Horner's syndrome are birth trauma (forceps), cardiothoracic surgery, vertebral anomalies, and congenital tumors (i.e., neuroblastoma in the cervical chain). Unless the history for presumed trauma is clear or the child is older and healthy so as to preclude an underlying neoplasm, investigation for neuroblastoma is mandated (see E).

B. Anisocoria of greater than 2 mm with the smaller pupil on the side of the ptosis establishes the diagnosis in children and infants. The asymmetry is greater in the dark. There is a lag of dilation of the affected side in the dark. This implies that the anisocoria is maximum at 5 seconds compared with 15 seconds. This can be assessed by Polaroid photos. However, children tend not to be co-operative, making the test difficult. Epinephrine 0.1% in both eyes reveals a denervation supersensitivity in postganglionic cases and causes a dilation of the affected side but not of the normal pupil. Cocaine 4% dilates the normal side but not preganglionic and often not postganglionic Horner's pupil. Hydroxyamphetamine 1% dilates the pupil if the postganglionic neurons are intact.

At times the ptosis is so small or variable that it is not noticed. At other times elevation of the lower lid gives the appearance of a narrow palpebral fissure (inverted ptosis). Because children cry with eye drops, cocaine and Paredrine tests are less reliable in children than in adults. For this reason the work-up depends upon clinical findings and history more than in adults.

C. Most cases of childhood Horner's syndrome are congenital and thought to represent birth trauma. If the child is older and the Horner's syndrome clearly has been present since near birth, the risk of undetected neuroblastoma has been ruled out by the long time interval and birth trauma can be assumed to be the cause. Heterochromia develops late and is a sign of congenital Horner's syndrome. Unless clear evidence of a traumatic birth exists, such as deformed skull or brachial plexus injury, all congenital cases should have chest radiography, and CT of head and neck looking for mass lesions in the cervical chain region, and 24-hour urine vanillymandelic acid (VMA) analysis should be done.

D. The biggest risk for neuroblastoma is in the older child with a clearly new onset of acquired Horner's syndrome. A similar work-up is indicated. If the child has had cardiovascular or neck surgery, the cause is clear and a work-up is not indicated. Cardiovascular surgery is the most common cause of late acquired Horner's syndrome in children.

E. Tests should be done to rule out neuroblastoma or other tumors in the region of the sympathetic cervical chain and lesions in the CNS capable of causing central Horner's syndrome.

References

Jaffe N, Cassady R, Filler RM, et al. Heterochromia and Horner syndrome associated with cervical and mediastinal neuroblastoma. J Pediatr 1975; 87:75.

Kardon RH, Denison CE, Brown CK, Thompson HS. Critical evaluation of the cocaine test in the diagnosis of Horner's syndrome. Arch Ophthalmol 1990; 108:384.

Sauer C, Levinsohn MW. Horner's syndrome in childhood. Neurology 1976; 26:216.

Shewmon, DA. Unilateral straight hair in congenital Horner syndrome due to stellate ganglion tumor. Ann Neurol 1983; 13:345.

Taylor D. Pupil anomalies and reactions. In: Taylor D, ed. Pediatric ophthalmology. Boston: Blackwell, 1990:566.

Weinstein J, Zweifel TJ, Thompson HS. Congenital Horner's syndrome. Arch Ophthalmol 1980; 98:1074.

Woodruff G, Buncic JR, Morin DJ: Horner's syndrome in children. J Pediatr Ophthalmol Strabismus 1988; 25:40.

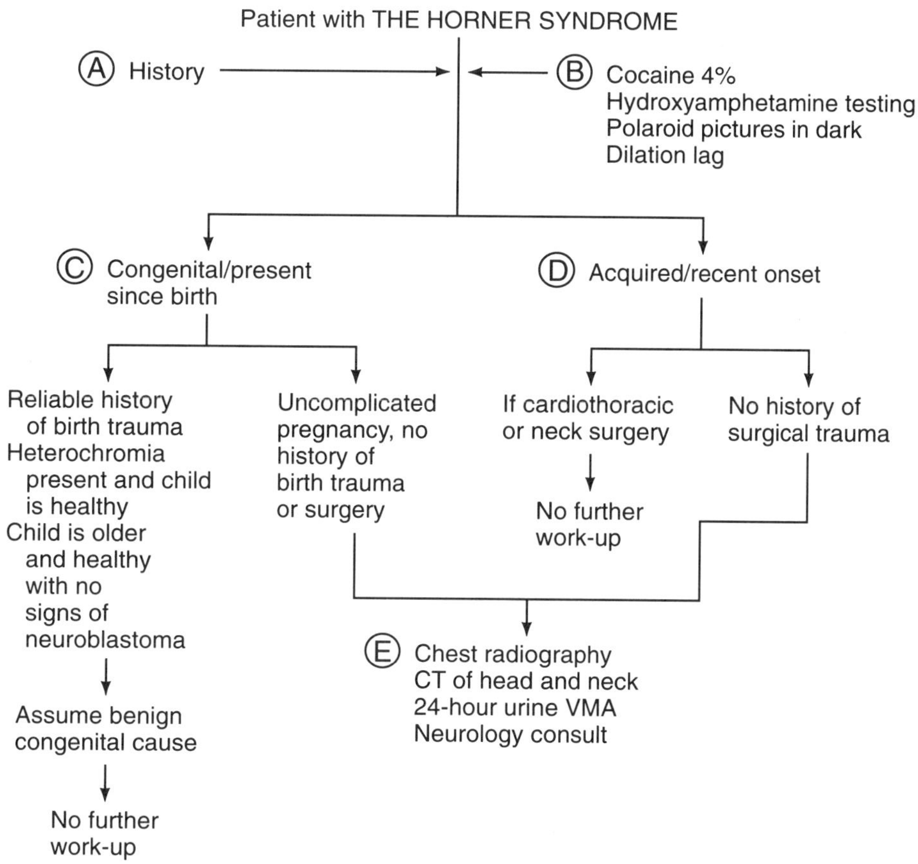

Patient with THE HORNER SYNDROME
(A) History
(B) Cocaine 4%
Hydroxyamphetamine testing
Polaroid pictures in dark
Dilation lag
(C) Congenital/present since birth
(D) Acquired/recent onset
Reliable history of birth trauma
Heterochromia present and child is healthy
Child is older and healthy with no signs of neuroblastoma
Assume benign congenital cause
No further work-up
Uncomplicated pregnancy, no history of birth trauma or surgery
If cardiothoracic or neck surgery
No further work-up
No history of surgical trauma
(E) Chest radiography
CT of head and neck
24-hour urine VMA
Neurology consult

PARTIAL CATARACT

Arlene V. Drack, M.D.
Ronald V. Keech, M.D.

A. A careful history of maternal illness, pregnancy, medication or drug use during pregnancy, and maternal trauma as well as birth trauma should be taken. The age at which the cataract(s) or decreased vision was first noticed should be ascertained as accurately as possible. Any systemic symptoms and medication use are also important, with emphasis on a failure to thrive, renal disease, hearing loss, skin conditions, and steroid use. A careful family history of poor vision, ocular surgery, or other congenital defects should be elicited.

B. A complete ocular examination should be performed using methods appropriate for the age of the child. Pupils are examined for responsiveness to light and for an afferent defect. Nystagmus is noted, if present, and the corneal diameters are estimated. A slit-lamp examination is performed to evaluate corneal clarity, anterior chamber depth, iris configuration, and cataract morphology. Glaucoma and other ocular disorders must be ruled out. Indirect ophthalmoscopy, or ultrasonography if there is no view of the posterior segment of the eye, helps to rule out a mass (e.g., retinoblastoma), retinal detachment, or other pathology that precludes a good outcome. In some cases sedation may be necessary to do a full examination. Family members should also have ocular examinations to detect incomplete penetrance or the carrier states of hereditary conditions.

C. Anterior segment dysgenesis must be excluded if the lens opacity is anterior. In this group of disorders there are often iris strands to the lens or cornea, corneal haze, and glaucoma. There may be associated ocular and systemic anomalies that suggest a hereditary condition such as Rieger syndrome. An anterior cataract may be associated with a persistent pupillary membrane (Fig 1) in which iris strands arise from the collarette. In this case, a mydriatic may aid in breaking the strands and improving vision. Patients with bilateral anterior lenticonus, particularly if acquired after birth, should be evaluated for renal disease and hearing loss (Alport syndrome). Approximately 8% of anterior polar lens opacities have a positive family history.

D. Congenital rubella typically presents with a dense nuclear cataract but may be lamellar. Galactosemia may present with nuclear, lamellar, or "oil droplet" appearance. Mannosidosis is associated with sutural cataracts, but such cataracts are often idiopathic. Children on hyperalimentation and premature infants can develop lens vacuoles, which are usually transient. Colored flecks and white punctate opacities are seen in myotonic dystrophy (but may not present until early adulthood), serum calcium abnormalities, and female carriers of Lowe syndrome and Stickler syndrome. Lamellar cataracts may be developmental (often with "riders") or associated with hypoglycemia, diabetes mellitus, and a variety of other disorders. A greenish sunflower appearance is characteristic of Wilson disease. Consultation with a pediatrician is recommended to rule out associated conditions. Nuclear cataracts may have an increased incidence of microphthalmos and glaucoma. Hereditary cataracts may also be partial.

E. Posterior lenticonus often begins with a clear, rounded lens that induces high myopia and later opacifies, although the opacity may be present at birth. Ninety percent of cases of posterior lenticonus are unilateral. Posterior subcapsular cataracts are typically associated with corticosteroid use, atopy, or inflammation and are bilateral; the cause should be vigorously sought. Persistent hyperplastic primary vitreous must be considered with any posterior lens opacity. Mittendorf's dot is a congenital posterior lens opacity that is a remnant of the attachment of the hyaloid artery. These are rarely visually significant.

F. Visual acuity should be assessed using preferential looking, fixation and following responses, or optotypes as appropriate for the age of the child. Differences between the eyes and changes in acuity with differing illumination should be noted. Anterior opacities are generally less visually debilitating than posterior opacities. Small (<3 mm) opacities are also less likely to interfere with vision, but careful acuity testing should be done to confirm this. Only the visual acuity assessment in an individual child can determine the treatment path to follow.

G. The potential for good vision following cataract surgery in children is related to the age of the patient when the opacity developed and the length of time the opacity has been present. Patients with lens opacities that have been present for several months or years have a worse prognosis than patients with cataracts of shorter duration. The presence of strabismus or unsteady fixation may suggest a poor prognosis in patients with unilateral or asymmetric bilateral cataracts. Safety glasses should be prescribed without further intervention for children with poor potential for visual improvement. This includes children over 6 months of age with dense monocular congenital cataracts and older children with monocular cataracts present for a prolonged period. Cataract surgery is also contraindicated if the parents are unwilling or unable to comply with postoperative optical correcton and occlusion therapy. The prognosis for vision following cataract surgery is good in children who are older (visually mature) at the onset of the cataract, in those for whom the cataract is present for a short duration,

(Continued on p. 35.)

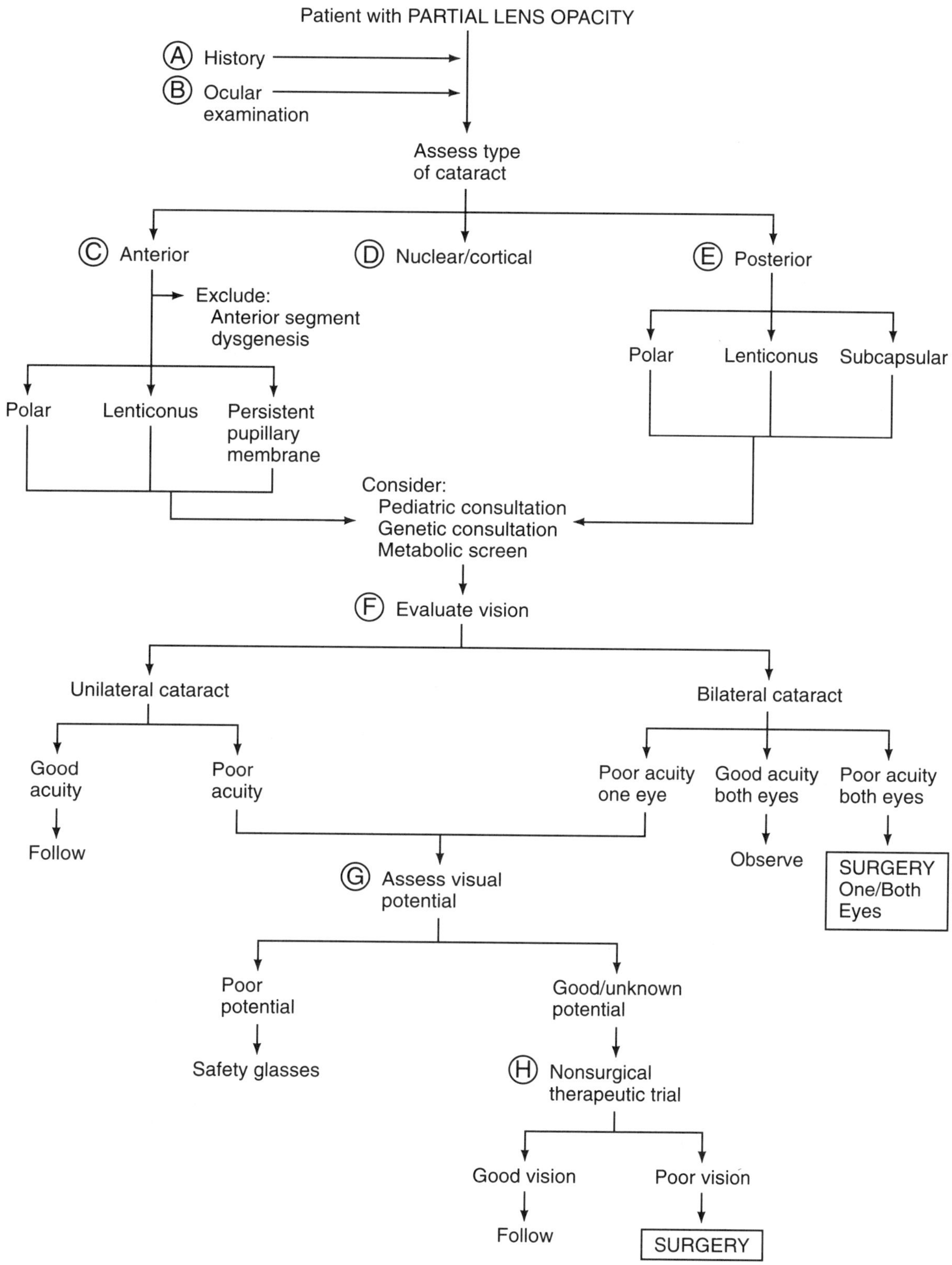
Patient with PARTIAL LENS OPACITY
(A) History
(B) Ocular examination
Assess type of cataract
(C) Anterior
(D) Nuclear/cortical
(E) Posterior
Exclude:
Anterior segment dysgenesis
Polar
Lenticonus
Persistent pupillary membrane
Polar
Lenticonus
Subcapsular
Consider:
Pediatric consultation
Genetic consultation
Metabolic screen
(F) Evaluate vision
Unilateral cataract
Bilateral cataract
Good acuity
Poor acuity
Follow
Poor acuity one eye
Good acuity both eyes
Poor acuity both eyes
Observe
SURGERY One/Both Eyes
(G) Assess visual potential
Poor potential
Good/unknown potential
Safety glasses
(H) Nonsurgical therapeutic trial
Good vision
Poor vision
Follow
SURGERY

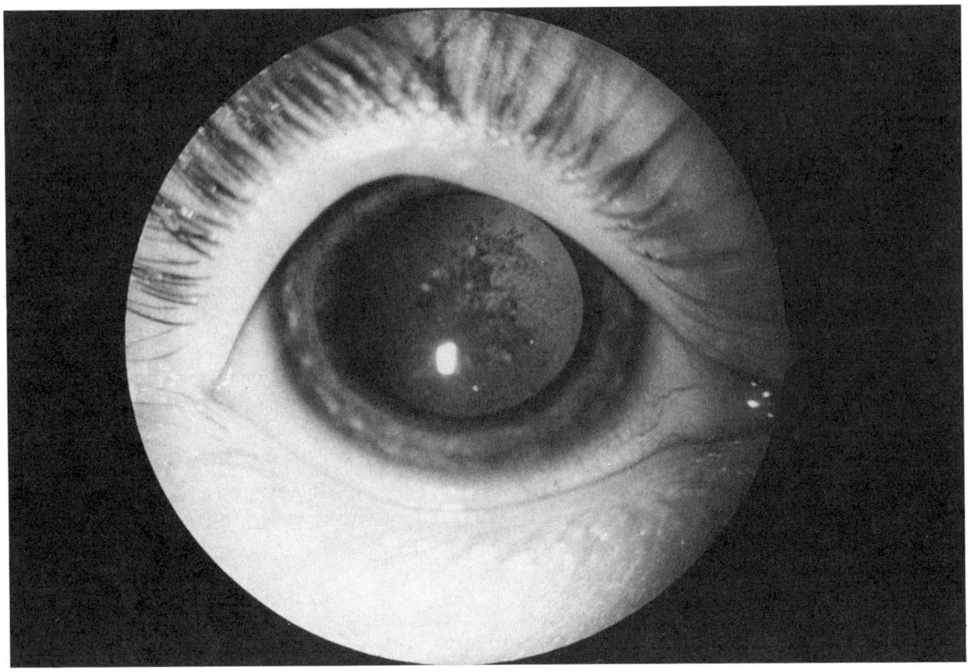

Figure 1 Persistent pupillary membrane with anterior opacity.

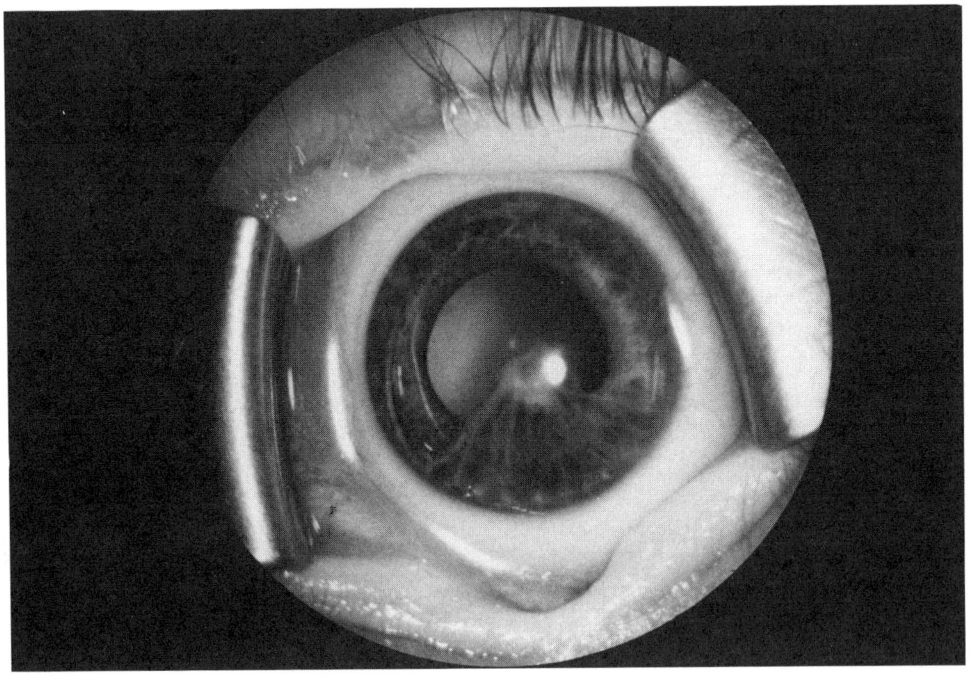

Figure 2 Partial cataract best seen with retroillumination.

when there are no other ocular abnormalities, and when the lens opacity is less than 3 mm in diameter. In older children, the potential acuity measurement or laser interferometry may provide useful information regarding the visual prognosis.

H. Children with monocular partial cataracts may have visual loss due to amblyopia. When the role of amblyopia is unclear, a trial of occlusion therapy may be warranted. In some cases, the vision improves and surgery can be avoided. Small axial and polar lens opacities can cause significant visual loss through a normal pupil but allow a clear visual image when the pupil is dilated. In these cases, a mydriatic eye drop may provide excellent vision without the need for surgery.

References

Bercovitch L, Donaldson DD. The natural history of congenital sutural cataracts. J Pediatr Ophthalmol Strabismus 1982; 19:108.

Jaafar MS, Robb RM. Congenital anterior polar cataract. A review of 63 cases. Ophthalmology 1984; 91:249.

Keech RV, Tongue A, Scott WE. Complications after surgery for congenital and infantile cataracts. Am J Ophthalmol 1989; 108:136.

Levin AV, Edmonds JA, Nelson LB, et al. Extended wear contact lenses for the treatment of pediatric aphakia. Ophthalmology 1988; 95:1107.

Sabates R, Krachmer JH, Weingeist TA. Ocular findings in Alport's syndrome. Ophthalmologica 1983; 186:203.

COMPLETE CATARACT

Arlene V. Drack, M.D.
Ronald V. Keech, M.D.

A. The age of the patient when the cataract(s) or decreased vision was first noticed should be ascertained. The pregnancy history and birth history should be elicited, with an emphasis on parental age, maternal illness (especially exanthematous), drug or medication use during pregnancy, and birth trauma. A complete review of systems should be performed. Approximately 40% of acquired pediatric cataracts are secondary to trauma. Between 8 and 33% of pediatric cataracts are hereditary. A careful family history of poor vision, ocular surgery, or other congenital defects should be elicited. Autosomal dominant is the most common inheritance pattern, but autosomal recessive and X-linked pedigrees have also been described.

B. A complete ocular examination should be performed using methods appropriate for the age of the child. Visual acuity can be assessed using preferential looking, fixation and following responses, or optotypes. Differences in acuity between the eyes and changes in acuity with differing illumination are noted. Pupils are examined for a response to light and afferent defect. Nystagmus is noted, if present, and corneal diameters are measured. A slit-lamp examination (portable for infants) is used to evaluate corneal clarity, anterior chamber depth, iris configuration, and the morphology of cataract. Glaucoma and other ocular disorders must be ruled out. The presence of a mass (e.g., retinoblastoma), retinal detachment, or other pathology that precludes a good visual outcome should be ruled out by indirect ophthalmoscopy or ultrasonography. In some cases sedation may be necessary to do a full examination. Family members should also have ocular examinations to detect incomplete penetrance or carrier states of hereditary conditions.

C. Pediatric consultation should be obtained, and screening for metabolic, infectious, genetic, and structural causes should be considered (see p 116 and Table 1). Most children with metabolic derangements have systemic signs, with the exception of galactokinase deficiency. This can be detected by urine-reducing substances following the ingestion of milk or by red blood cell enzyme studies. Unaffected heterozygote mothers may have affected children with normal galactose metabolism. In congenital cataracts, TORCH titers should be done to rule out intrauterine infection with toxoplasmosis, rubella, cytomegalovirus, and herpes. A lens aspirate can also be sent for culture if rubella is suspected. Infants with more than one congenital anomaly or a strong family history should be considered for chromosomal analysis. CT of the head and orbits should be considered if there is deformity of the globe and/or developmental delay.

D. Unless the cause is apparent, congenital cataracts should be evaluated in consultation with a pediatrician, as mentioned in C. Both congenital and acquired cataracts may be confused with persistent hyperplastic primary vitreous (PHPV), which may first present with a shallow anterior· chamber followed by a lens opacity. A blood vessel usually extends from the posterior lens capsule to the posterior pole or peripheral retina. Retinoblastoma may also present with an opaque lens in infancy or childhood. Prompt recognition of this condition may be lifesaving.

E. A specific cause or associated factor can be found in approximately 50% of pediatric cataracts. Acquired cases, in general, have a better prognosis than congenital because the visual fixation response may

TABLE 1 Pediatric Cataracts: Causes and Associated Conditions

- I. Intrauterine infection
  - Rubella
  - Toxoplasmosis
  - Herpes simplex
  - Cytomegalovirus
  - Varicella
- II. Metabolic
  - Galactosemia
  - Galactokinase deficiency
  - Hypoparathyroidism
  - Pseudohypoparathyroidism
  - Diabetes mellitus
  - Hypoglycemia
  - Hyperalimentation (vacuoles)
  - Mannosidosis
- III. Drug-induced
  - Corticosteroids
  - Chlorpromazine
  - Ergot
  - Naphthalene
  - Triparanol
- IV. Inflammatory
  - Juvenile rheumatoid arthritis
  - Sarcoidosis
  - Pars planitis
  - Atopy
- V. Trauma
- VI. Genetic/syndromes
  - Autosomal dominant
  - Autosomal recessive
  - X-linked recessive
  - Down syndrome (trisomy 21)
  - Trisomy 13
  - Trisomy 18
  - Turner syndrome
  - Lowe syndrome
- VI. Genetic/syndromes (cont'd)
  - Hallerman-Streiff syndrome
  - Alport syndrome
  - Cri du chat syndrome
  - Cerebrotendinous xanthomatosis
  - Marinesco-Sjogren syndrome
  - Myotonic dystrophy
  - Rothmund-Thomsom syndrome
  - Cockayne syndrome
  - Incontinentia pigmenti
  - Stickler syndrome
  - Craniofacial syndromes
  - Zellweger syndrome
  - Wilson syndrome
  - Hallgren syndrome
  - Laurence-Moon-Bardet-Biedl syndrome
  - Chondrodysplasia punctata
  - Refsum disease
  - Congenital ichthyosis
  - Sclerodactyly
  - G-6-PD deficiency
  - Rubinstein-Taybi syndrome
- VII. Prematurity (vacuoles)
- VIII. Radiation
- IX. Ocular disease
  - Retinitis pigmentosa
  - Aniridia
  - Persistent hyperplastic primary vitreous (PHPV)
  - Leber congenital amaurosis
  - Retinopathy of prematurity

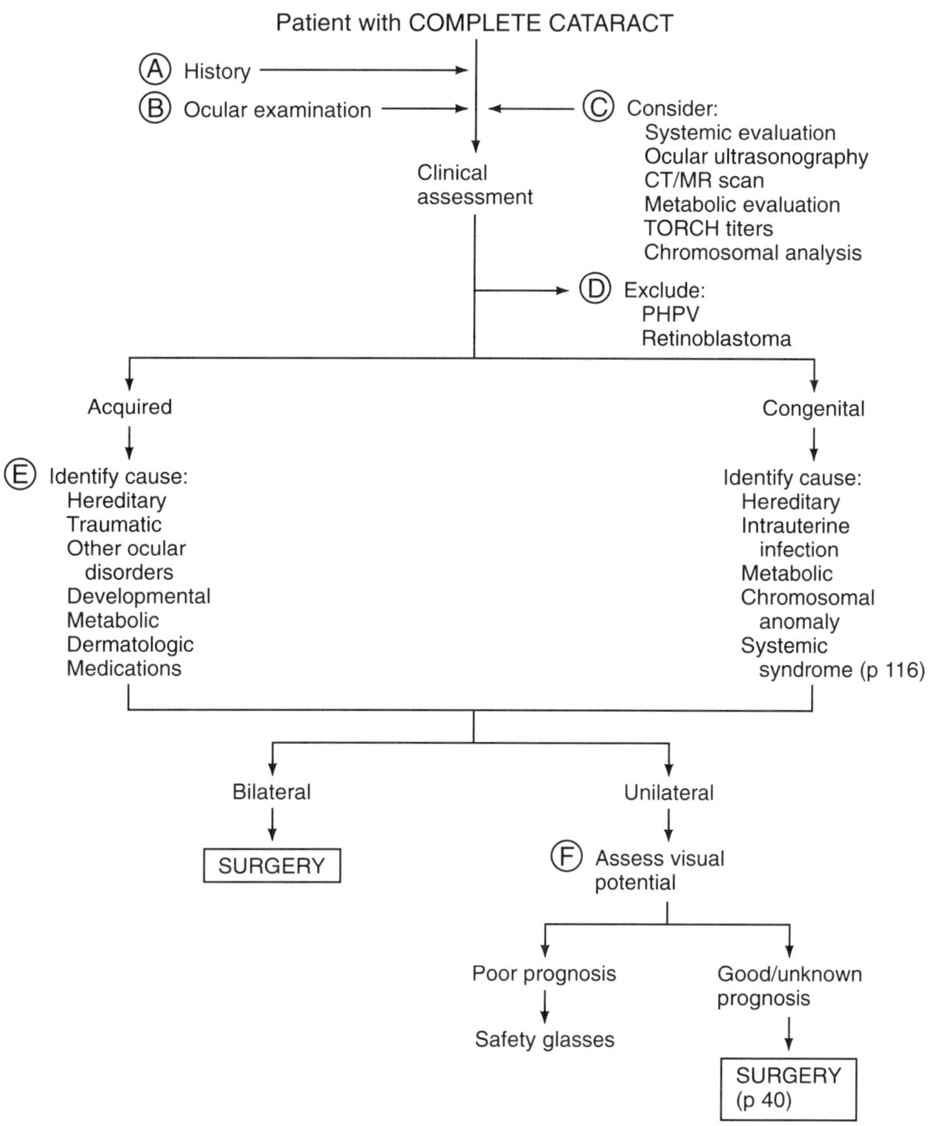

have developed before the opacity became dense. Although these cataracts may be hereditary or developmental, other causative factors must be sought. Trauma, either accidental or through child abuse, should be suspected. A variety of other eye diseases as well as treatment with corticosteroids, chemotherapeutic agents, or irradiation may secondarily cause cataract.

F. The potential for good vision following cataract surgery in children is related to the age of the patient when the opacity developed and the length of time the opacity has been present. Patients with lens opacities that have been present for several months or years have a worse prognosis than patients with cataracts of shorter duration. The presence of strabismus or unsteady fixation may suggest a poor prognosis in patients with unilateral or asymmetric bilateral cataracts. Safety glasses should be prescribed without further intervention for children with poor potential for visual improvement. This includes children over 6 months of age with monocular congenital cataracts and older children with acquired monocular cataracts present for a prolonged period. Cataract surgery is also contraindicated if the parents are unwilling or unable to comply with post-surgical optical correction and occlusion therapy. The prognosis for vision following cataract surgery is good in children who are older (visually mature) at the onset of the cataract, in those for whom the cataract is present for a short duration, in those who have no other ocular abnormalities, and in those whose lens opacity is less than 3 mm in diameter. In older children, potential acuity meter (PAM) testing or laser interferometry may provide useful information regarding the visual prognosis.

References

Drummond GT, Scott WE, Keech RV. Management of monocular congenital cataracts. Arch Ophthalmol 1989; 45:197.

Kohn BA. The differential diagnosis of cataracts in infancy and childhood. Am J Dis Child 1976; 130:184.

Lambert SR, Akmaya L, Taylor D. Detection and treatment of infantile cataracts. Int Ophthalmol Clin 1989; 29:51.

Merin S. Congenital cataracts. In: Goldberg's genetic and metabolic eye disease. 2nd ed. Boston: Little, Brown & Co., 1986:369.

Winder AF. Laboratory screening in the assessment of human cataract. Trans Ophthal Soc UK 1981; 101:127.

DISLOCATED LENS

Gerhard W. Cibis, M.D.

A. Interest in the dislocated lens may stem from finding it on ophthalmic examination, but more commonly the reverse occurs. It is specifically looked for when particular disease conditions are suspected. As in all suspected genetic disorders, the parents and siblings of patients should be examined for similar traits. Dilated pupil examination is mandatory, as subtle subluxations can be missed. Look for sectorial flattening or "notching" of the lens rim similar to a lens coloboma in areas of absent or decreased zonular tension. Before dilation look for iridodonesis (tremulousness of the iris due to lack of support by the subluxated lens), an early sign of subluxation and loose zonules. After dilation, also look for phakokinesis.

B. Trauma, even without predisposing factors, is the single most common cause of ectopia lentis. As with all ectopia lentis, glaucoma, retinal detachment, cataracts, and dislocation into the vitreous are complications. Vision therapy, especially for amblyogenic factors, is necessary. Glasses to correct astigmatism and bifocals for near focus are needed. When the dislocation is sufficient, patients may be impossible to refract because they look through the edge of the lens to achieve varying refractive powers. If this is associated with untreatable amblyopia, surgery is needed. Some patients respond best to an aphakic refraction looking around the lens. In those situations surgery is not needed unless other factors are present such as glaucoma or threatened subluxation. With modern vitrectomy instruments the surgery is far less daunting than in the past, but significant complications are still prevalent. Retinal detachment or dislocation of the lens or large lens particle into the vitreous occurs. Intraocular lenses can be placed with sulcus fixation or into the anterior chamber.

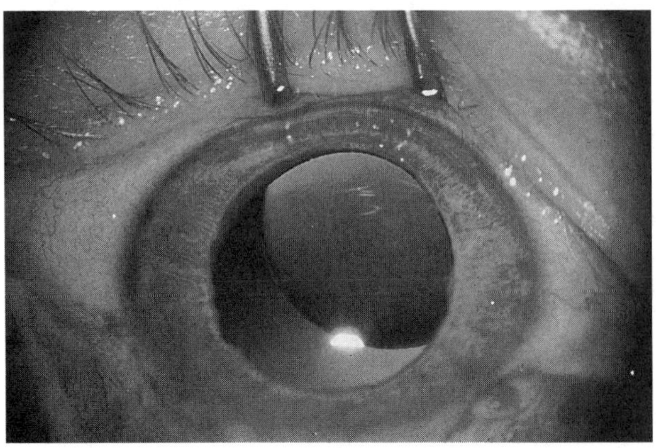

Figure 1 Congenitally dislocated lens, unknown cause.

C. Lens dislocation unassociated with any syndrome or other cause is called simplex. Dislocation may occur later in life than childhood.

D. Dislocation of lens and pupil occurs in 20% of simplex cases. Microspherophakia is present.

E. Marfan syndrome is characterized by arachnodactyly, loose jointedness, scoliosis, and anterior chest deformities along with aortic dilation. Fifty to 80% of Marfan patients have dislocation early in life. It is generally not progressive. It is bilateral and usually the lens dislocates superior temporally. Myopia, retinal detachment, peripheral retinal degeneration, anomalous chamber angles, and iris transillumination are common. The globe is commonly enlarged, diagnosed by ultrasound axial length measurements.

F. Homocystinuria is much rarer than Marfan syndrome but has similar clinical appearance. Like lysinemia and sulfite oxidase deficiency, it can be detected biochemically. Retardation occurs in 50% of cases. It is the manifestation of several enzyme deficiencies in the same metabolic pathway. There is a pyridoxine-responsive type. The sodium-nitroprusside test is used to screen urine for this disorder. Thrombotic vascular occlusions are a significant threat to the survival of these patients and must be taken into consideration for anesthetic procedures. Antiplatelet aggregation treatment can prevent thrombi formation (see p 308). Lens dislocation is classically inferior, opposite to the superior temporal dislocation seen with Marfan syndrome.

G. The Weill-Marchesani physique is pyknic, the opposite of Marfan syndrome and homocystinuria. Microspherophakia, lenticular myopia, ectopia lentis, shallow anterior chamber, and secondary glaucoma are the ophthalmic findings. The anteroposterior increase in diameter accounts for the high myopia. Glaucoma is an acute phakogenic phenomenon. Prophylactic laser iridotomy to prevent pupillary block by the lens is indicated. Microspherophakia is a prerequisite to making the diagnosis of Weill-Marchesani syndrome.

H. Hyperlysinemia is diagnosed by showing elevated plasma levels of lysine on paper chromatography or spectrophotometry. Sulfite oxidase deficiency has increased urinary excretion of S-sulfocysteine, taurine, sulfite, and thiosulfate. Mental retardation is common.

I. Therapy for prevention of amblyopia is of utmost importance and the most common need of these patients. Good refraction and patching are needed far more often than surgery.

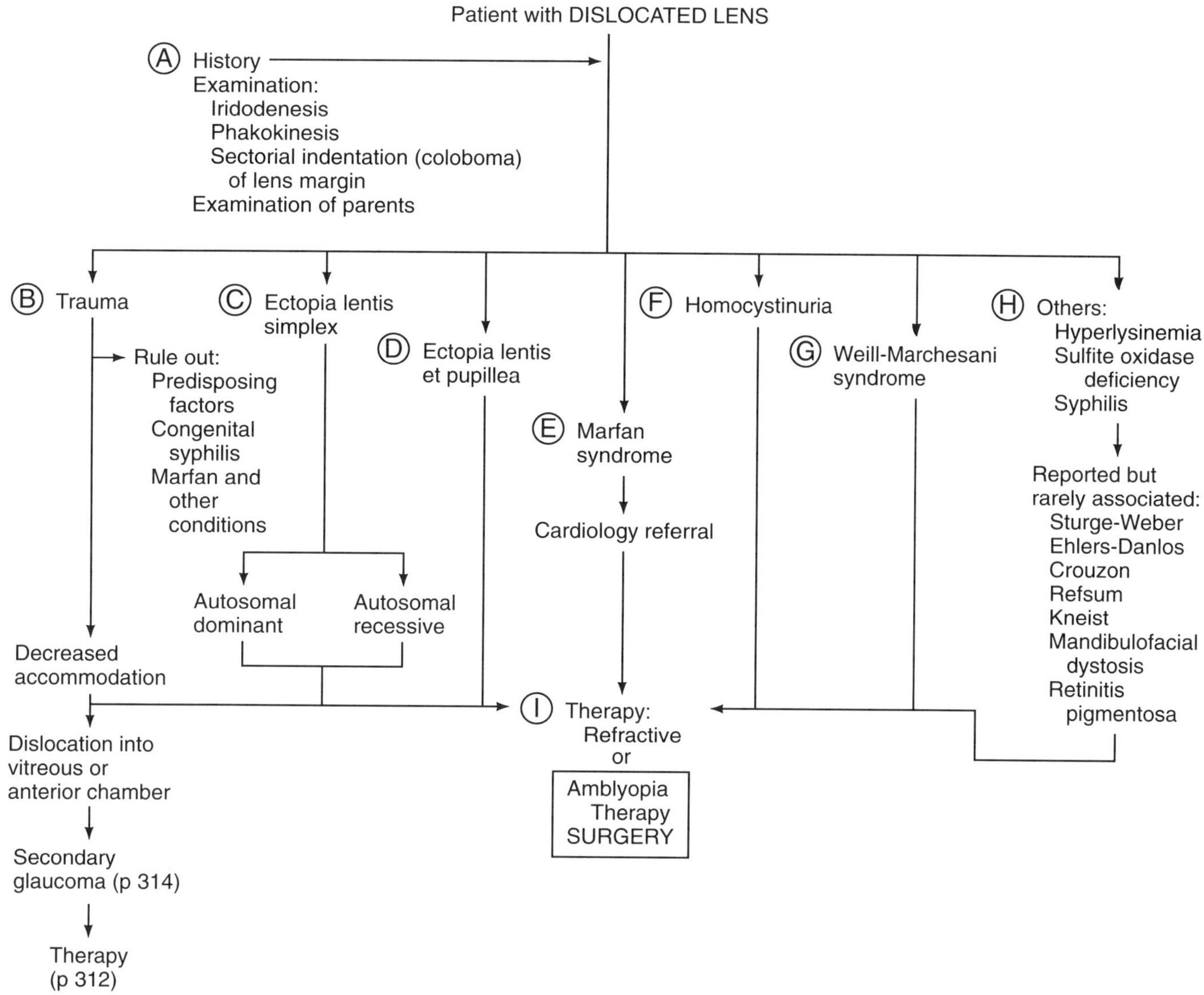

References

Gold DH, Weingeist TA, eds. The eye in systemic disease. Philadelphia: JB Lippincott, 1990.

Nelson LB, Maumenee IH. Ecotopia lentis. In: Renie WA, ed. Goldberg's genetic and metabolic eye disease. 2nd ed. Boston: Little Brown & Co, 1986:389.

SURGICAL ISSUES IN PEDIATRIC CATARACT CARE

Robert W. Lingua, M.D.

The work-up and etiologic consideration of pediatric cataracts have been addressed in preceding chapters. This chapter deals strictly with the surgical care of children with cataracts.

A. Regardless of laterality, prompt clearing of the visual axis with immediate optical correction offers the optimal chance for visual recovery. The particular procedure depends on the patient's age (ability to cooperate), risk of amblyopia, and expected ocular growth and reactivity to the surgery and implanted material.

B. In the infant less than 6 months of age who presents with a dense cataract, the only option to successfully clear the visual axis and have it remain clear during the critical period of vision development is the lensectomy-vitrectomy with total posterior capsulectomy. This eliminates any possibility of reopacification of capsule or remnants during a period when even mild amounts of occlusion could result in permanent vision loss. No peripheral irridectomy is required because the anterior segment has only a single chamber.

C. In the infant older than 6 months of age, it is usually difficult to date the time of onset of the cataract. It may well have been present during the critical period of vision development, in which case a maximum acuity of 20/200 is usually the case. Later-onset cataracts have a much better vision potential. The presence of strabismus or nystagmus at the time of presentation usually presages a poor visual outcome and is more consistent with a long-standing cataract. These patients have passed the critical period of vision development and, although no longer susceptible to deprivation amblyopia, are still susceptible to functional amblyopia. Prompt management is recommended. However, in these cases the major modification in approach is to preserve the necessary architecture for a secondary implant at a later age, should this be desired by the family or required because of failure with other optical devices. A central posterior capsulectomy of 4 mm with the automated cutter is sufficient, and a shallow anterior vitrectomy is performed to eliminate the chance of reopacification across an anterior vitreous face. A generous discission is not an equivalent procedure because it preserves the necessary architecture for re-opacification of the visual axis due to proliferation of retained cellular elements. It can also lead to strands of vitreous to the wound, causing persistent iritis, and moves in the direction of discissions that have a higher incidence of retinal detachment. A peripheral irridectomy is performed to avoid secondary glaucoma due to iridocapsular adhesions.

D. The child who is 3 years of age has undergone most of his ocular growth and the eye is less reactive. Children in this age group who present with progressively opacifying lamellar cataracts, traumatic cataracts, or cataracts of long-standing duration without strabismus or nystagmus can be considered for primary intraocular lens (IOL) implantation. Additional important criteria for eligibility include the ability to examine the patient with the slit lamp for careful postoperative examination as well as preoperative IOL power calculations. In these cases, the lensectomy can be performed with a 6-mm anterior capsular opening, a 4-mm posterior capsular opening, and a shallow anterior vitrectomy. With the use of viscoelastic material, intracapsular placement is feasible. A peripheral iridectomy is added. Postoperatively these patients are tapered from an initial regimen of hourly steroids until all anterior chamber reactivity has ceased. One should consider hospitalization for close postoperative care and medication compliance.

E. The patient who is more than 6 years of age can be approached as an adult with extracapsular cataract extraction and primary IOL implantation without capsulectomy. Because the child is still susceptible to amblyopia, cataracts should also be promptly removed. Opacifications that begin during the period of visual immaturity and persist beyond 10 years of age have a high association with postoperative diplopia and horror fusionis.

F. Infants less than 6 months of age and any other child for whom an intraocular lens is inappropriate can be corrected with contact lenses. Silicon, gas-permeable, and hard lenses offer a wide range of flexibility for the appropriate power and fit.

G. Contact lens failures are particularly difficult to manage in pediatric aphakia. No one single procedure is available to rescue these children from a high incidence of amblyopia. Epikeratophakia should be considered. In monocular cases, full aphakic eyeglasses can be prescribed for use half time to preserve vision (although of course not binocularity) until the patient is contact lens compliant or visually mature. In binocular cases, aphakic glasses are usually well accepted. Anterior segment surgeons who are adept at sewing in a sulcus IOL have been consulted for assistance in their care.

H. Patients who have received an IOL are screened postoperatively for anisometropia, precipitate on the IOL, or strabismus, all of which can lead to amblyopia. Anisometropia should be kept to less than 1½ diopters at distance and near. Lens precipitates can often be sufficiently managed with topical steroids if recognized early.

I. All children who have undergone cataract surgery require follow up every 3 to 4 months to rule out late-onset primary glaucoma and secondary glau-

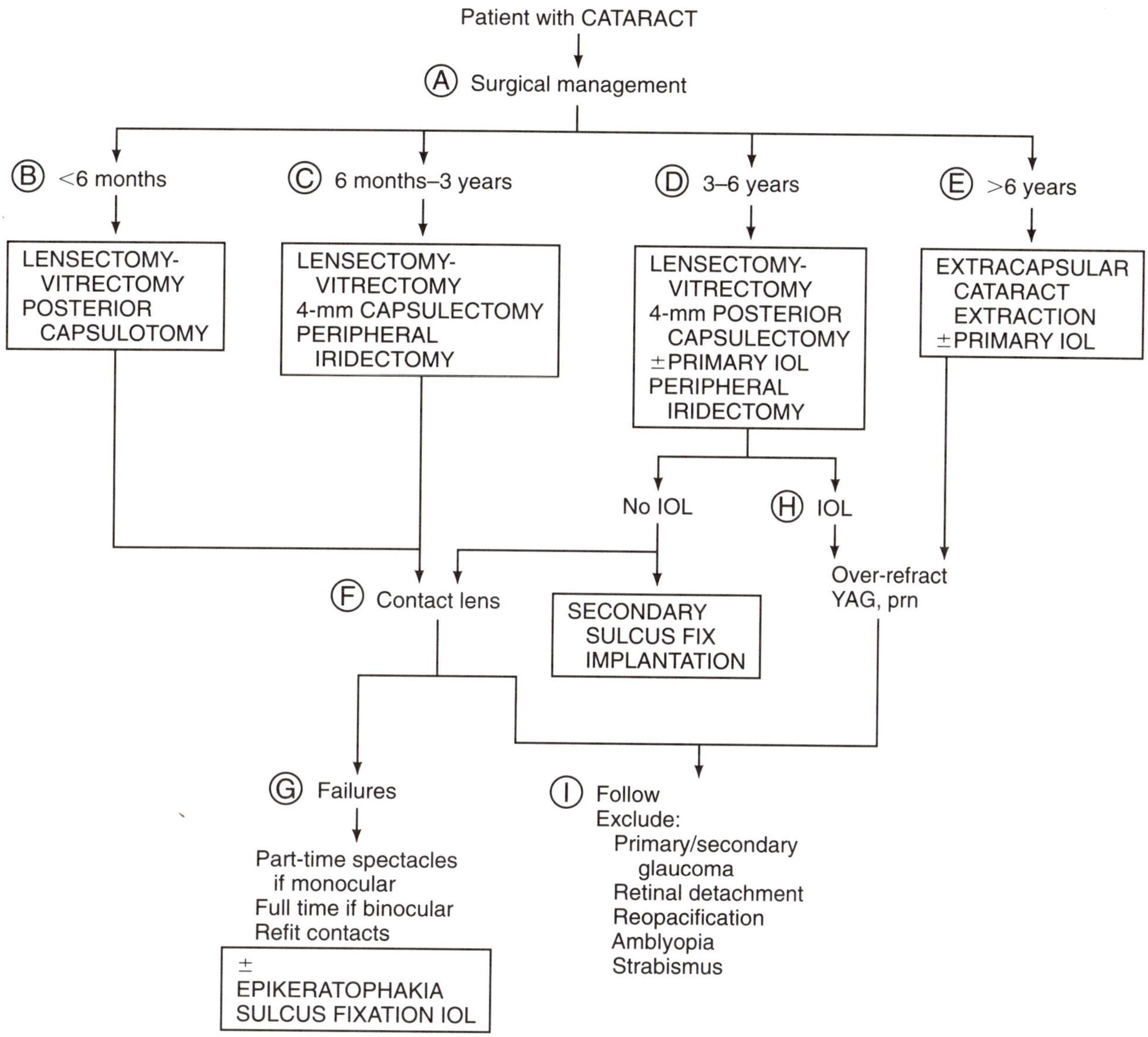

coma. If indirect ophthalmoscopy was not possible preoperatively, it should be performed postoperatively for assistance in diagnosis and to rule out associated anomalies of the optic nerve or foveal differentiation. Especially in the case of monocular cataracts, patching needs to be done and is usually continued to age 6 to 9 years (visual maturation) to optimize visual acuity.

References

Chrousos GA, Parks MM, O'Neill JF. Incidence of chronic glaucoma, retinal detachment, and secondary membrane surgery in pediatric aphakic patients. Ophthalmology 1984; 91:1238.

Dahan E, Salmenson BD. Pseudophakia in children: precautions, technique, feasibility. J Cataract Refract Surg 1990; 16:75.

Hiles DA. Cataract surgical indications in children. Cataract 1984; 1:8.

Hoyt CT. Treatment of congenital cataracts. In: Fraunfelder F, ed. Recent advances in ophthalmology. 7th ed. Liverpool: Sidney I Davidson, 1985:97.

Lingua R. Infantile cataract surgery. In: Jaffe NS, ed. Atlas of ophthalmic surgery. New York: Gower Medical Publications, 1989:134.

Parks MM. Visual results in aphakic children. Am J Ophthalmol 1982; 94:441.

CONTACT LENSES IN PEDIATRIC APHAKIA

Max S. Mancillas, O.D.

The pediatric aphakic eye requires correction of its refractive error as soon as possible. Corrections are most commonly done today with contact lenses. Fitting contact lenses to these eyes has several goals: (1) selecting the appropriate power; (2) selecting the lens that provides the best physiologic fit to ensure proper corneal metabolism; and (3) watching for, treating, and solving all contact lens–related ocular health problems. All doctors involved must remember that amblyopia is always a problem, and time without contact lenses for these children could easily mean losing any advances made in amblyopia treatment.

A. Once the decision to fit contact lenses has been made, the type of contact lens to trial fit must be addressed. Soft lenses are the most frequent selection, but the number of pediatric soft lenses available is limited. The most common soft lens chosen is a silicon lens. Gas-permeable (GP) rigid lenses are also an option and, unlike the limited number of pediatric soft lenses available, the majority of GP plastics can be manufactured to any pediatric parameters prescribed.

B. The main advantage to trial fitting with anesthesia is the ability to try a number of lenses in a short period of time and to take accurate keratometry measurements, if needed. Should a keratometer not be available and keratometry measurements are deemed a requirement, they may be obtained by trial and error fitting of rigid GP lenses, looking for an "apical alignment" fit. GP lenses should be fit with a slight apical touch pattern. Soft lenses should be fit as flat as possible, avoiding edge stand-off and excess movement. Both types of lenses should center well, provide good pupil coverage, and show good lag or movement upon blinking, which is simulated by manually opening and closing the eye. If a nonsilicon soft lens is used, fluorescein must be avoided. The disadvantage to trial fitting under anesthesia is that the over-refraction and fitting are often incorrect because of retinoscopy off axis due to the deviation of the eyes under anesthesia.

C. Trial fitting without anesthesia is the preferred method, as this allows the fitter to assess centering and lens movement more accurately. Keratometry measurements are not usually obtainable in this situation but in general are not required. The fitting philosophy here remains unchanged. GP lenses should have a slight apical touch and soft lenses should fit as flat as possible, avoiding edge stand-off and excess movement.

D. Initially an over-refraction is performed with a trial contact lens in place. The power of the trial lens should approximate that of the refraction, thus avoiding possible miscalculations secondary to large over-refractions and variable vertex distance. The power of the ordered contact lens (if it is a soft lens) is equal to the trial lens power + sphere power of the over-refraction. If the child is less than 3 years of age, we add an additional 3 diopters to fit for near, as this is the most important visual dimension in this age group. This same formula is used for GP lenses, provided that the trial lens has the same base curve (BC) to be ordered. Otherwise, the final power needs an additional adjustment based upon the dioptric change between the trial lens BC and the BC ordered.

E. The diameter of pediatric soft lenses is established and unchangeable for most manufacturers. If the diameter can be ordered, it should be between 9.5 and 12 mm. A GP lens diameter should be between 6.5 and 7.5 mm.

F. At the dispensing, parents are instructed about insertion, removal, and care of the lens as well as an initial wearing schedule, usually 4 to 8 hours the first day, adding 1 to 2 hours each following day. If the dispensed contact is approved for extended wear use, which it probably should be, removal during naps is not required. Removal at the end of the day is strongly recommended. Parents should also be asked to watch for potential problems as evidenced by conjunctival injection and signs of patient intolerance (rubbing of the eye). Most importantly, this visit allows parents to gain confidence with lens handling and reassurance that they will not harm their child.

G. Initial follow-up should occur 3 to 7 days after the original dispensing visit. Many times, follow-up visits coincide with postoperative visits so no additional time is required from the parents. Wearing time and parental observations and concerns are discussed and all questions are answered at these visits.

H. The general fit is assessed at each visit, and the definition of a good fit continues to be the same as that used at the initial fitting. Deviations from acceptable movement and/or centration must be compensated for by appropriate changes in the base curve, diameter, and if possible, optic zone size, center thickness, and peripheral curve radius and width.

I. With contact lens in place, an over-refraction is checked. An over-refraction (−3.00) in the child less than 3 years old is desirable, as discussed in D. Small discrepancies in refraction can be compensated for with glasses. Bifocals may be necessary for the older child. Spectacles are also required to correct astigmatic errors. Should the unoperated eye have a significant myopic refractive error, the aphakic eye can be overplused by approximately 3 diopters. This creates a Gallilean telescope effect, thereby decreasing anisometropia. In addition, should there be a large anisometropic over-refraction, the power of the contact lens should be altered first and second.

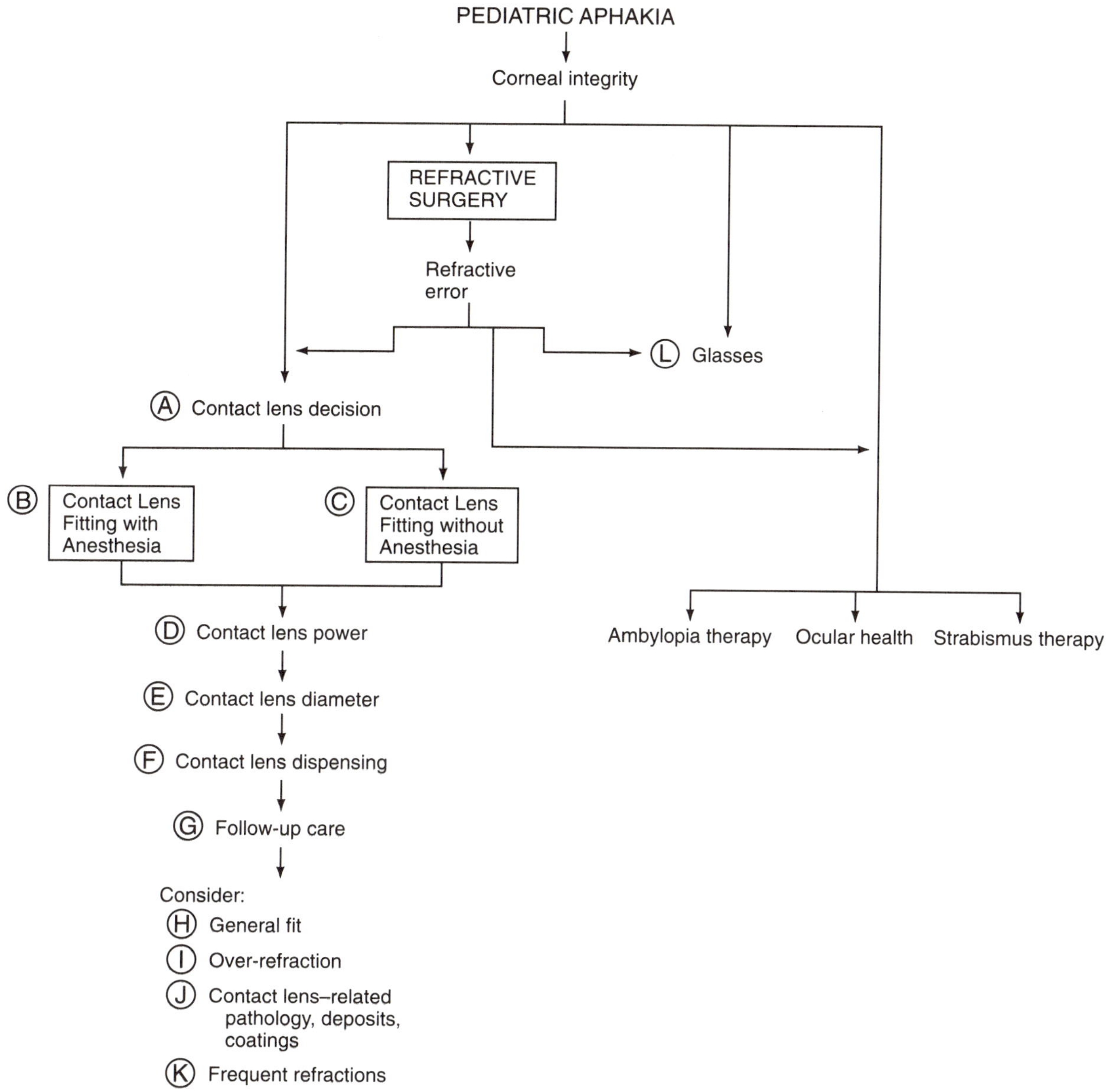

J. Contact lens–related pathology must be treated vigorously and deposits and coatings eliminated so that time out of the contact lens is kept to a minimum. For these reasons, daily-wear lenses rather than extended-wear lenses and regular replacement are preferred.

K. Because the eye grows as the child grows, frequent over-refractions are necessary to make sure the lens power selection is correct.

L. Aphakic spectacles should be fit only for bilateral aphakics. Otherwise, spectacle correction is not tolerated owing to the large anisometropia that occurs with the unilateral aphake.

References

Edmonds SA. Contact lens management of aphakic children. Contact Lens Forum 1990; 8:15.

Gold R, Simon J, Sak RD. Contact lens fitting in the aphakic infant. Ophthalmology Annual 1988.

Pollard ZF. Contact lens therapy for pediatric aphakes. Contact Lens Forum 1987; 8:26.

OPTIC ATROPHY IN CHILDHOOD

Karen S. Shimshak, M.D.

A. Childhood optic antrophy (OA) visual deficits include progressive visual acuity loss, sluggish pupillary light reaction, visual field defects, color vision loss, a reduced sense of brightness, and sometimes nystagmus. Ophthalmoscopy reveals OA ranging from mild (temporal disc pallor) to severe with a totally white optic nerve. Numerous forms and causes of OA constitute a diagnostic challenge. Determination of an identifiable cause or family history is critical.

B. With bilateral, symmetric, insidious vision loss, a hereditary form should be considered. Familial incidence may be difficult to establish because the many forms of OA occur with variable patterns of transmission, penetrance, and clinical severity. It may occur as an isolated event or in association with progressive nervous system degenerations.

C. Two forms of dominant OA (DOA) are described based upon the severity of the disease. The severe or congenital form presents with vision loss to 20/200 in the first decade of life, often associated with achromatopsia and nystagmus. In the mild, infantile form, vision loss progresses slowly to the 20/30 to 20/70 level with temporal disc pallor, cecocentral enlargement of the blind spot, and acquired tritan (blue-yellow) dyschromatopsia. DOA with progressive vision loss to the 20/30 to 20/70 range is seen with congenital or progressive hearing loss and may be associated with Friedreich's ataxia. DOA with hearing loss and ophthalmoplegia is seen with progressive loss of muscular function causing ptosis, ataxia, and insidious loss of vision.

D. Recessive OA occurs as part of a multisystem disorder affecting the CNS. These should be distinguished from secondary OA resulting from primary CNS diseases. Behr syndrome involves incomplete OA in infancy in association with neurologic abnormalities, including mental deficiency, Babinsky, hypertonia, gait spasticity, and ataxia. Wolfram (DIDMOAD) syndrome associates the childhood onset of OA with diabetes mellitus, diabetes insipidus, and hearing loss. GAPO syndrome refers to the association of growth retardation, alopecia, pseudoanodontia, and slowly progressive OA. Opticocochleodentate syndrome is a fatal disease that includes profound OA leading to blindness with severe neurologic abnormalities including spastic quadriparesis, hearing loss, and mental deficiency. Rosenberg and Chutorian described a sex-linked recessive OA in males coupled with hearing loss and progressive polyneuropathy resembling Charcot-Marie-Tooth disease. Infantile OA with neurologic abnormalities and mental deficiency described by Went may be included in this spectrum of disease. Opticoacoustic atrophy with dementia is a sex-linked recessive syndrome of progressive OA, with hearing loss, and dementia presenting in the second to third decade of life. OA associated with deafness and distal amyotrophy is described by Iwashita.

E. Leber's OA is characterized by the acute loss of central vision during the second or third decade of life, usually affecting males (14% affected are women). Loss of vision is rapid in the affected eye to the 20/200 level, followed by vision loss in the other eye within a few weeks to months. Muscle biopsy shows aggregates of enlarged mitochondria. Leber's OA may be related to defective cyanide metabolism by the enzyme rhodanese. Transmission is by maternal mitochondrial DNA mutation through cytoplasmic inheritance; thus, affected males are unable to transmit the disease. Only carrier women can transmit the disease.

F. The neurodegenerative syndromes such as Dawson's disease, Leigh's disease, and Hallervorden-Spatz syndrome should be considered in addition to those discussed as a part of the hereditary ataxia syndromes in D.

G. Inborn errors of metabolism including abetalipoproteinemia, Batten's ceroid lipofuscinosis, gangliosidosis, homocystinuria, mucopolysaccharidosis, hypophosphatasia, and Krabbe's disease are to be considered in the differential diagnosis of patients with OA.

H. Children with acquired OA atrophy may retain nearly normal vision or present with a monocular or bilateral visual deficit with acute or slowly progressive dimming of central vision, a visual field defect, reduced color vision, and pupils poorly reactive to direct light. OA results from loss of optic nerve axons, leaving only the glial connective tissue of the nerve remaining. The nerve may appear pale or white without the normal small superficial blood vessels that feed the optic disc. The insult can occur at the level of the retinal nerve fiber layer or optic disc, in the pregeniculate retrobulbar pathways of the optic nerve, chiasm, or optic tract, or in the postgeniculate visual pathways. The progression of optic nerve pallor depends upon the cause and the location of the offending lesion or insult. In many cases a cause can be identified when a thorough history and physical examination are obtained. This evaluation should include any history of significant head or birth trauma, inflammation or infection, nutritional deficiencies, intake of toxins, hydrocephalus, or familial OA. Neuroimaging studies may be required to confirm the suspected cause. If a cause is not readily identified, neuroimaging studies must be performed to rule out a tumor.

I. OA may occur from compression of the optic nerve due to orbital or optic canal fractures, orbital hemorrhage, intraneural and extraneural edema of the optic nerve fibers, or a projectile foreign body such as a BB pellet or bullet lodged in the orbital apex. Contusion,

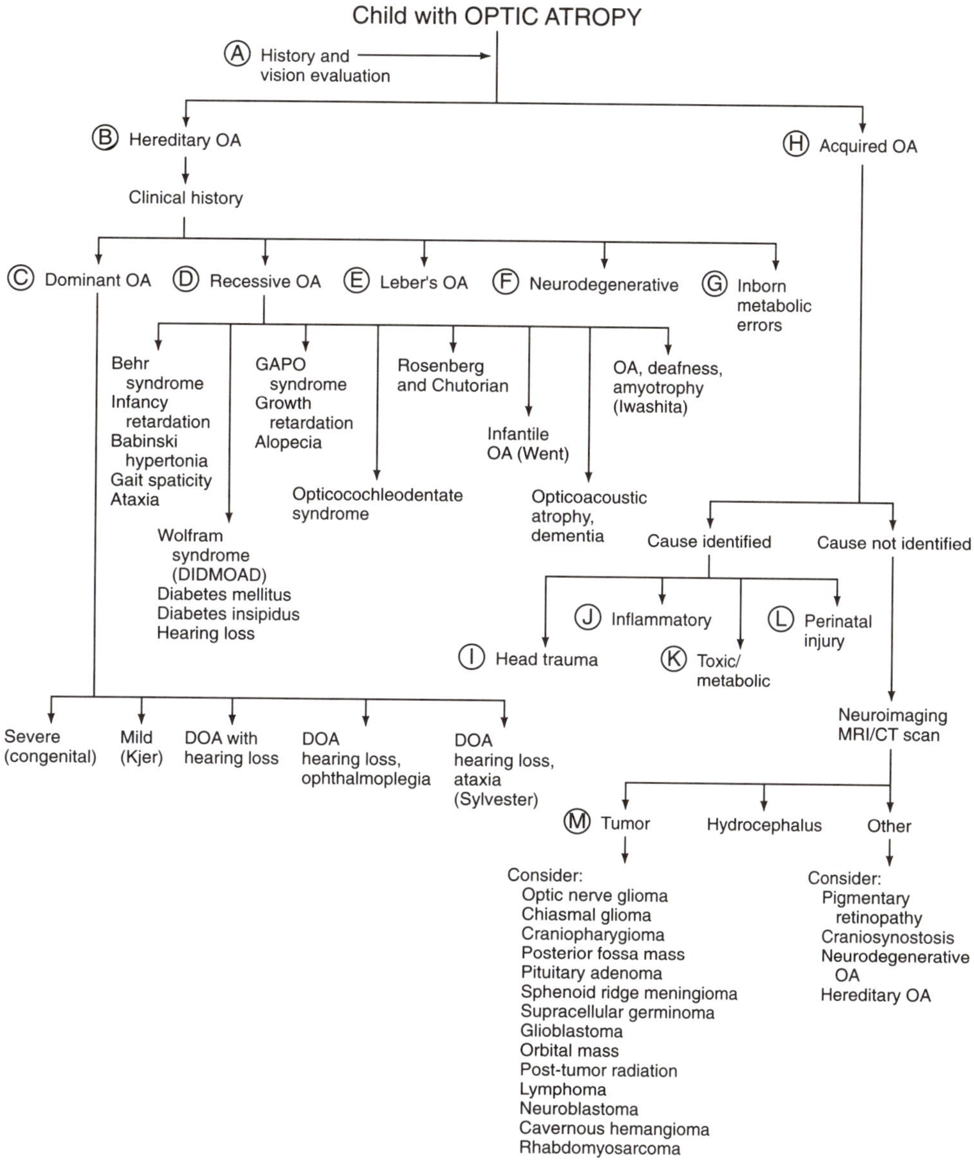

stretching, and shearing forces within the optic nerve result in OA.

J. Postinflammatory OA results from optic neuritis. Viral or bacterial meningoencephalitis, orbital cellulitis, severe sinusitis, infiltration of the optic disc by infections such as sarcoidosis, tuberculosis, cryptococcosis, toxoplasmosis, toxocariasis, cytomegalovirus, or coccidioidomycosis are the cause. Postneuritic OA resulting from demyelinating diseases such as multiple sclerosis, Schilder's disease, and Devic's disease is less commonly seen in children.

K. Toxins, including lead, thallium, sulfonamide, streptomycin, ethambutol, and chloramphenicol, and nutritional deficiencies, including those of thiamine and vitamin B_{12}, can produce bilateral, slowly progressive vision loss with a bilateral cecocentral visual field defect. The optic disc may atrophy if the insult is long-standing. If the cause is corrected, vision may recover.

L. Perinatal insult including prematurity of less than 31 weeks' gestation, anoxia, intrauterine or perinatal infection, birth trauma with intracranial hemorrhage, or gestational drug and alcohol exposure can result in OA in infancy.

M. Slowly progressive monocular vision loss seen in the setting of OA is typical of an orbital or prechiasmal compressive lesion.

References

Glaser JS. Neuro-ophthalmology. Philadelphia: JB Lippincott, 1990:106.

Merlin S. Inherited eye diseases—diagnosis and clinical management. New York: Marcel Dekker, 1991:323.

Repka MX, Miller NR. Optic atrophy in children. Am J Ophthalmol 1988; 106:191.

Sergott RC. Pediatric neuro-ophthalmology. In: Nelson LB, ed. Pediatric ophthalmology. 3rd ed. Philadelphia: WB Saunders, 1991:472.

OPTIC NERVE HYPOPLASIA

Luis C. F. de Sa, M.D.
William V. Good, M.D.
Creig S. Hoyt, M.D.

Optic nerve hypoplasia (ONH) is a developmental nonprogressive anomaly in which there is a diminished number of axons within the affected nerve. It results from an excessive loss of axons in the involved nerve before its full development. Several predisposing factors have been described, including maternal anticonvulsant ingestion, low maternal age, and maternal alcohol or drug abuse. Clinically, ONH manifests according to degree of severity and bilaterality. It can present as an isolated defect without any symptoms in milder cases or can be associated with strabismus, poor visual development, and nystagmus.

A. The diagnosis is based on *direct ophthalmoscopy* (indirect ophthalmoscopy does not provide enough magnification) to evaluate the optic discs. Segmental or partial ONH may be difficult to distinguish from normal nerves. The characteristic funduscopic features are (1) small size of the optic nerve, (2) double pigmentary ring sign, which surrounds the small disc, (3) abnormal nerve fiber layer, (4) tortuosity of the blood vessels, and (5) tilting of the optic nerve head. Usually electrodiagnostic tests are not necessary, although visual evoked potentials can be useful to estimate visual function at an early age. Neuroradiologic evaluation can provide information regarding the optic nerve and chiasma size but usually is performed to evaluate associated conditions. Other ocular disorders associated with ONH are albinism, aniridia, and coloboma.

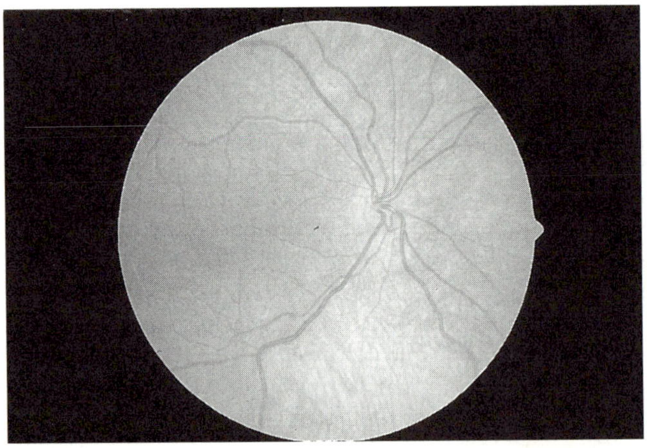

Figure 1 ONH, showing the double ring sign and poor fundus reflexes due to lack of nerve fiber layer.

B. Once the diagnosis of ONH is made, it is important to consider separately unilateral and bilateral cases. Unilateral ONH is less frequent and less commonly associated with systemic abnormalities than bilateral cases.

C. In bilateral cases, a good history should be obtained regarding general health as well as neurologic status because of the frequent association with endocrine and neurologic disturbances (58.5% to 64.7%). Bilateral segmental ONH and/or good vision is much less frequently associated with endocrine/neurologic disease.

D. Among the neurologic disturbances, septo-optic dysplasia (de Morsier syndrome) can be associated with ONH and includes absence of the septum pellucidum, partial or complete agenesis of the corpus callosum, and dysplasia of the third ventricle. Other neurologic abnormalities include anencephaly, porencephaly, cerebral atrophy, hydranencephaly, colpocephaly, and encephalocele. Congenital tumors (glioma, craniopharyngioma) are rarely associated with ONH.

E. History of neonatal jaundice, hypoglycemia, apnea, or seizure followed by failure to thrive or delayed development can be signs of an endocrine disturbance. About two thirds of patients with de Morsier syndrome can present with some form of pituitary hypofunction. Deficiency of growth hormone is considered to be the most prevalent endocrine abnormality but presents in children over 2 years of age. In children less than 2 years, look for diabetes insipidus, abnormalities of cortisol production, and hypoglycemia. Follow yearly in endocrinology for the first 5 years, then every other year through puberty. Endocrine evaluation should be done upon referral and again 3 years later.

F. Counseling should be provided to all families.
   1. Genetics: rarely autosomal recessive.
   2. Warn families of prenatal risk factors.
   3. Bilateral ONH with nystagmus improves, but special resources are required at school according to visual acuity.

G. Patching should be considered in cases of unilateral or asymmetric ONH with strabismus because part of the visual deficit can be caused by superimposed amblyopia.

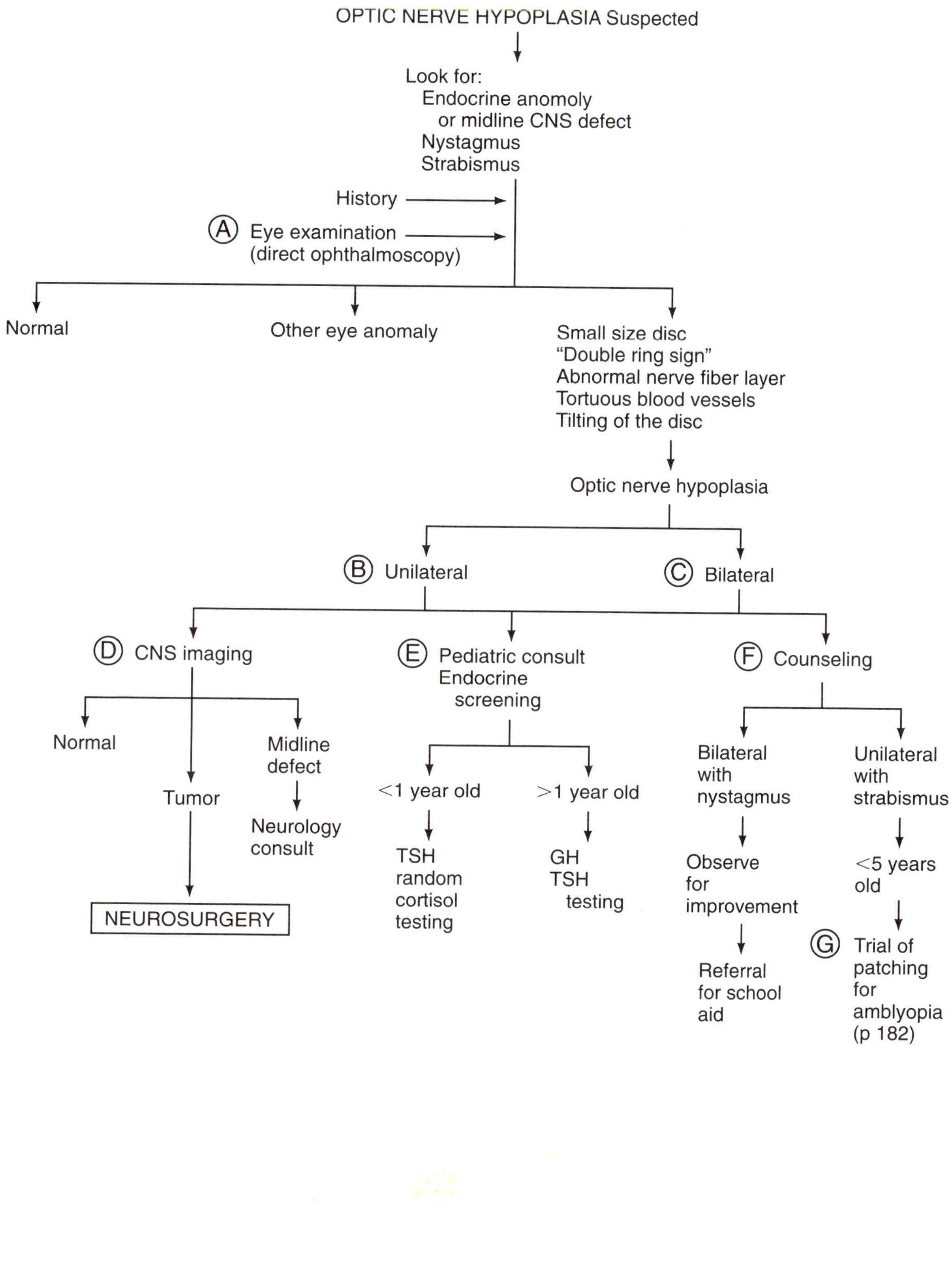

References

Jacobs M, Taylor D. The systemic and genetic significance of congenital optic disc anomalies. Eye 1990; 5:470.

Lambert SR, Hoyt CS, Narahara H. Optic nerve hypoplasia. Surv Ophthalmol 1987; 32:1.

Roberts-Harry J, Green SH, Wilshaw HE. Optic nerve hypoplasia: associations and management. Arch Dis Child 1990; 65:103.

Skarf B, Hoyt CS. Optic nerve hypoplasia in children. Association with anomalies of the endocrine and CNS. Arch Ophthalmol 1984; 102:62.

COLOBOMA OF THE UVEA

Mette Warburg, M.D.

A. Coloboma means mutilation; it indicates that a portion of the eye is lacking. Uveal colobomata may present as coloboma of iris, choroid, or optic nerve or as cystic coloboma or microphthalmos with cyst.

B. Congenital colobomata are embryologic defects of closure of the embryonic fissure of the eye. They are therefore typically situated downwards nasally. Expressivity is highly variable. The microphthalmos-coloboma complex may present as anophthalmos, microphthalmos, cystic colobomatous eye, or coloboma of the choroid and optic nerve or only the iris. Acuity varies from no perception of light to normal, according to the extent of the lesion.

The morning glory syndrome, or megalopapilla, and optic disc hypoplasia may be manifestation of uveal colobomata. In the morning glory syndrome, the optic nerve head is large and glial hyperplasia is seen in the center. The vessels emerge peripherally from the glial tuft. In optic nerve hypoplasia the disc is small, the nerve fiber layer may be deficient, and the retinal vessels are usually tortuous. There is a double contour of the nerve head.

C. History should include inquiry into consanguinity, pregnancy, twinning, systemic disorders, and ocular malformations in relatives. Ocular malformations in the family must be examined. Illness or medication during pregnancy must be elucidated.

D. Genetic colobomata may be familial or sporadic. New germ-line mutations of dominant disorders have a 50% risk of recurrence in sibs and offspring; consanguinity may disclose a recessive mutation with a 25% risk of recurrence in full siblings. If there are familial cases, an effort should be made to see all those affected in order to explore the variable range of manifestation of both ocular and systemic lesions.

E. The most common type of coloboma is the autosomal dominant uveal coloboma. This has a very variable expressivity within the same family, as described in B. There are more than 40 different genetic syndromes with coloboma. The phenotypes are different, and careful systemic examination and a comprehensive family history can often identify them. Counseling of the family requires a precise diagnosis.

F. Deletions or breaks of chromosomes and duplications of parts of chromosomes give rise to malformations. Colobomata may be observed in deletions and duplications of almost all chromosomes. The cat-eye syndrome with mild mental retardation and coloboma of the iris is a tetrasomy or trisomy of chromosome 22. Trisomy 13 is a common lethal malformation syndrome of the eye, digits, kidneys, and brain. High-resolution karyotypes are advisable in patients with colobomata associated with two other congenital anomalies. Parents of affected children must be examined if counseling is to take place.

G. Prenatal environmental or teratologic causes of colobomata are poorly understood; different genetic backgrounds may cause different responses to the drugs ingested by the pregnant mother. The extension of the malformations also depends on the time, dosage, and duration of degradation of the drug.

H. Closure of the embryonic fissure takes place at 36 to 40 days after conception. Drugs inducing colobomata are taken prior to this time, but the action of the drug may continue and give rise to later malformations. Few drug-related colobomata have been described.

I. Maternal disease resulting in uveal coloboma is extremely rare.

J. An association is a nonrandom concurrence of several malformations that are not pathogenetically related or known to have the same principal cause. In associations, the cause is rarely known. It is not inherited and, so far, teratologic causes have been described in only a few. Colobomata are commonly but not always present in CHARGE, VATER, and Goldenhar (oculo-auriculo-vertebral, or OAV) associations. Their features are listed in Table 1.

K. Colobomata may be acquired postoperatively after complicated surgery for cataract or after perforating traumas. These are usually situated at 12 o'clock or where the object hit the eye.

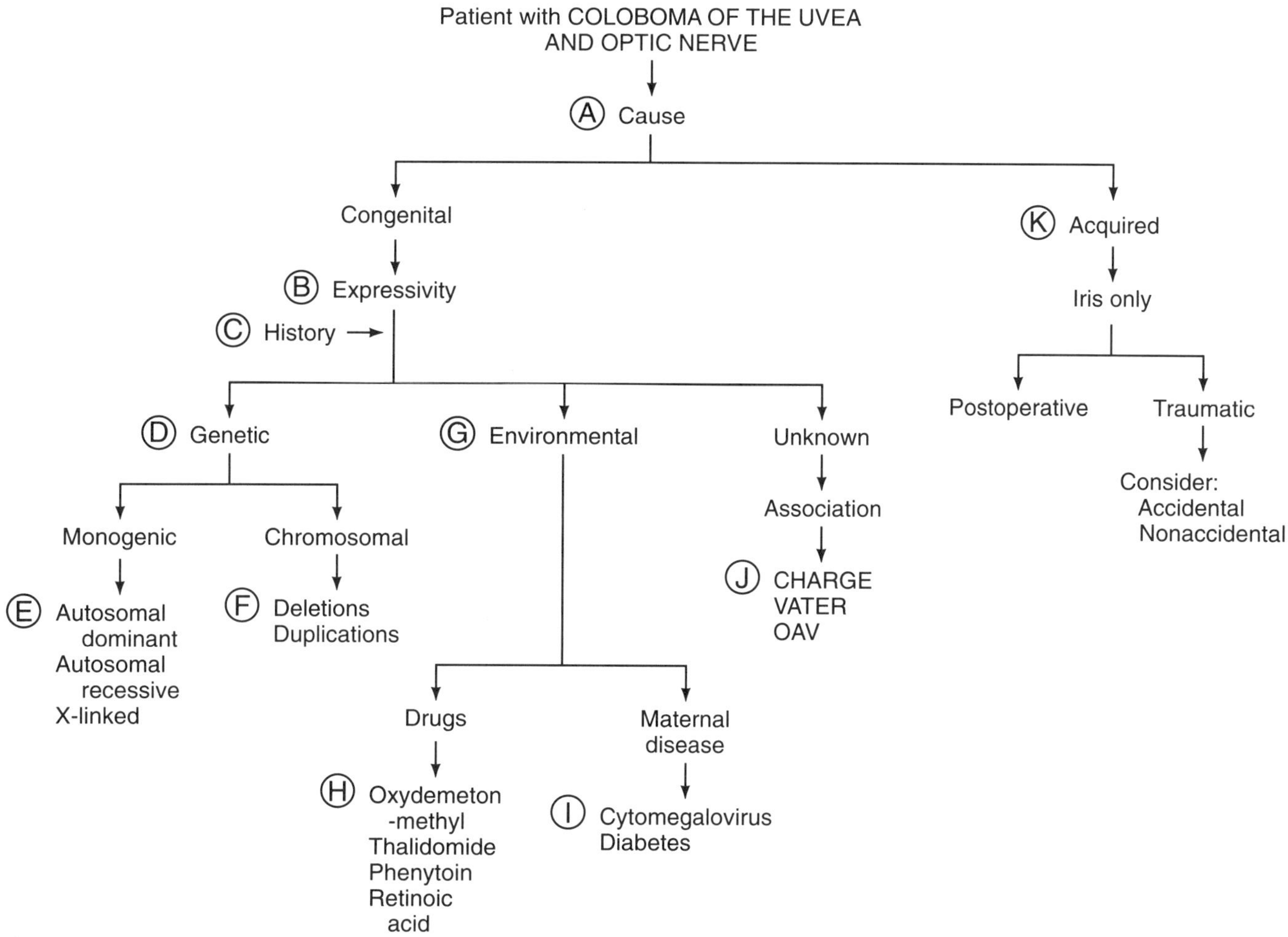

TABLE 1 CHARGE, VATER, and Goldenhar (OAV) Associations

CHARGE	*VATER*	*OAV*
***C**oloboma*	***V**ertebral anomalies and ventricular septal defect*	*Oculo:* Microphthalmos complex (see C), ptosis, epibulbar epidermoid
***H**eart disease*		*Auriculo:* Malformed ears, preauricular tags, hearing loss
***A**tresia choanae*	***A**nal atresia*	*Vertebral:* Cervical spine fusions, spina bifida, congenital heart disease, macrostomia, cleft palate, abnormal cranial base, hemifacial microsomia
***R**etarded growth and development*	***T**racheo-**E**sophageal fistula*	
***G**enital hypoplasia*	***R**adial and renal dysplasia*	
***E**ar anomalies, hearing loss*		

References

Gorlin RJ, Cohen MM, Levin LS. Syndromes of the head and neck. 3rd ed. Oxford: Oxford University Press, 1990.

Stromland K, Miller M, Cook C. Ocular teratology. Surv Ophthalmol 1991; 35:429.

Warburg M. An update on microphthalmos and coloboma. A brief survey of genetic disorders with microphthalmos and coloboma. Ophthal Paediatr Genet 1991; 12:57.

Warburg M, Friedrich U. Coloboma and microphthalmos in chromosomal aberrations. Ophthal Paediatr Genet 1987; 8:105.

PAPILLEDEMA

Peter C. Kohler, M.D.

A. When one encounters a patient with swollen optic discs, the most important initial diagnosis to consider is papilledema (Fig. 1). By definition, papilledema is optic nerve swelling due to elevated intracranial pressure (ICP). *Pseudopapilledema* is a term used for optic disc swelling, or the appearance of swelling, in the absence of raised ICP. (Note, some reserve the term *pseudopapilledema* for cases of anomalous elevation of the discs in the absence of any disc swelling, as occurs with high hyperopia.) In the evaluation of a patient with swollen optic nerves, it is important to look for neurologic signs or symptoms (e.g., headache, diplopia, nausea, vomiting, transient episodes of loss of vision, focal neurologic deficits). If any are present, it must be assumed that true papilledema exists and an emergent diagnostic evaluation with cranial CT should be done. In the absence of neurologic signs or symptoms, one can proceed with the work-up of pseudopapilledema. True papilledema can exist without symptoms.

B. Ophthalmologic examination, besides looking for extracranial palsies, can include visual field testing when possible to document an enlarged blind spot or neurologic defects that would indicate an intracranial lesion. Visual acuity tends to remain normal with papilledema but is affected with optic neuritis, as is color vision. Examine the optic nerve with red-free light to look for infarcts and swelling of the nerve fiber layer and dilation of surface capillaries. In true papilledema the disc margins are not visible. The peripapillary retina is swollen and edematous, and venous pulsations are absent. The optic cup is obliterated (Fig. 2). Drusen frequently show a delay in the visual evoked response (see p 274), which is rare with papilledema.

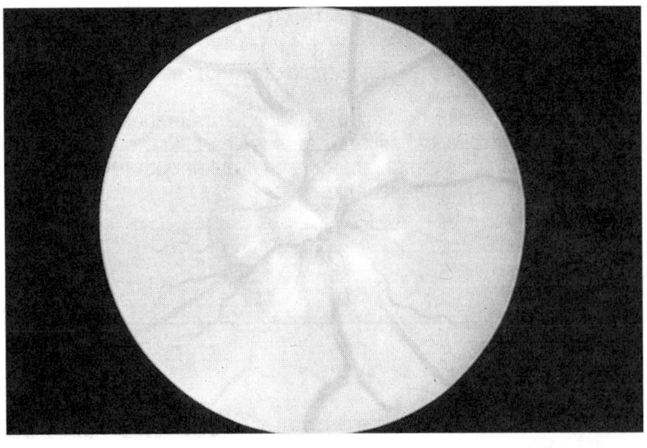

Figure 1 Papilledema secondary to intracranial tumor. The lid margins are obliterated. Vessels disappear segmentally under swollen and infarcted nerve fibers. Disc surface capillaries are dilated, giving the disc a ruddy appearance. Disc and retinal hemorrhages may be present.

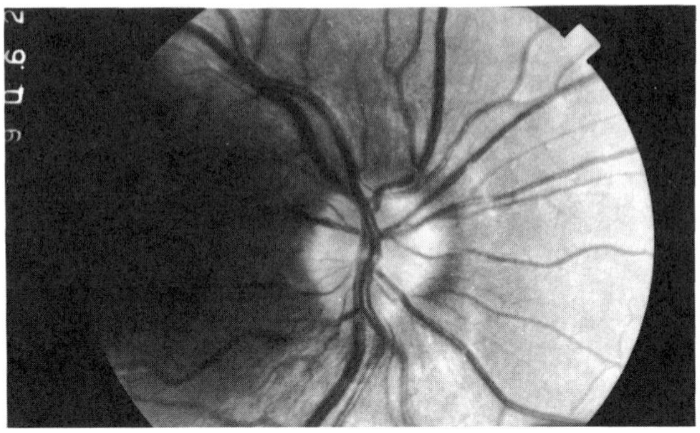

Figure 2 Pseudopapilledema due to drusen. The nerve margins, optic cup, and venous pulsations are preserved. There are no dilated surface capillaries or nerve fiber infarcts as with true papilledema (see Fig. 1).

C. A cranial CT with contrast should be performed prior to lumbar puncture to rule out an intracranial mass lesion.

D. Neurosurgical consultation should be obtained in the presence of an intracranial mass lesion.

E. Lumbar puncture (LP) can be performed when cranial CT is normal or demonstrates small ventricles. Opening pressure should be recorded and CSF sent for analysis.

F. The diagnosis of pseudotumor cerebri requires four criteria: increased ICP, normal or small ventricles by CT, normal CSF, and papilledema. Headache and transient episodes of vision loss are the main symptoms. Diplopia secondary to sixth cranial nerve palsy, visual field loss, tinnitus, dizziness, nausea, or vomiting can occur. This occurs predominantly in young females. Many conditions are associated with pseudotumor cerebri, including obesity, pregnancy, and the use of medications such as tetracycline, oral contraceptives, nalidixic acid, and vitamin A. Systemic steroid withdrawal has also been implicated. The extent and progression of visual loss as measured by serial testing of visual function, perimetry, and visual acuity should dictate patient management. Treatment includes weight loss, discontinuing possible causative medications, and diuretics. Surgical intervention with lumboperitoneal shunt or optic nerve decompression is reserved for medical treatment failures.

G. If an initial LP reveals a normal ICP and the diagnosis of pseudotumor cerebri is still strongly suspected, a repeat LP may be considered. ICP can fluctuate, giving a normal value on one isolated examination.

(Continued on p. 52.)

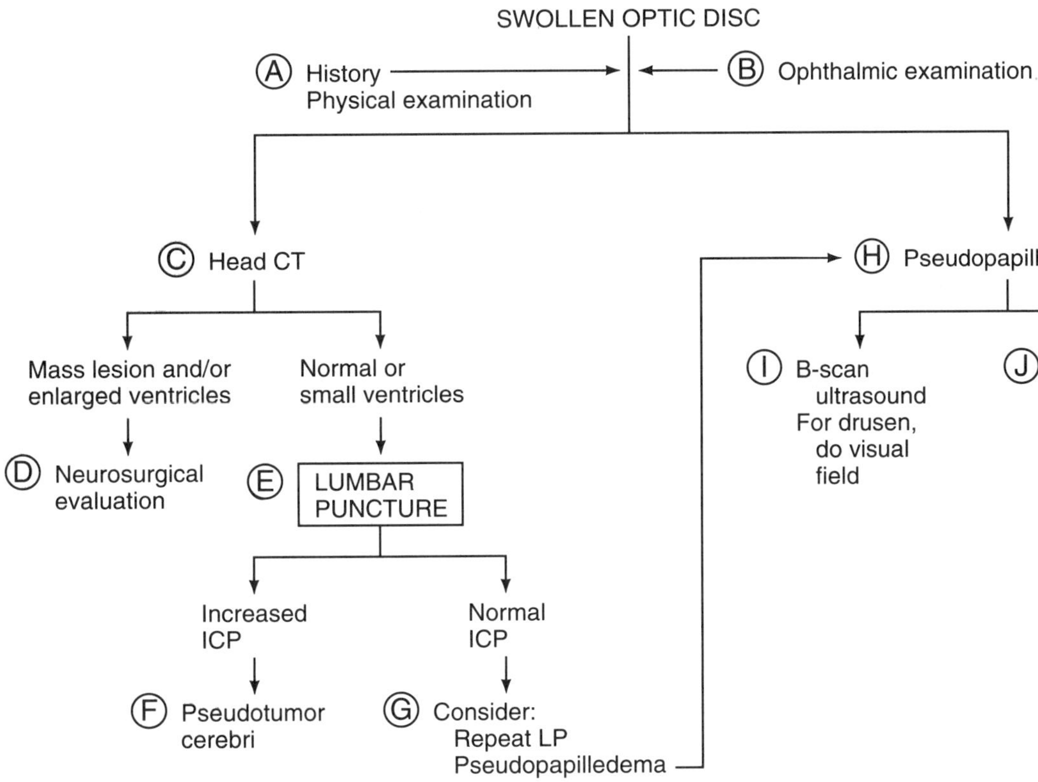
SWOLLEN OPTIC DISC
(A) History
Physical examination
(B) Ophthalmic examination
(C) Head CT
Mass lesion and/or enlarged ventricles
(D) Neurosurgical evaluation
Normal or small ventricles
(E) LUMBAR PUNCTURE
Increased ICP
(F) Pseudotumor cerebri
Normal ICP
(G) Consider:
Repeat LP
Pseudopapilledema
(H) Pseudopapilledema
(I) B-scan ultrasound
For drusen, do visual field
(J) Consider:
Ocular disease
Orbital disease
Systemic disease
(Table 1)

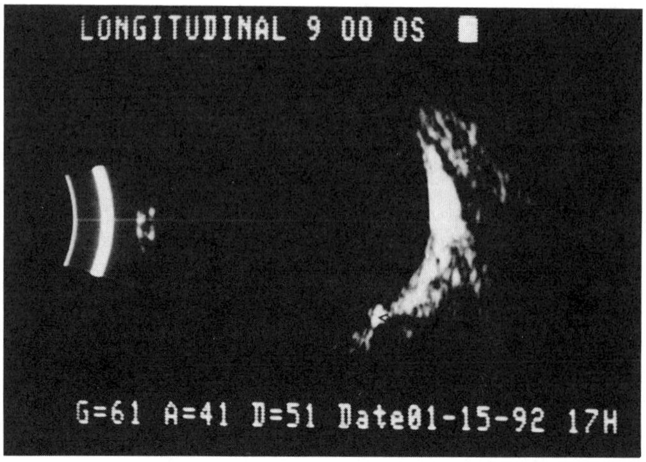

Figure 3 Same eye as in Figure 2. Ultrasonography at "normal" gain shows optic nerve head and three drusen.

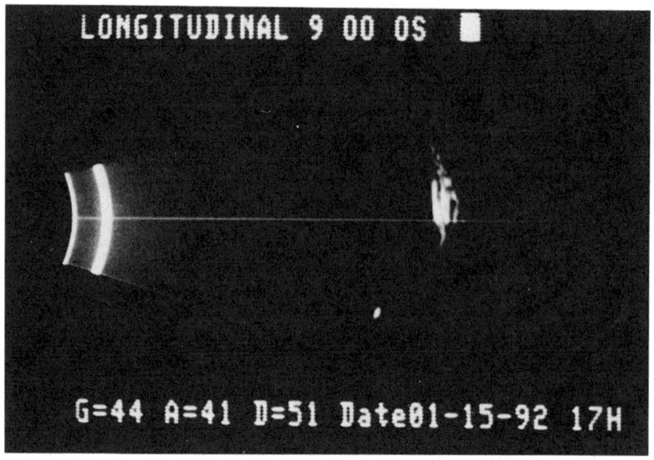

Figure 4 Ultrasonography of the same eye as in Figures 2 and 3 with gain turned down. Loss of sclera except where perpendicular to the axis of the globe. The drusen remain visible owing to high reflectivity of the calcification.

TABLE 1 Ophthalmoscopic Appearance

	Papilledema	*Pseudopapilledema*
Spontaneous venous pulsations	Absent	May be present
Central disc cup	Present	Absent
Disc vessels branching	Telangiectasias	Anomalous
NFL hemorrhages	Present	Rare
Disc margins	Blurred	Irregular
Hyaline bodies	Absent*	May be seen

*Axoplasmic crystals may form with chronic papilledema, resembling drusen.

TABLE 2 Causes of Optic Disc Swelling

I. Ocular Disease
    - Uveitis
    - Hypotony
    - Retinal vein occlusion

II. Orbital Disease
    - Optic nerve inflammation (e.g., retrobulbar neuritis)
    - Primary optic nerve tumors (e.g., hemangioma, glioma)
    - Metastatic optic nerve tumors
    - Orbital tumors
    - Dysthyroid orbitopathy

III. Systemic Disease
    - Diabetes mellitus
    - Lymphoma
    - Leukemia
    - Anemia
    - Hyposomia
    - Hypertension
    - Cranial arteritis

Data from Glaser JS. Neuro-ophthalmology. In: Duane TD, ed. Clinical ophthalmology. Vol 2. Hagerstown: Harper and Row, 1978:32.

H. Pseudopapilledema can refer to any condition resulting in a true or apparent swelling of the optic disc(s) in the setting of a normal ICP. However, many reserve the term pseudopapilledema for cases of anomalous disc elevation without true edema (e.g., optic disc drusen, simple hyperopia, persistent hyaloid tissue). Certain funduscopic characteristics help distinguish between true papilledema and anomalous elevation (most commonly optic disc drusen) (Table 1). The presence of spontaneous pulsations of the major disc veins is an important sign, present in approximately 80% of normal eyes. According to one study, if it is present, the ICP is below 200 ± 25 mm H_2O.

I. Optic disc drusen are acellular laminated concretions of unknown cause, often partially calcified. The presence of calcification allows B-scan ultrasonography to be a helpful diagnostic tool. While viewing the nerve head, the gain is decreased, thus losing the image of normal tissue. The calcified drusen remains hyperintense (Figs. 3 and 4). Drusen are also seen with orbital CT scanning. Optic disc drusen are typically bilateral and have an incidence of 0.3% to 2.0%. They are thought to be asymptomatic but may have transient visual effects. Loss of central acuity is rare. Visual field abnormalities are common, most often representing nerve fiber bundle defects, but are not pathognomonic. Their cause is unknown but they are thought to be the result of slowed axoplasmic nerve flow at the lamina cribrosa.

J. Optic disc swelling, in the absence of elevated ICP or anomalous elevation, may be of ocular, orbital, or systemic origin (Table 2). A careful history and physical examination help direct the work-up. To evaluate orbital disease, both axial and coronal thin-section CT or MR scanning are important.

References

Glaser JS. Neuro-ophthalmology. In: Duane TD, ed. Clinical ophthalmology. Vol 2. Hagerstown: Harper and Row, 1978:20.

Friedman AJ, Beckerman B, Gold DH, et al. Drusen of the optic disc. Surv Ophthalmol 1977; 21:375.

Walsh TJ, Garden J, Gallagher B, eds. Obliteration of retinal venous pulsations. Am J Ophthalmol 1969; 57:954.

RETINOPATHY OF PREMATURITY

Merrill L. Stass-Isern, M.D.

Retinopathy of prematurity (ROP), formerly known as retrolental fibroplasia, is a disease of abnormal vasoproliferation of the retina. The mesenchymal tissue, which is the precursor of retinal vasculature, reaches the ora serrata nasally at approximately 8 months' gestation and temporally 1 to 2 months later. When this process is altered by premature birth and oxygen therapy, neovascularization develops. This neovascularization may stop or regress at any time. If it progresses, it can lead to fibrovascular proliferation, vitroretinal traction, and retinal detachment. ROP seems to be inversely proportional to gestational age and weight. Oxygen therapy also appears to play a role, but the exact nature still remains undetermined. There also seems to be a direct correlation with the degree of illness of the child. The International Classification of Acute Stages of Retinopathy of Prematurity should be used when following children with ROP. It should be remembered that ROP is a very dynamic disease. The untrained observer should not be fooled by the child at 4 to 6 weeks who has no ridge or line, but whose retinal vasculature has not reached the ora serrata. This immature retina may indeed just be evolving and in the very early stages of the disease. Examination techniques:

1. Dilation: Cyclomydril (cyclopentolate 0.2% plus phenlyephrine 1%) to both eyes, 1 drop; repeat after 5 minutes. Administer one-half hour prior to examination.
2. Equipment:
   Lid speculum
   Scleral depressor
   Indirect ophthalmoscope
   20 or 28 lenses
3. Monitor: A neonatal intensive care unit nurse should hold the child and monitor the infant's general health during the examination. If necessary, a heart monitor and O_2 saturation monitor should be in place.

A. The American Academy of Pediatrics recommends examination of all high-risk infants (less than 36 weeks' gestation or birth weight less than 2000 grams, who have received oxygen therapy) at 4 to 6 weeks or at the time of discharge from the nursery. ROP is rare in infants with a birth weight greater than 2000 grams. Risk increases as gestational age and birth weight decrease. Those weighing less than 1250 grams and born at less than 28 weeks are especially vulnerable.

B. Prethreshold disease was described in the CRYO-ROP study as Zone 1, any stage; Zone 2, stage 2 (ridge) with "plus" disease; or Zone 2, stage 3 (ridge with extraretinal fibrovascular proliferation.) Plus disease was defined as dilated or tortuous vessels in the posterior pole. There may be increased vitreous haze. This may be accompanied by "anterior segment plus disease," which is dilation of the iris vasculature and pupillary rigidity.

C. Threshold disease was defined in the CRYO-ROP study as a level of severity at which the risk of blindness approaches 50%. There must be at least five contiguous or eight cumulative sectors (clock hours) of stage 3 ROP in zone 1 or 2, in the presence of plus disease.

D. Children with regressed ROP have a higher incidence of strabismus, amblyopia, and high refractive errors. Therefore, frequent examinations are necessary in their early years. Regressed advanced disease can cause peripheral and posterior retinal changes. Therefore, periodic examinations are necessary. Tractional retinal detachments, retinal folds, and dragging of the macula can occur.

E. It is the choice of the surgeon, neonatologist, and pediatric anesthesiologist whether topical anesthesia, local infiltration, local infiltration with sedation, or paralysis and general anesthesia are used. If local topical anesthesia is used, the child should be monitored by a neonatologist. If a general anesthetic is used, most children should be monitored postoperatively for 24 hours. Conjunctival peritomy may or may not be used. Cryotherapy may be applied with a standard retinal probe, cataract probe, or any number of the new pediatric ROP probes. The technique used by the CRYO-ROP study was a row of applications at the ora serrata, followed by more posterior applications. The applications are contiguous and single, rather than repeated and overlapping. The end point for each freeze is sudden whitening of the retina; freeze time is usually 2 to 3 seconds. Cryotherapy should be carried out until the entire anterior avascular retina has been treated to the anterior edge of the ridge. This usually averages 50 treatment spots. Treatment does not extend posterior to the ridge or anterior to pars plana. The cryoprobe should be completely withdrawn from the fornices at intervals of 5 minutes or less to avoid any prolonged ocular

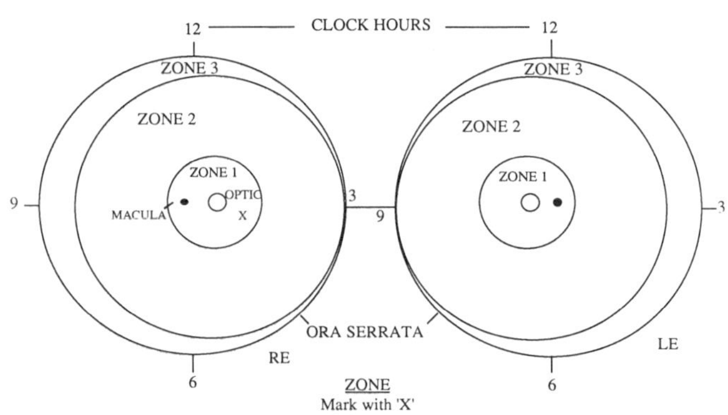

Figure 1 Drawing of zones according to the international classification.

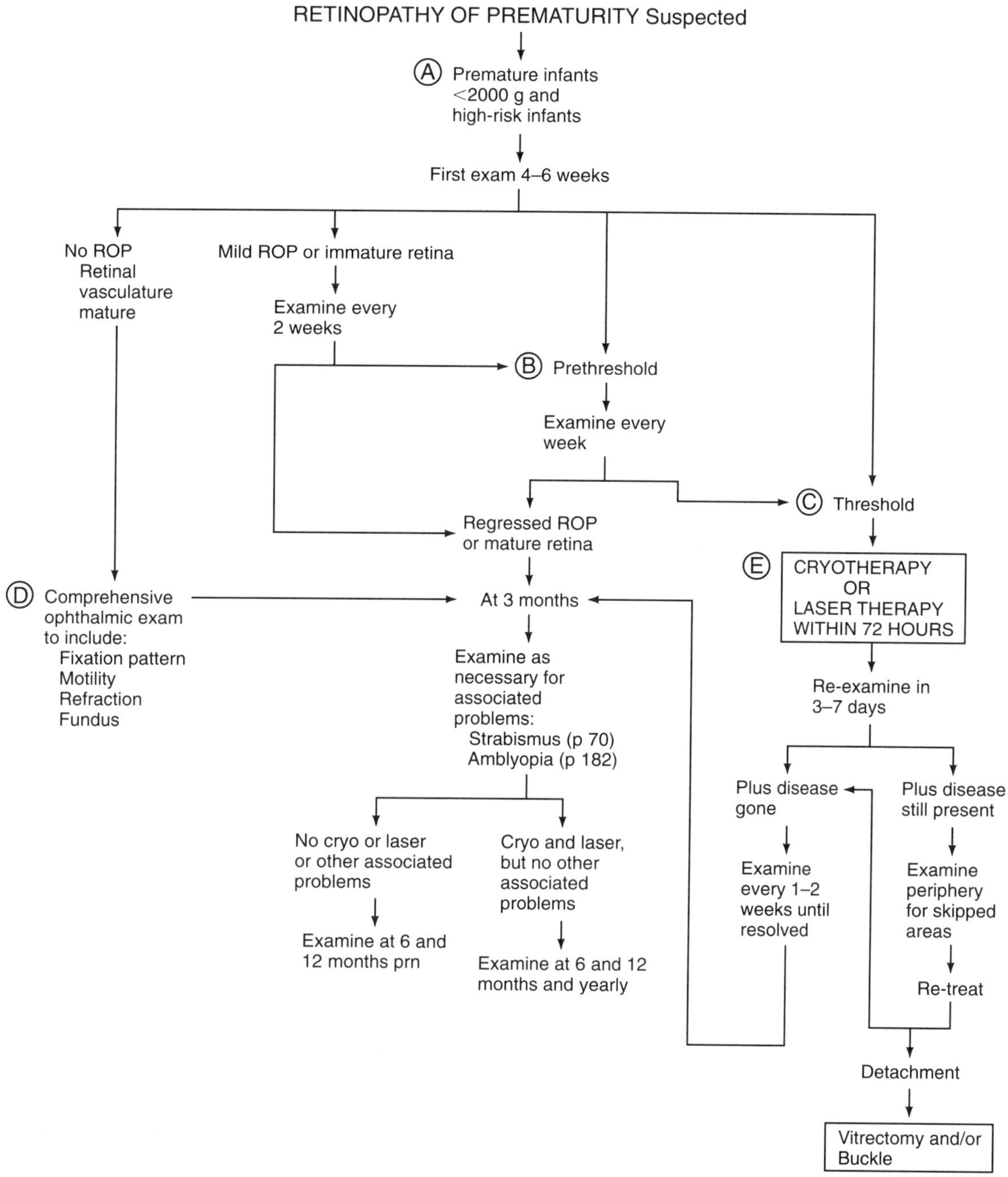

hypertension and compromise of central retinal artery flow. Any systemic complications (i.e., cyanosis, bradycardia, or apnea) should be treated by the anesthesiologist or neonatologist and treatment continued only if approved by one of these physicians. Recent literature reports equal efficacy in treating threshold ROP with the indirect diode and argon laser. The theory behind therapy is that avascular retina peripheral to the ridge is destroyed, thereby eliminating a vasoproliferative factor. The ridge itself need not be treated.

Moderate to severe swelling of the eyelids and conjunctival hemorrhage are expected 48 to 72 hours following treatment. They subside over 5 to 7 days. Postoperative medicines include Homatropine, 2% twice a day, and an antibiotic steroid combination ointment twice a day. Indirect ophthalmoscopy should be performed at 3 to 7 days. If plus disease still exists with skipped areas peripherally, these should be watched closely and treatment considered.

References

Committee for the Classification of Retinopathy of Prematurity: An international classification of retinopathy of prematurity. Arch Ophthalmol 1984; 102:1130.

Cryotherapy for Retinopathy of Prematurity Cooperative Group: Multicenter trial of cryotherapy for ROP. Arch Ophthalmol 1988; 106:471.

Iverson DA, Treese MT, Orgel IK, Williams GA. Laser photocoagulation for threshold retinopathy of prematurity (letter to editor). Arch Ophthalmol 1991; 109:1342.

Landers MB III, Toth CA, Semple HC, Morse LS. Treatment of retinopathy of prematurity with Argon laser photocoagulation. Arch Ophthalmol 1992; 110:44.

MACULAR COLOBOMA

Brian L. Lee, M.D.
John R. Heckenlively, M.D.

Macular coloboma refers to an uncommon, nonprogressive congenital retinochoroidal disorder that presents as poor vision since birth. Fundus examination reveals characteristic bilateral round circumscribed atrophic lesions at the macula. The term *coloboma* is used to denote an absence of ocular tissue. Whereas coloboma of the iris, lens, choroid and retina, or optic nerve is ascribed to the failure of fusion of the embryonic fissure of the optic cup, the cause of macular coloboma is unknown but is not the result of a similar arrest of normal eye development. Because of the inappropriate tendency to group macular coloboma with the other types of coloboma, terms such as *bilateral macular dysplasia, atypical coloboma of the macula,* and *macular staphyloma* have been used in the literature to refer to macular coloboma.

A. Macular coloboma appears to have a strong hereditary component. Pedigrees of pure macular coloboma consistent with autosomal dominant and autosomal recessive inheritance patterns have been documented. The degree of penetrance is not known.

B. Two major ophthalmologic patterns exist, although there is considerable overlap. The first form is the "pigmented" type, in which a mass of pigment covers the macular region through which retinal vessels are seen to course. Underneath, patches of bare, nonectatic sclera and choroidal vessels can be seen. The second form, the "nonpigmented" type, demonstrates both clumping of pigment and halting of retinal vasculature at the margin of the macular lesion, within which ectatic, or posteriorly excavated, sclera is visualized. It has been speculated that these forms reflect a difference in the temporal initiation of the pathogenetic insult. Ophthalmologic appearance of the lesion may vary even within families.

C. A large percentage of cases of macular coloboma are actually postinflammatory scar secondary to intrauterine or later acquired chorioretinitis. A unilateral lesion or additional lesions of similar character distributed peripheral to the macula strongly indicate this possibility. Chorioretinitis from infection by *Toxoplasma gondii,* the agent of toxoplasmosis, acquired by ingestion of undercooked meat containing *T. gondii* tissue cysts or cat feces containing oocysts, is most often implicated. Intrauterine ocular toxoplasmosis has never been documented in nontwin siblings owing to maternal immunity after initial infection. Healed ocular infections with cytomegalovirus, *Toxocara canis, Toxocara cati,* and *Treponema pallidum* may leave behind a similar ocular finding. Serologic tests are available (Sabin-Feldman dye or ELISA testing).

D. Macular coloboma is untreatable. However, it is important to be aware of certain uncommon but possible associated ocular and systemic defects. Keratoconus or cataracts may be found or may develop. A host of skeletal dysmorphologies along the extremities, ranging from flexion and size abnormalities of digits to dwarfism, have also been reported. In general, however, proper management for a patient with pure macular coloboma includes low vision care and genetic counseling for the family.

E. Numerous reports have documented the presence of highly subnormal electroretinograms (ERGs) in the face of macular coloboma, a condition in which the lesion is focal. Concomitant peripheral retinal disease may account for this finding. In particular, macular coloboma may be a feature of a form of Leber's congenital amaurosis (see p 68) with nystagmus, severely reduced vision, and extinguished ERGs in infancy) or progressive cone-rod dystrophy (with night blindness in early adulthood and ultimately very poor ERGs).

F. Other retinochoroidal disorders of noninfectious etiology may mimic macular coloboma in ophthalmologic appearance. These include chorioretinal coloboma and advanced stages of certain macular dystrophies. Chorioretinal colobomata (see p 48) can be differentiated from macular colobomata by their location on the inferonasal aspect of the retina. The importance of making the distinction lies in the former condition's high risk for retinal detachment and hemorrhage.

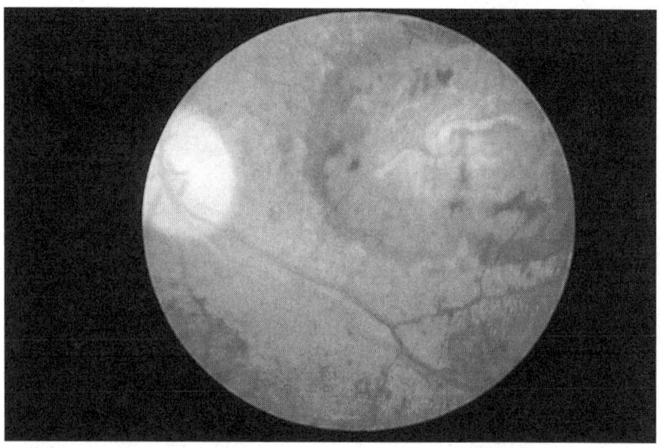

Figure 1 Congenital macular coloboma and pigmentary retinopathy in a 17-year-old man with count finger vision and nystagmus.

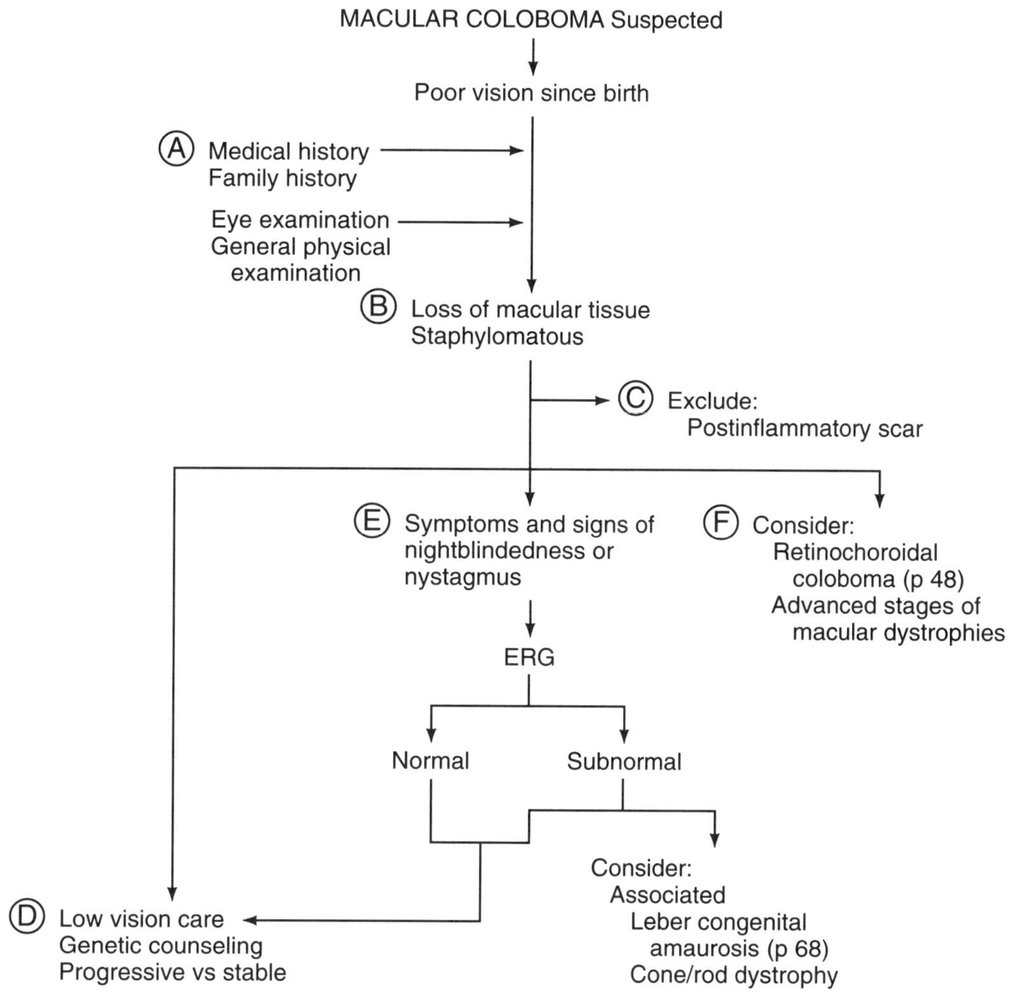

Certain dystrophies of the macula may culminate in atrophy of the retinal pigment epithelium and choroid, leaving behind eyegrounds with a colobomatous appearance. An example is North Carolina dystrophy, which, unlike many macular dystrophies, has an extremely young age of onset and a rapid progression. A critical distinction is that this and other macular dystrophies are progressive, whereas macular coloboma is stationary. Vestiges of a less advanced stage of these dystrophies, such as drusen-like deposits, may still be present in the affected individual and family.

References

Heckenlively JR, Foxman SG, Parelhoff ES. Retinal dystrophy and macular coloboma. Documenta Ophthalmol 1988; 68:257.

Moore AT, Taylor DS, Harden A. Bilateral macular dysplasia ('colobomata') and congenital retinal dystrophy. Ophthalmol 1985; 69:691.

Pasman FMH, Pinckers A. Hereditary macular coloboma. Ophthalm Paediatr Genet 1982; 2:67.

Primo SA. Macular coloboma. J Am Optom Assoc 1990; 61:373.

MACULAR DYSTROPHIES IN CHILDHOOD

Gerhard W. Cibis, M.D.

A maculopathy is usually found as part of the examination of a child with vision problems. At other times the positive family history leads to examination of the child. Whenever an index case is found, good family history and examination of the family members are indicated.

A. Macular coloboma is discussed in the previous chapter. Hereditary causes are listed in Table 1. When unilateral, TORCH is most likely. When bilateral, inherited retinal disease needs to be considered. The electroretinogram (ERG) is critical in the differential diagnosis.

B. When the condition is present from birth and bilateral, nystagmus develops. Color vision evaluation can be helpful in the differential diagnosis, being most affected in cone dystrophies but somewhat affected in Stargardt dystrophy, especially in the late stages. The Stargardt ERG cone responses are nearly normal, whereas they are distinctly abnormal in cone dystrophy.

C. Vision in Stargardt dystrophy decreases before much maculopathy is evident. Fluorescein angiography may show transmission defects before changes are seen by direct ophthalmoscopy. Flavimaculatus flecks block choroidal transmission, unlike drusen, which allow transmission. The flecks fade with time and new ones appear. In the area of the faded flecks, a pigment epithelial defect transmits choroidal fluorescence. In Stargardt dystrophy, therefore, fluorescein transmission does not correspond to the flavimaculatus flecks but to where flecks used to be. Stargardt dystrophy is most commonly inherited as autosomal recessive, but large pedigrees of dominant inheritance are reported.

D. Best disease has typical and atypical appearances in the same pedigree. The classic "egg yolk" can rupture to give a "scrambled eggs" appearance or leave a maculopathy with scarring and pigmentary changes difficult to distinguish from other forms of pigmentary and even senile maculopathies. The flat electro-oculogram (EOG) is the hallmark of Best disease. Expression is variable, and carriers with normal fundi can be identified on the basis of the flat EOG. The EOG also differentiates true Best disease from pseudo-Best disease.

E. Plicated macula, also described as spokes of a wheel, usually represents schisis in the macula. Sex-linked recessive juvenile schisis shows a negative ERG with a very low amplitude b-wave but present a-wave. The ERG is normal in dominantly inherited familial retinoschisis. It is flat in the Goldmann-Favre syndrome, which is a vitreodegenerative syndrome (see p 216). Dominant cystoid macular edema can look like the plications of schisis.

F. Bull's eye maculopathy is a ring of depigmentation surrounding a central area of hyperpigmentation. It is associated with a number of conditions (Table 2).

G. There are a number of pigmentary dystrophies usually referred to according to the pattern that the pigment resembles (see Table 3).

H. Crystalline maculopathies are listed in Table 4. Although rare, the clinically most relevant of these is Sjögren-Larson syndrome with mental retardation, congenital ichthyosis, and spastic diplegia. Electrophysiology is normal. A metabolic workup is indicated with crystalline retinal deposits if the diagnosis is not clear.

TABLE 1 Hereditary Causes of Macular Coloboma

Leber congenital amaurosis
Retinitis pigmentosa
Idiopathic infantile hypercalcuria
North Carolina dystrophy

TABLE 2 Conditions Associated with Bull's Eye Maculopathy

Cone dystrophy
Cone/rod dystrophy
Batten disease (lipofuscinosis)
Lawrence-Moon-Bardet-Bied
Hallervordern Spatz
Olivopontocerebellar atrophy

(Continued on p. 60.)

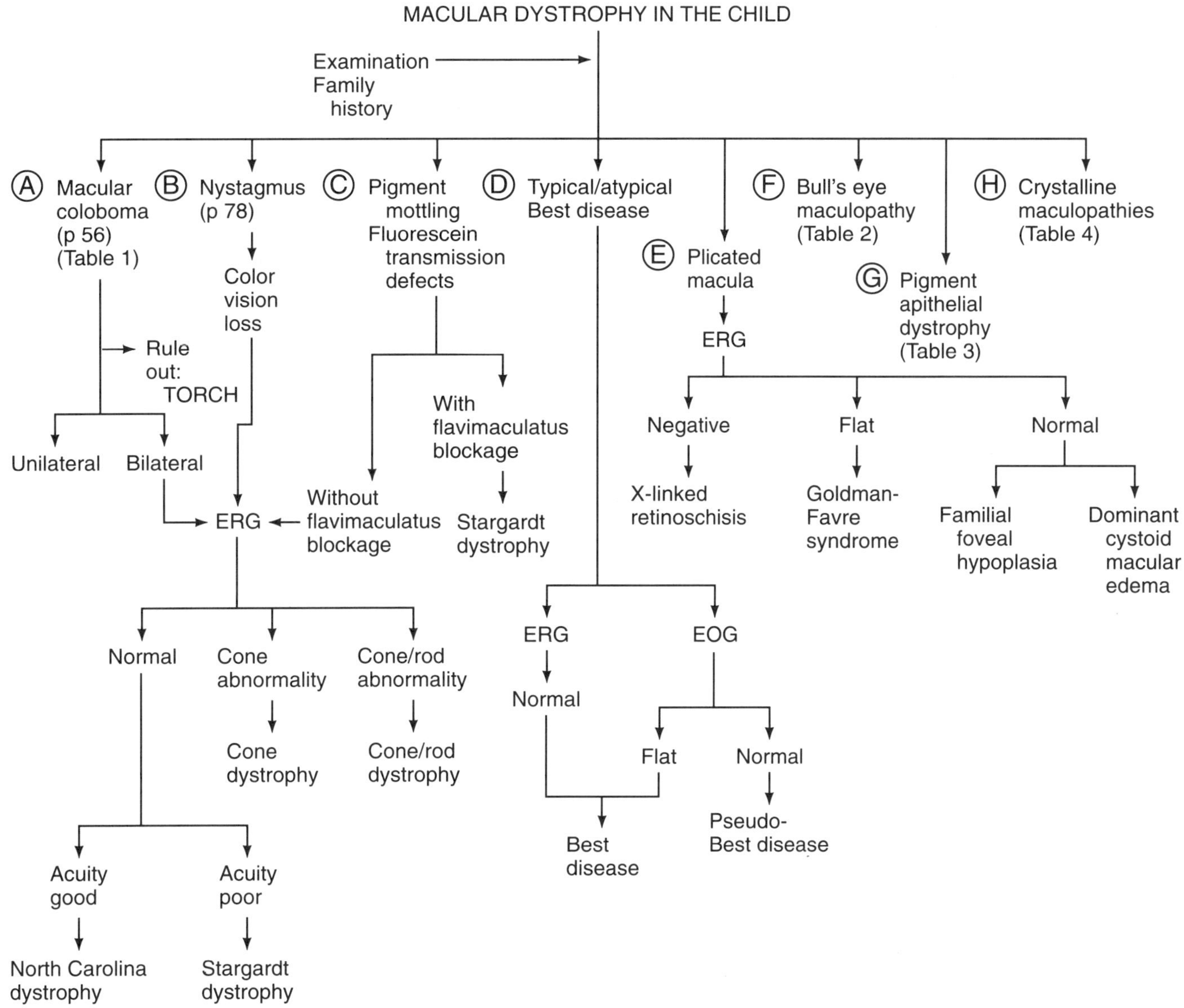
MACULAR DYSTROPHY IN THE CHILD
Examination
Family history
(A) Macular coloboma (p 56) (Table 1)
Rule out: TORCH
Unilateral
Bilateral
(B) Nystagmus (p 78)
Color vision loss
(C) Pigment mottling Fluorescein transmission defects
Without flavimaculatus blockage
With flavimaculatus blockage
Stargardt dystrophy
ERG
Normal
Cone abnormality
Cone/rod abnormality
Cone dystrophy
Cone/rod dystrophy
Acuity good
Acuity poor
North Carolina dystrophy
Stargardt dystrophy
(D) Typical/atypical Best disease
ERG
EOG
Normal
Flat
Normal
Best disease
Pseudo-Best disease
(E) Plicated macula
ERG
Negative
Flat
Normal
X-linked retinoschisis
Goldman-Favre syndrome
Familial foveal hypoplasia
Dominant cystoid macular edema
(F) Bull's eye maculopathy (Table 2)
(G) Pigment apithelial dystrophy (Table 3)
(H) Crystalline maculopathies (Table 4)

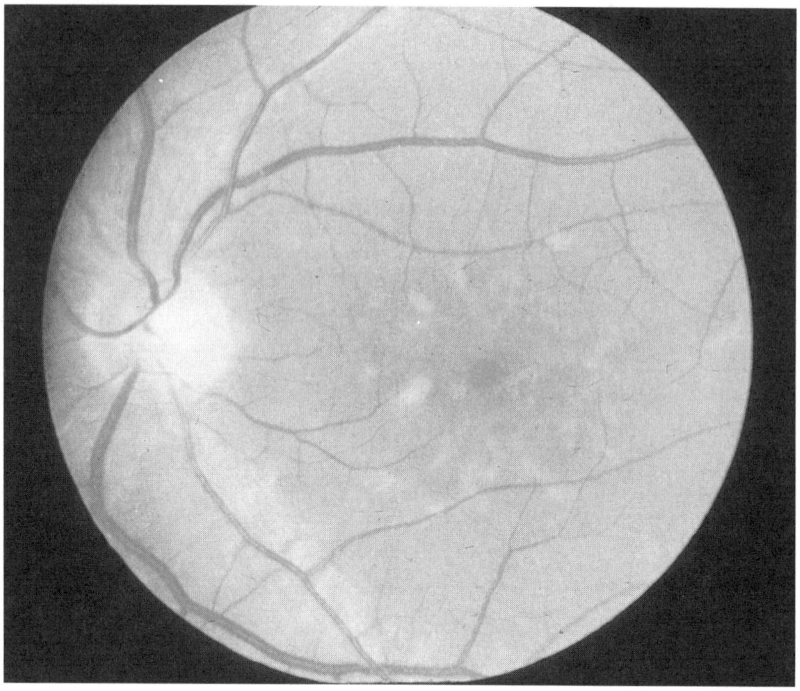

Figure 1 Fundus flavimaculatus with macular degeneration of Stargardt.

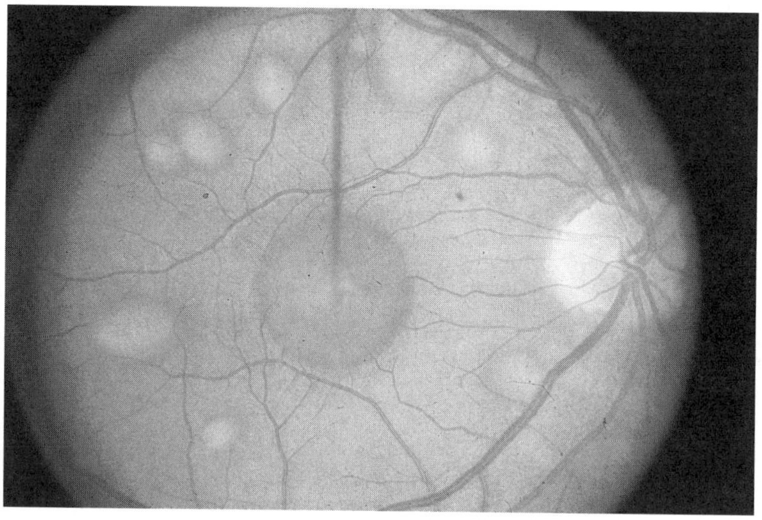

Figure 2 Multiple vitelliform lesions (Best disease).

TABLE 3 Pigment Epithelial Dystrophy

Butterfly
Reticular
Fundus pulverulentus
Central areolar pigment epithelium (CAPE)
Benign concentric anular

TABLE 4 Crystalline Maculopathies

Sjögren-Larson syndrome
Oxalosis Bietti syndrome
Crystalline dystrophy
Cystinosis
Tamoxife retinopathy
Canxanthine retinopathy

References

Cibis GW, Morey M, Harris DJ. Dominantly inherited macular dystrophy with flecks (Stargardt). Arch Ophthalmol 1980; 98:785.

Fishman GA. Electroretinography and inherited macular dystrophies. Retina 1985; 5:172.

Moore A. Inherited macular dystrophies. In: Taylor D, ed. Pediatric ophthalmology. Boston: Blackwell, 1992: 407.

BRAIN-RETINA NEUROEMBRYODYSGENESIS

Gerhard W. Cibis, M.D.

A. Embryologically, the retina is an extension of the brain. Ocular primordia of the neural plate are the earliest precursor cells for eye development. Very early genetic, chromosomal, or teratogenic influences acting on the neural plate, tube, and crest cells may influence retina, eye, and brain development. As the retina is part of the embryonic brain, the findings of associated malformations of the eye and brain are common. Colobomata of the optic disc or retina, abnormal disc size, and retinal pigmentary changes often predict brain defects. However, many individuals have gross anomalies of brain formation without clinically evident eye defects. In such cases, the disorderly development of the retina may be reflected in the electroretinogram (ERG).

B. In our experience, both dark- and light-adapted responses as well as oscillatory potentials can be variably affected. Characteristically, the ERGs are increased in implicit time with decreased amplitude but may be extinguished, highly attenuated, or "negative." A negative ERG is defined as a waveform with the amplitude of the B wave less than that of the A wave for the same response. It is most often associated with congenital stationary night blindness (CSNB) and is described as a Schubert-Bornschein–type ERG. The negative ERG seen with brain-retina neuroembryodysgenesis is not a classic Schubert-Bornschein type as seen in CSNB. The similarity of such ERGs to those of CSNB indicates a possible defect in neural transmission which may not be seen on histologic examination.

Our experience of extinguished, highly attenuated, and negative ERGs associated with congenital developmental brain anomalies leads us to reject the existence of a "type II" congenital amaurosis of Leber (see p 68). We restrict ourselves to considering congenital amaurosis of Leber as only the congenitally extinguished ERG with normal brain and eye findings except for tapetoretinal changes.

As genetic mapping advances, genetic subsets of brain-retina neuroembryodysgenesis will be identified. At that point, other cases will be more clearly seen to be caused by environmental factors such as intrauterine infections or teratogens such as alcohol or cocaine. The combination of early developmental brain defects and an abnormal ERG excludes perinatal insult as a cause. Developmental defects of the corpus

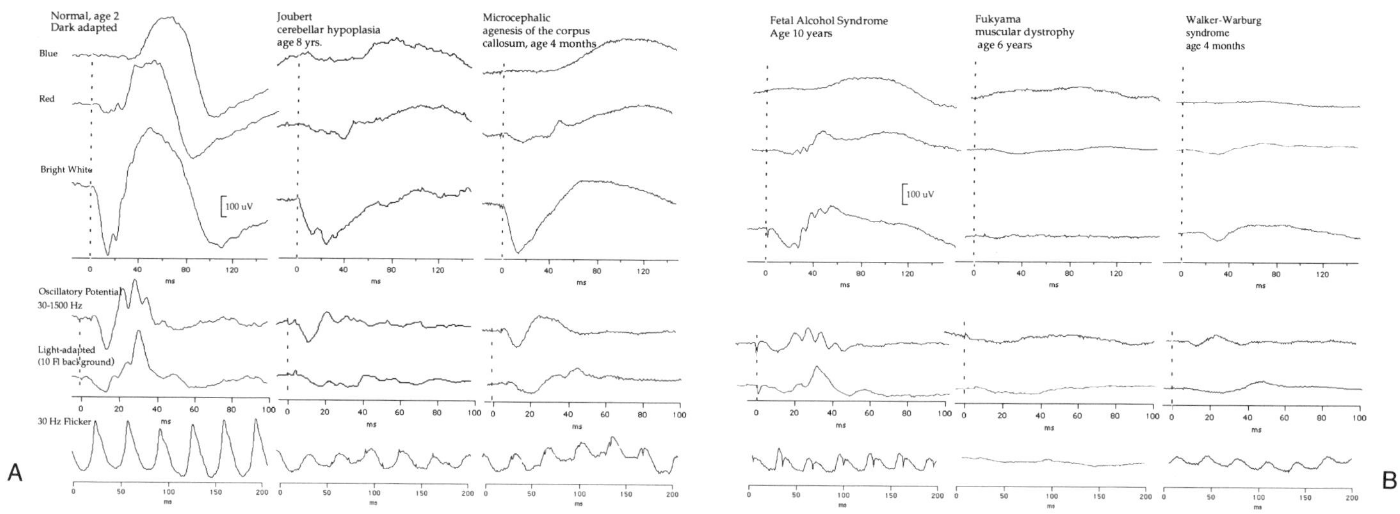

Figure 1 Representative ERG in brain-retina neuroembryodysgenesis.

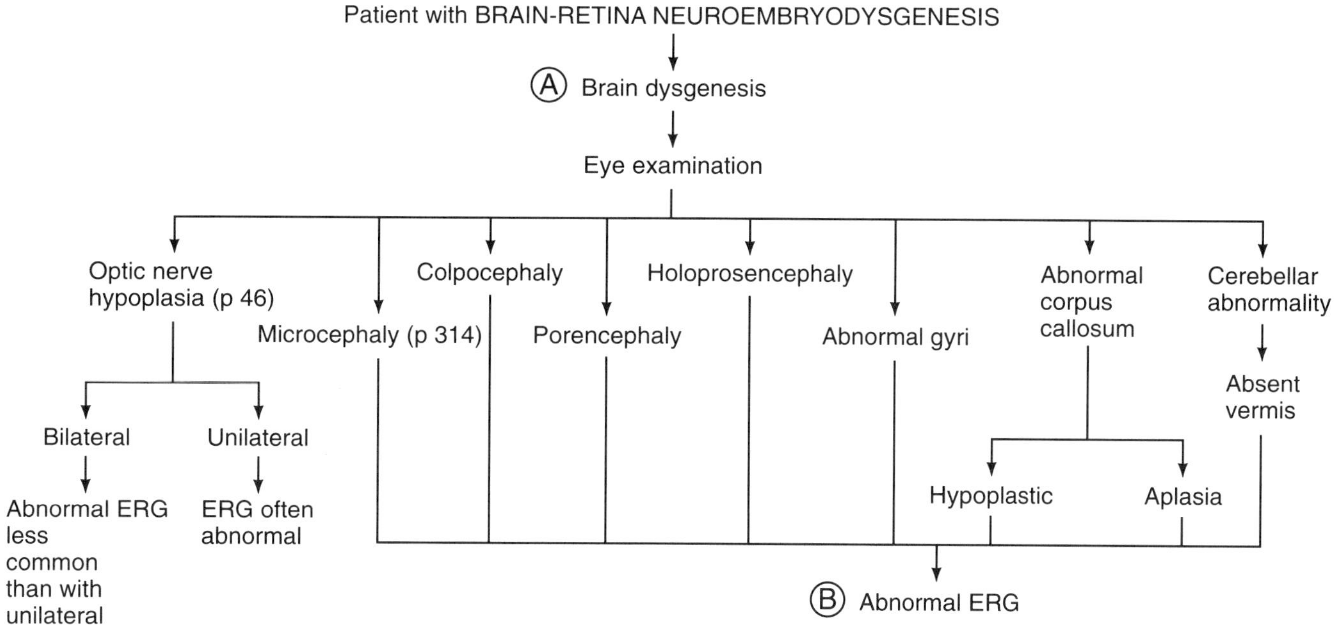

TABLE 1 Brain-Retina Neuroembryodysgenesis Conditions

Trisomy 13
Senior-Lockton syndrome
Walker-Warburg syndrome
Eye-muscle
Fukyama muscular dystrophy
Joubert syndrome
Dandy Walker malformation spectrum
CHARGE syndrome (p 46)
VACTER syndrome (p 46)
Morning glory syndrome
Ocular colobomata (p 46)
Fetal alcohol syndrome (p 94)
Ring 21
Trisomy 18
Peters' anomaly
Microphthalmos (p 18)
Zellweger syndrome

callosum, cerebrum, and cerebellum, especially the vermis, occur in the first trimester, but not later than the second trimester.

Brain-retina neuroembryodysgenesis is a descriptive term and not a diagnosis (Table 1). The label points to a disruption of early embryonic events in the formation of neural brain and retina. Within this group of patients there is undoubtedly a spectrum of genetic, metabolic, and unknown causes. A full work-up including ERG to search for the underlying pathogenesis is indicated.

References

Cook CS, Nowotny AZ, Sulik KK. Fetal alcohol syndrome. Arch Ophthalmol 1987; 105:1576.

Ripps H. Night blindness revisited: From man to molecules. Proctor Lecture. Invest Ophthalmol Vis Sci 1982; 23:588.

Warburg M, Friedrich U. Coloboma and microphthalmos in chromosomal aberations; chromosomal aberrations and neural crest cell developmental field. Ophthalmic Paediatri Genet 1987; 8:105.

THE INFANT AND TODDLER

"MY BABY DOESN'T LOOK AT ME"

Andrea M. Scalise-Gordy, D.O.
Edward G. Buckley, M.D.

A. Important points are prematurity, birth weight below 1200 grams, fetal distress, anoxic events, and birth trauma. Failure to reach developmental milestones may indicate neurologic abnormalities. History of a seizure disorder, cerebral palsy, or chromosomal abnormalities helps to identify potential underlying causes.

B. Normal newborn infants follow faces. A widening of lid fissures when room lights are extinguished indicates the presence of at least light perception. By age 2 months, infants should follow lights and high-contrast toys. Assessment of vision can be achieved in some infants using an optokinetic nystagmus drum. Creating a vertical nystagmus denotes visual acuity of 20/400 or better.

C. Ocular motility disturbances may be the underlying cause of a child's apparent visual inattention. Such entities as gaze palsies, bilateral third nerve palsy, or congenital fibrosis syndrome can give this impression owing to abnormal following movements. The infant with congenital fibrosis syndrome may present with a severe restriction of eye movements, often with the eyes fixed in down gaze, and a bilateral ptosis, giving the appearance of decreased visual acuity. Severe CNS abnormalities or ocular motor palsies can cause the eyes to deviate tonically into one gaze position, with an inability to generate voluntary eye movements. When this is accompanied by other neurologic defects, such as poor head control, visual field defects, or the inability to communicate effectively, the infant can appear to have extremely poor visual acuity. Placing objects in line with the deviated visual axis may elicit responses indicating normal or nearly normal vision.

D. Nystagmus (p 80) is a sign of decreased vision, and greater than 90% of these infants have underlying identifiable abnormalities of the anterior visual pathway. The onset is usually at birth or shortly after, when central foveal fixation should develop. Some infants may exhibit wandering or roving eye movements before the onset of frank nystagmus. The nystagmus may be pendular or jerk, and the direction may be characterized as horizontal, vertical, rotatory, oblique, or circular. The characteristics may vary with different fields of gaze, and this should be noted at the time of the examination.

E. Bilateral congenital ptosis is rare, and if severe may cause profound occlusion amblyopia. These children often develop abnormal chin-up head positions to preserve vision, and surgical correction can usually restore good vision.

F. Abnormalities of the anterior segment (pp 20, 24, 32) that cause profound visual loss are easily visible with minimal magnification. These include corneal opacification due to congenital glaucoma, Peters anomaly, and congenital hereditary corneal dystrophy, as well as leukokoria due to congenital cataracts, persistent hyperplastic primary vitreous, and inflammatory disease.

G. Posterior segment: The vast majority of patients with severe visual problems have an abnormal funduscopic appearance. This can range from retinoblastoma or retinal detachment (due to retinopathy of prematurity) to very subtle findings such as mild pigmentary disturbances or vascular attenuation. These infants may exhibit a sluggish or paradoxical pupillary response (pupil constricts in darkness). Oculodigital signs (persistent rubbing of the eyes) and photophobia may be additional symptoms leading to a suspicion of retinal disease. Examination under anesthesia (EUA) may be necessary if satisfactory visualization cannot be achieved in an office setting (p 310).

Optic nerve abnormalities may be associated with midline CNS defects such as an absent septum pellucidum, agenesis of the corpus callosum, and hypopituitarism. A CT or MRI scan can identify these abnormalities (see pp 46, 284).

H. An electroretinogram (ERG) (see p 294) may be helpful in determining the cause of decreased visual acuity with nystagmus and a seemingly normal ocular examination in infants. The three most commonly diagnosed conditions exhibiting these findings and having an abnormal ERG are Leber's congenital amaurosis, congenital achromatopsia, and congenital stationary night blindness (CSNB). The ERG in Leber's amaurosis is nonrecordable or highly attenuated. In achromatopsia, only the cone-mediated ERG is markedly attenuated or nonrecordable; the rod-mediated ERG is usually normal. CSNB has a rod-mediated ERG showing a normal "a" wave but an attenuated "b" wave, and the cone-mediated ERG may be abnormal as well.

I. High refractive errors may result in the appearance of significant visual loss. Spectacle correction usually alleviates the symptoms. Amblyopia is rarely a problem with symmetric refractive errors.

J. Cortical visual impairment or developmental delay is a diagnosis of exclusion. Failure to show evidence of visual awareness with normal ocular examinations and the absence of nystagmus suggest this diagnosis. These children may often have a history of prematurity and be slow reaching other developmental milestones. Delayed myelination of the optic nerve fibers and visual cortex is believed to be the underlying cause. Vision is often normal by age 6 months. An ERG is indicated in infants who fail to show visual improvement with observation.

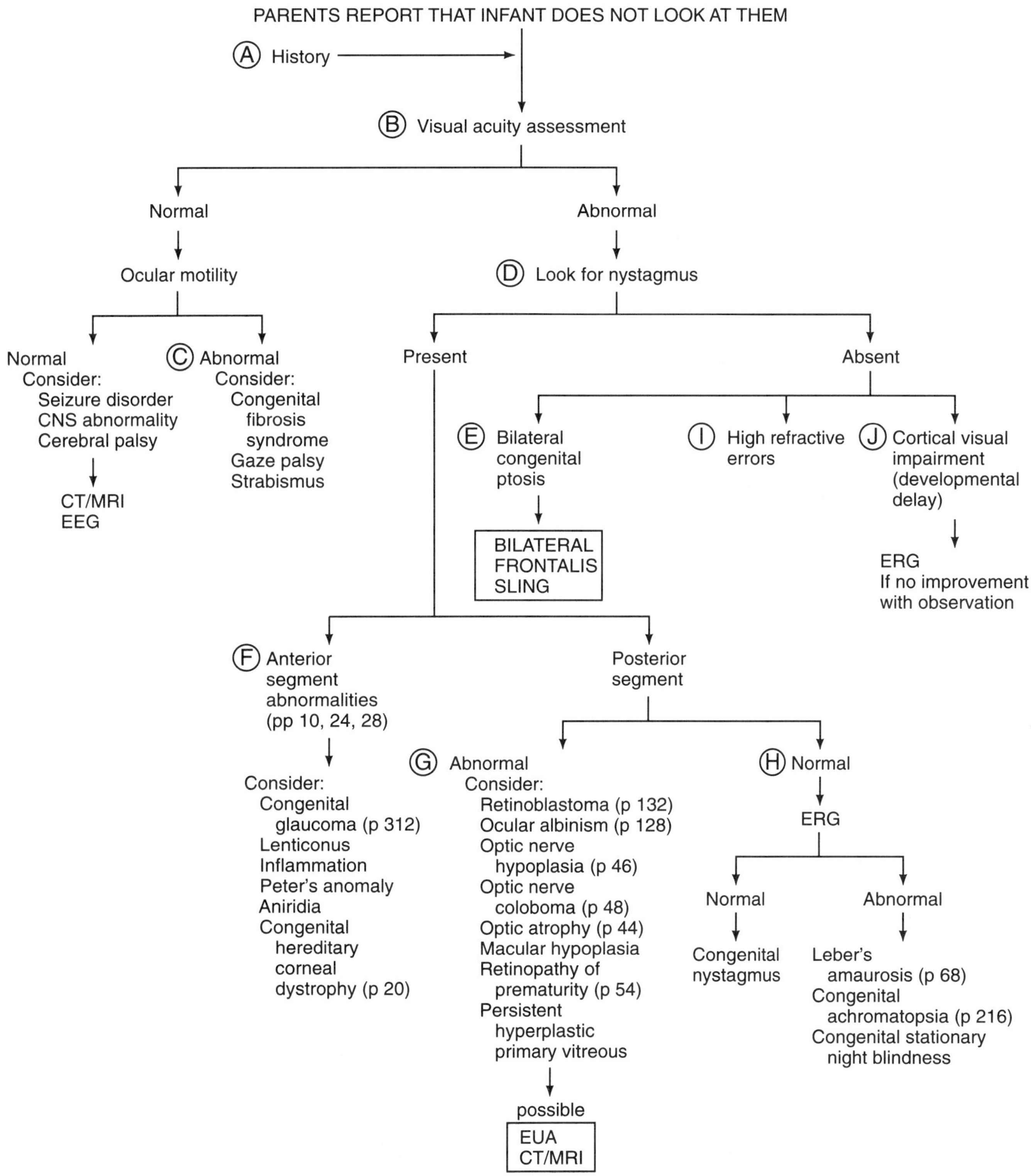

References

Buckley EG. The clinical approach to the pediatric patient with nystagmus. Int Pediatr 1990; 5:225.

Hoyt CS, Jastrzebski G, Marg E. Delayed visual maturation in infancy. Br J Ophthalmol 1983; 67:127.

Hoyt CS, Nickel BL, Billson FA. Ophthalmological examination of the infant. Developmental aspects. Surv Ophthalmol 1982; 26:177.

Kivlin JD, Bodnar A, Ralston CW, Hunt S. The visually inattentive preterm infant. J Pediatr Ophthalmol Strabismus 1990; 27:190.

Lambert SR, Taylor D, Kriss A. The infant with nystagmus, normal appearing fundi; but an abnormal ERG. Surv Ophthalmol 1989; 34:173.

Weleber RG, Tongue AC. Congenital stationery night blindness presenting as Leber's congenital amaurosis. Arch Ophthalmol 1981; 105:360.

BLIND INFANT WITH EXTINGUISHED ELECTRORETINOGRAM

Gerhard W. Cibis, M.D.

An apparently blind child at birth with sluggish pupillary responses has an extinguished electroretinogram (ERG). Deciding which of such children have congenital amaurosis of Leber (CAL) and which do not is very problematic. The question was defined historically by the clinical description of Leber in 1861 and the later introduction of the ERG. It must be redefined today as molecular biology and imaging technology further differentiate these cases. McKusic lists at least six possible genes that cause this syndrome. Fraser and Friedmannvin calculated that there may be as many as 17 different gene loci for this condition. Should the term be an umbrella to include all the different genetic paths proceeding to blindness at birth with an extinguished ERG or should it be limited to a more precise definition? We support the latter.

Henkes, in 1963, accepted three possibilities for the pathogenesis of CAL: retinal aplasia or "agenesis neuroepithelialis"; a "dysgenesis neuroepithelialis" in which the retina is histologically intact but functionally defective; and an "abiotrophy" or tapetoretinal degeneration beginning even in utero, as originally suggested by Leber. Such an all-inclusive classification was appropriate for that time but is no longer adequate, in our opinion. Retinal agenesis and dysgenesis are often associated with brain and metabolic abnormalities detectable by modern biochemical and imaging techniques. *We therefore recommend reserving the term CAL for cases without evidence for metabolic or brain abnormalities. Chromosomal abnormalities and syndromes such as Meckel syndrome are already excluded from the diagnosis.*

A. Because CAL is a progressive tapetoretinal degeneration beginning in utero, pigmentary changes are typically not present at birth but develop over time.

B. The area of associated findings raises the greatest problem as to prior inclusion as a subset of CAL. Renal dysplasia (Senior-Lockton syndrome) has long been accepted as a subset, as was Joubert syndrome. MRI and metabolic screenings to rule out peroxisomal disorders such as Zellweger syndrome and neonatal adrenoleukocorticodystrophy are needed for every patient suspected of being blind with an extinguished ERG.

C. The question of mental retardation or neurologic defects associated with CAL arose when Schappert-Kimmijser, examining patients from mental retardation institutions, found CAL cases with flat ERG among them. In contrast, Alstroem and Olson found that 10% of intelligent, neurologically intact children in Swedish schools for the blind had a congenital type of blindness that fit Leber's description. They described late keratoconus. From MRI it is now clear that a large number of developmental brain abnormalities can be associated with an abnormal, even flat ERG (brain-retina neuroembryodysgenesis) (p 62). Certain syndromes such as Walker-Warburg lissencephaly clearly fit this and historically are not confused with CAL. Joubert syndrome at one time was included as a subset of CAL.

D. It is our experience that optic nerve hypoplasia (ONH) (see p 46) can occur from defects anywhere in the developing visual system and may be associated with numerous causative agents—genetic, teratogenic, infectious, and mechanical. We therefore consider ONH to exclude CAL.

E. It is this author's opinion, as well as that of others, that the diagnosis of congenital amaurosis of Leber should be reserved for the child who presents with profound visual loss present at or shortly after birth, nystagmus, poorly reactive pupils, and an extinguished ERG. A pigmentary retinopathy may develop with time, and keratoconus may develop later in life. A macula coloboma may be present and there is a higher incidence of hyperopia. Most patients with CAL have some degree of vision (light perception) and normal intelligence. Visual aids and special education need to be provided for these children.

References

Alstroem CH, Olson O. Heredoretinopathia congenitalis monohybridia recessiva autosomalis. Hereditas (LUND) 43:1.

Fraser GR, Friedmannvin AL. The causes of blindness in childhood. The Baltimore: Johns Hopkins Press, 1967.

Heher KL, Traboulsi EI, Maumenee IH. The natural history of Leber's congenital amaurosis. Ophthalmology 1992; 99:241.

Henkes HE, Verduin PC. Dysgenesis or abiotrophy? A differentiation with the help of the electroretinogram (ERG) and electro-oculogram (EOG) in Leber's congenital amaurosis. Ophthalmologica 1963; 145:144.

Leber T. Ueber retinitis pigmentosa und angeborene amaurose. Graefes Arch Ophthal 1867; 15:1.

McKusick VA. 20040, 20410, 26690, 26692. In: Mendelian inheritance in man. 8th ed. Baltimore: Johns Hopkins University Press, 1988:804.

Schappert-Kimmijser, Henkes HE, van den Bosch J. Amaurosis congenita (Leber). Arch Ophthalmol 1959; 61:211.

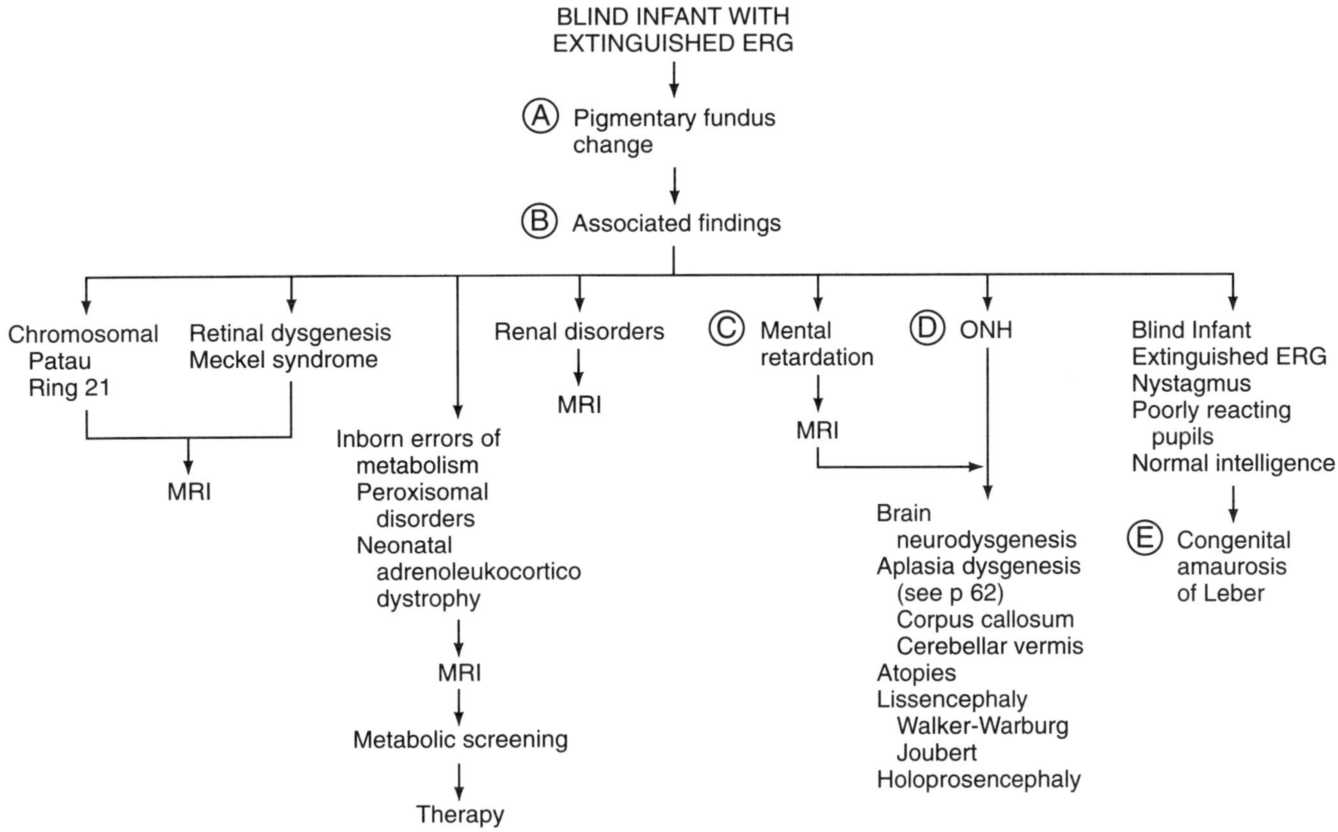
BLIND INFANT WITH EXTINGUISHED ERG
Ⓐ Pigmentary fundus change
Ⓑ Associated findings
Chromosomal
Patau
Ring 21
Retinal dysgenesis
Meckel syndrome
MRI
Inborn errors of metabolism
Peroxisomal disorders
Neonatal adrenoleukocortico dystrophy
MRI
Metabolic screening
Therapy
Renal disorders
MRI
Ⓒ Mental retardation
MRI
Ⓓ ONH
Brain neurodysgenesis
Aplasia dysgenesis
(see p 62)
Corpus callosum
Cerebellar vermis
Atopies
Lissencephaly
Walker-Warburg
Joubert
Holoprosencephaly
Blind Infant
Extinguished ERG
Nystagmus
Poorly reacting pupils
Normal intelligence
Ⓔ Congenital amaurosis of Leber

INFANTILE ESOTROPIA SYNDROME

Gerhard W. Cibis M.D.

A. The term *infantile esotropia* (ET), specifically the infantile esotropia syndrome, was coined by Lange to replace "congenital esotropia." Most infantile esotropia is not truly congenital, i.e., appearing at birth. Rather, the syndrome manifests usually in the first 2 to 3 months of life. Infantile ET includes all esotropias that begin in the first 6 months of life. A number of commonly associated characteristics may appear over time. Some of these point to a defect in the fusion mechanism. These include dissociated vertical divergence (DVD), nystagmus, and optokinetic nystagmus (OKN) asymmetry. This explains why the best surgical result that can be achieved is microtropia with peripheral, but probably never central, fusion. Cases that have central fusion following surgery most likely are misdiagnosed sixth nerve palsies.

B. The differentiation of true infantile ET from mimicking conditions is important. Pseudoesotropia, common in infants because of their wide nasal bridge and epicanthal folds, is best detected by analyzing the Hirschberg reflex. The Brueckner method is excellent for this purpose (p 304). The syndromes of Duane and Moebius have associated findings that differentiate them (Table 1). Abduction is often limited in infantile ET. When this occurs, a short period of patching or stimulating the vestibular system by spinning the child reveals intact lateral rectus function.

C. The angle of deviation may vary in the first several months but usually by 6 months settles into a large steady deviation. When there is variability, especially after 6 months of age, an accommodative component must be ruled out. Oblique dysfunction giving a V pattern is common but may not be present at the time of presentation. Many secondary characteristics of the syndrome such as DVD and inferior oblique overaction (IOO) develop later.

TABLE 1 Differential Diagnosis

Condition	*How to Detect or Treat*
Pseudostrabismus	Rule out with Hirschberg and cover test
Accommodative ET	Cycloplegia; wear full prescription 3 months
VI nerve palsy	Patch, observe, vestibular stimulation (spin child)
Duane co-contraction syndrome	Defective abduction, narrowing palpebral fissure
Moebius syndrome	Look for feeding problems, facial palsy

D. Usually infantile ET has a normal amount of hyperopia for age. If the hyperopia is less than 3 to 4 diopters and the onset occurs before 6 months of age with a classic large angle, I do not try glasses before surgery. When there is variability to the angle or onset is after 6 months of age, a trial of glasses is appropriate. When more than 4 diopters of hyperopia exists, I usually try glasses. At least a 3-month trial is appropriate to determine if all or only part of the esotropia can be corrected. The higher the hyperopia, the more likely glasses will be needed after surgery to keep the eyes aligned and avoid recurrence of the deviation. Fully accommodative esotropia can unquestionably develop prior to 6 months of age.

E. Associated findings do not always exist at the time of presentation. Surgical correction of a DVD or IOO should be done at the time the ET is surgically corrected (p 234). Presence of occlusion nystagmus is diagnostically useful, but no therapy is necessary. Occasionally it can be the source of difficulty when patching for amblyopia. Penalization may work better than occlusion in such cases.

F. Amblyopia is rare prior to surgery in infantile ET. This is because the large angle allows for cross fixation, decreasing the incidence of amblyopia. If amblyopia is suspected, a short period of part-time patching usually reveals alternation. If the patient is microtropic after surgery, the danger of amblyopia development exists.

G. Surgery is the treatment of choice for infantile ET. Post-surgical results are maintained by glasses, phospholine iodide drops, and patching. Unlike a late-onset, partially accommodative ET, the surgery comes first. It is important to make parents aware of the difference in handling these different types of strabismus so they don't think surgery is being rushed. The choice of surgery varies with different schools of thought. Certainly all agree it need not be done in stages. All aspects that need correcting should be addressed at the time of surgery. This means recession for IOO or DVD. Bimedial recessions and recession resection are equivalent. The type of incision should be left to the preference of the surgeon, as should how to measure or whether to do "en bloc" recessions. One method has not proven better than another. The same is true for whether one operates on the fixing or the nonfixing eye. My personal preference for alternating ET is to do bimedials; however, when one eye is primarily deviated, I perform an R+R on the deviated eye.

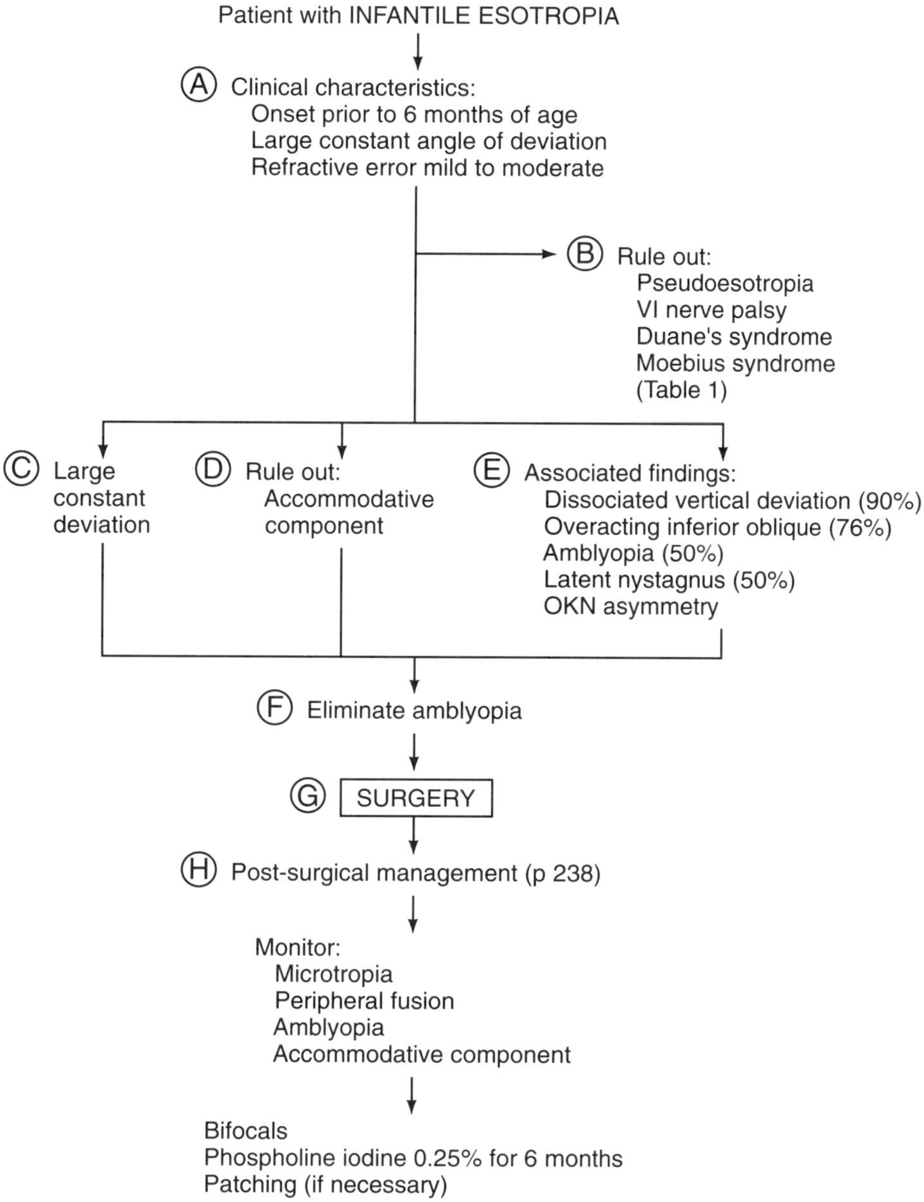

Early or late surgery once meant before or after 2 years of age. In the United States the argument now is whether surgery before 6 months of age gives better results than surgery after 6 months. This debate is fueled by the finding that fusion develops by 3 to 4 months of age. Does alignment prior to that time help ultimate outcome? In my experience, children are rarely referred before 4 months of age.

H. Post-surgical management is as important for the ultimate outcome as the surgery (p 238). Without good post-surgical management, the surgical recurrence rate triples. Monitor for any deviations above microtropia and intervene when that occurs. Bifocal glasses are useful for high AC/A ratio. I use phospholine iodide 0.25% for 6 months if it works. To stimulate peripheral fusion (binocularity), do not patch unless necessary. For this reason amblyopia, when present, should be eliminated preoperatively. If post-surgical amblyopia develops, I start with part-time patching. To prevent amblyopia, it may be necessary to patch a markedly dominant eye several hours a day.

References

Christenson GN, Rouse MW. Management of infantile-onset esotropia. J Am Optom Assoc 1990; 7:559.

Helveston EM. Atlas of strabismus surgery. St. Louis: CV Mosby, 1985.

Lang J. Strabismus. Trans. by GW Cibis. Thorofare, NJ: Slack, 1983.

Parks MM. Atlas of strabismus surgery. Philadelphia: Harper & Row, 1983.

Von Noorden GK. Binocular vision and ocular motility: Theory and management of strabismus. St. Louis: CV Mosby, 1990.

PSEUDOSTRABISMUS

Trudi R. Grin, M.D.

In pseudostrabismus the patient has the appearance of having strabismus (a misalignment of the visual axes), when in fact the eyes are straight. Pseudoesotropia, or false crossing, is the most common type, but pseudoexotropia and pseudohypertropia can also occur. These are secondary to prominent or abnormal epicanthal folds, facial asymmetries, increased or decreased interpupillary distance, or angle kappa.

A. Before examining an infant or child with possible strabismus, the family must be questioned regarding neonatal history, birth weight, history of retinopathy of prematurity (ROP), and presence or absence of birth defects, particularly craniofacial abnormalities. Severe ROP can lead to temporal macular dragging, displacing the visual line. This may result in a pseudoexotropia. Craniofacial anomalies are associated with hypertelorism, which may cause a patient to appear exotropic, although true exotropia may also occur. In pseudoesotropia the parents often describe the crossing as intermittent and more prominent in lateral gaze.

B. Infants often have a wide, flat nasal bridge, prominent or asymmetric epicanthal folds, and a reduced interpupillary distance. These features may create the appearance of esotropia when the eyes are actually straight. Pseudoexotropia may occur in a child with an increased interpupillary distance and/or hypertelorism. Facial asymmetries or orbital tumors may cause a lid fissure or the globe itself to appear higher on one side than the other, creating the impression of a hypertropia.

C. The corneal light reflex test is a useful screening technique, especially in infants and uncooperative patients, to assess the presence or absence of strabismus and to estimate the degree of misalignment. A bright penlight is held directly in front of the patient; as the patient fixates on the light, the location of the light reflex on the corneas is noted. Normally, the corneal light reflex is centered or slightly nasal to the center of the cornea. If the light reflex is decentered temporally, an esotropia may exist. If the light reflex is decentered nasally, an exotropia may be present. Each millimeter of decentration corresponds to 7 degrees or 14 prism diopters of ocular deviation of the visual axis. However, a number of limitations of this test may lead to erroneous results. Accommodation is not controlled, pupil size may affect measurements, errors could be made owing to poor fixation, and small deviations could be missed.

D. Whenever possible, cover testing should be performed in all patients with suspected strabismus. This is the most accurate method for determining if strabismus is present and for measuring the deviation. If a movement of the eye is noted on cover testing, then strabismus is present. If a patient has an abnormal corneal light reflex and cover testing is normal, then angle kappa (Fig. 1) must be present.

E. Angle kappa may produce pseudostrabismus, may make an existing ocular deviation appear worse, or may mask a deviation. Angle kappa is caused by the failure of the visual and pupillary axis to coincide. Clinically, angle kappa is measured by observing the relationship of the corneal light reflex to the center of the pupil. The simplest way to determine angle kappa is to have the patient fixate on a light held 1 foot in front of the patient's right eye while the left eye is covered. The examiner interprets the position of the light reflex on the cornea with his or her line of sight directly behind the light. If the light reflex is centered, there is no angle kappa. If the light reflex is decentered nasally, the fovea is temporal to the pupillary axis and positive angle kappa exists. If the light reflex is decentered temporally, the fovea is nasal to the pupillary axis and a negative angle kappa is present. The test is then repeated for the opposite eye.

F. A small positive angle kappa is seen in many normal individuals. In the absence of true strabismus, positive angle kappa simulates exotropia. Most commonly it is due to temporal displacement of the macula, as seen in advanced ROP. If an existing exotropia is present, a positive angle kappa causes the exotropia to appear greater than it is. An existing esotropia is decreased in appearance with a positive angle kappa.

G. A negative angle kappa is less common and may be seen as a variant of normal. It can also occur as a result

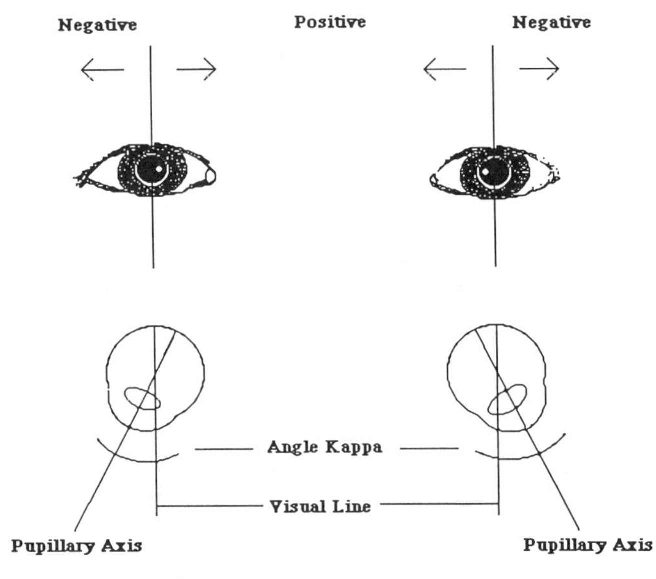

Figure 1 Angle kappa.

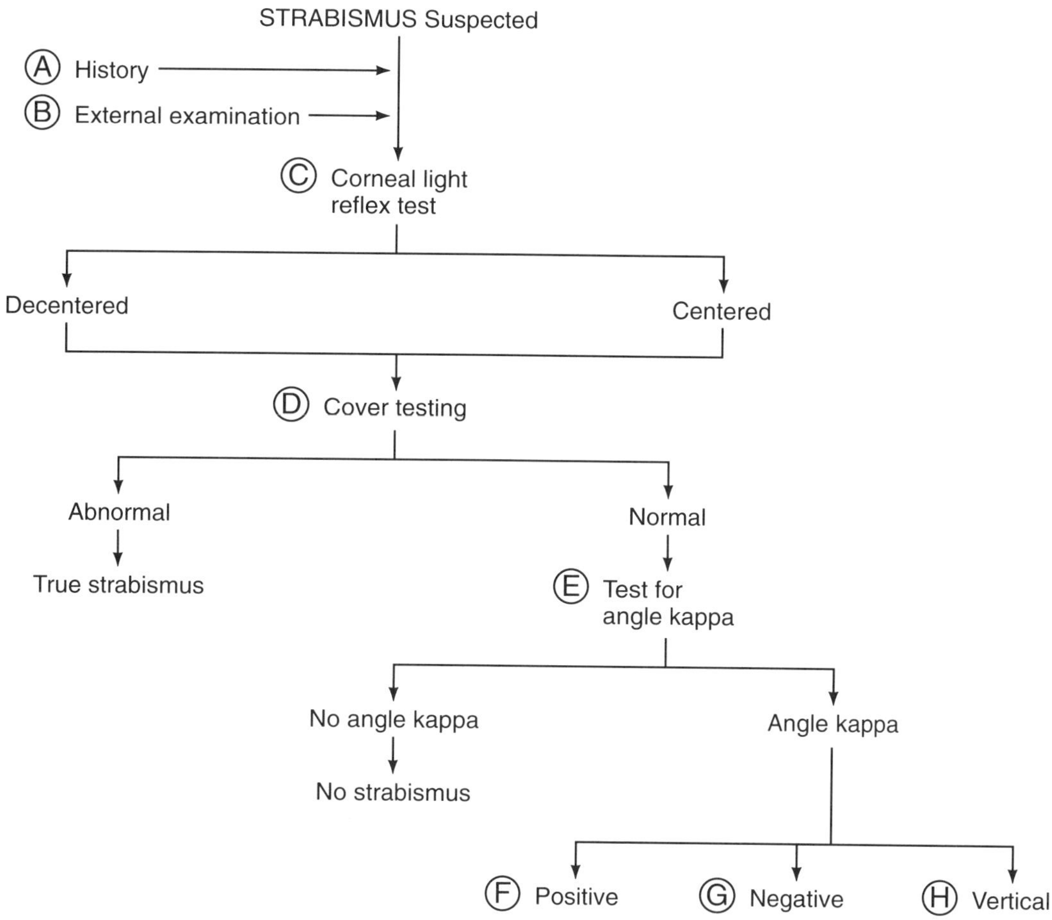

of nasal displacement of the macula or may be seen in high myopes. A negative angle kappa simulates esotropia, causing an existing esotropia to appear greater than it is. Conversely, exotropia is decreased in appearance with a negative angle kappa.

H. Vertical angle kappa simulates a hyperdeviation and is very rare. It is caused by superior or inferior displacement of the macula from scar tissue.

References

Cibis GW, Waeltermann JM. Rapid strabismus screening for the pediatrician. Clin Pediatr 1986; 25:304.

Manley DR. Strabismus: clinical presentation and surgical procedures. In: Harley RD. Pediatric ophthalmology. 2nd ed. Philadelphia: WB Saunders, 1983:217.

Von Noorden GK. Binocular vision and ocular motility. St. Louis: CV Mosby, 1990:162.

DUANE'S SYNDROME

Joseph H. Calhoun, M.D.

A. Duane's syndrome is nearly always a congenital defect, occurring more often in females and more often involving the left eye. A limitation of movement of one or both eyes tends to occur in several characteristic clinical patterns. Electromyographic (EMG) studies, initially by Huber, provided evidence of anomalous innervation patterns in the affected horizontal muscles which are typical for each clinical type. A few autopsies showed absence of the abducens nucleus and nerve. The lateral rectus muscles were innervated by branches from the oculomotor nerve.

B. Type I Duane's syndrome is the most common. Clinically there is little or no abduction and some evidence of simultaneous firing of the medial and lateral rectus muscles on adduction that is detected by any or all of the following: limited adduction (exotropia in field of medial rectus, reduced near point of convergence), narrowing of the fissure, and retraction of the globe. In primary position there may be orthotropia, esotropia, or exotropia with a corresponding compensatory face turn. By EMG the medial rectus is normal. The lateral rectus has little to no activity on attempted abduction but fires on adduction, accounting for the characteristic clinical findings.

C. With Type II Duane's syndrome, there is little or no adduction and the abduction is normal or nearly so. Narrowing of the fissure and/or retraction of the globe occurs on attempted adduction. Often there is exotropia in the primary position with the corresponding compensatory face turn. By EMG the medial rectus is normal, but the lateral rectus fires on both adduction and abduction, accounting for the reduced adduction.

D. Type III Duane's syndrome exhibits significant limitation of both adduction and abduction with some narrowing of the fissure and retraction of the globe on attempted adduction. Frequently there is exotropia in the primary position. By EMG there is simultaneous firing of both the medial and lateral rectus muscles on attempted adduction or abduction.

E. In a small percentage of patients, Duane's syndrome may occur in each eye. Usually it is Type I on each side, but other combinations may occur.

F. In many patients there is an obvious movement upward (upshoot) and/or downward (downshoot) on adduction or attempted adduction (depending on the type). This is most commonly seen in Type I. If this upshoot or downshoot is cosmetically significant, treatment may be indicated. Weakening the inferior oblique for upshoot or the superior oblique for downshoot is almost never helpful. This phenomenon may be caused by the horizontal rectus muscles simultaneously firing and acting like a bridle, pulling the eye up or down as soon as the eye is out of the horizontal plane. Surgical approaches vary. Limiting the vertical slipping of the horizontal rectus muscles by posterior fixation sutures on each has been successful. Splitting the lateral rectus muscle into a Y and attaching the split ends at the upper and lower border of the insertion or recessing the appropriate muscle for the face turn may help the upshoot or downshoot.

G. In all types of Duane's syndrome, vertical movements in straight up and down gaze are usually normal. However, there is frequently a different horizontal position of the eyes in up or down gaze. Commonly a divergence in up gaze produces a V pattern. Less often there is a divergence in down gaze, producing an A pattern. Least common is convergence in up or down gaze. Weakening the inferior oblique for the V or the superior oblique for the A pattern is of little benefit. Treatment should be limited to aligning the eyes in the primary position.

H. Abnormal compensatory head positions to align the eyes—nearly always face turns in the horizontal plane—are common. In Type I the face turn is usually toward the involved eye, reflecting the underaction of the lateral rectus. In Types II and III the face turn is usually in the opposite direction, toward the underacting medial rectus. Frequently the face turn is of such magnitude that treatment is warranted. Regardless of the type of Duane's syndrome, if the involved eye is esotropic, the medial rectus should be recessed, and if the involved eye is exotropic, the lateral rectus should be recessed. Some report success for the esotropia in Type I Duane's syndrome with a full vertical rectus muscle transposition adjacent to the lateral rectus.

I. Patients with Duane's syndrome may have a higher incidence of anisometropia and amblyopia. Duane's syndrome may be seen with a wide variety of craniofacial anomalies that are obvious to external inspection. However, neural deafness seems to occur with a higher frequency in these patients.

References

Molarts AB, Rosenbaum AL. Vertical rectus muscle transposition surgery for Duane's syndrome. J Pediatr Ophthalmol Strabismus 1990; 27:171.

O'Malley ER, Helveston EM, Ellis FD. Duane's retraction syndrome-plus. J Pediatr Ophthalmol Strabismus 1982; 19:161.

Pressman SH, Scott WE. Surgical treatment of Duane's syndrome. Ophthalmology 1986; 93:29.

Raab EL. Clinical features of Duane's syndrome. J Pediatr Ophthalmol Strabismus 1986; 23:64.

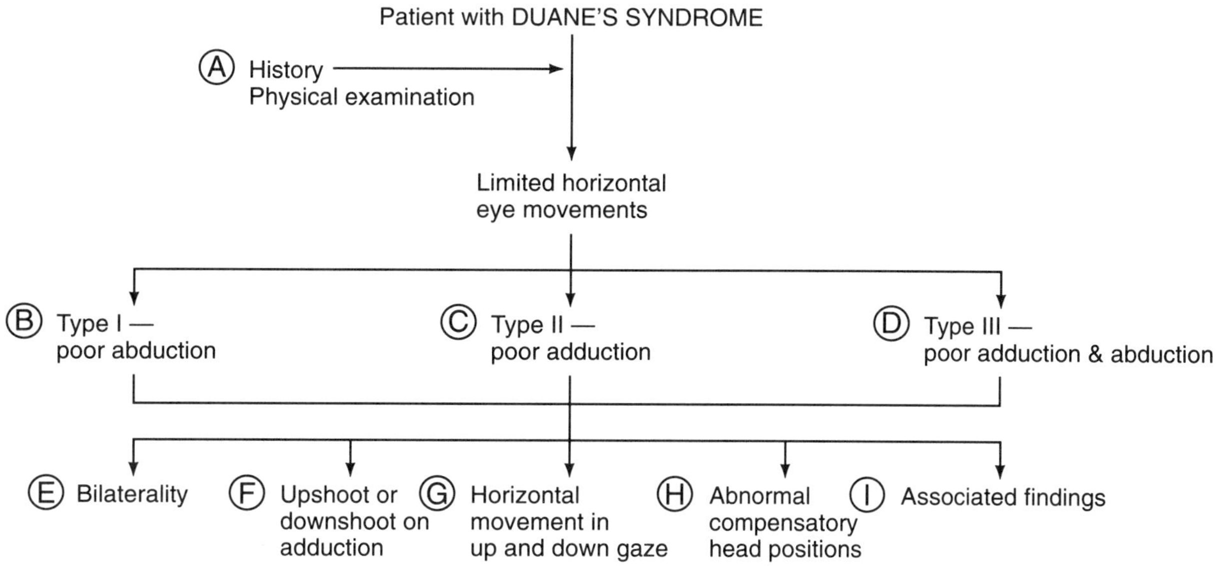

Patient with DUANE'S SYNDROME
(A) History
Physical examination
Limited horizontal eye movements
(B) Type I — poor abduction
(C) Type II — poor adduction
(D) Type III — poor adduction & abduction
(E) Bilaterality
(F) Upshoot or downshoot on adduction
(G) Horizontal movement in up and down gaze
(H) Abnormal compensatory head positions
(I) Associated findings

INTRODUCTION TO NYSTAGMUS AND ABNORMAL EYE MOVEMENTS SIMULATING NYSTAGMUS

Merrill L. Stass-Isern, M.D.

Nystagmus traditionally has been divided into two types based on the clinical impression of the waveform: pendular—when the oscillations appear to have equal speed in either direction, or jerk—when movement in one direction appears to be faster. However, often these are clinically difficult to distinguish and can be assessed only by accurate waveform recordings. Furthermore, the classic thinking that pendular nystagmus is associated with congenital sensory nystagmus and that jerk is associated with congenital motor nystagmus is often incorrect and simplistic. Therefore, we do not separate these in the following chapters.

The ensuing chapters on nystagmus are first divided according to timing of the appearance of the nystagmus, because the child's age at the time of onset of the nystagmus has different implications as to cause and prognosis. They are further subdivided according to direction—horizontal, vertical, and so fourth, which also have different implications.

A. We first must distinguish abnormal nystagmus from normal, or physiologic, nystagmus. Physiologic nystagmus appears with fatigue, end point gaze, and caloric and optokinetic testing. Next we need to ask when the nystagmus appeared. Any nystagmus detected beyond 4 months of age should be considered acquired until proven otherwise. Also of critical importance is the investigation of the family's ocular history. Inquire if any other members have nystagmus or poor vision—this may lead to the diagnosis of a hereditary eye disease associated with nystagmus (i.e., autosomal dominant, inherited, congenital motor nystagmus). Prenatal, perinatal, and neonatal history is also important, as certain conditions acquired during one of these periods may lead to an abnormality of the eye and poor vision, such as congenital toxoplasmosis with macular lesions. Symptoms of vestibular dysfunction, such as vertigo, tinnitus, and nausea can also be helpful in pinpointing the diagnosis. Attention should be paid to investigating any use of drugs because many produce nystagmus at therapeutic or toxic levels. A history of head trauma, seizures, or neurosurgical intervention may help define a neuroanatomic abnormality. Some forms of congenital sensory nystagmus with retinal abnormalities are part of a generalized syndrome. Therefore, any obvious nonocular structural abnormality may also be helpful in pinpointing the diagnosis. Finally, after the examination, the nystagmus may be classified into one of the broad categories of congenital (p 80), acquired (p 78), or abnormal eye movements simulating nystagmus described below.

B. Congenital oculomotor apraxia is usually first noticed by the parents because the child cannot look around the room (failure to make saccades). Later, when head control develops, instead of using saccades to shift their eyes, they move their head in the direction of attention at a high velocity. With this the eye is swept over into extreme deviation in the opposite direction (by virtue of the vestibulo-ocular reflex). Head rotations overshoot the intended target, enabling the contraversively deviated eye to fixate the target. Once fixation has occurred, the head rotates back to bring the eyes into the straight-ahead position. This may be familial. CNS defects such as porencephaly and hypoplasia of the corpus callosum and cerebrum may be associated. Occasionally a brain stem lesion may mimic this.

C. Opsoclonus consists of rapid, involuntary, chaotic, repetitive, unpredictable conjugate saccadic eye movements in all directions which persists during sleep. Most commonly it is seen with myoclonic encephalitis or neuroblastoma. Rarely it is secondary to drugs.

D. In ocular bobbing the eyes repeatedly move downward from the primary position and remain for a few seconds, then drift back. It is readily distinguished from downbeat nystagmus. The jerks may be disconjugate in the two eyes, and the eyes often remain deviated for several seconds. It is indicative of a brain stem dysfunction.

E. Ocular dysmetria is manifested by either a binocular conjugate undershooting or overshooting of saccades followed by a to-and-fro saccadic oscillation. It is secondary to a cerebellar dysfunction.

F. Ocular myoclonus is a continuous, usually to-and-fro, pendular oscillation occurring with synchronous movements of the face, palate, or extremity. These usually indicate damage in the myoclonic triangle formed by the ipsilateral red nucleus, inferior olivary nucleus, and contralateral dentate nucleus of the cerebellum and their interconnecting fiber tracts.

References

Cogan DG. Ocular dysmetria, flutter like oscillations of the eyes, and opsoclonus. Arch Ophthalmol 1954; 51:318.

Hoyt CS. Neonatal opsoclonus. J Pediatr Ophthalmol 1977; 14:274.

Susac JO, Hoyt WF, Daroff RB, Lawrence W. Clinical spectrum of ocular bobbing. J Neurol Neurosurg Psychiatry 1977; 33:771.

Nakada T, Kwee IL. Oculopalatal myoclonus. Brain 1986; 109:431.

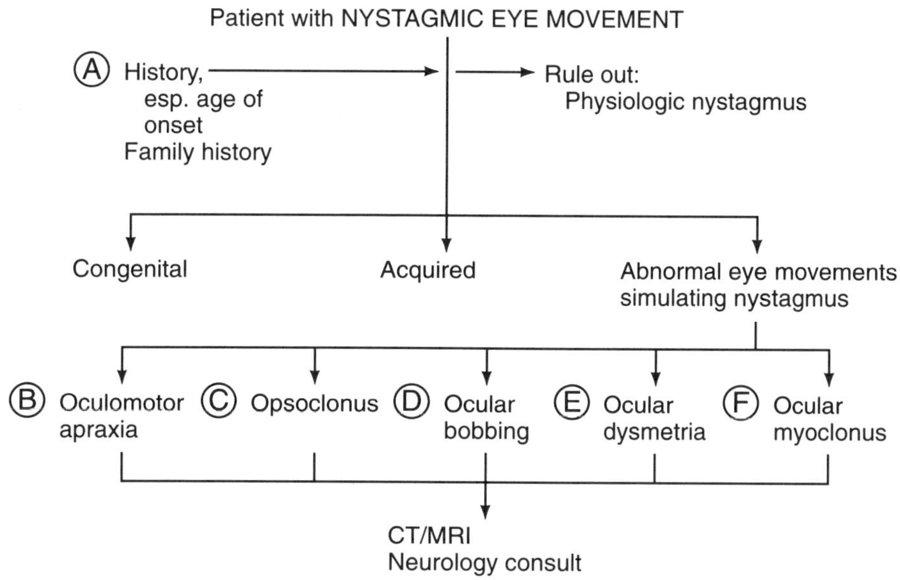

Patient with NYSTAGMIC EYE MOVEMENT
Ⓐ History, esp. age of onset
Family history
Rule out:
Physiologic nystagmus
Congenital
Acquired
Abnormal eye movements simulating nystagmus
Ⓑ Oculomotor apraxia
Ⓒ Opsoclonus
Ⓓ Ocular bobbing
Ⓔ Ocular dysmetria
Ⓕ Ocular myoclonus
CT/MRI
Neurology consult

ACQUIRED NYSTAGMUS

Merrill L. Stass-Isern M.D.

A. Acquired nystagmus is classified as any nystagmus appearing beyond 4 months of age. The birth history is important. The child's development as well as past illnesses, surgeries, or medications need to be reviewed. A family history of any eye disorders must be obtained. The form of nystagmus, presence of vision, pupillary responses, optokinetic nystagmus (OKN), and ophthalmoscopy are next.

B. Unilateral or asymmetric nystagmus may be associated with congenital sensory or motor nystagmus. If the onset occurred after 4 months of age, however, one must consider other causes. A complete ocular examination and CT or MR scanning should be performed.

C. Occasionally a child with uniocular poor vision secondary to an acquired structural abnormality has monocular nystagmus—that is, vitreous hemorrhage—long standing from child abuse; cicatricial retinopathy of prematurity, and so forth. If no structural ocular problems are found, one must consider chiasmal or parachiasmal pathology, usually optic nerve or chiasmal gliomas. The afferent visual pathway needs to be carefully evaluated. Many times afferent pupillary defects or optic nerve abnormalities accompany these problems.

D. Once an ocular examination and CT or MR scan are found to be normal, electroretinography (ERG) is performed to eliminate a sensory visual defect.

E. Visual sensory defects that have been found to produce asymmetric nystagmus include rod monochromatism, cone dystrophy, and any other generalized disorder of the rods and cones. Appropriate treatment and genetic counseling are in order.

F. Spasmus nutans is a diagnosis of exclusion. It should be reserved for those children who present with:
   1. Acquired small-amplitude, rapid, horizontal nystagmus, monocular or asymmetric in nature.
   2. Head nodding.
   3. Anomalous head positions.
   4. Normal ocular examination not suggestive of any type of neurologic or ocular cause for the underlying symptoms.
   5. A normal ERG.
   6. Appearance by 12 months of age and resolution by age 36 months. If symptoms persist past this, a visual sensory disorder or intracranial abnormality should be suspected.

G. Vestibular nystagmus is secondary to dysfunction of the vestibular end-organ, nerve, or nuclear complex within the brain stem. Vertigo usually co-exists. End-organ causes include labyrinthitis, Meniere's syndrome, vascular disorders, and trauma. Nuclear causes include brain stem lesions such as neoplasms and demyelinating disorders.

H. Periodic alternating nystagmus (PAN) is a condition in which the horizontal nystagmus periodically changes direction. PAN may be congenital or acquired. The congenital variety can be seen with albinism. Numerous conditions have been associated with PAN, including CNS trauma, vascular problems, encephalitis, posterior fossa tumors, drugs. However, particular attention should be paid to abnormalities of the craniocervical junction.

I. Downbeat nystagmus is nystagmus in the primary position with the fast phase beating downward. This type of nystagmus is suggestive of a disorder in the craniocervical junction such as Arnold-Chiari malformation or spinocerebellar degeneration.

J. Upbeat nystagmus is usually indicative of a structural disease. Brain stem pathology is common.

K. When nystagmus is conjugate, both eyes moving in the same direction, drugs are the most common cause, especially sedatives, anticonvulsants, and barbiturates. If there is no drug history, look at the cerebellum.

L. With dissociated nystagmus, the eyes move in opposite directions. It usually implies a posterior fossa lesion.

References

Antony JH, Ouvrier RA, Wise G. Spasmus nutans. A mistaken identity. Arch Neurol 1980; 37:373.

Bogousslavsdy J, Regli F, Hungerbuler JP. Downbeat nystagmus. Neuroophthalmology 1980; 1:137.

Cogan DG. Dissociated nystagmus with lesions in the posterior fossa. Arch Ophthalmol 1963; 70:361.

Dehaene I, Van Zandijcke M. See-saw jerk nystagmus. Neuroophthalmology 1984; 4:261.

King RA, Nelson LB, Wagner RS. Spasmus nutans: A benign clinical entity? Arch Ophthalmol 1986; 104:1501.

Lavery MA, O'Neill JF, Chu FC, Martyn LJ. Acquired nystagmus in early childhood: A presenting sign of intracranial tumor. Ophthalmology 1984; 91:425.

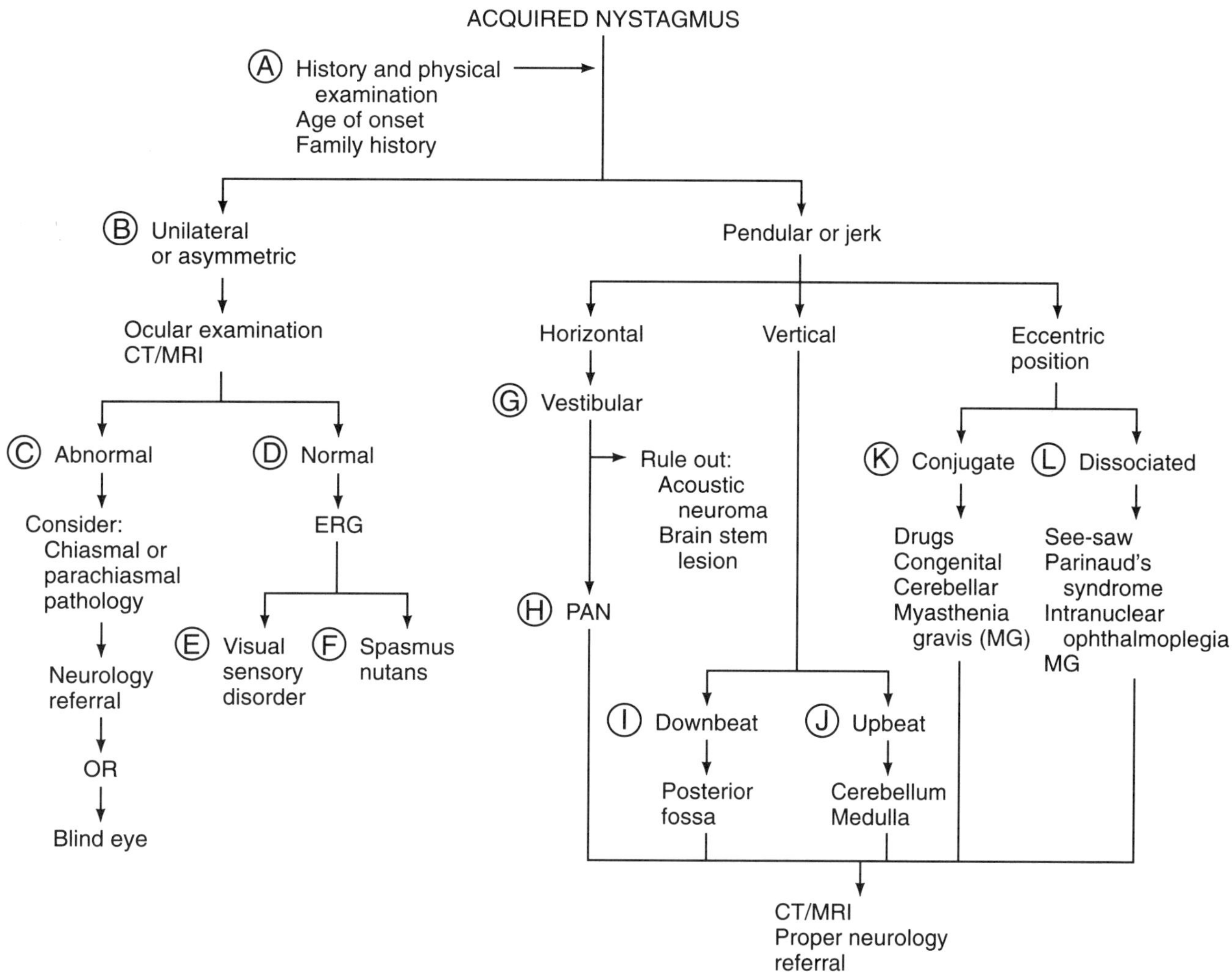
ACQUIRED NYSTAGMUS
(A) History and physical examination
Age of onset
Family history
(B) Unilateral or asymmetric
Ocular examination
CT/MRI
(C) Abnormal
Consider:
Chiasmal or parachiasmal pathology
Neurology referral
OR
Blind eye
(D) Normal
ERG
(E) Visual sensory disorder
(F) Spasmus nutans
Pendular or jerk
Horizontal
(G) Vestibular
Rule out:
Acoustic neuroma
Brain stem lesion
(H) PAN
Vertical
(I) Downbeat
Posterior fossa
(J) Upbeat
Cerebellum
Medulla
Eccentric position
(K) Conjugate
Drugs
Congenital
Cerebellar
Myasthenia gravis (MG)
(L) Dissociated
See-saw
Parinaud's syndrome
Intranuclear ophthalmoplegia
MG
CT/MRI
Proper neurology referral

CONGENITAL NYSTAGMUS

Gerhard W. Cibis, M.D.
Merrill L. Stass-Isern, M.D.

The terminology for nystagmus occurring within the first 6 to 12 months of life is largely misunderstood and confusing. For the purpose of simplification we will divide such nystagmus into the following three main groups:

1. Sensory defect nystagmus (SDN), previously labeled congenital sensory nystagmus, in which there is a proven sensory impairment.
2. Congenital idiopathic nystagmus (CIN), previously labeled congenital motor nystagmus, in which there is no visual or neurologic impairment.
3. Neurologic nystagmus (NN) which is secondary to a neurologic disease.

The distinctions are important as the three have different etiologies, treatments, and prognoses. Latent and manifest latent nystagmus are a subdivision of CIN; slow, pendular nystagmus of the blind is a subgroup of SDN.

A. Evaluation of the infant must be methodical and complete. Inquire about family history of nystagmus or ocular disease. Investigate birth history. Assess development, past illnesses, and surgeries. Check for prescribed and nonprescribed medications. Evaluate the form of the nystagmus, visual acuity, pupillary responses, optokinetic nystagmus stimulation, and ophthalmoscopy. Look for iris transillumination defects, which occur in albinism. Evaluate for strabismus, seen frequently in congenital nystagmus.

B. NN is from central nervous system lesions, including tumors. It may be unilateral or highly asymmetric. Any visual pathway pathology can produce nystagmus. Imaging is mandatory. NN may present as seesaw nystagmus with vertical dissociated eye movement or rotary component (falling eye extorts; rising eye intorts). It usually implies a large congenital tumor such as a craniopharyngioma or glioma. Nystagmus beating downward in the primary position suggests a disorder of the craniocervical junction, such as Arnold-Chiari malformation. Congenital familial vertical nystagmus is rare.

C. If the ocular examination is normal with normal-appearing fundi, a retinal disorder must be eliminated before assuming CIN. Electroretinography (ERG) is mandatory. If ocular examination and ERG are normal, a diagnosis of CIN can be made. If either is abnormal, the assumption is SDN. Imaging is optional with CIN if there are no other neurologic signs and is not needed if the ERG provides the diagnosis. Most patients with CIN obtain the best visual acuity in the null region (decreased oscillations) and this may be associated with a particular gaze or converging angle. With attempted fixation, the nystagmus is usually exaggerated. Inversion of the optokinetic reflex is present in approximately 70% of patients with CIN. For example, when the optokinetic stimulus presented to a patient with CIN, the nystagmus may be opposite in direction from what would be anticipated if the OKN simply summated the ongoing nystagmus. Patients with CIN do not experience oscillopsia, and the nystagmus disappears with sleep. Head oscillations and a superimposed latent component may be present.

D. Children with CIN or SDN develop a head turn to the point of least nystagmus, or null point. This is also true for albinos. If this a significant cosmetic, social, or functional problem (education, driving), a Kestenbaum procedure is recommended. The eyes are moved in the direction of the face turn. This shifts the null position more into a primary position. Face turns tend to develop after 1 year of age as the intellectual interest in smaller detail increases and by 3 years of age are usually prominent, needing surgery. Older patients, either for comfort or because of embarrassment, do not normally adopt the head-turn position unless forced to. Therefore when the patient is reading vision charts, the turn becomes greater as the letters become smaller and it is therefore maximum at the smallest letter size they can read. Yoke prisms shift the image in the direction of the apex of each prism, shifting the null point in the direction of the face turn. Prisms are prescribed base in the direction of the face turn, opposite the direction of the eye shift (null position). Yoke prisms can handle small degrees of turn. Surgery is needed for large head turns. Maximum prisms that are practical are 10 to 12 diopters per eye. Inducing convergence with bilateral base-out prisms or over-minus lenses is of limited help in our experience. Fresnel prisms blur vision, however, and may be useful as a trial.

E. The incidence of SDN to CIN is about 9:1. It is important to search for an underlying sensory defect before labeling a child as CIN as the visual prognosis and genetic counseling differ considerably.

F. Latent nystagmus is not present under binocular viewing conditions but develops in both eyes during

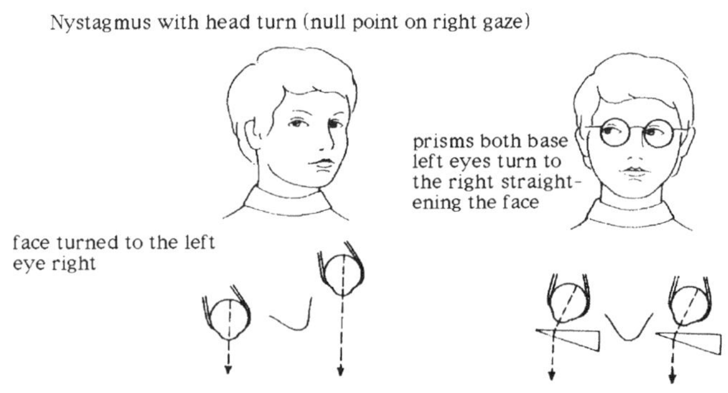

Figure 1 Placement of yoke prisms. In this example, patient's face is left and eyes are right. Base left prisms (direction of face turn) shifts image to apex of prism (patient's right), allowing reduction in face turn.

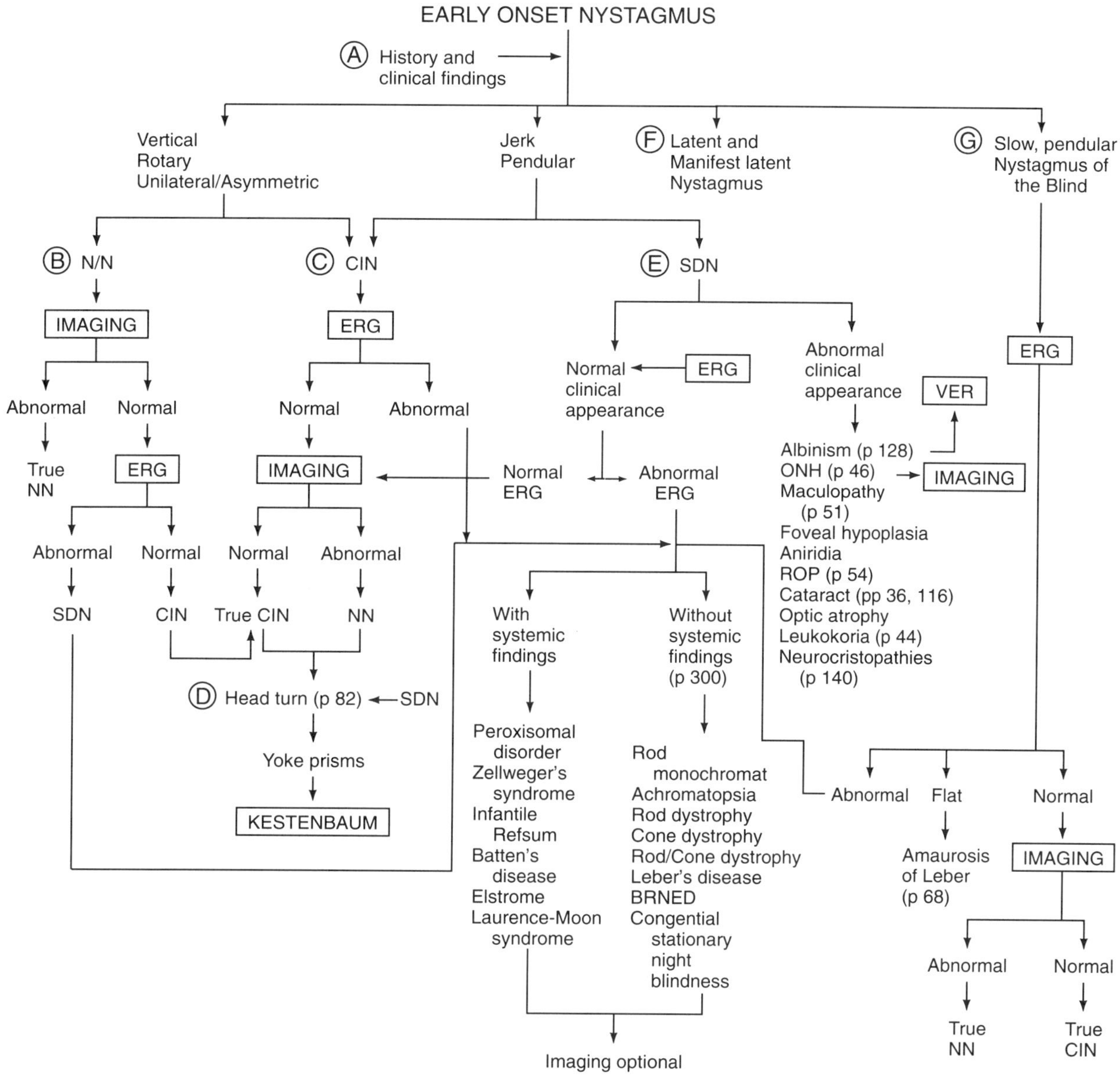

monocular viewing (with either eye covered or blurred or with reducing image brightness). The nystagmus is jerk-like with the fast phase in the direction of the viewing eye. Although a congenital condition, it is usually not seen until a first eye examination or visual screening when monocular vision is tested. Manifest latent nystagmus occurs when nystagmus is present with both eyes open but only when one eye is being used for vision. The nystagmus is jerk type with the fast phase in the direction of the viewing eye. Patients usually have a horizontal tropia and more than 50% also have a hypertropia. The image suppression in the deviating eye is analogous to an occlusion (as in latent nystagmus), causing the nystagmus to manifest. Neither ERG nor imaging study is needed with strabismus associated with latent nystagmus.

G. Nystagmus of the blind is a slow, pendular searching movement. If the ERG is flat, it is amaurosis of Leber. If the ERG is abnormal, the diagnosis is made by the characteristic waveforms. If it is normal, presumably the blindness is cortical (NN) and imaging studies are needed.

References

Casteels I, Harris CM, Shawkat F, Taylor D. Nystagmus in infancy. Brit J Ophthalmol 1992; 76:435.

Daroff RE, Troost BD, Dell'Osso LF. Nystagmus and saccadic intrusions and oscillations. In: Glaser JS, ed. Neuroophthalmology. Hagerstown: Harper and Row, 1990; 325.

Lambert SR, et al. The infant with nystagmus normal appearing fundi but an abnormal ERG. Surv Ophthalmol 1989; 34:73.

Nelson LB, Ervin-Mulvey LD, Calhoun JH, et al. Surgical management of abnormal head position in nystagmus: The augmented modified Kestenbaum procedure. Brit J Ophthalmol 1984; 68:96.

von Noorden GK, Munoz M, Wong SY. Compensatory mechanisms in congenital nystagmus. AJO 1987; 104:387.

TORTICOLLIS

Gerhard W. Cibis, M.D.

A. Torticollis is a head tilt or unnatural position of the head. Ninety percent of pediatric cases are ocular in origin. Only a minority can be ascribed to nonocular causes such as a stiff sternocleidomastoid muscle. A few are skeletal or orthopedic in origin. A careful ophthalmic examination establishing an ocular cause can save the patient unneeded orthopedic surgery and should be done before such surgery in all cases. Torticollis can be neurogenic, caused by irritation of the spinal accessory nerve from tumors. Ocular torticollis serves to compensate for hyperphoria or paresis of one or more of the vertically acting extraocular muscles. These can be congenital or acquired in nature. It is differentiated from nonocular causes by lack of true sternocleidomastoid contracture and signs of hypertropia, torsional strabismus, or abnormal ocular movements. Patching one eye should eliminate the need for a head tilt caused by an ocular problem.

B. Fourth nerve palsy, seen as underaction of the superior oblique, overaction of the antagonist inferior oblique, and hypertropia with torticollis is common congenitally. Birth trauma is thought to be the underlying cause. Torticollis is often the earliest sign. The hypertropia may be small at first but builds with time, so patients do not present until older ages. At that time, review of earlier photos often reveals the congenital nature of the torticollis. Familial superior oblique palsy with torticollis exists. Acquired fourth nerve palsies from trauma occur in children as they do in adults. Surgical correction of one side may unmask a similar problem on the other side. Bilateral but asymmetric fourth nerve palsies can sometimes be recognized by observing the degree of torsion in the fundi. Care should be taken to try to measure a reversal in the hypertropia on extreme side gaze left from right.

With acquired torticollis from trauma, it is best to wait at least 6 months for recovery of the weakened nerve. As long as the torticollis is present there is no danger of amblyopia because the head tilt allows for binocular vision and is adopted to maintain binocularity. Parents should be warned that disappearance of the head tilt may not be a good sign (the patient may be amblyopic and suppressing) and calls for re-examination. Similarly, in congenital cases in which the patient is uncooperative, even though waiting brings no hope of improvement, one can safely wait to better assess motility and make a surgical plan as long as fusion and binocularity are present. We therefore may see a child at 1 year of age but defer surgery for congenital fourth nerve palsy until a more cooperative 3 years of age.

C. The most common cause of head tilt in the pediatric age group is double vertical dissociation (DVD) (see p 234). Usually the tilt is toward the more upward deviating side. DVD is a common component of the infantile esotropia syndrome and may not be clinically apparent until long after the horizontal deviation presents and even after horizontal surgery has been successfully accomplished. Because infantile esotropia is so common, torticollis secondary to DVD associated with infantile esotropia is the most common pediatric cause of head tilt. DVD less commonly is seen as part of exotropia. Anything that prevents binocularity in the first year of life can result in DVD with torticollis. This includes unilateral blindness from whatever cause, cataract and cataract surgery, and strabismic or deprivational amblyopia.

D. Vertical nystagmus, more rare than horizontal, can result in a chin tilt, up or down position, which may be asymmetric, thereby causing a horizontal tilt as well. Therapy is similar to horizontal face turns, namely Kestenbaum procedures to improve the position of the null point.

E. Face turns from classic causes such as nystagmus or horizontal muscle palsies can have a tilt associated with the turn. These need to be differentiated from purely vertical muscle palsies and classic torticollis. *Note:* A mnemonic for remembering how patients tilt their heads:

IS SO
IS = *I*nferior *S*ame
SO = *S*uperior *O*pposite

Reference

Dunn DW, Epstein LG, eds. Torticollis. In: Decision Making in Child Neurology. Toronto, BC Decker, 1987:68.

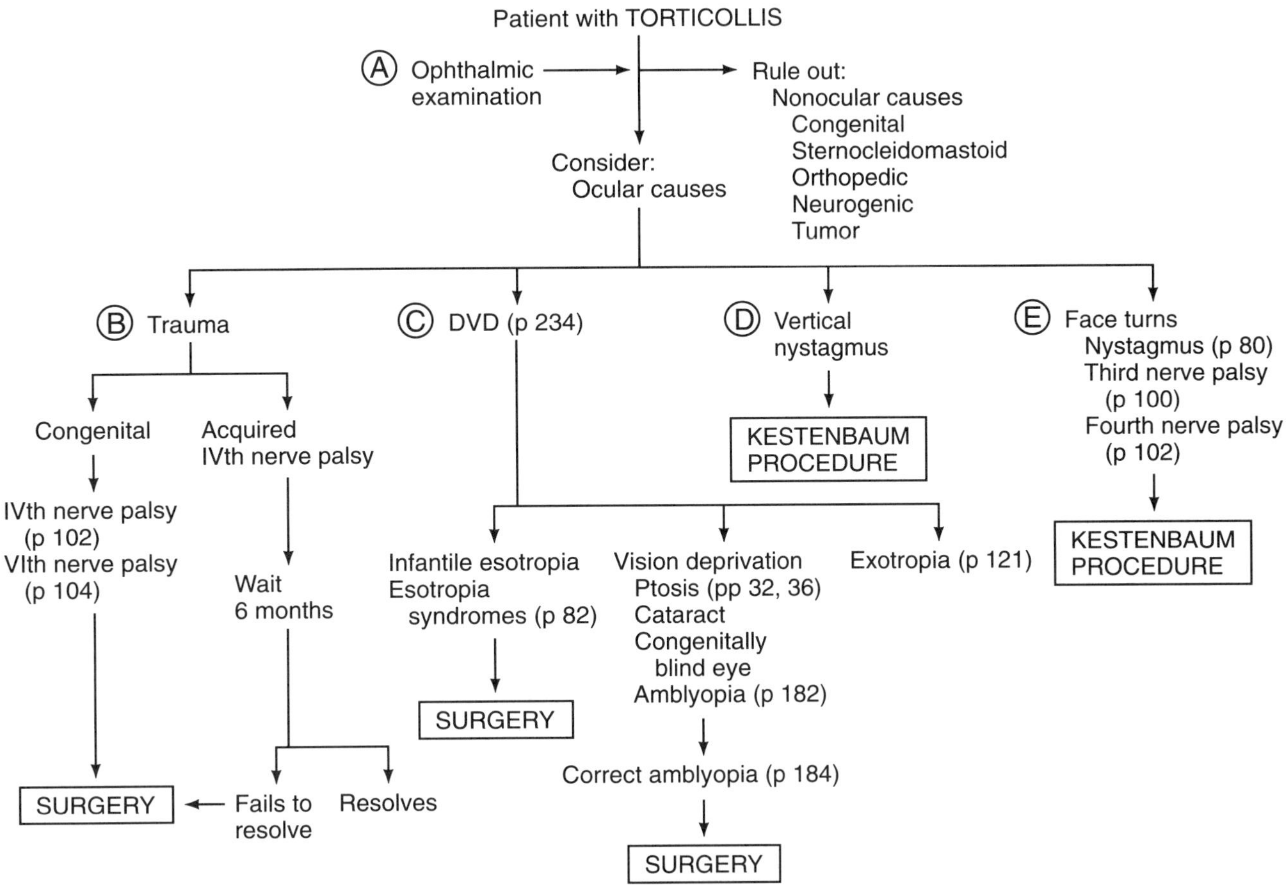
Patient with TORTICOLLIS
Ⓐ Ophthalmic examination
Rule out:
Nonocular causes
Congenital
Sternocleidomastoid
Orthopedic
Neurogenic
Tumor
Consider:
Ocular causes
Ⓑ Trauma
Congenital
IVth nerve palsy (p 102)
VIth nerve palsy (p 104)
Acquired IVth nerve palsy
Wait 6 months
Fails to resolve
Resolves
SURGERY
Ⓒ DVD (p 234)
Infantile esotropia
Esotropia syndromes (p 82)
SURGERY
Vision deprivation
Ptosis (pp 32, 36)
Cataract
Congenitally blind eye
Amblyopia (p 182)
Correct amblyopia (p 184)
SURGERY
Exotropia (p 121)
Ⓓ Vertical nystagmus
KESTENBAUM PROCEDURE
Ⓔ Face turns
Nystagmus (p 80)
Third nerve palsy (p 100)
Fourth nerve palsy (p 102)
KESTENBAUM PROCEDURE

HEAD NODDING OR BOBBING

Merrill L. Stass-Isern, M.D.

A. When taking a history of a child with head nodding, it is particularly important to find out the age of onset, duration, and associated symptoms. If the onset occurred after the age of 12 months through the teen years and was associated with other neurologic, nonocular findings, degenerative diseases, intracranial tumors, and essential tremors should be eliminated. Congenital nystagmus may be associated with head nodding or shaking, as a compensatory response to the nystagmus which improves the visual acuity. Although said to be present at birth, its presence is usually not noticed until several weeks of age. If, however, the age of onset was before age 12 to 18 months but after the neonatal period and associated with ocular findings, one must rule out chiasmal and parachiasmal pathology, visual sensory disorders, and spasmus nutans. Medications at any age may cause a tremor or head nodding, usually associated with systemic findings. Such drugs include phenothiazines, theophylline, amphetamines, and other CNS stimulants. When performing the ocular examination, watch particularly for the presence of nystagmus.

B. If ocular involvement has been eliminated, appropriate neurologic referral is necessary. Neurodegenerative diseases, intracranial tumors, medications, essential tremors, benign childhood tics, and the bobble head doll syndrome should all be considered. Tics usually do not have the repetitive rhythmic quality seen with other neurologic disorders and can be voluntarily suppressed. In the bobble head doll syndrome, there are jerky head movements reminiscent of a doll's head that sets atop a spring. A third ventricular cyst is the most common cause of this syndrome.

C. By far the most commonly encountered ocular finding associated with head nodding is nystagmus (see p 76). It should be classified into jerk or pendular and its amplitude, frequency, and direction recorded. The position of gaze in which the nystagmus occurs should be noted. Head positions, although less common, are another important associated finding with head nodding; position and ability to neutralize the nystagmus (null point) should be noted. Whether the nystagmus is bilateral or unilateral is particularly important in helping to establish this cause.

D. Myoclonus with eye and head movement, although not likely to be confused with head nodding and nystagmus, should be mentioned for the sake of completeness. It is characterized by continuous, rhythmic, to-and-fro pendular oscillation, usually in the vertical plane. Coexisting movements of other nonocular structures, most frequently the soft palate, are what really distinguish this from pendular nystagmus. Isolated palatal myoclonus is actually much more common than the palatal-ocular variety.

E. Many patients with congenital nystagmus report an improvement of vision with head nodding (see p 152). Patients with typical motor defect nystagmus show jerk nystagmus in gaze to either side with the fast component in the direction of gaze. There may be a "null" or neutral point, where the eyes are relatively stable, with the eyes either straight ahead or eccentrically directed (thus giving a head tilt or turn).

The nystagmus of sensory defect is commonly pendular, although it can become more jerk type on gaze to either side. Head turns or tilts and head nodding may also be associated. Congenital ideopathic and sensory defect nystagmus are addressed in other chapters.

F. CT and MRI of the head should be obtained to rule out any intracranial pathology. Special attention should be paid to the chiasm and optic nerves, the most common sites of origin.

G. Electroretinograms (ERG) should be obtained using corneal electrodes and standardized Ganzfeld stimulation.

H. Spasmus nutans is a diagnosis of exclusion. It should be reserved for only those children who present with the following:

1. Acquired small-amplitude, rapid, horizontal nystagmus, monocular or asymmetric in nature
2. Head nodding
3. Anomalous head positions
4. Normal ocular examination not suggestive of any type of neurologic or ocular cause for the underlying symptoms
5. A normal ERG
6. The appearance of symptoms by age 12 months and resolution by age 36 months. If symptoms persist past this, a visual sensory disorder or intracranial abnormality should be suspected.

I. Several visual sensory disorders have been reported to produce a spasmus nutans–like syndrome. Such examples are rod-cone dystrophy and rod monochromatism. Obtaining an ERG is most important because visual sensory disorders are not transient and benign as is spasmus nutans. The expected visual potential and long-term prognosis are distinctly different.

J. Acquired monocular nystagmus—horizontal, vertical, or rotary; asymmetric vision; afferent pupil defects; abnormalities of the optic nerve; any associated systemic neurologic abnormalities; and atypical age of onset are the most common findings mistakenly confused with spasmus nutans. Therefore, any child with any one or all of these findings should be suspected first of having chiasmal or parachiasmal pathology such as glioma or arachnoid cyst.

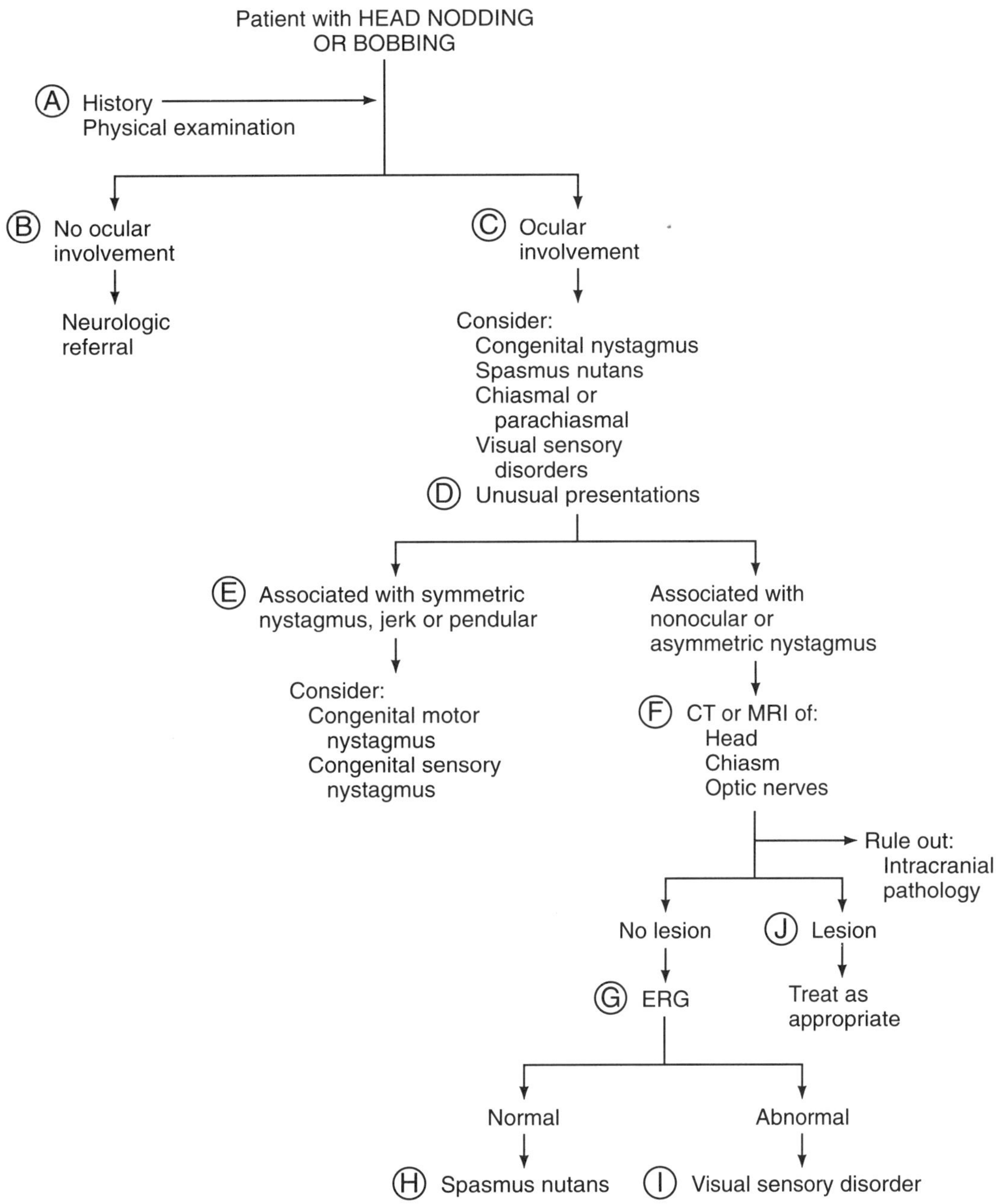

References

Dell'Osso LF, Daroff RB, Troost BT. Nystagmus and saccadic intrusions and oscillations. In: Glaser JS. Neuroophthalmology. Philadelphia: JB Lippincott, 1990:325.

King RA, Nelson LB, Wagner RS. Spasmus nutans: a benign clinical entity? Arch Ophthalmol 1986; 104:1501.

Taylor D. Pediatric ophthalmology. Vol 1. Cambridge: Blackwell Scientific Publications, 1990:612.

PHOTOPHOBIA

Richard W. Hertle, M.D.

A. Photophobia ("fear of light") presents in infancy with behavioral responses such as irritability, frequent eye closure, tearing, blinking, and burying the head. In addition, older children usually complain that the light bothers their eyes. Important aspects of the history include duration of symptoms, any suspected trauma or exposure to environmental toxins, allergens, and medications. Specific questions about coincidental systemic conditions should be asked, because the parents may not think they are related. It is useful to ask specifically when the child appears photophobic. Does he or she play in sunshine, or just complain about certain lights. Some parents bring children in with complaints of photophobia related just to the car seat, to a certain lamp at home, and so forth. What parents may interpret as light sensitivity may not be so. Finally, information about familial eye disease should be obtained, specifically blindness, cataracts, glaucoma, and nystagmus.

B. The age of the patient is very important in the differential diagnosis because congenital and developmental conditions that lead to photophobia are often indicators of severe ocular disease.

C. The ocular examination is the cornerstone of diagnosis. All attempts should be made to evaluate the infant's or child's vision. Fluorescein evaluation of the ocular surface and slit-lamp examination of the anterior segment are integral parts of the evaluation. The lids should be inspected carefully and everted to search for hidden foreign bodies. Office examination also includes a dilated intraocular examination for lens, vitreous, optic nerve, and fundus abnormalities. If there is a suspicion of glaucoma or hereditary eye disease, intraocular pressure measurements and electrophysiologic investigations may be carried out. An examination under anesthesia (EUA) may be needed. Look for microscopic nystagmus, iris transillumination, and pale fundi.

D. During the examination, a broad classification of inflammatory versus noninflammatory ocular disease is considered. This helps in the initial differential diagnosis. Inflammatory conditions are commonly acute and related to trauma or infections. Noninflammatory conditions are more often chronic, congenital, or developmental.

E. Lid abnormalities are readily apparent and inflammatory conditions such as blepharitis or deformities such as trichiasis usually cause photophobia secondary to corneal irritation.

F. Corneal abnormalities represent the most frequent reason for photophobia in infancy and childhood. It is imperative to rule out sight-threatening conditions first. Congenital glaucoma often presents with tearing and photophobia without corneal clouding. Corneal enlargement, raised intraocular pressure, myopia, increased axial length, and an enlarged cup/disc ratio are accompanying signs. Infectious keratitis is characterized by conjunctival hyperemia, corneal edema, infiltration, and fluorescein staining, often accompanied by an anterior chamber reaction and confirmed by microbiologic investigation. Corneal dystrophies, inflammatory noninfectious keratitis, abrasions, and foreign bodies are also evaluated with these techniques. Treatment of these disorders is specifically related to the diagnosis.

G. Iridocyclitis is often asymptomatic in childhood but may also present with pain, photophobia, and conjunctival hyperemia. This is the case with the seronegative spondyloarthropathies, herpetic eye disease, and vasculitides. A partial cataract or subluxed lens may cause photophobia secondary to diffraction and edge glare. These lens abnormalities may be related to systemic diseases. These disorders are treated with anti-inflammatory agents and surgery.

H. Some noninflammatory posterior segment diseases such as cone dystrophies and albinism may cause photophobia. Electrophysiology is valuable in making these diagnoses (see p 294). Inflammatory posterior segment disease is important because it usually represents an ocular manifestation of a systemic disease. Any posterior segment inflammation should alert the ophthalmologist to begin a systemic evaluation, including pediatric referral.

I. Strabismus, particularly intermittent exotropia, may be responsible for frequent eye closure (see p 228) simulating photophobia. This is diagnosed by ocular motility examination. Unfortunately this does not always disappear with treatment of the exotropia.

J. Systemic conditions such as meningitis and encephalitis may demonstrate photophobia without ocular abnormalities. These can be recognized by their associated systemic signs and symptoms. Meningeal irritation, fever, nausea, headache, and mental status changes alert the physician that a more serious condition exists and emergency pediatric referral can be made. Lastly, patients with dry eye and fair-skinned children often complain about light sensitivity in the absence of ocular abnormalities. Some individuals are light sensitive with no abnormalities of the eye or visual system. In some cases light sensitivity improves with age; in others, family history often reveals a parent who is light sensitive.

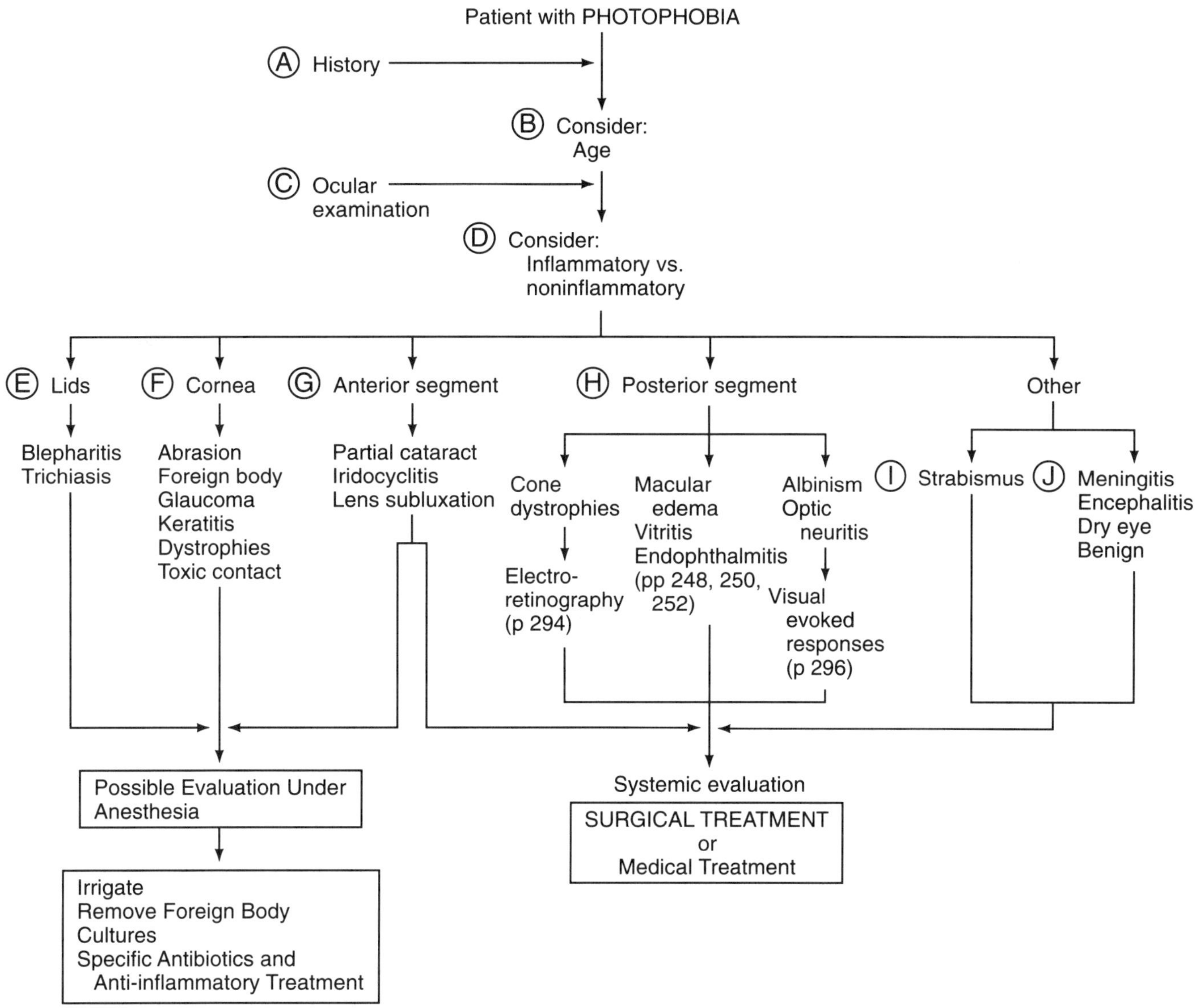

References

Day S. Photophobia. In: Taylor D, ed. Pediatric ophthalmology. Vol 1. Cambridge: Blackwell Scientific Publications, 1990:679.

Morin JD, Coughlin WR. Corneal changes in primary congenital glaucoma. Trans Am Ophthalmol Soc 1980; 78:123.

Omerod LD, Murphree AL, Gomez DS, et al: Microbial keratitis in children. Ophthalmology 1986; 93:449.

Sharpe LT, van Norrend D, Nordby K. Pigment regeneration, visual adaptation and spectral sensitivity in the achromat. Clin Vis Sci 1988; 101:361.

Wang M, Chryssanthou G. Monocular eye closure in intermittent exotropia. Arch Ophthalmol 1988; 106:941.

CLOSING ONE EYE

Eugene M. Helveston, M.D.

A. When a patient presents to the ophthalmologist with one eye closed, the first diagnostic step should be to inspect the lid for swelling, tumor, and levator function and then lift the lid to inspect the eye beneath. This initial step focuses the subsequent examination, which in turn leads to a diagnosis and finally an appropriate treatment program.

B. When the eye is abnormal beneath the closed lid, reflex closure can be inferred.

C. An abnormal cornea can be caused by infection, including epidemic keratoconjunctivitis (EKC), herpes simplex keratitis, and bacterial ulceration. EKC is ordinarily treated symptomatically. Frequent lubricating drops may be useful. Herpes simplex keratitis may be treated by a variety of techniques, including specific antiviral agents, debridement, and in certain cases a combination of antiviral and steroid medication. Bacterial ulcers should be cultured and then treated with frequent instillation of specific concentrated antibiotics.

D. Metabolic corneal disease can manifest with crystals or other deposits that indicate the need for a specific metabolic work-up.

E. Trauma to the cornea can range from superficial corneal erosion to corneal laceration with or without the presence of a foreign body and/or iris prolapse. Corneal abrasions should be treated with antibiotic, analgesic, dilatation, and patching. Foreign bodies should be removed from the cornea and or the cul-de-sac. A corneal laceration should be treated surgically unless it is self-sealing.

F. An abnormal conjunctiva can be the result of conjunctivitis. A purulent discharge suggests a bacterial cause and should be treated with antibiotic after culture if the process is virulent or recurrent. Viral conjunctivitis, often associated with a watery discharge, is treated symptomatically with lubricating drops. Trauma to the conjunctiva is treated by antibiotics, patch, and repair if it is extensive.

G. Anterior chamber abnormalities include anterior uveitis, which is characterized by flare and cell with miosis and ciliary flush. This is treated with topical steroids and cycloplegic drops. Decreased pigment of the iris indicates albinism that may be ocular (in males) or universal, of varying degrees of severity, and occuring with manifest nystagmus. This is treated with dark glasses.

H. If the eye beneath the lid is normal, a determination is made whether the lid closure is voluntary or involuntary. If lid closure is voluntary the patient should be asked about diplopia. If no diplopia is present and the eye beneath is completely normal, idiopathic photophobia may be diagnosed and dark glasses prescribed, but the patient should be observed for pathology not evident at the initial examination.

I. If the patient describes diplopia, it should be determined whether this diplopia is monocular or binocular. Monocular diplopia is tested with pinhole glasses. If the diplopia disappears with the placement of the pinhole, further efforts are made to determine the cause for the diplopia. This may be due to one or more of the following: (1) corneal scar or irregularities, (2) polycoria, (3) reduplication of the lens nucleus, and (4) retinal abnormalities. When possible, the cause for the monocular diplopia is eliminated, but frequently this is not possible.

Binocular diplopia should be evaluated by determining whether fusion potential is present. If the patient is able to demonstrate fusion potential, the strabismus should be carefully measured and the cause determined. The diplopia may be treated with one or more of the following: (1) prism, (2) spectacles, (3) surgery, and (4) oculinum. For a short-term measure, such patients can be patched. If no fusion potential is present, the patient should be treated with occlusion or should be encouraged to suppress the double image.

J. Involuntary lid closure with a normal eye can be subdivided.

K. If the lid is normal the patient may have an intermittent exotropia, closing the eye usually in bright sunlight and out of doors. This can be treated successfully with surgery to align the eyes. If blepharospasm is the cause for the lid closure, oculinum can be successful.

L. If the lid is abnormal, it should be evaluated for levator function. If there is levator insufficiency, differentiation should be made between neural and mechanical causes. A neural deficiency causing complete closure of the eye is treated with a frontalis suspension. Mechanical ptosis can be treated with repair of an aponeurosis dehiscence. Crutch glasses have limited use. Most cases of unilateral ptosis result in incomplete lid closure of one eye but nonetheless require treatment to ensure symmetry and restoration of normal peripheral visual field.

Lid swelling or enlargement should be differentiated between those that are inflamed and those that simply have increased bulk. Inflamed lids causing closure are usually the result of preseptal cellulitis (see p 152). This is treated with specific antibiotic, usually parenterally. Tumors of the lid causing closures, such as would occur with neurofibromatosis, are treated with debulking. Hemangioma is treated with intralesional steroids and observation. Excision or debulking should be reserved for special circumstances.

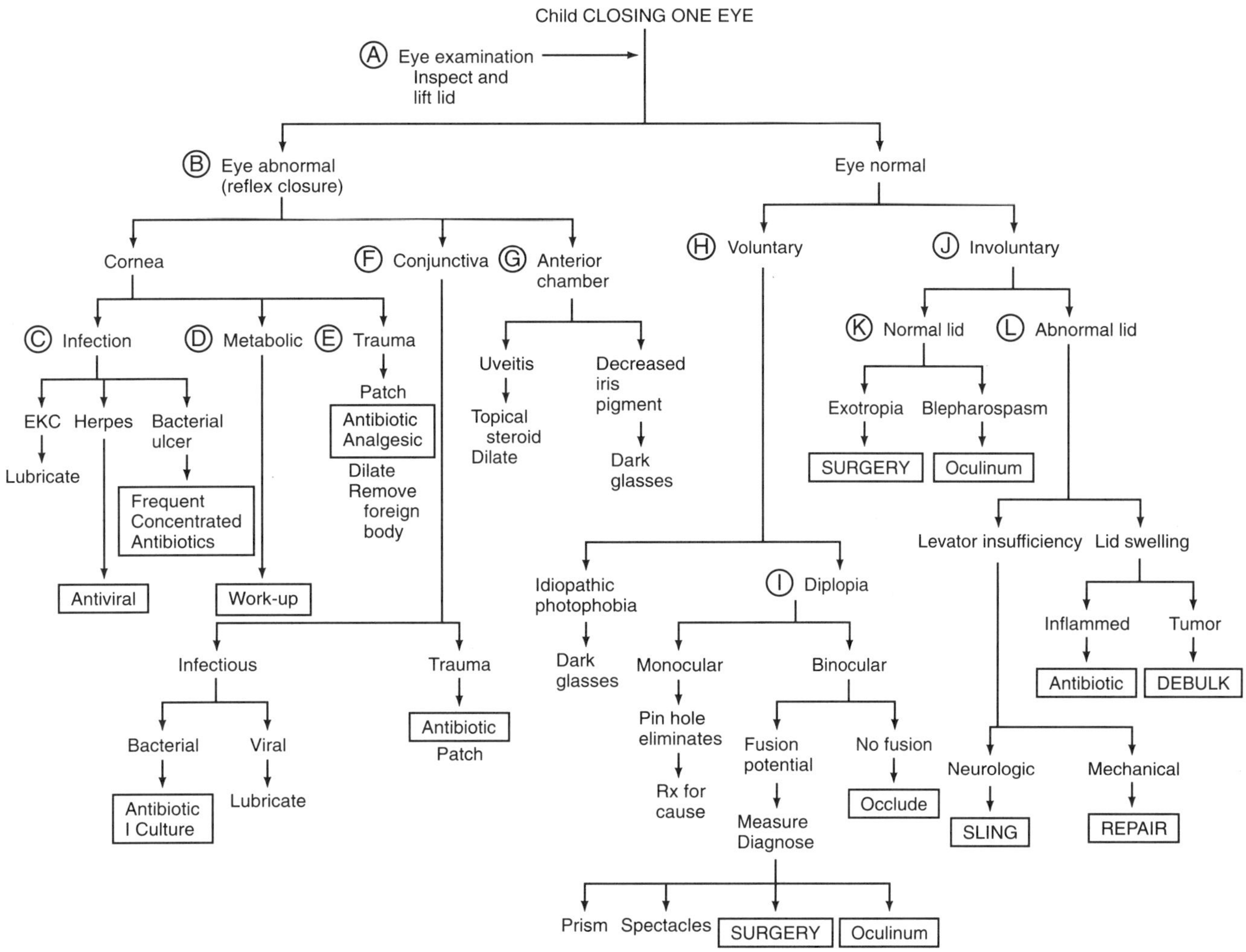

Any time lid closure of one eye occurs in a child in the amblyopia-prone years (approximately under 5 years) measures should be taken to give the eye beneath at least part-time visual stimulation to support proper visual development.

References

Wang FM, Chryssanthou G. Monocular eye closure in intermittent exotropia. Arch Ophthalmol 1988; 106:941.

Wiggens RE, VonNoorden GK. Monocular eye closure in sunlight. Pediatr Ophthalmol Strabismus 1990; 27:16.

ABNORMAL BLINKING

Forrest D. Ellis, M.D.

Blinking is a physiologic phenomenon initiated by inhibition or relaxation of innervation to the levator palpebrae superioris muscles and by contracture of the palpebral portion of the orbicularis oculi, thereby producing closure of the eyelids. Blink reflexes are absent in infancy but develop along with an infant's ability to maintain eyelid opening. Blinking is divided into spontaneous, reflex, and voluntary types. Normal blink rates vary from 12 to 60 per minute. Variation in rate occurs with the level of awareness and with the emotional state of the individual. Increased awareness results in an increase in the spontaneous blink rate as does a heightened emotional state, whereas depressive states cause a decrease in the blink rate. These variations apparently coincide with and reflect the physiologic range of activities of the basal ganglia and the reticular formation. A normal spontaneous blink lasts for about 0.2 second and a normal voluntary blink lasts for about 0.4 second.

A. The blink rate may be too fast or too slow. Patients are more likely to complain about blinking too rapidly rather than the less noticeable slowing of the blink rate, although either condition may be pathologic in origin.

B. Decreased spontaneous blink rates result from overall depression of the CNS, from more specific abnormalities of neural, muscular, or endocrine function such as Parkinson's disease, hyperthyroidism, or myasthenia gravis, reflecting dopamine, cholinergic, adrenergic, or myoneural junction abnormalities.

C. Decreases in reflex blinking are important signs of serious disease processes.

D. Decreased sensitivity of the afferent arms of the blink reflex may reflect decreased sensitivity of cranial nerves I, II, V, and VIII, either focally or secondary to the activity level of the CNS, being globally depressed with increase in comatose or drugged states and regionally or globally depressed by increased intracranial pressure or brain stem lesions. Focal depression of the optic pathways near the superior colliculi may result in loss of the dazzle reflex (lid closure in response to a bright light) and the pupillary light reflexes despite the presence of good vision, indicating a mesencephalic lesion. A decrease in optic nerve function may result in loss of the menace reflex, although blind persons continue to have normal spontaneous blink rates. A decrease in eighth nerve function or brain stem connections results in loss of the startle reflex.

E. Cranial nerve VII, the efferent arm of the blink reflex, may be unable to activate the orbicularis if nerve function is depressed, either focally or globally.

F. Prolonged lid closure must be differentiated from a decrease in the blink rate. Prolonged lid closure generally is voluntary or due to irritability of the seventh cranial nerve. Essential blepharospasm is characterized by episodic uncontrollable lid closure, often with the involvement of other facial muscles (Meige syndrome). Tardive dyskinesia may produce forced lid closure, whereas apraxia may prevent spontaneous lid opening. Voluntary lid closure may be difficult to differentiate from blepharospasm.

G. A pathologic increase in the blink rate may result from stimulation or irritation of the meninges or of cranial nerves I, II, V, VII, or VIII. The more common disorders are those producing irritation of cranial nerve V, such as conjunctival, corneal, or anterior segment irritation or inflammation. Corneal irregularities or opacities may scatter light and produce increased blinking via retinal pathways.

H. The seventh cranial nerve may be irritated at any site but especially in the posterior fossa where hemifacial spasm may be produced. Myokymia is a more localized irritability of the nerve or the orbicularis muscle, often unilateral, which results in a visible contracture of individual muscle bundles, usually beneath the eye. This condition is more likely to be seen in young persons and is not likely to be confused with essential blepharospasm.

I. Structural abnormalities of the eye or deficiencies in pigmentation may result in a high blink rate due to excessive light entering the eye or to scatter of the light. Abnormalities may be subtle or not visible to the examiner, so that tests of function such as color vision or electroretinography (ERG) may be necessary to demonstrate cone dysfunction.

J. Children may develop tics or habit spasms that are annoying to parents and occasion ophthalmologic examination. In the absence of demonstrable abnormalities, the conditions are almost always benign and self-limited. Other more serious but incompletely understood disorders such as Tourette's and Rett's syndrome are characterized by repetitive behavior that often includes frequent blinking.

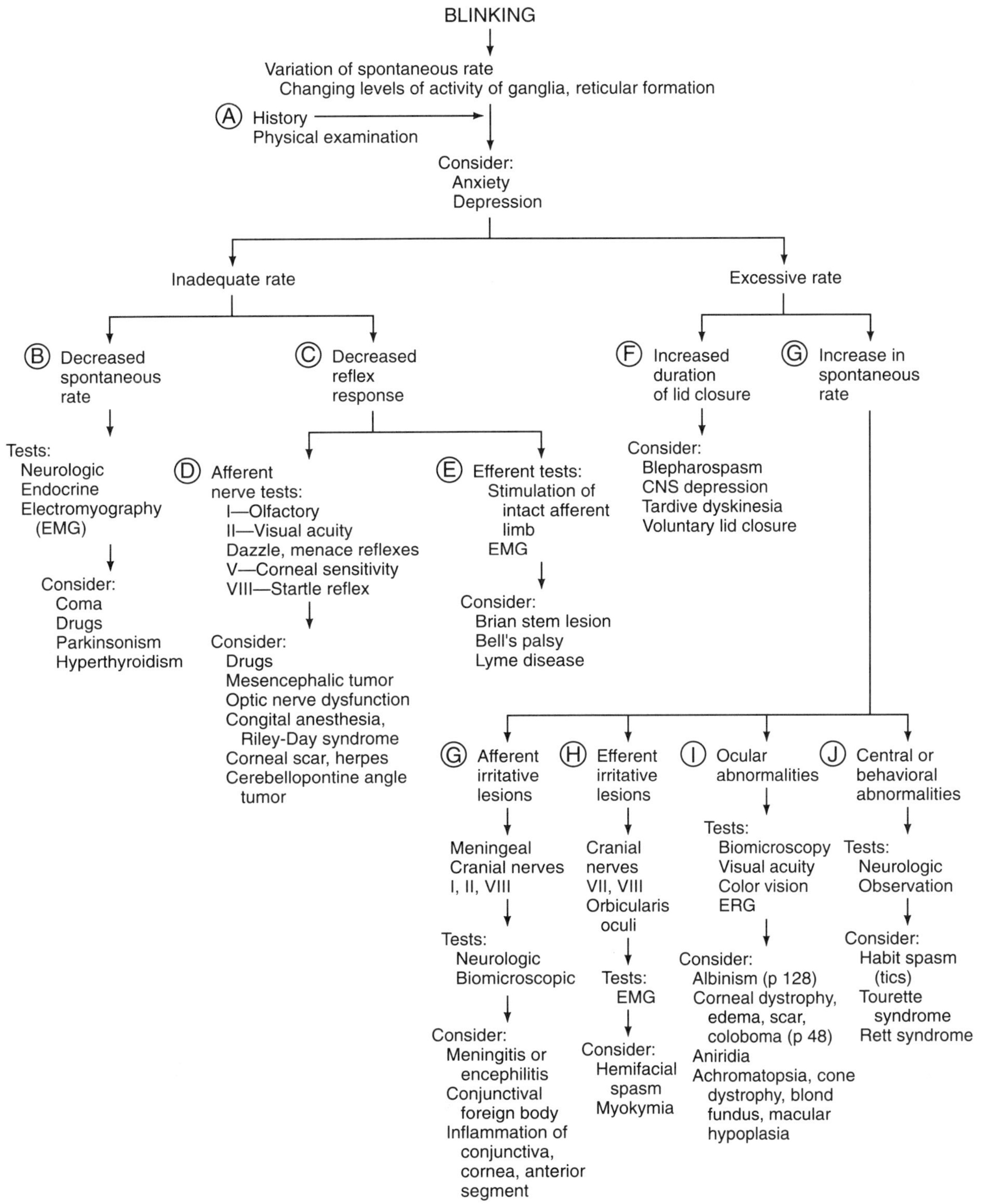

References

Adler FH. Physiology of the eye. St. Louis: CV Mosby, 1965.

Balaban MT, Anthony BJ, Graham FK. Prestimulation effects on blink and cardiac reflexes of 15 month human infants. Dev Psychobiol 1989; 22:115.

Gorke W, Felix S, Severien C. Apparent central facial paralysis in Lyme-borreliosis. Klin Paediatr 1989; 201:467.

Hatanaka T, Yasuhara A, Kobayashi Y. Electoencephalog Clin Neurophysiol 1990; 76:39.

Moller AR, Janetta PJ. Physiological abnormalities in hemifacial spasm studied during microvascular decompression operations. Exp Neurol 1986; 93:584.

Vrabec TR, Levin AV, Nelson LB. Functional blinking in childhood. Pediatrics 1989; 83:967.

Walsh TJ. Neuro-ophthalmology, clinical signs and symptoms. Philadelphia: Lea & Febiger, 1992.

INTRAUTERINE INFECTIONS

Scott R. Lambert, M.D.

A. If an intrauterine infection is suspected, the mother should be asked whether she had a flulike illness or a rash during the pregnancy and whether she has a history of genital herpes. Her rubella antibody status should also be ascertained. Inquiries should also be made into exposure to cats or the ingestion of undercooked meat during pregnancy.

B. Infants with intrauterine infections are generally small for gestational age, with jaundice, hepatosplenomegaly, thrombocytopenia, and anemia. They are also usually delayed developmentally. Intracranial calcification and microcephaly are also commonly present (Fig. 1). A variety of dermatologic abnormalities may be present. Vesicles are frequently present on children with herpes simplex infections. Desquamation of the palms of the hands and soles of feet often occurs in children with congenital syphilis. Hypotropic limbs and cicatricial scarring may occur in children with the congenital varicella syndrome. Hearing loss and cardiac abnormalities commonly occur in children with the congenital rubella syndrome.

C. Ophthalmologists are frequently asked to examine children with suspected intrauterine infections while they are hospitalized. The anterior chamber should be examined whenever possible with a hand-held slit lamp. The corneas should be checked for epithelial defects using fluorescein. The fundi should be examined using ophthalmoscopy. Careful attention must be paid not only to the posterior pole, but also to the periphery.

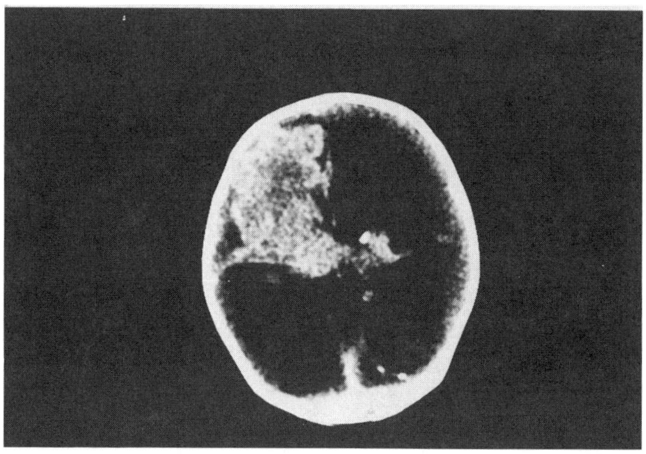

Figure 1 Porencephaly with intracranial calcification in a newborn with the congenital varicella syndrome.

D. Corneal abnormalities may occur in children with both congenital herpes simplex and cytomegalovirus (CMV) infections. Corneal dendrites may be seen in children with congenital herpes simplex infections. Children with congenital CMV infections may have complete opacification of the cornea or central corneal opacities resembling Peters anomaly.

E. Cataracts are frequently present in children with congenital rubella syndrome. Most commonly they consist of opacification of the central nucleus with a surrounding clear zone. Infants with congenital toxoplasmosis and varicella infections may also have cataracts, particularly if there is an underlying vitritis.

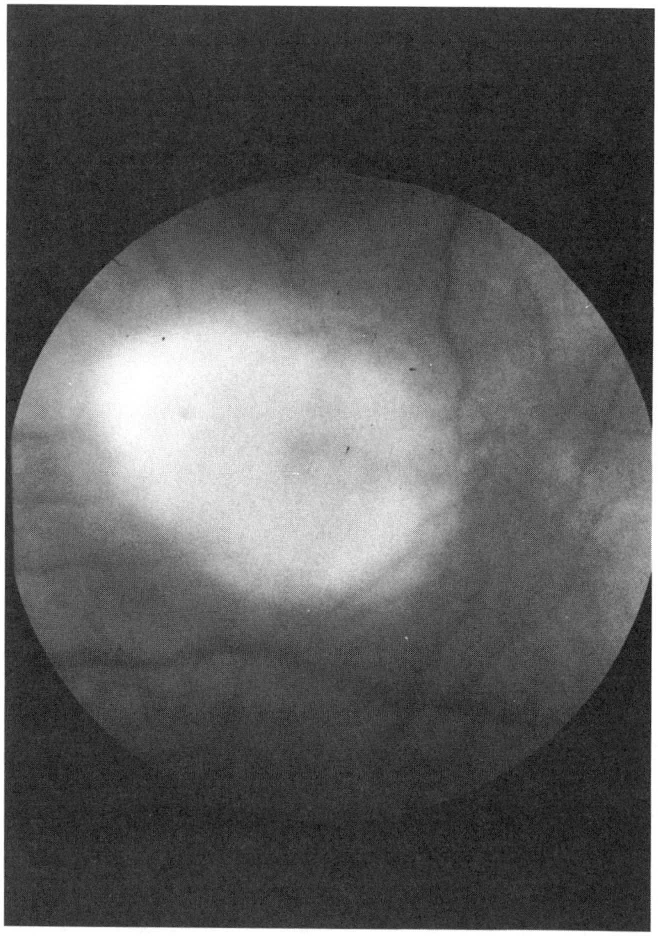

Figure 2 Macular chorioretinitis and vitritis in a newborn infant with congenital toxoplasmosis.

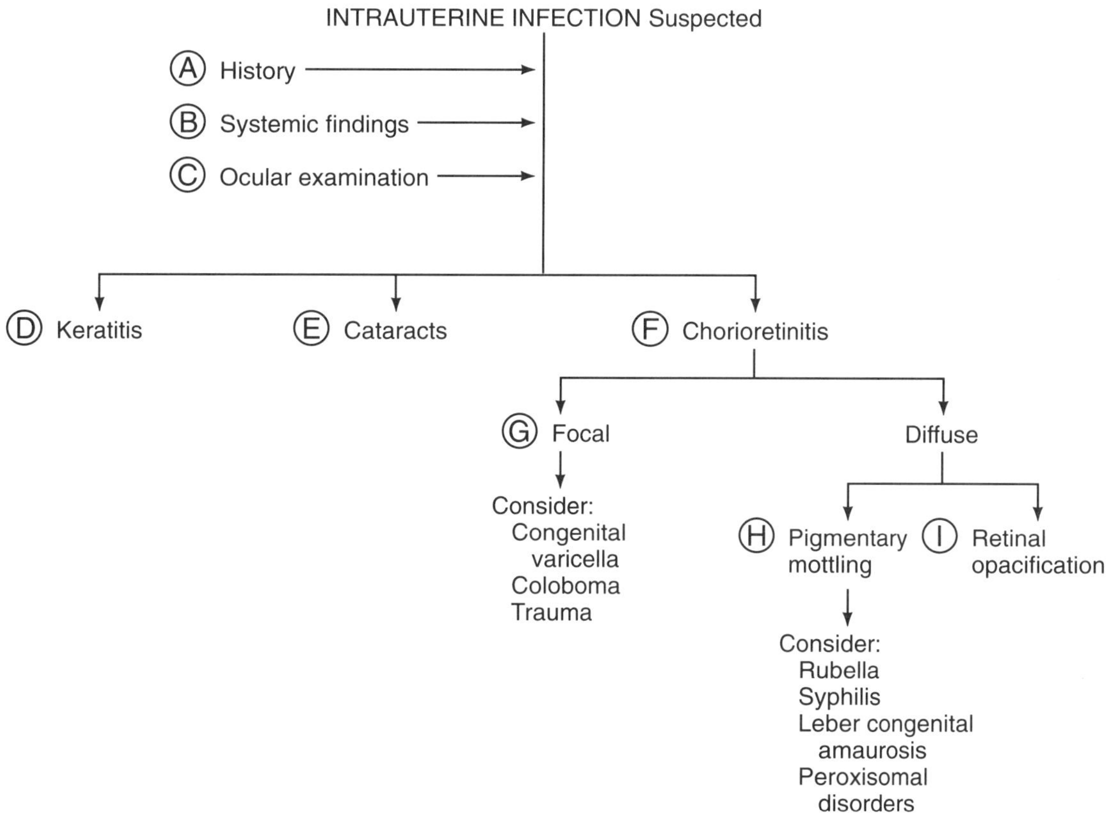

F. Chorioretinitis is one of the most common findings in children with intrauterine infections. It is usually bilateral and may be focal or diffuse. The overlying vitreous may or may not be involved.

G. Focal lesions involving the macula may occur with toxoplasmosis, varicella, or CMV infections. Seventy to 80% of children with congenital toxoplasmosis develop chorioretinitis, but the chorioretinitis is not always present at birth. When present at birth, it frequently has a yellowish appearance (Fig. 2). Over time, the lesions usually become depigmented and develop a surrounding halo of pigmentation. Congenital varicella infections may also be associated with chorioretinitis. The chorioretinal scar is usually more heavily pigmented in children with congenital varicella infections. Chorioretinitis occurs in 5 to 30% of children with clinically apparent CMV infections. In addition to these disorders, one should also consider the possibility that the lesion represents a chorioretinal coloboma. Chorioretinal colobomata (see p 48) are always located in the inferotemporal quadrant. Trauma may also result in focal chorioretinal scars.

H. Diffuse pigmentary mottling may also be seen. This is frequently referred to as a salt-and-pepper retinopathy. It is most commonly seen after intrauterine rubella or syphilis infections. Similar findings may also be seen in children with Leber's congenital amaurosis and peroxisomal disorders.

I. Complete retinal opacification may occur in children with congenital herpes simplex infections. This most commonly occurs in children with CNS involvement. This is frequently a preterminal finding.

References

Cibis GW. Herpes simplex retinitis. In: Blodi FC, ed. Herpes simplex infections of the eye. Edinburgh: Churchill Livingstone, 1984:57.

Koppe JG, Loewer-Sieger DH, DeRoever-Bonnet H. Results of 20-year follow-up of congenital toxoplasmosis. Lancet 1986; 1:254.

Lambert SR, Taylor D, Kriss A, et al. Ocular manifestations of the congenital varicella syndrome. Arch Ophthalmol 1989; 107:52.

Wolff SM. The ocular manifestations of congenital rubella. Trans Am Ophthalmol Soc 1972; 70:577.

FETAL ALCOHOL SYNDROME

Marilyn T. Miller, M.D.

A. A diagnosis of fetal alcohol syndrome (FAS) is not a laboratory diagnosis. It is a combination of physical findings and supportive history of heavy alcohol consumption by the mother during pregnancy. Without both, it remains only a presumptive diagnosis. Most children with FAS are products of clearly alcoholic mothers who consumed 6 or 7 drinks a day during at least the early weeks of pregnancy. An important evolving concept is that some children do not meet the classic FAS criteria but show a variety of types of malformations. Many have fetal alcohol effects (FAE). It has been suggested that binge drinking could result in a wide group of adverse effects, depending on the time of insult and level of alcohol and modified by genetic and environmental factors. However, these children may not show the classic spectrum of anomalies.

Although FAS or FAE may be strongly suspected by the history and physical findings, other evaluations such as chromosome anomalies and radiologic tests, when indicated, may be appropriate if the diagnosis is not clear.

B. The systemic findings most associated with a history of high alcohol intake during gestation are as follows:

1. Growth retardation in both weight and height that persists in the postnatal period.
2. CNS dysfunction, including intellectual defects, microcephaly, and hyperactivity.
3. Characteristic craniofacial anomalies, including telecanthus (increased distance between the medial canthi) with shortened palpebral fissures, flat philtrum (the area between the nose and the lip), short upturned nose, thin vermillion border of the upper lip, epicanthal folds, and ptosis.
4. Additionally, there is an increased frequency of abnormalities of the cardiovascular and urogenital system and other organs.

C. Routine examination reveals most of the reported ocular manifestations of FAS. The external examination should include observations of intercanthal distances, palpebral fissure height and width, and interpupillary distance (corrected for strabismus). Ptosis, a frequent finding, is often unilateral or asymmetric. Another common finding is epicanthal folds. Children with FAS are at a significantly greater risk for strabismus, amblyopia, high refractive errors, and optic nerve disease. Although it is not usually necessary, a sedated examination or examination under anesthesia (EUA) is occasionally appropriate when significant pathologic findings are suspected. This is usually to obtain either the intraocular pressure or to do an adequate evaluation of an abnormal optic nerve.

D. Estimation of visual acuity, which is often decreased, is important. It usually requires methodology appropriate for the retarded child (pp 298, 304). This frequently requires multiple visits, but it is important because these children need special schooling and the degree of visual impairment is important for placement.

E. Strabismus is a common finding in FAS children, with reported frequencies near 50%. The type does not appear remarkable, although comitant esotropia is the most frequently reported form. The treatment follows the usual principles of amblyopia therapy, proper refractive correction, and surgical intervention at a later age, if necessary. Because children with FAS have more associated ocular malformations, such as high refractive errors and optic nerve problems, which may be asymmetric, the treatment of amblyopia is more complex. Refractive errors are not distributed normally. More patients have high myopia or hyperopia, astigmatism, and anisometropia.

F. The most serious and frequent ocular anomaly relates to malformations of the optic nerve. This is usually in the form of hypoplasia but may just be abnormally appearing nerves and vasculature on the disc. Some reduction in visual acuity, although not necessarily profound, usually exists, and some degree of nystagmus with the more serious cases. A common finding—but not one with visual impairment implications—is increased tortuosity of the retinal vessels. Testing of visual evoked potential (VEP) is indicated in the case of suspected or confirmed optic nerve anomaly. It may help in estimating visual prognosis or the need for amblyopia treatment.

G. Anterior segment anomalies have been noted in many children with FAS. The incidence is probably less than 10%. The malformations have ranged from posterior embryotoxon to severe corneal opacification with perforation in the neonatal period. The most typical developmental malformation is the Peters anomaly. The malformation may be unilateral or bilateral, with visual impairment ranging from minimal to severe. Some patients may require corneal transplantation, especially if the anomaly is bilateral. As with other anterior segment anomalies, glaucoma can be present at any time and ocular tension must be monitored (p 120). It is not unusual to see a moderately severe anomaly in one eye and a posterior embryotoxon in the other, supporting the concept of a stepladder distribution of anterior segment anomalies (p 140). One explanation of this severe but infrequent associated finding is that it is due to a binge drinking effect in a very narrow critical time period.

H. Other ophthalmologic problems such as cataracts have been reported to occur in a relatively low incidence in children with FAS, but certainly higher than one would expect in the general population.

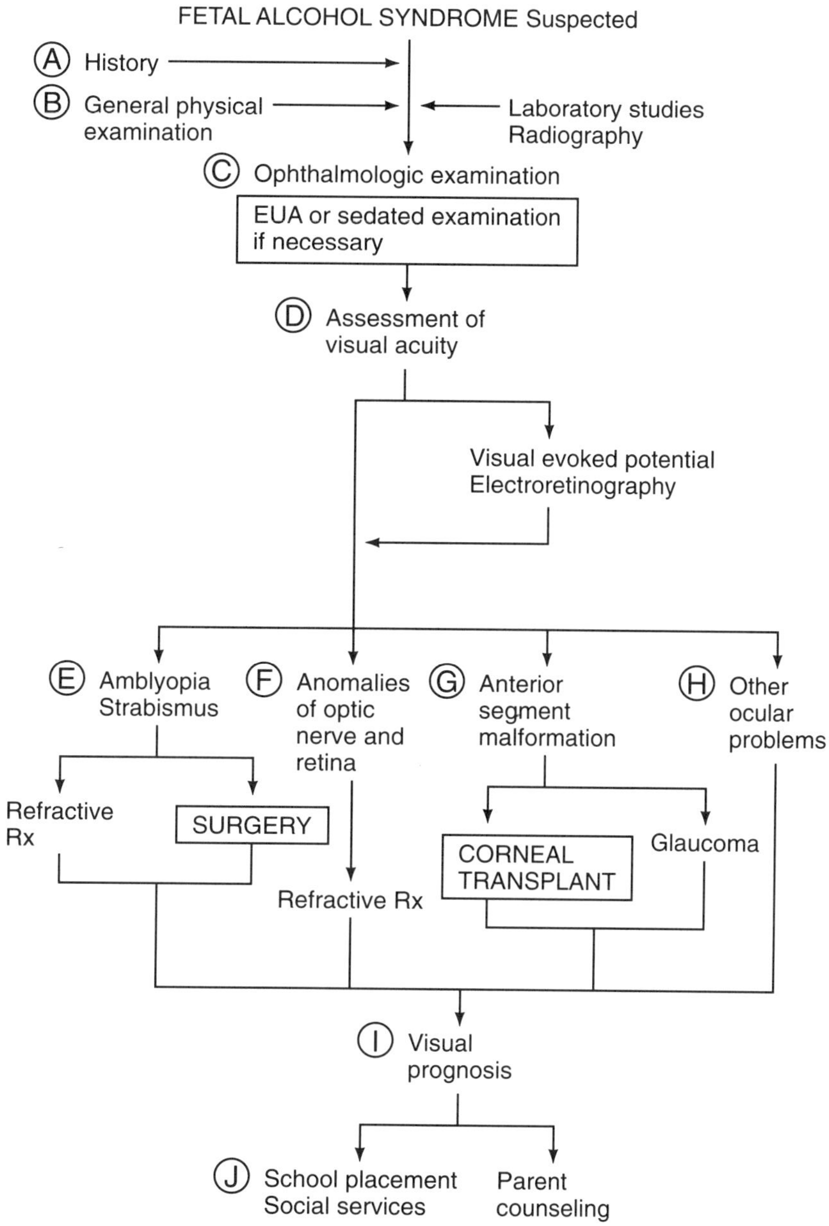

Nystagmus may be present, usually secondary to optic nerve hypoplasia. Ptosis, which is frequently asymmetric, is common and may require cosmetic surgery but is generally not a functional concern.

I. It is the ophthalmologist's responsibility to discuss the child's visual prognosis, and information must be shared with the pediatrician, the family, and the school or social service responsible for the child's education.

J. It is imperative that the families of children with FAS receive support from social services beginning at an early point. These children have special needs and require adjustments in their learning situations. The pediatrician usually arranges this counseling, but the ophthalmologist should share in this responsibility.

References

Clarren SK, Smith DW. The fetal alcohol syndrome. N Engl J Med 1978; 298:1063.

Gorlin RJ, Cohen MM, Levin LS. In: Syndromes of the head and neck. Oxford: Oxford University Press, 1990:16.

Hanson JW, Jones KL, Smith DW. Fetal alcohol syndrome: Experience with 41 patients. JAMA 1976; 235:1485.

Miller M, Israel J, Cuttone J. Fetal alcohol syndrome. J Pediatr Ophthalmol Strabismus 1981; 18:6.

Miller MT, Epstein RJ, Sugar J, et al. Anterior segment anomalies associated with the fetal alcohol syndrome. J Pediatr Ophthalmol Strabismus 1984; 21:8.

Streissugth AP, Dase JM, Clarren SK, et al. Fetal alcohol syndrome in adolescent and adults. JAMA 1991; 265:1961.

Stromland K. Ocular abnormalities in the fetal alcohol syndrome. Acta Ophthalmol 1985; 63:171.

Waring GO, Rodrigues MM, Laibson PR. Anterior chamber cleavage syndrome. A stepladder classification. Surv Ophthalmol 1975; 20:3.

PEDIATRIC HUMAN IMMUNODEFICIENCY VIRUS INFECTION AND OCULAR DISEASE

Andrea R. Sperduto, M.D.
Yvonne J. Bryson, M.D.

Human immunodeficiency virus (HIV) infection is an increasingly important disease entity in children today. Limited information is available about HIV and its relationship to ocular disease. This is particularly true in children, in whom the incidence of ocular disease related to HIV is much less than in adults. HIV infection results in progressive T-cell and B-cell dysfunction, resulting in depressed cellular as well as humoral immunity. T-cell dysfunction is directly related to a progressive decrease in CD4+ T-helper cell numbers. B-cell dysfunction is reflected by both hypergammaglobulinemia and abnormal responses to a variety of antigens. This leads to increased susceptibility to viral, fungal, parasitic, and bacterial systemic and ocular infections.

A. Presence of ocular symptoms such as decreased visual acuity, loss of a visual field, or floaters in an HIV-infected patient is an indication for urgent referral to an ophthalmologist for a complete ophthalmic examination. These symptoms are often difficult to assess in a young child or infant, so one must rely on the presence of systemic manifestations of an opportunistic infection to alert one to the possibility of the presence of ocular disease.

B. The diagnosis of ocular disease is based primarily on clinical observation. Confirmatory evidence can at times be obtained by tissue biopsy, but often this is not possible. Serum titers of various infectious agents have been used as collaborating evidence for diagnosis.

C. Routine periodic eye examinations by an ophthalmologist in pediatric patients with HIV infection is probably not cost effective because the incidence of ocular manifestations is approximately 20%, far less than that found in adults (50 to 73%). It is recommended that ophthalmic screening be performed in all pediatric HIV patients who have (1) symptoms suggesting eye involvement, (2) disseminated opportunistic infections, or (3) encephalopathy.

D. Particular disseminated opportunistic infections are thought to result in ocular disease in children as well as in adults with HIV infection. Ocular toxoplasmosis is thought to result from newly acquired infection or from dissemination of organisms from nonocular sites. The appearance of retinitis with disseminated cytomegalovirus (CMV) infection is more common in children than in adults.

E. Encephalopathy has been reported in children with AIDS in 50 to 90% of cases. In one series it was reported that 50% of children with encephalopathy had positive ocular findings. It therefore seems reasonable to perform ocular examinations on all children with encephalopathy.

F. Cotton wool spots are the most common ocular finding in patients with AIDS. They are found in 25 to 53% of adults and only 8% in children with ocular manifestations. Cotton wool spots are thought to be due to a microvascular infarct of the nerve fiber layer, which leads to edema in the retinal layer without significant loss of visual function in the surrounding retina. Usually these spontaneously regress in 4 to 8 weeks. The cause is unknown. Vision is usually not significantly affected unless a retinal arterial or venous occlusion occurs. These must be differentiated from CMV retinitis, which progresses over 4 to 8 weeks.

G. CMV retinitis is the most common intraocular infection. It has been found in 5% of HIV-infected children, compared with 12 to 26% of adults. Presenting signs and symptoms include floaters, decreased visual acuity, and loss of a visual field. The pathogenesis of CMV retinitis is thought to be a cell-to-cell viral advance across the surface of the retina. Infected retinal cells become edematous and appear white when visualized after edema resolves; the remaining atrophic retina has pigment stippling. Retinal hemorrhages occur frequently. Symptoms are determined by the area of retina that is involved. Peripheral lesions are often asymptomatic except for complaints of floaters due to a vitreitis. Lesions involving the optic nerve or macula result in loss of vision. CMV retinitis is not associated with photophobia, pain, or erythema of the eye. Diagnosis is usually based upon the depressed immune status of the patient and the clinical appearance of the fundus. Disease often progresses to involve both retinas. Although the overall incidence of CMV retinitis in pediatric HIV patients is lower than in adults, the appearance of retinitis in children with disseminated CMV is more frequent than in adults. Ganciclovir is currently being used as the first-line drug for treatment. The usual recommended dosage for patients with normal renal function who are not neutropenic or thrombocytopenic is 5 mg/kg q12h IV for 2 weeks, followed by a lifetime maintenance dose of 5 mg/kg/day IV. A second intravenous drug, foscarnet, is also available for treatment of CMV retinitis and is usually used in ganciclovir-resistant CMV infections.

H. Varicella-zoster (VZV) and herpes simplex (HSV) viruses can infect and destroy retinal tissue, but the disease progression is typically more fulminant and acute than in CMV retinitis. Clinically it can be

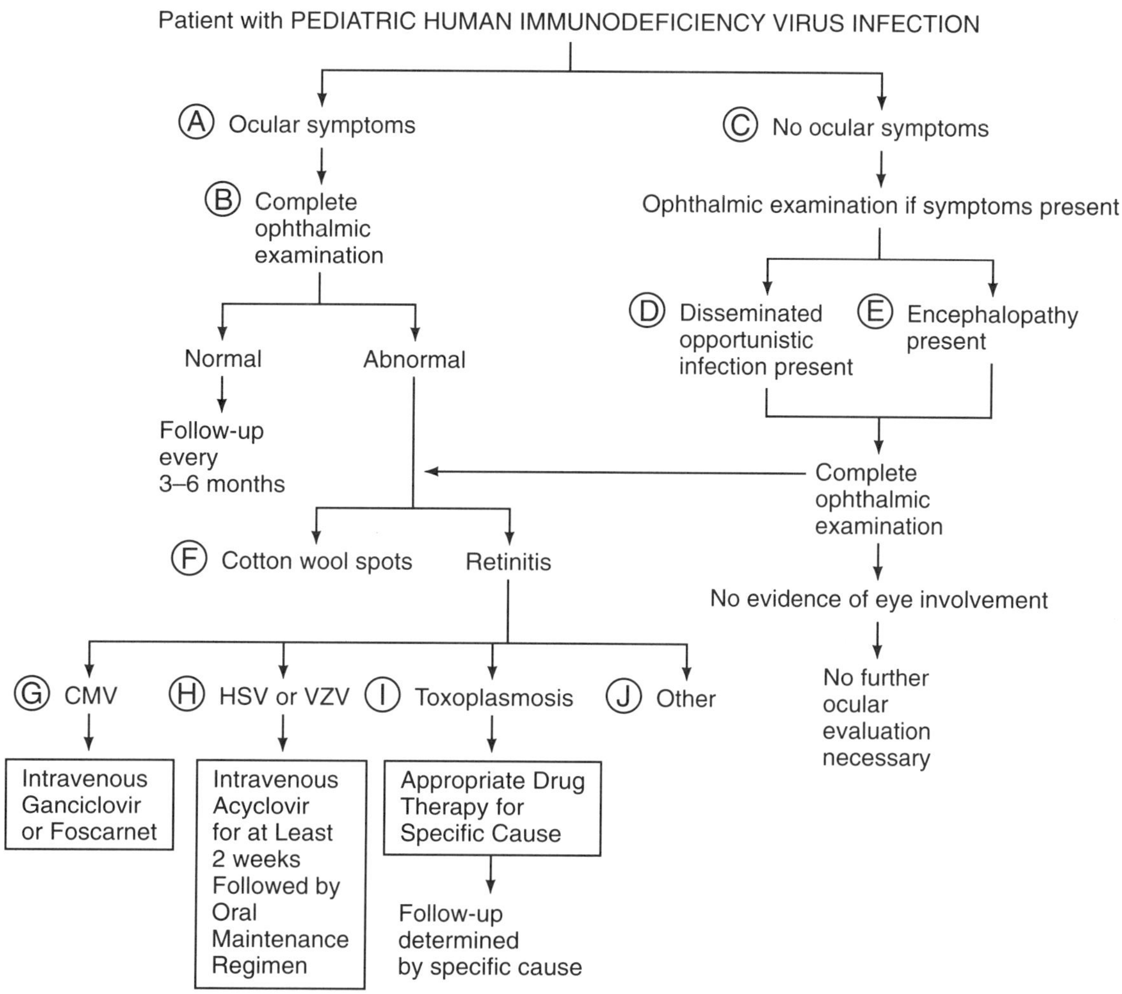

difficult to differentiate these lesions from those of CMV. Diagnosis sometimes requires retinal or vitreous biopsies. Signs and symptoms are the same as those found in CMV retinitis. Treatment of choice is acyclovir intravenously at a dose of 10 mg/kg q8h for HSV and 12.4 mg/kg q8h for VZV for a minimum of 2 weeks, followed by an oral maintenance regimen.

I. Retinochoroiditis due to toxoplasmosis is most typically found in someone with reactivation of *Toxoplasma gondii* cysts following dissemination to the retina. Characteristically, one sees localized retinal necrosis near a chorioretinal pigmented scar. Typically, the vitreous contains more inflammation than is found in CMV retinitis. In addition, retinal hemorrhages are rarely found, in contrast to CMV. Presenting symptoms include complaints of blurred vision and floaters. Treatment involves combination therapy and typically includes pyrimethamine, folinic acid, and sulfadiazine orally, followed by a suppression regimen.

J. Candidal infections of the retina are usually secondary to dissemination. Lesions can be single or multiple and appear fluffy and yellow-white. If left untreated, they enlarge. Candidal endophthalmitis is associated with significant vitreitis but not with retinal hemorrhages. Syphilis can also result in a retinitis. This is associated with an inflammatory reaction of the vitreous in contrast to CMV retinitis. Less commonly, *Cryptococcus, Mycobacterium avium* complex, *Pneumocystis carinii,* and *Mycobacterium tuberculosis* can cause a retinitis.

References

Dennehy PJ, Warman R, Flynn JT, et al. Ocular manifestations in pediatric patients with acquired immunodeficiency syndrome. Arch Ophthalmol 1989; 107:978.

Jabs DA, Enger L, Bartlett JG. Cytomegalovirus retinitis and acquired immunodeficiency syndrome. Arch Ophthalmol 1989; 107:75.

Palestine AG, Bloom JN. The diagnosis of cytomegalovirus retinitis. Ann Intern Med 1988; 109:963.

Palestine AG, de Smet M. Retinitis and ophthalmic problems. In: Pizzo PA, Wilfert CM, eds. Pediatric AIDS, the challenge of HIV infection in infants, children and adolescents. Baltimore: Williams & Wilkins, 1991:336.

Pepose JS, Holland GN, Nestor MS, et al. Acquired immune deficiency syndrome pathogenic mechanisms of ocular disease. Ophthalmology 1985; 92:472.

NEUROLOGIC IMPAIRMENT IN PEDIATRIC OPHTHALMOLOGY

Luis C. F. de Sa, M.D.
William V. Good, M.D.
Creig S. Hoyt, M.D.

A. The brain is vulnerable to a variety of injuries in childhood. Malformations during embryogenesis, infection, trauma, vascular events such as hemorrhage or ischemia, and metabolic derangements are the main causes of brain dysfunction. Clinically, brain dysfunction can manifest as motor impairment or delay in development varying from mild language/hearing disorder to severe mental retardation. *Cerebral palsy* is the term used for patients with a nonprogressive brain dysfunction. This should be termed static encephalopathy and usually is characterized by motor impairment associated with or without intellectual deficit. Brain dysfunction can also present with ocular manifestations including eye movement disorders and/or vision handicap.

B. *Delayed visual maturation* (DVM) is the term used to describe infants who present with poor or no visual responsiveness but whose vision subsequently improves. DVM is classified into four types: Type I—DVM as an isolated defect, Type II—DVM associated with neurodevelopmental abnormalities, Type III—DVM with nystagmus or albinism, and Type IV—DVM associated with serious ocular disease. Vision in these patients starts to improve between 10 and 28 weeks postnatally but can take longer. Generally Type I patients recover normal vision, Type III patient reach the lower end of the acuity range, and Type IV patients do not achieve normal visual acuity. The pathogenesis of DVM is unknown. It is hypothesized that the extrageniculostriate visual system (colliculus-pulvinar-parietal) is abnormal. This visual system is used by neonates and is concerned with detection, location, and orientation responses. When the geniculostriate system (fovea, optic tracts, radiation, and occipital cortex) becomes functional, vision improves in infants with DVM.

C. Cortical blindness refers to visual impairment resulting from injury of the geniculostriate system. The term *cortical visual impairment* (CVI) is preferable because most children have some residual vision. It is manifested clinically by reduced vision, absence of nystagmus (and optokinetic nystagmus), intact pupillary light responses, and normal ocular examination. After cortical injury, most children recover some vision. Neuroradiologic tests can localize the damaged areas. Prognosis for recovery of vision is better if occipital lobes are damaged than if damage occurs to optic radiations. Recently PET (positron emission tomography) and SPECT (single photon emission tomography) scanning have been used in neuropediatrics to evaluate brain areas that appear normal on CT and MR scanning. Visual evoked potential (VEP) has its limitations. Although it can provide information on visual recovery, it may be intact in some cortically blind infants.

D. There are different classes of eye movements: saccades, smooth pursuit, vestibular, optokinetic, vergences, visual fixation, and some forms of nystagmus. Each one has its function, although all these movements are harmonious and coordinate, depending on the environment and visual task. All are generated and regulated by different parts of the brain. Some abnormalities of eye movements are specific and diagnostically localizing. Lesions of the frontal cortex can impair saccades; lesions of the occipital cortex can impair smooth pursuit; brain stem lesions can cause several different eye movement disorders depending on the site of injury (e.g., vertical nystagmus).

E. A complex interaction between sensory and motor eye coordination is controlled by different parts of the brain, permitting ocular alignment. A disruption in this relation causes misalignment of the eyes (i.e., strabismus). Some forms of strabismus are caused by paralysis of the nerves that supply the extraocular muscles (III, IV, and VI). These nerves can be damaged anywhere from nuclei in the brain stem to the peripheral innervation of extraocular muscles.

F. When potential for re-establishment of fusion can be demonstrated, surgery on the extraocular muscles or administration of botulinum toxin is indicated. When the lesion involves the fusion center or the fusion mechanism is disrupted and cosmesis is not of concern, surgery should be avoided. The best treatment to alleviate diplopia is fogging one of the eyes. Surgery is also indicated for cosmetic goals.

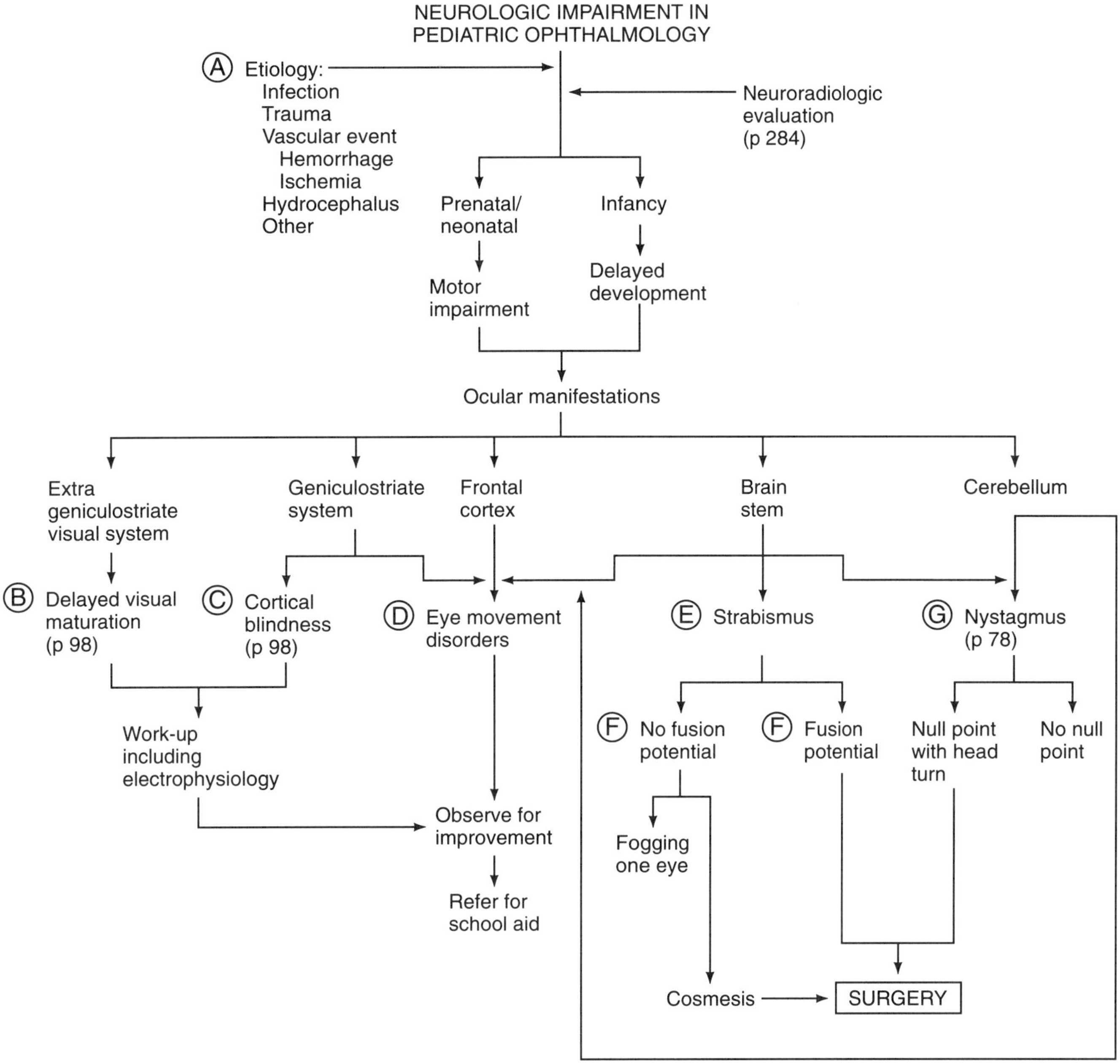

G. Nystagmus is a repetitive oscillation of the eyes that can be present as an initial slow phase followed by a fast phase (jerk nystagmus) or by two phases opposite in direction but equal in velocity (pendular nystagmus). It can be physiologic, as in response to optokinetic and vestibular stimuli or in extreme positions of gaze. A variety of pathologic types of nystagmus occur. Different neurologic regions have been related to these types of nystagmus, including cerebral hemispheres, brain stem, visual pathways, cerebellum, medulla, and neuromuscular junction. Occasionally, patients with nystagmus (usually congenital) present with a head turn that is caused by the presence of a null zone, an area where the frequency and amplitude of nystagmus diminishes and visual acuity improves. In these cases, surgery can be performed to move the null zone and alleviate the head turn.

References

Hoyt CS. Optic nerve and cortical blindness. In: Isemberg SJ, ed. The eye in infancy. Chicago: Year Book, 1989:336.

Leigh RJ, Zee DS. The neurology of eye movements. 2nd ed. Philadelphia: FA Davis, 1991.

Tresidder J, Fielder AR, Nicholson J. Delayed visual maturation: Ophthalmic and neurodevelopmental aspects. Dev Med Child Neurol 1990; 32:872.

THIRD NERVE PALSY

Jonathan M. Holmes, B.M., B.Ch.
Monte A. Del Monte, M.D.

A. Third nerve palsy should be distinguished from a double elevator palsy and inferior rectus fibrosis syndrome. An intact Bell's phenomenon may be elicited in double elevator palsy and is absent in third nerve palsy. Forced ductions are positive in a fibrosis syndrome. Pupillary involvement may also be present in third nerve palsies.

B. Congenital third nerve palsy is the most common form of third nerve palsy in children. It is usually associated with evidence of aberrant regeneration. Amblyopia may occur in the involved or uninvolved eye, and when treating amblyopia, care should be taken to maintain fixation with the nonpalsied eye, because fixation with the palsied eye results in a larger secondary deviation. There may be a history of birth trauma in a child with congenital third nerve palsy, and other neurologic abnormalities, such as paraparesis, may be present. Consultation with a pediatrician or pediatric neurologist should be obtained.

C. Acquired third nerve palsies in childhood are most commonly traumatic. The ophthalmologist should be aware of the possibility of child abuse. Inflammatory causes are often related to an infection such as meningitis, chickenpox, or infectious mononucleosis. Neoplasms are less common; brain stem gliomas usually present with multiple cranial nerve palsies. Other neoplasms may present with isolated third nerve palsy such as sarcomas and lymphomas. Therefore, neuroradiologic studies are recommended. Third nerve palsies may occur in association with headache lasting hours or days, described as ophthalmologic migraine. Cyclic ophthalmoplegia is rare, with cycles lasting 2 to 5 minutes. Aneurysms may cause isolated third nerve palsies in older teenagers and adults; therefore, angiography should be considered. Common adult causes of third nerve palsy such as diabetic microvascular pathology, pituitary adenoma, and metastatic tumors are extremely rare in children.

D. Ptosis repair may be urgently required in young children with severe unilateral or bilateral ptosis to prevent amblyopia. A frontalis sling procedure is usually performed. Attention should be paid to postoperative corneal exposure, particularly because Bell's phenomenon is impaired in third nerve palsy. If aberrant regeneration results in lid elevation on adduction, then resecting the medial rectus and recessing the lateral rectus muscles of the contralateral eye may improve the lid and eye position of the affected eye. The amount of surgery can be evaluated preoperatively by placing prisms over the nonpalsied eye.

E. Although good cosmetic alignment in primary position can be accomplished in most patients, surgery should be undertaken cautiously in patients with complete palsy and good monocular vision, because elevation of the lid and imperfect realignment without useful singular binocular visual field may produce incapacitating diplopia. Preoperative prism adaptation testing (preoperative neutralization of the manifest deviation with Fresnel prisms) at home is helpful in determining the likelihood of patient satisfaction and of elimination of diplopia with surgery. Fortunately, because of the development of suppression, the incidence of diplopia in patients with onset before age 8 years is so small that it need not be a consideration.

F. It is impossible to restore normal ocular motility to the affected eye when there is no recovery, but alignment and fusion in the primary position may be improved, allowing some small area of single binocular visual field. A large recess/resect procedure with vertical (usually upward) transposition of both tendons may result in an acceptable eye position. Transposing the superior oblique tendon, with or without fracturing the trochlea, has been reported to change the superior oblique into an adductor. However, transposing the superior oblique tendon may result in abnormal movements of the eye postoperatively (e.g., elevation or adduction of the eye in attempted down gaze), which may be cosmetically unacceptable compared with the normal movements of the unaffected eye.

References

Harley RD. Paralytic strabismus in children. Etiology, incidence and management of the third, fourth and sixth nerve palsies. Ophthalmology 1980; 87:24.

Miller NR. Solitary oculomotor nerve palsy in childhood. Am J Ophthalmol 1977; 83:106.

O'Donnell FE, Del Monte MA, Guyton DL. Simultaneous correction of blepharoptosis and exotropia by strabismus surgery in aberrant regeneration of the oculomotor nerve: A new simplified ptosis correction for selected cases. Ophthal Surg 1980; 11:695.

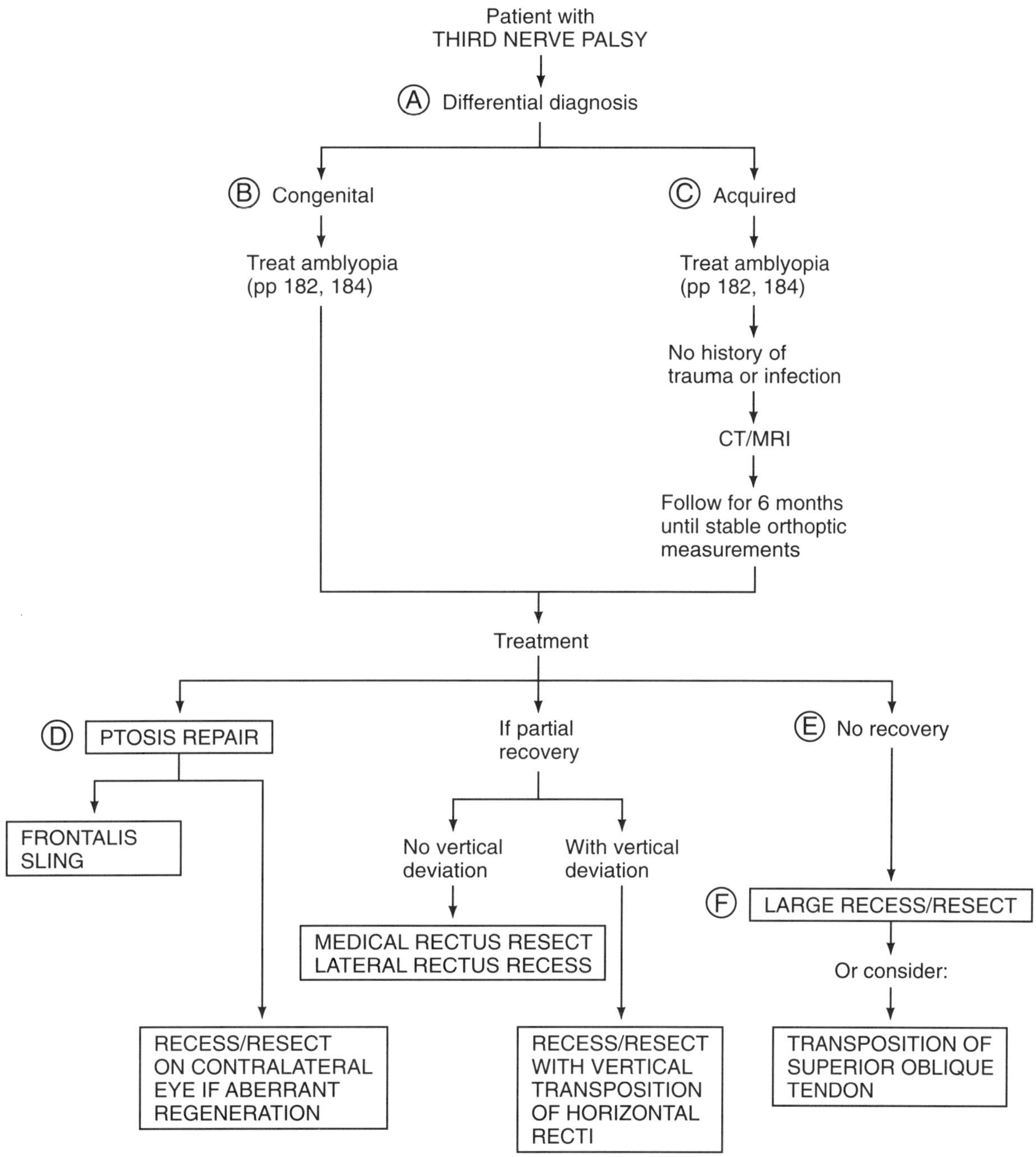
Patient with
THIRD NERVE PALSY
(A) Differential diagnosis
(B) Congenital
(C) Acquired
Treat amblyopia
(pp 182, 184)
Treat amblyopia
(pp 182, 184)
No history of
trauma or infection
CT/MRI
Follow for 6 months
until stable orthoptic
measurements
Treatment
(D) PTOSIS REPAIR
If partial
recovery
(E) No recovery
FRONTALIS
SLING
No vertical
deviation
With vertical
deviation
(F) LARGE RECESS/RESECT
MEDICAL RECTUS RESECT
LATERAL RECTUS RECESS
Or consider:
RECESS/RESECT
ON CONTRALATERAL
EYE IF ABERRANT
REGENERATION
RECESS/RESECT
WITH VERTICAL
TRANSPOSITION
OF HORIZONTAL
RECTI
TRANSPOSITION OF
SUPERIOR OBLIQUE
TENDON

FOURTH NERVE PALSY

Jonathan M. Holmes, B.M., B.Ch.
Monte A. Del Monte, M.D.

A. Congenital fourth nerve palsies usually become apparent when an infant develops sufficient head control to demonstrate a head tilt. Straightening the head from the tilted position usually demonstrates the hyperdeviation of the affected eye. Treatment may be delayed until the infant can be fully evaluated, provided that bifoveal fixation is maintained. However, delaying surgery until late childhood may result in permanent musculoskeletal changes.

B. Acquired fourth nerve palsy in children is most commonly caused by closed head trauma. In these cases bilateral palsies are common. Postinfectious palsies do occur, however. In the absence of a history of trauma or infection, neuroradiologic studies should be performed to rule out posterior fossa tumors. Vascular and diabetic fourth nerve palsies, common in adults, are not found in children.

C. Bilateral fourth nerve palsy should be suspected if there is excyclotropia of more than 10 degrees measured by the double Maddox rod test. The excyclotropia is usually worse in downgaze. Bilateral fourth nerve palsy should also be suspected if there is a V pattern of greater than 20 prism diopters (p.d.), if there is a chin-down position rather than a head tilt, or if there is a reversal of the hyperdeviation in one of the oblique gaze positions.

D. For hyperdeviations of greater than 15 p.d. in primary position, where the hyperdeviation is greater in upgaze or across the entire lateral field, a two-muscle operation is necessary. First an inferior oblique weakening procedure should be performed, then either a contralateral inferior rectus (IR) recession or an ipsilateral superior oblique tuck should be performed. The superior oblique tuck may result in an iatrogenic Brown syndrome and is technically more difficult to perform. The inferior rectus recession is easier to control and in older teenagers may be performed on an adjustable suture. However, a significant head tilt may be better corrected with a superior oblique tuck.

E. The asymmetric bilateral superior oblique palsy may be corrected with a superior oblique (SO) tuck on the hyper deviated side and a Harada-Ito procedure on the other. The Harada-Ito procedure may also be performed on an adjustable suture to tailor the amount of vertical and torsional correction.

References

Price NC, Vickers S, Lee JP, Fells P. The diagnosis and surgical management of acquired bilateral superior oblique palsy. Eye 1987; 78.

Kushner BJ. The diagnosis and treatment of bilateral masked superior oblique palsy. Am J Ophthalmol 1988; 105:186.

Reynolds JD, Biglan AW, Hiles DA. Congenital superior oblique palsy in infants. Arch Ophthalmol 1984; 102:1503.

Scott WE, Kraft SP. Classification and surgical treatment of superior oblique palsy. Trans New Orleans Acad Ophthalmol 1986; 15.

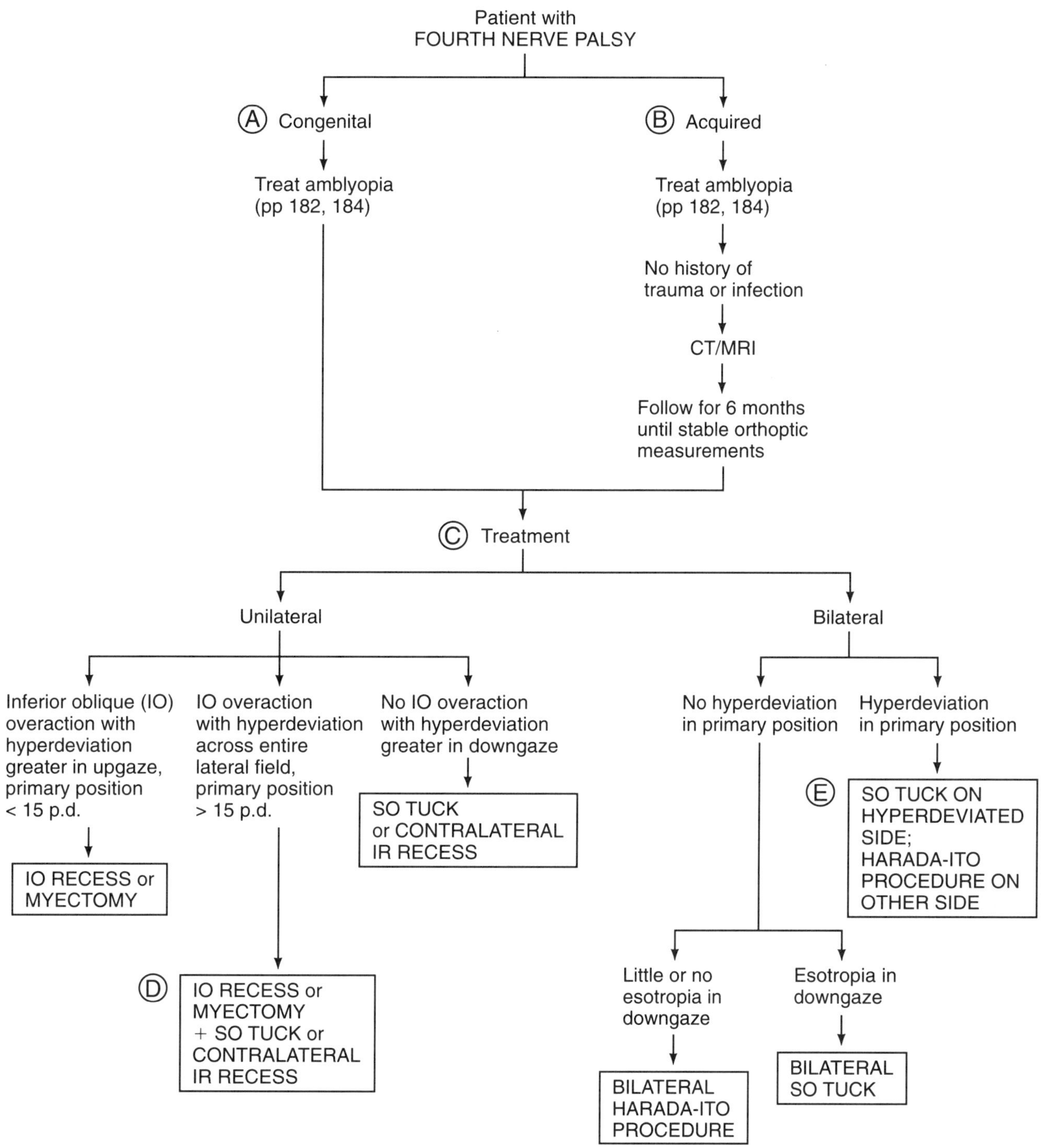
Patient with
FOURTH NERVE PALSY
(A) Congenital
Treat amblyopia
(pp 182, 184)
(B) Acquired
Treat amblyopia
(pp 182, 184)
No history of
trauma or infection
CT/MRI
Follow for 6 months
until stable orthoptic
measurements
(C) Treatment
Unilateral
Inferior oblique (IO)
overaction with
hyperdeviation
greater in upgaze,
primary position
< 15 p.d.
IO RECESS or
MYECTOMY
IO overaction
with hyperdeviation
across entire
lateral field,
primary position
> 15 p.d.
(D)
IO RECESS or
MYECTOMY
+ SO TUCK or
CONTRALATERAL
IR RECESS
No IO overaction
with hyperdeviation
greater in downgaze
SO TUCK
or CONTRALATERAL
IR RECESS
Bilateral
No hyperdeviation
in primary position
Little or no
esotropia in
downgaze
BILATERAL
HARADA-ITO
PROCEDURE
Esotropia in
downgaze
BILATERAL
SO TUCK
Hyperdeviation
in primary position
(E)
SO TUCK ON
HYPERDEVIATED
SIDE;
HARADA-ITO
PROCEDURE ON
OTHER SIDE

SIXTH NERVE PALSY

Jonathan M. Holmes, B.M., B.Ch.
Monte A. Del Monte, M.D.

A. True congenital sixth nerve palsy is rare and should be distinguished from Duane's syndrome Type I (see p 74). Transient unilateral sixth nerve palsy of the newborn is a recognized entity. It is not associated with any neurologic abnormality and usually gradually resolves within the first 3 months of life. Close follow-up is necessary, and if improvement does not occur within 3 months, a CT or MR scan should be performed. Congenital sixth nerve palsy also occurs in the context of the Moebius syndrome.

B. Acquired sixth nerve palsies in children are most commonly benign isolated palsies, usually associated with a preceding infection. These may be recurrent and last from 3 to 12 weeks. However, acquired sixth nerve palsy may be caused by tumor; therefore, "benign isolated sixth nerve palsy" is a diagnosis of exclusion which can be made only after a full neurologic work-up has been completed. Pontine gliomas are the most frequent tumors causing sixth nerve palsy, but there are usually other cranial nerve or brain stem signs at the time of presentation. Other tumors causing sixth nerve palsies in children include astrocytomas, medulloblastomas, and neuroblastomas. Other causes of acquired sixth nerve palsy in childhood include hydrocephalus, traumatic head injury, and inflammatory causes such as meningitis and varicella. Diabetic microvascular and aneurysmal sixth nerve palsies, more common in adults, are extremely rare in children.

C. Determination of the presence or absence of residual lateral rectus function is critical in planning surgery. Partial lateral rectus recovery can be documented by the presence of abduction past the midline, positive active force generation, and normal or nearly normal saccadic velocities on abduction compared with adduction. If residual lateral rectus function is demonstrated, then a recess/resect procedure will be effective; if not, a transposition procedure is required.

D. Some patients with partial lateral rectus recovery demonstrate marked incomitance with increasing esotropia in gaze into the field of action of the palsied lateral rectus. This incomitance can be reduced or eliminated by performing a recess/resect procedure on the palsied eye to correct the primary position deviation and, at the same time (or later), a posterior fixation suture on the yoke medial rectus of the normal eye to progressively weaken it in gaze toward the field of action of the palsied lateral rectus.

E. Transposition procedures include full tendon transfer of the superior and inferior recti to the lateral rectus or the Jensen muscle-splitting procedure. The medial rectus may be recessed at the time of the transposition and immediate postoperative binocularity may be achieved, particularly if adjustable sutures are used. The injection of botulinum toxin into the medial rectus prior to or at the time of surgery may be performed instead of recession, reducing the risk of anterior segment ischemia from a three-muscle operation. However, botulinum completely paralyzes the medial rectus and results in a large postoperative exotropia. This exotropia gradually decreases in amplitude over several months, but the advantage of immediate binocularity is lost. If a three-muscle procedure is performed, then fornix conjunctival incisions should be used, if possible, to maintain the limbal conjunctival circulation and reduce the risk of anterior segment ischemia.

References

Riesner SH, Perlman M, Ben-Tovin N, et al. Transient lateral rectus paresis in the newborn infant. J Pediatr 1971; 78:461.

Rucker CW. The causes of paralysis of the third, fourth and sixth cranial nerves. Am J Ophthalmol 1966; 61:293.

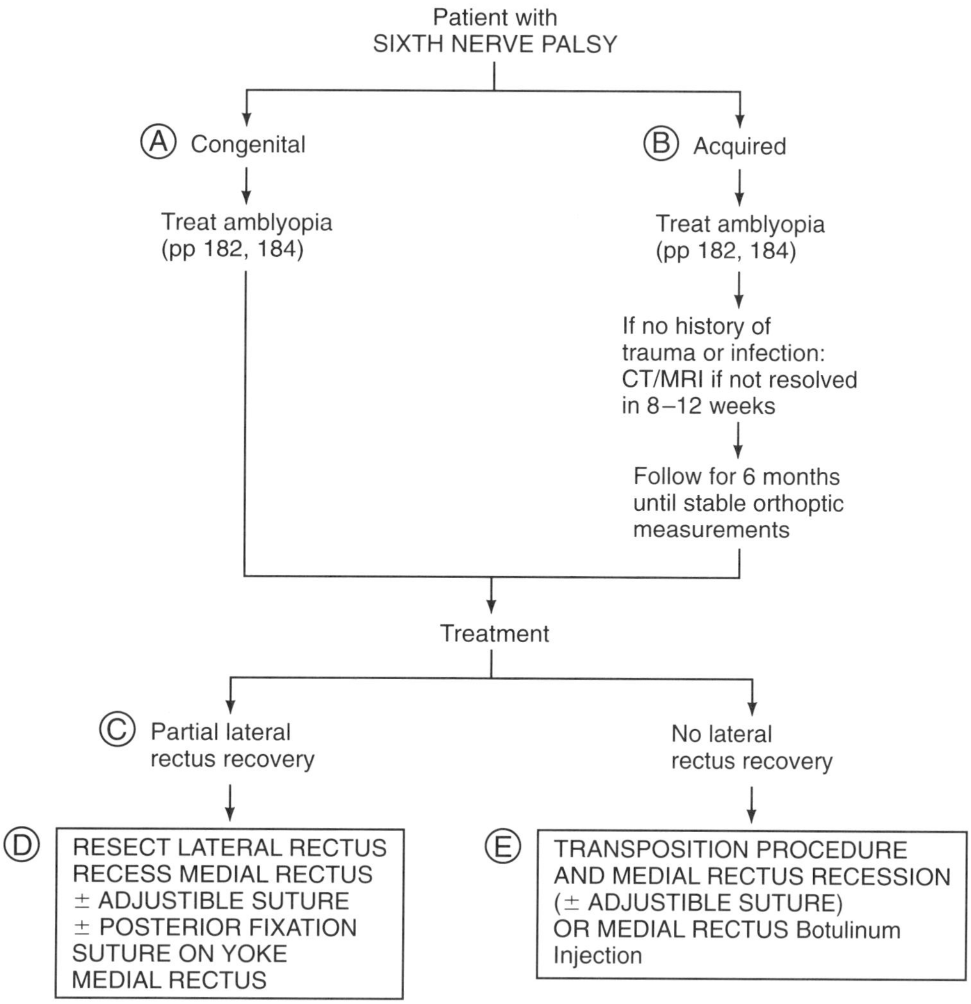
Patient with
SIXTH NERVE PALSY
(A) Congenital
Treat amblyopia
(pp 182, 184)
(B) Acquired
Treat amblyopia
(pp 182, 184)
If no history of
trauma or infection:
CT/MRI if not resolved
in 8–12 weeks
Follow for 6 months
until stable orthoptic
measurements
Treatment
(C) Partial lateral
rectus recovery
No lateral
rectus recovery
(D) RESECT LATERAL RECTUS
RECESS MEDIAL RECTUS
± ADJUSTIBLE SUTURE
± POSTERIOR FIXATION
SUTURE ON YOKE
MEDIAL RECTUS
(E) TRANSPOSITION PROCEDURE
AND MEDIAL RECTUS RECESSION
(± ADJUSTIBLE SUTURE)
OR MEDIAL RECTUS Botulinum
Injection

ACQUIRED VISUAL DEFECTS IN THE OLDER CHILD

J. Raymond Buncic, M.D.

Although older children commonly complain of bilateral decrease in vision if it occurs at least subacutely, chronic progressive visual loss may evolve so gradually that deterioration of visual behavior becomes an early clue, possibly the earliest, that a serious visual problem exists. This behavioral change—"he never used to have problems but now he holds things close, runs into walls, cannot seem to see"—is all the more dramatic when previous vision and eye examinations have been normal. Such a history indicates serious bilateral visual acuity and field loss.

A. The intent of the visual history and ocular examination is to define, first of all, the anatomic level of visual loss (i.e., ocular, retro-ocular, intracranial) before investigating and treating the problem appropriately. Although most serious problems occur on a purely afferent basis, occasionally a recent motor or strabismus disorder can produce significant functional visual difficulty.

B. Each ocular globe requires a complete cycloplegic examination and refraction to ensure the degree of corrected vision and anatomic integrity. The presence of paralytic strabismus can be ascertained by direct observation and prism cover management. Oculomotor instability in the form of nystagmus or dysmetric syndromes may be part of the greater picture involving both the afferent and efferent systems or an isolated problem in itself.

C. When the ocular examination is normal, special attention should be paid to the pupillary reactions. Bilateral anterior afferent loss may produce sluggish pupils with no relative afferent pupillary defect (RAPD). Regardless of the degree of visual loss, a RAPD exists only when the loss is asymmetric. Briskly reactive pupils can be found in cerebral and cortical visual loss or in cases of malingering or nonorganic loss. Sometimes pupillary reactions in a child can be misleading, that is, sluggish because of generalized increase in sympathetic tone, or confusion with the miosis due to convergence.

D. The presence of other signs such as proptosis and strabismus suggest a retrobulbar or orbital problem. Bilateral optic gliomas of the optic nerve or chiasm can produce serious visual loss with little or no optic atrophy at first. Bilateral orbital tumors compressing the optic nerves (e.g., lymphangioma, histiocytosis) are uncommon. Neuroimaging (CT or MR) usually reveals orbital, chiasmal, or retrochiasmal pathology when present. With negative neuroimaging studies, the visual loss should be corroborated with a visual evoked potential (VEP). A normal VEP suggests a nonorganic visual loss; this impression can usually be verified clinically by follow-up examination. In general, follow-up assessments are suggested in these cases to reassure all concerned that no organic problem exists. Retrobulbar neuritis is less common than bilateral papillitis in children but can and does occur. Children's optic neuritis problems tend to respond well to treatment with corticosteroids.

E. Abnormalities of globes (corneal disease, uveitis, glaucoma, cataracts) are readily apparent (see appropriate chapters). Similarly, vitreoretinal disease may be obvious as well clinically, but occasionally early maculopathy and retinal dystrophies require prolonged observation and investigation with fluorescein angiography and electroretinography (ERG) to secure the diagnosis (see appropriate chapter).

F. Optic nerve abnormalities can result from both ocular and retro-ocular disease. Bilateral optic atrophy indicates a slow destructive process. Familial forms of atrophy generally do not produce dramatic behavioral changes, although the visual acuity is sometimes moderately to severely reduced. Compressive lesions of the optic nerve and chiasm should be ruled out completely with neuroimaging and suspicious cases monitored. A CT scan identifies the calcium in craniopharyngiomas in most cases. MRI is superior to CT in showing the full extent of gliomatous involvement of the visual pathways intracranially. Postedema optic atrophy may be the result of any long-standing papilledema (raised intracranial pressure) as with hydrocephalus, brain tumors, and benign intracranial hypertension (BIH). Again, neuroimaging almost always elucidates the cause, although lumbar puncture may be necessary to demonstrate raised intracranial pressure in BIH. The presence of other CNS signs and symptoms may suggest a neurodegenerative disorder, sometimes familial. Postneuritic and post-traumatic optic atrophy rarely pose a diagnostic problem in this age group because the history is usually clear cut. Neurologic consultation is most often indicated in these cases. Disc edema, on the other hand, can represent either a bilateral papillitis or an atrophic form of long-standing papilledema, with bilateral visual loss. Generally, in cases of bilateral optic atrophy or disc edema with visual loss, CT or MRI in consultation with a neurologist is indicated.

G. Uncommonly, confusion, disorientation, and difficulty with gait can arise from acute onset of paralytic strabismus, mimicking to some degree a primary visual afferent problem. Similarly, some forms of acquired coarse nystagmus or dysmetria syndromes (e.g., opsoclonus) can produce similar visual difficulties. Clinical examination should elucidate the role of these factors. Again, neuroimaging and appropriate follow-up with a neurologist are usually indicated.

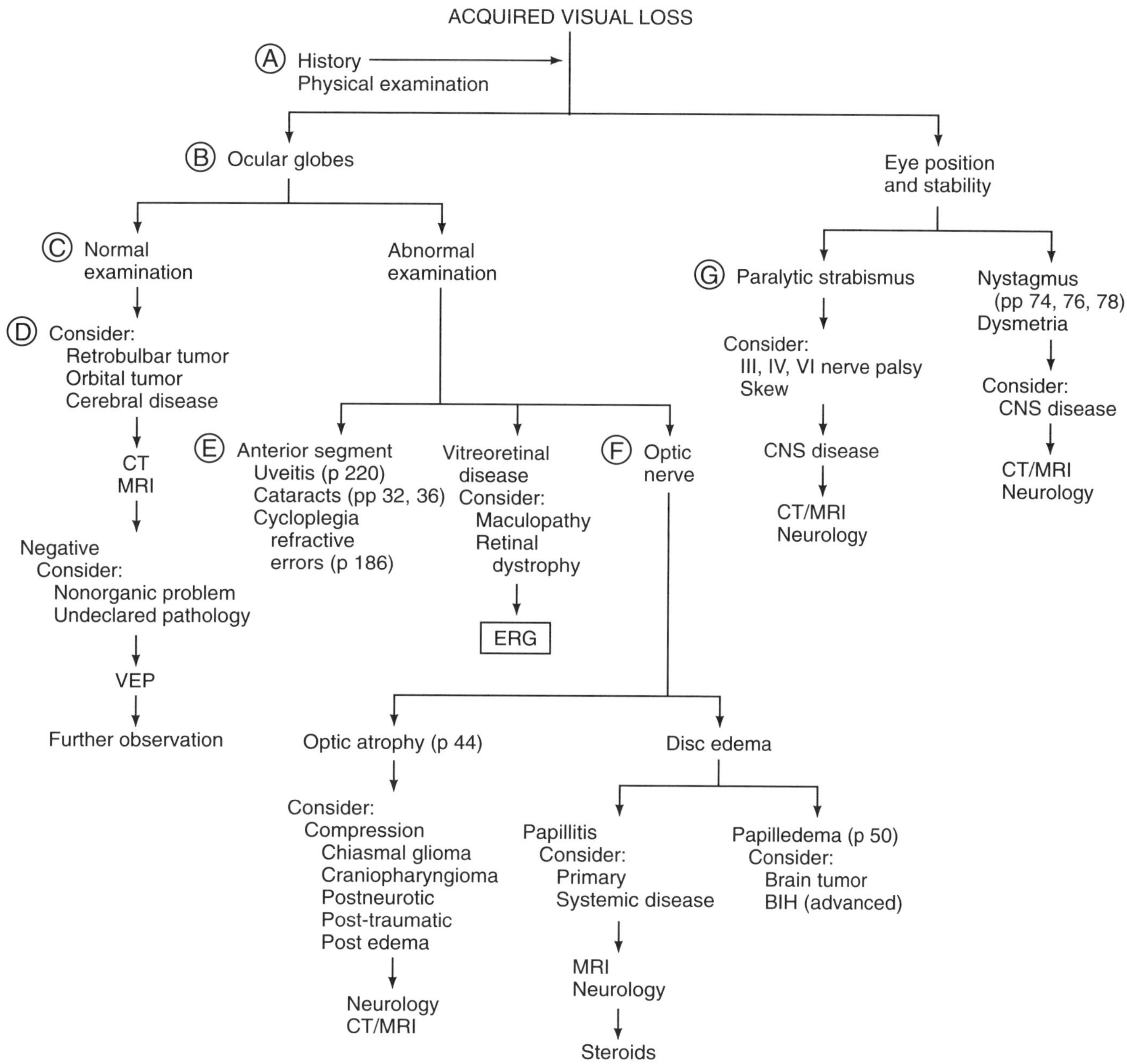

References

Buncic JR, Lloyd L. In: Crawford JS, Morin JD, eds. The eye in childhood. 2nd ed. New York: Grune and Stratton, 1983:395.

Harley RD. Pediatric ophthalmology. Philadelphia: WB Saunders, 1983.

Taylor D. Pediatric ophthalmology. London: Blackwell, 1990.

OCULAR SIGNS OF CHILD ABUSE

Andrea Cibis Tongue, M.D.

The injuries sustained by children who are subjects of willfully inflicted trauma are essentially the same as those resulting from accidental trauma. Nonaccidental trauma as the cause of injuries is a diagnosis of exclusion, the primary diagnosis when the injuries are not compatible with the clinical findings from the alleged trauma.

A. History of events leading to medical care and a clinical history of the signs and symptoms are of utmost importance because the diagnosis is based on the incompatibility of the history given with the clinical observation. Exact documentation of the history is important because changes and inconsistencies, as they relate to the supposed trauma, strongly suggest child abuse. With no history of trauma or diseases that could possibly cause the clinical findings, nonaccidental trauma is most likely.

B. A thorough clinical evaluation and complete physical examination are mandatory in cases of suspected child abuse.

C. Particular attention is directed to the detection of bruises and dermatographic imprints, such as bite marks, outlines of belt buckles, electric cords, irons, and so forth. The mouth should be examined for tears of the frenulum and the genital area for signs of sexual abuse.

D. Skeletal surveys with a search for subtle metaphyseal and rib injuries should be performed in all children under 2 years of age and should be considered in those between 2 and 5 years of age. In the absence of clinical signs of skeletal injury, skeletal surveys are of little value in children older than 5 years. In addition to complete skeletal surveys, skeletal scintigraphy may be helpful in detecting early periosteal elevation and subtle shaft and rib fractures.

E. In cases of CNS injury, MRI is more sensitive than CT in identifying subdural hematomas, cerebral edema, white matter injuries, and cortical contusions. MRI is also more sensitive in estimating the age of the hemorrhage. CT is superior in showing subarachnoid hemorrhage and may be the procedure of choice in the acutely ill child because it is less complicated to perform in an unstable child and is useful in imaging the calvaria, chest, and abdomen during the examination. Detection of injuries of varying ages, associated skull fractures, and other systemic signs of injuries point to severe trauma as the cause.

F. The most common ocular findings of nonaccidental trauma in infants and toddlers is intraocular hemorrhage. Hemorrhages may be unilateral but are most often bilateral and may involve all layers of the retina, vitreous, and subhyaloid space, as well as the choroid, sclera, optic nerve, and optic nerve sheath. Vitreous hemorrhages are probably secondary to the breakthrough of blood through the hyaloid face. Hemorrhages may be so severe that they cause retinal necrosis. Retinoschisis and elevation of the hyaloid face by blood cause hemorrhagic dome-shaped elevations. Circumferential retinal folds are not uncommon and are usually temporal and perimacular.

G. Although these fundus findings are described primarily in children who have sustained CNS injuries from shaking and/or battering, it has not been established with any absolute certainty that they are pathognomonic for shaking or severe anteroposterior acceleration-deceleration forces on the head and eyes. The finding of retinal hemorrhages does not establish a diagnosis of child abuse. It is important that one not attribute the finding of retinal hemorrhage in infants solely to child abuse. Correlation with other clinical findings and the history is critical. Severe accidental trauma that causes CNS injuries with subdural hemorrhages, cerebral edema, and subarachnoid hemorrhages may be associated with retinal hemorrhages. Bleeding dyscrasias, leukemia, acute postoperative or intraoperative hypotonia with cataract extractions, and normal vaginal deliveries are some conditions that can be associated with retinal hemorrhages in the absence of any trauma. CT scans may be negative in children with CNS injuries. MR scans should be performed when retinal hemorrhages are seen in a child with suspected head trauma and negative CT scan.

H. Other signs in injuries described in infants and children with the shaken baby syndrome are subconjunctival hemorrhages, posterior subcapsular cataracts, angle recession, and pigment adhesions of the anterior lens. Choroidal tears may be seen.

I. Postmortem examination of the eyes may identify these abnormalities. Postmortem hemosiderin stains may be helpful in dating the hemorrhages.

J. The morbidity of infants surviving the CNS and associated ocular injuries depends primarily on the severity of the injuries sustained. Localized and diffuse cortical infarcts and atrophy cause a spectrum of neurologic deficits. Impaired vision is usually the result of optic atrophy, retinal atrophy, and gliosis. Amblyopia may occur if macular or vitreous hemorrhages occur or persist for a longer period of time in one eye. Persistence of severe unilateral vitreous hemorrhage in an otherwise neurologically intact infant should lead to consideration of vitrectomy to avoid amblyopia. Severe vitreous hemorrhages may not clear for months. Usually they are associated with other ocular damage such as macular and optic nerve atrophy.

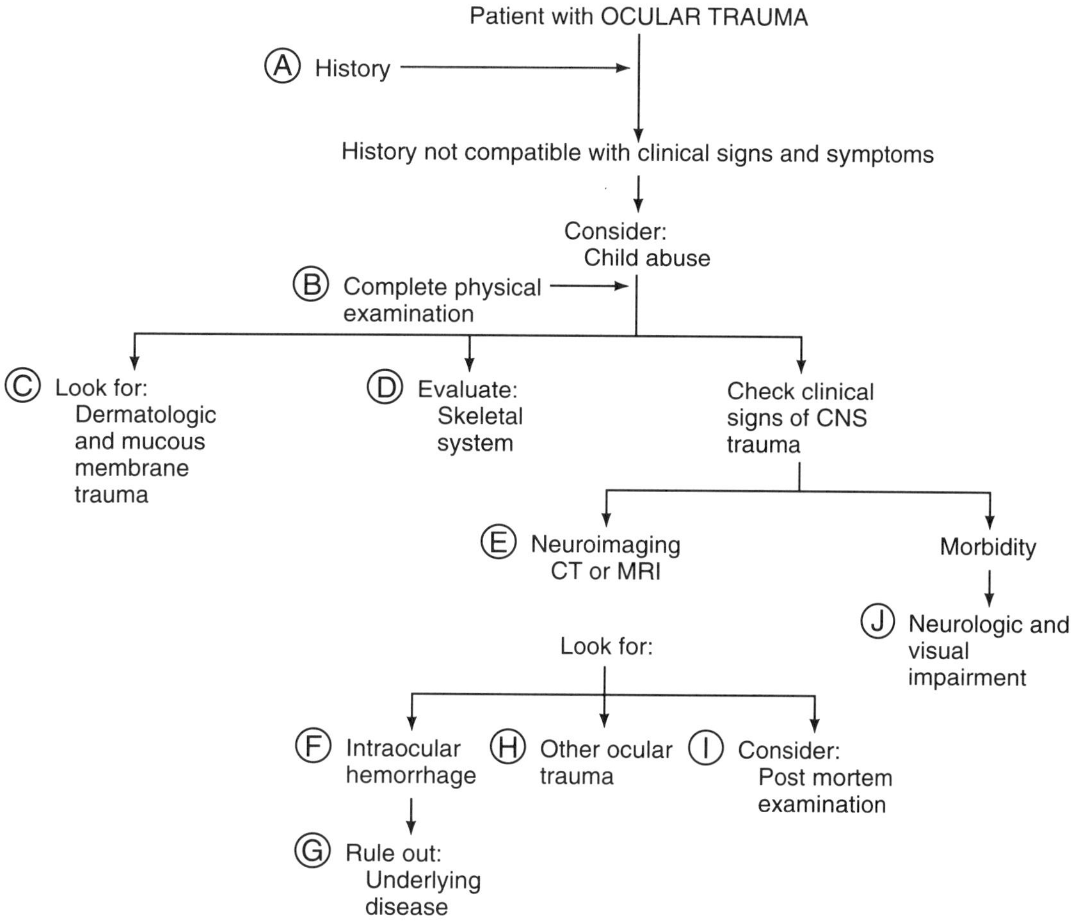

Nonaccidental trauma to the eye unassociated with CNS injuries is much rarer than the above-detailed condition. Hyphemas, subluxated lenses, cataracts, retinal detachments, vitreous hemorrhages, choroidal ruptures, conjunctival hemorrhages, periorbital chemosis, and ecchymosis unexplained by accidental trauma or a disease process should lead to the diagnosis of nonaccidental trauma. Glaucoma may be one of the sequelae in a traumatized eye.

References

Ball WS. Non-accidental craniocerebral trauma (child abuse): MR imaging. Radiology 1989; 173:609.

Duhaime AC, et al. Head injury in very young children: Mechanisms, injury types, and ophthalmologic findings in 100 hospitalized patients younger than 2 years of age. Pediatrics 1992; 90:179.

Elner SG, Elner VM, Arnall M, Albert D. Ocular and associated systemic findings in suspected child abuse. A necropsy study. Arch Ophthalmol 1990; 108:1094.

Greenwald MJ, Weiss A, Oesterele CS, Friendly DS. Traumatic retinoschisis in battered babies. Ophthalmology 1986; 93:619.

Massicotte SJ, Folberg R, Torcyznski E. Vitreoretinal traction and perimacular retinal folds in the eyes of deliberately traumatized children. Ophthalmology 1991; 98:1124.

MICROCEPHALY

Gerhard W. Cibis, M.D.

A. The prenatal and postnatal history is critical in evaluating the possible causes of microcephaly. Microcephaly may be apparent at birth, especially in hereditary cases, but may not be evident for some time as the growth of body and head become disproportional. Postnatal causes include meningitis, intraventricular hemorrhage, and trauma. Prenatal causes include viral infection, radiation, and teratogens such as fetal alcohol and cocaine use early in pregnancy.

B. Inherited microcephaly, usually with retardation, occurs with autosomal recessive and autosomal dominant inheritance.

C. Examination includes measurement of head size and body length. Evaluation for chorioretinitis should be done to look for signs of TORCH.

D. Brain imaging differentiates between the various causes. Although plain films can show calcifications, they miss a great deal of structural detail better appreciated with CT scanning. MRI is ideal. Myelination patterns, differentiations between gray and white matter, and atopies consisting of gray matter islands erroneously isolated in white matter are appreciated only by MRI. CT gives only a hint of agenesis of the corpus callosum, whereas MRI shows the corpus in detail. Microgyria, polygyria, and macrogyria are best appreciated with MRI.

E. Microcephaly vera exists when there are no structural abnormalities. The brain appears normal in every detail except that it is small (more than two standard deviations below the mean) compared with body size. Microcephaly vera usually is not associated with strabismus or poor vision.

F. In proportional microcephaly, the head is smaller than average but is in proportion to body size, which is also small. True dwarfism and failure to thrive fit into this category. There may be underlying infectious, genetic, or teratogenic causes. However, the head (brain) size is not disproportionate as with true microcephaly. It is the neurologic damage of infection, teratogen, chromosomal anomaly, or genetic defect that leads to retinal, optic nerve, or brain (strabismus) ocular manifestations. Retardation is common.

G. Intrauterine viral and other infections occurring early in embryogenesis lead to structural brain abnormalities that include agenesis of the corpus callosum optic nerve hypoplasia (ONH), microgyria, and polygyria as well holoprosencephaly and lissencephaly. Differentiation from genetic or teratogenic causes for the same structural brain anomalies lies in the presence of brain calcifications in the case of TORCH syndrome. Chorioretinal pigmentary changes reflective of inflammation are helpful as well. Electroretinography (ERG) in such early destructive lesions may be diminished or even absent. However, it often is simply attenuated with normal latencies. This is in comparison with brain-retina neuroembryodysgenesis, in which abnormal brain and retinal development is reflected in delayed and distorted ERG patterns (see p 62).

H. Prematurity and other postnatal stress frequently leads to intraventricular hemorrhages. Although this often results in hydrocephalus, it not uncommonly results in the opposite—microcephaly.

I. Early influences in the blastula gastrula stage of development affect both brain and retina. This is true of genetic factors, including allelic disease and chromosomal defects. Certain teratogens, alcohol and cocaine among them, have the same effect. This results in retinal and brain neurodysgenesis expressed as ONH, retinal pigmentary changes, ERG anomalies associated with brain dysgenesis (agenesis of corpus callosum, holoprosencephaly, lissencephaly, macrogyria and microgyria, atopia, migrational disorders, and cerebellar dysgenesis). These can be found by MRI and ERG testing.

References

Harbord MG, Lambert SR, Kriss A, et al. Autosomal recessive microcephaly, mental retardation with nonpigmentary retinopathy and a distinctive electroretinogram. Neuropediatrics 1989; 20:139.

Manning FJ, Bruce AM, Berson EL. Electroretinograms in microcephaly with chorioretinal degeneration. Am J Ophthalmol 1990; 109:457.

McKusick VA, Stauffer M, Knox DL, Clark DS. Chorioretinopathy with hereditary microcephaly. Arch Ophthalmol 1966; 75:597.

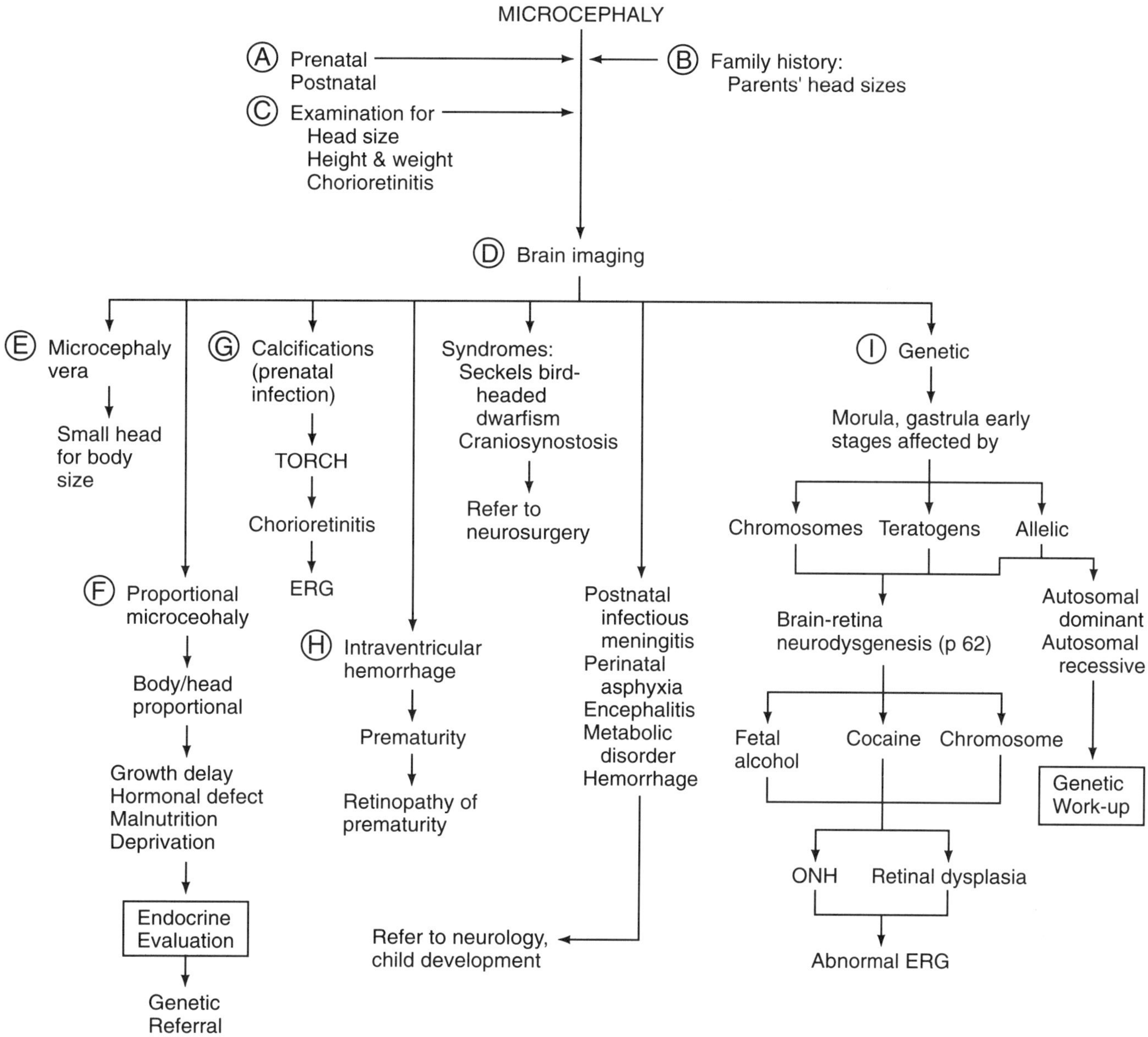
MICROCEPHALY
(A) Prenatal
Postnatal
(B) Family history:
Parents' head sizes
(C) Examination for
Head size
Height & weight
Chorioretinitis
(D) Brain imaging
(E) Microcephaly vera
Small head for body size
(F) Proportional microceohaly
Body/head proportional
Growth delay
Hormonal defect
Malnutrition
Deprivation
Endocrine Evaluation
Genetic Referral
(G) Calcifications (prenatal infection)
TORCH
Chorioretinitis
ERG
(H) Intraventricular hemorrhage
Prematurity
Retinopathy of prematurity
Syndromes:
Seckels bird-headed dwarfism
Craniosynostosis
Refer to neurosurgery
Postnatal infectious meningitis
Perinatal asphyxia
Encephalitis
Metabolic disorder
Hemorrhage
Refer to neurology, child development
(I) Genetic
Morula, gastrula early stages affected by
Chromosomes
Teratogens
Allelic
Brain-retina neurodysgenesis (p 62)
Autosomal dominant
Autosomal recessive
Genetic Work-up
Fetal alcohol
Cocaine
Chromosome
ONH
Retinal dysplasia
Abnormal ERG

GENETIC EYE DISEASE: THE ANOMALY CHECKLIST

Barbara K. Hecht, Ph.D.
Frederick Hecht, M.D.

A significant proportion of children's eye disease is due to genetic disorders and malformations. Although some malformations are of unknown etiology or teratogic origin, the clinical approach to them is identical to that used with genetic anomalies.

A. The history should serve two purposes with regard to the physical examination: It should lead into the physical examination and provide clues to areas of interest; after the physical examination has been done, one should return to the history to verify it and supplement it.

B. The family history (p 2) permits the identification of heritable conditions. The family history impacts on the physical examination. For example, if the family history is positive for glaucoma, the patient's pressures should be monitored. Conversely, if the patient's pressures are elevated, one should return to the family and the family history in search of other relatives with glaucoma.

C. The checklist provided here is an example. You may wish to add or subtract items and develop your own checklist.

The interpupillary distance is measured with a transparent millimeter rule, as is the palpebral fissure length. Both measurements are then compared with normal values for children of that chronologic age. Ocular hypotelorism, for example, can be an outward sign of holoprosencephaly. Ocular hypertelorism is often found in the Noonan syndrome and is a common anomaly in children born to mothers exposed to teratogens such as aminopterin, hydantoin (Dilantin), and retinoic acid (Accutane). Short palpebral fissures are a hallmark of fetal alcohol and Williams syndromes (with prominent lips and cardiovascular anomaly). Graphs to check the normal interpupillary and palpebral fissure distances are contained in many textbooks, including *Smith's Recognizable Patterns of Human Malformations* (see References below).

Interpupillary distance:	Hypertelorism	_____	Hypotelorism	_____		
Palpebral fissures:	Short	_____	Slanted up	_____	Slanted down	_____
Supraorbital ridges:	Prominant	_____	Shallow	_____	Absent	_____
Eyebrows:	Bushy	_____	Synophrys	_____	Medial flare	_____
	Arched	_____	Hypoplastic	_____	Absent	_____
Eye lids:	Ptosis, unilat	_____	Fused	_____	Notched	_____
	Ptosis, bilat	_____	Hemangioma	_____		
Eye lashes:	Long	_____	Curly	_____	Hypoplastic	_____
Inner canthi:	Epicanthus, unilat	_____	Epicanthus, bilat	_____	Lateral displaced	_____
Lacrimal ducts:	Obstructed	_____	Excess tearing	_____	Decreased tearing	_____
Eye muscles:	Esotropia	_____	Exotropia	_____		
Eye movements:	Nystagmus	_____	Wandering	_____		
Globes:	Prominent	_____	Myxedema	_____	Microphthalmia	_____
Sclerae:	Blue	_____	Telangiectasia	_____	Scarred	_____
Conjunctivae:	Dermoid	_____	Telangiectasia	_____		
Corneas:	Macrocornea	_____	Microcornea	_____	Keratoconus	_____
Pupils:	Irregular	_____	Asymmetric	_____	Unreactive	_____
Iris:	Coloboma	_____	Speckled	_____	Hypoplastic	_____
Pressure:	Glaucoma, unilat	_____	Glaucoma, bilat	_____		
Retina:	Coloboma	_____	Mass	_____	No red reflex	_____
	Dysplastic	_____	Degeneration	_____	Abn. pigmentation	_____
Optic nerve:	Bulging	_____	Hypoplastic	_____	Atrophic	_____
Refraction:	Myopia	_____	Hyperopia	_____	Astigmatism	_____
Lens:	Cataract, unilat	_____	Cataract, bilat	_____	Dislocated	_____

Figure 1 Sample checklist for anomalies of the eyes and orbital region.

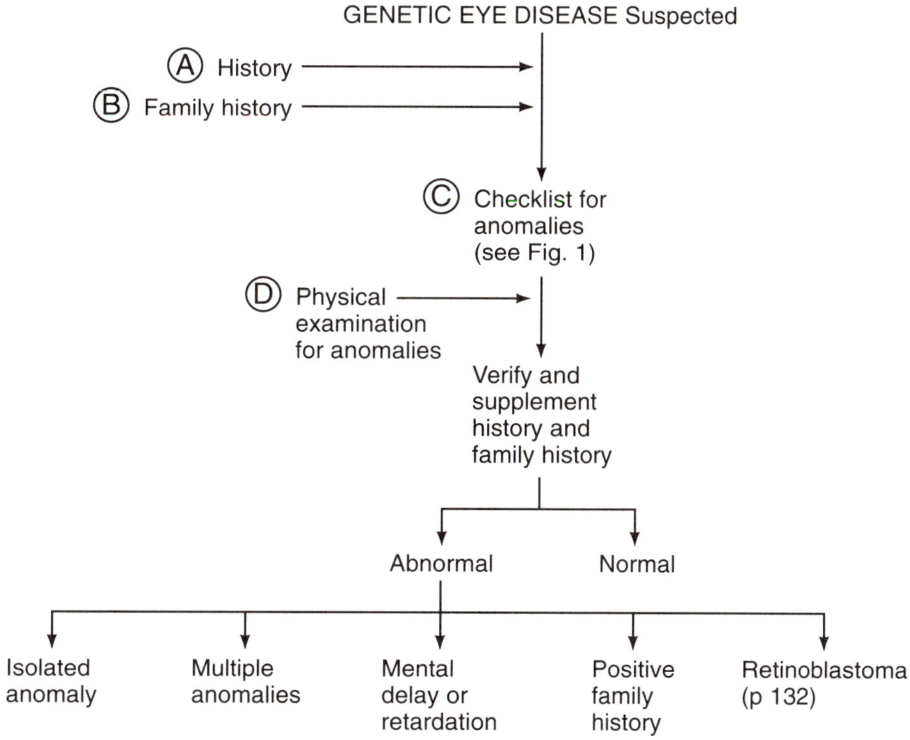

Additional measurements can be taken within the context of pediatric ophthalmology. These include the head circumference and ear length. There is also nothing that says an ophthalmologist is not allowed to look at the ears to see if they are low-set, backwards rotated, or malformed (as in the Treacher Collins syndrome) or to look at the nasal bridge to see if it is low (as in achondroplasia), broad (as in generalized gangliosidosis), or prominent (as in trisomy 9 mosaicism). Similar considerations apply to the shape and size of the nose itself, the philtrum (the area between the nose and the upper lip), the lips, the mouth, the teeth, the midface, the chin, and so forth. The basic issue is whether the eyes and other anatomic structures are normal or abnormal. If abnormal, the next issue is whether there is a single, isolated anomaly or evidence of multiple anomalies, mental retardation, or other ominous findings.

Note that a number of findings in the checklist given here represent chapters in this book—for example, coloboma (p 122) corneal size abnormalities (p 18), cataracts (p 116), and nystagmus (pp 76, 78, 80). It is imperative to use a systematic approach to examining the patient to detect and record not just one abnormality but multiple abnormalities. The essence of clinical genetics is the clinical component. Clinical genetics is a vital part of pediatric ophthalmology.

D. The physical examination for anomalies of the eye and orbital region can be greatly aided by an effective checklist.

References

Goodman RM, Gorlin RJ. The malformed infant and child. An illustrated guide. New York: Oxford University Press, 1983.

Gorlin RJ, Cohen MM, Levin LS. Syndromes of the head and neck. 3rd ed. New York: Oxford University Press, 1990.

Jones KL. Smith's recognizable patterns of human malformation. Philadelphia: WB Saunders, 1988.

GENETIC EYE DISEASE: DIFFERENTIAL DIAGNOSIS

Barbara K. Hecht, Ph.D.
Frederick Hecht, M.D.

The eye is a window into genetic disease and malformation syndromes. The approach to genetic disease of the eye is facilitated by the use of a checklist for anomalies of the eyes and orbital region (p 10). This checklist combines the history of the patient, the genetic family history (p 2), and the physical examination directed specifically and efficiently at the detection of anomalies. All this information is used in the differential diagnosis.

A. Epicanthal folds are used here as an example of an anomaly. An epicanthal fold must of course be differentiated from the normal configuration of the Oriental eye, in which the fold is continuous with the pars orbitalis and hides a major part of the pars tarsalis. A true epicanthal fold is smaller, arises from the inner medial portion of the pars orbitalis, and sweeps down diagonally across the inner canthus. The embryologic origin of epicanthal folds is redundant skin due usually to depression of the nasal bridge and excess skin such as in cutis laxa.

B. Epicanthal folds can be seen in the United States in about 20% of normal children under the age of 10. They are frequently a familial finding and are especially common in children of Northern European descent.

C. Nonetheless, epicanthal folds are an anomaly because about 80% of normal children do not have them, and they are common in anomalous children.

D. The chromosome abnormalities listed here represent only a small sample of the cytogenetic aberrations associated with epicanthal folds. In Down syndrome, the epicanthal fold is a classic finding, together with Brushfield spots, and is seen in about 60% of patients under age 10 with Down syndrome in the United States. Turner syndrome is due to 45,X (also called X0) or structural rearrangements of the X chromosome. Extra X syndromes include XXXX and XXXXX in females and XXXY and XXXXY in males. Partial deletion of the short (p) arm of chromosome 4, the Wolf-Hirschhorn syndrome, is characterized by ocular hypertelorism, broad nasal bridge, and strabismus. Deletion of 5p causes the cat's cry (cri du chat) syndrome. Deletion of 13q is associated with sporadic retinoblastoma, multiple malformations, and mental retardation. Deletion of 18p is accompanied by ptosis, hypertelorism, low nasal bridge, and arhinocephalic holoprosencephaly. Suspicion of an underlying chromosome abnormality should prompt cytogenetic studies (p 124).

E. Epicanthal folds are a sign of maternal exposure to teratogens such as the antifolate aminopterin, methotrexate, anticonvulsants of the trimethadione family, and valproate. Verify teratogen exposure by checking with the mother's other physicians and pharmacies.

F. Women with undetected or untreated phenylketonuria (PKU) tend to have children with microcephaly, growth retardation, and structural defects such as epicanthal folds plus strabismus. If suspicious, test the mother for PKU.

G. Numerous single-gene disorders are associated with epicanthal folds. These genetic syndromes can be inherited as autosomal (nonsex chromosomal traits that are dominant or recessive) and as X-linked traits (on the X chromosome).

Autosomal dominant: Examples that are inherited in this way and associated with epicanthal folds are listed. The blepharophimosis syndrome causes lateral displacement of the inner canthi, ptosis of the eyelids, short palpebral fissures, and cupped ears. Freeman-Sheldon syndrome has the "whistling face" appearance and hypoplasia of the nasal wings, deep-set eyes with telecanthus, blepharophimosis, and strabismus. Stickler syndrome has a flat midface, myopia, increased risk of retinal detachment, and glaucoma. With an autosomal dominant gene, the risk is 50%.

Autosomal recessive: Esobar syndrome involves multiple pterygia (arthrogryposis) with eyelid ptosis, downslanted palpebral fissures, and ocular hypertelorism. It must be distinguished from the lethal multiple pterygium syndrome. Pena-Shokeir syndrome also causes arthrogryposis and hypertelorism (plus pulmonary hyperplasia). There is a strong connection between arthrogryposis and epicanthal folds. Smith-Lemli-Opitz syndrome affects the eyes with epicanthal folds, ptosis, strabismus, and cataracts. With autosomal recessive disorders, the risk for the next child is 25%.

X-linked: FG syndrome (an unfortunate name) presents with hypotonia, prominent forehead, epicanthal folds, and imperforate anus or anal stenosis. It carries a 50% risk for the patient's brothers. Carrier sisters can be asymptomatic.

H. Little is known about the cause of many malformations. Examples of mysterious disorders associated with epicanthal folds include Noonan syndrome with eyelid ptosis, hypertelorism, downslanting palpebral fissures, strabismus, nystagmus, keratoconus, and myopia; Rubenstein-Taybi syndrome with downslanted palpebral fissures and broad thumbs and big toes; and Weaver syndrome with big babies who have accelerated growth and advanced bone age plus hypertelorism and downslanted palpebral fissures.

I. Some disorders associated with epicanthal folds require biochemical tests. For possible Hurler syndrome, a progressive mucopolysaccharide disorder, the test is of white cell lysosomal alpha-L-iduronidase (an enzyme absent in this disease). Leroy I-cell disease is characterized by thin eyebrows, puffy eyelids, and

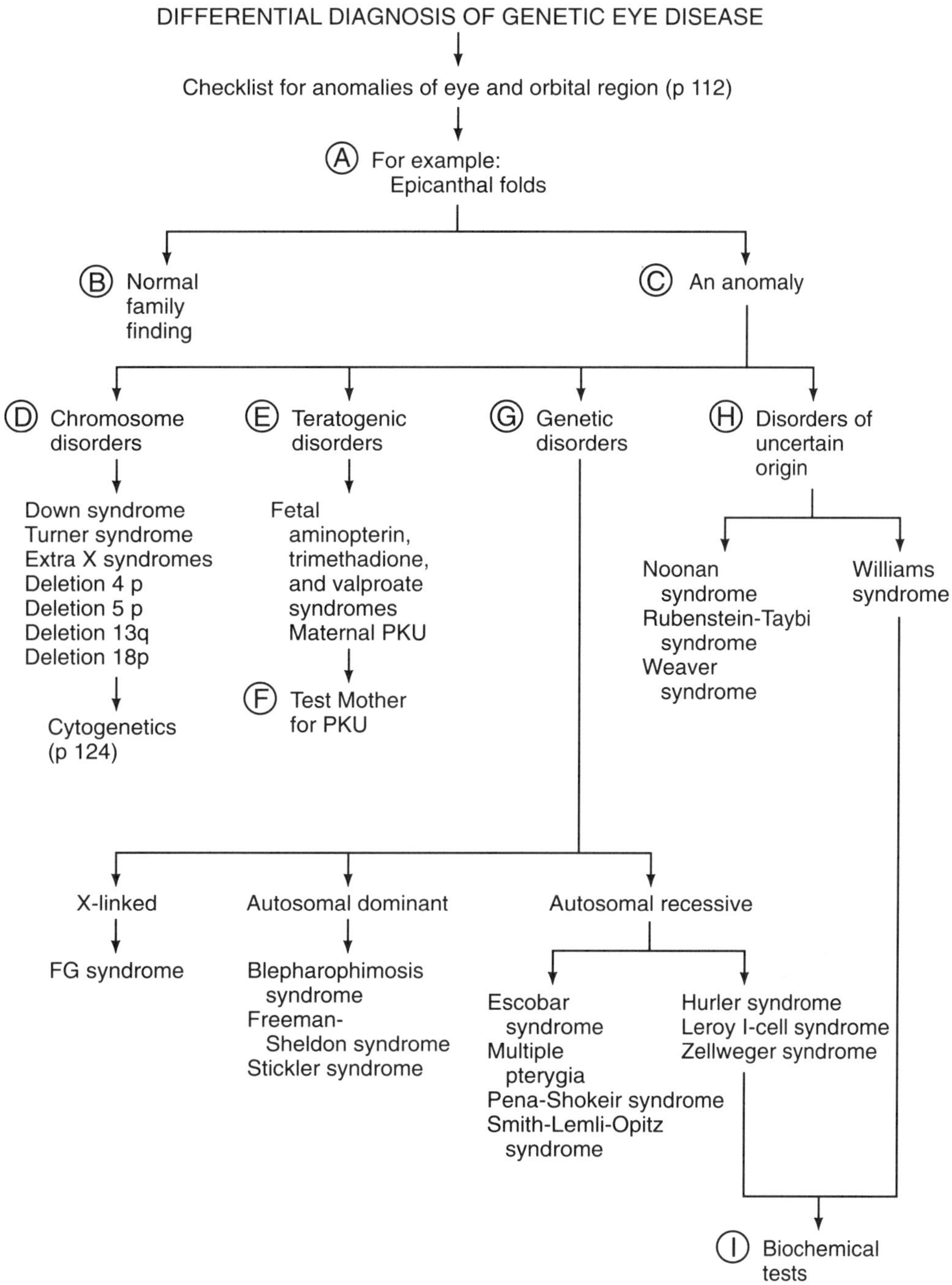

sometimes faint haziness of the cornea; tests measure lysosomal enzymes that are deficient in skin fibroblasts (and amniotic fluid cells) but increased in plasma and urine. Zellweger cerebrohepatorenal syndrome is accompanied by high forehead, shallow supraorbital ridges, and Brushfield iris spots; tests analyze the peroxisomal enzyme DHAP-AT (dihydroxyacetone phosphate acyltransferase), which is absent, and very long-chain fatty acids, which are increased. Williams syndrome has prominent lips, hoarse voice, medial eyebrow flare, periorbital fullness, short palpebral fissures, and blue eyes with stellate irises; hypercalcemia is uncommon, but delayed calcium clearance is common.

References

McKusick VA. Mendelian inheritance in man. Catalog of autosomal dominant, autosomal recessive and X-linked phenotypes. 9th ed. Baltimore: John Hopkins University Press, 1990.

Thompson MW, McInnes RR, Willard HF. Thompson and Thompson's genetics in medicine. 5th ed. Philadelphia: WB Saunders, 1991.

Vogel F, Motulsky AF. Human genetics: Problems and approaches. 2nd ed. Berlin: Springer-Verlag, 1986.

CATARACTS AND DYSMORPHOLOGY

Michael L. Begleiter, M.S.
David J. Harris, M.D.

A. Taking a history for the purpose of identifying a possible genetic problem is somewhat different from taking a history for the evaluation of disease in a given patient. It is important to collect a pregnancy, labor, and delivery history as well as information relating to the child's development. By obtaining a pedigree and asking the parents to give names and birthdates of their children, parents, and siblings, you force them to think about health problems present in their families. One should always inquire into the possibility of consanguinity.

B. Measure and plot on a growth chart the height, weight, and head circumference of the child. If historical information is available, plot that as well. Starting at the head or the feet and working your way to the other end, make a careful assessment of any other problems the child has. Note any variations in structure no matter how subtle. Obtain specific measurements if there is unusual eye spacing, limb lengths, or any other quantifiable differences in structure. These variations in structure or size may provide the clues to a syndrome diagnosis.

C. In the absence of any other clinical findings, it is necessary to distinguish children with isolated cataracts from those whose cataracts have a metabolic origin. Therefore, amino acid and galactosemia screening should be performed. In evaluating galactosemia, a Clinitest for reducing substances is not adequate. Either enzyme screening or a formal galactose-1-phosphate uridyl transferase assay should be performed because some newborns do not show reducing substances even when they have galactosemia. In screening for homocystinuria, make sure the patient is not receiving vitamin supplementation. A vitamin B_6–responsive form of homocystinuria can not be identified if the patient is getting extra vitamin B_6.

D. The diagnosis of galactosemia, homocystinuria, or any inborn error of metabolism is an indication to refer the patient to a genetics center experienced in managing children with metabolic disorders.

E. Children with cataracts, no other congenital malformations, and normal metabolic screening may have cataracts due to simple mendelian traits. The only way to establish this is to have documented in the family history the transmission of cataracts. Isolated congenital cataracts can be caused by autosomal dominant, autosomal recessive, or X-linked mechanisms. Appropriate genetic counseling should be offered to these families.

F. Every child with multiple congenital anomalies deserves a chromosome analysis. This study is performed for diagnostic purposes and to obtain information for reproductive counseling of the parents. One should strive to obtain high-resolution banding studies so that even minor alterations of chromosome structure are identified.

G. Once a chromosome anomaly has been identified, the family should be referred for genetic counseling and management of the child's nonophthalmologic problems.

H. The evaluation of children with multiple congenital anomalies and normal karyotypes is very difficult. The only way a syndrome diagnosis can be established is by identifying a unique malformation that allows you to sort the child's problems into a short list of possible syndromes. The list included here encompasses the described syndromes with cataract, multiple congenital anomalies, and normal chromosomes. After consulting one of the syndrome identification books listed in the references, you may be able to assign a diagnosis. Be careful not to overdiagnose. If the child does not fit an established category, he or she may need to be left unclassified.

I. Another category for consideration is children with cataracts and abnormalities in one other body system. By following the decision tree you may be able to establish a diagnosis. Again, do not overdiagnose and do not hesitate to say that the problems do not fit into a syndrome.

J. Children with short stature or limb abnormalities warrant radiographic study with skeletal surveys. The problems identified can be categorized by consulting a textbook of radiologic syndrome identification.

References

Aase JM. Diagnostic dysmorphology. New York: Plenum, 1990.

Gorlin RJ, Cohen MM, Levin LS. Syndromes of the head and neck. New York: Oxford University Press, 1990.

Jones KL. Smith's recognizable patterns of human malformation. Philadelphia: WB Saunders, 1988.

Taybi H, Lachman RS. Radiology of syndromes, metabolic disorders and skeletal dysplasias. Chicago: Year Book, 1990.

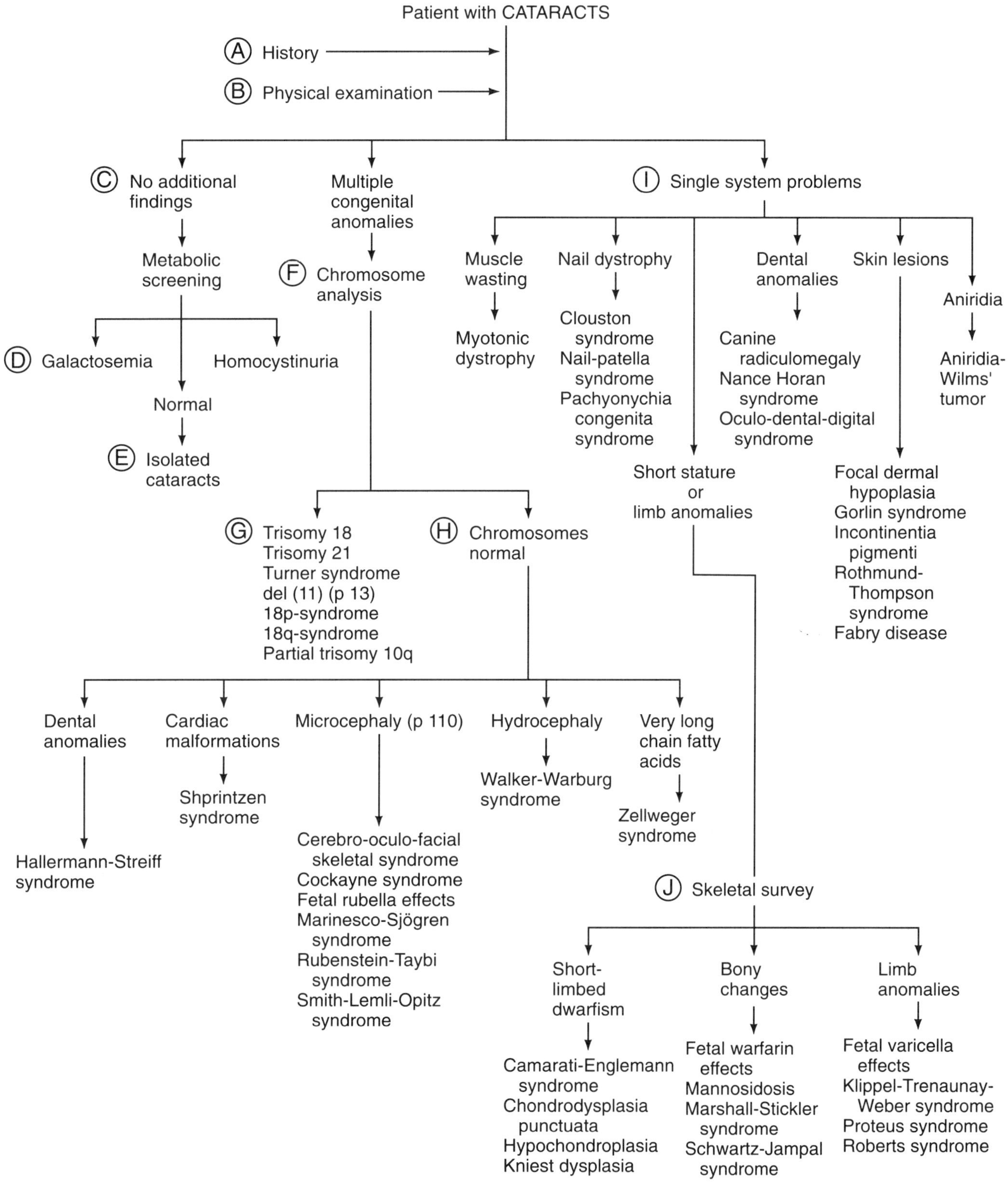
Patient with CATARACTS
(A) History
(B) Physical examination
(C) No additional findings
Metabolic screening
(D) Galactosemia
Homocystinuria
Normal
(E) Isolated cataracts
Multiple congenital anomalies
(F) Chromosome analysis
(G) Trisomy 18
Trisomy 21
Turner syndrome
del (11) (p 13)
18p-syndrome
18q-syndrome
Partial trisomy 10q
(H) Chromosomes normal
Dental anomalies
Hallermann-Streiff syndrome
Cardiac malformations
Shprintzen syndrome
Microcephaly (p 110)
Cerebro-oculo-facial skeletal syndrome
Cockayne syndrome
Fetal rubella effects
Marinesco-Sjögren syndrome
Rubenstein-Taybi syndrome
Smith-Lemli-Opitz syndrome
Hydrocephaly
Walker-Warburg syndrome
Very long chain fatty acids
Zellweger syndrome
(I) Single system problems
Muscle wasting
Myotonic dystrophy
Nail dystrophy
Clouston syndrome
Nail-patella syndrome
Pachyonychia congenita syndrome
Short stature or limb anomalies
Dental anomalies
Canine radiculomegaly
Nance Horan syndrome
Oculo-dental-digital syndrome
Skin lesions
Focal dermal hypoplasia
Gorlin syndrome
Incontinentia pigmenti
Rothmund-Thompson syndrome
Fabry disease
Aniridia
Aniridia-Wilms' tumor
(J) Skeletal survey
Short-limbed dwarfism
Camarati-Englemann syndrome
Chondrodysplasia punctuata
Hypochondroplasia
Kniest dysplasia
Bony changes
Fetal warfarin effects
Mannosidosis
Marshall-Stickler syndrome
Schwartz-Jampal syndrome
Limb anomalies
Fetal varicella effects
Klippel-Trenaunay-Weber syndrome
Proteus syndrome
Roberts syndrome

CORNEAL OPACITY AND DYSMORPHOLOGY

Michael L. Begleiter, M.S.
David J. Harris, M.D.

A. Taking a history for the purpose of identifying a possible genetic problem is somewhat different from taking a history for the evaluation of disease in a given patient. It is important to collect a pregnancy, labor, and delivery history as well as information relating to the child's development. By obtaining a pedigree and asking the parents to give names and birthdates of their children, parents, and siblings, you force them to think about any health problems present in their families. One should always inquire into the possibility of consanguinity.

B. Measure and plot on a growth chart the height, weight, and head circumference of the child. If historical information is available, plot that as well. Starting at the head or the feet and working your way to the other end, make a careful assessment of any other problems the child has. Note any variations in structure, no matter how subtle. Obtain specific measurements if there is unusual eye spacing, limb lengths, or any other quantifiable differences in structure. These variations in structure or size may provide the clues to a syndrome diagnosis.

C. Multiple congenital anomalies should always make one think of the possibility of a chromosome anomaly. A high-resolution banded chromosome analysis should be performed for the purpose of diagnosis; if an anomaly is identified, reproductive counseling is offered.

D. For children with multiple congenital anomalies and normal chromosomes, it is necessary to identify a unique malformation in order to establish a syndrome diagnosis.

E. Children with short stature, especially if there is shortening of the limbs, should have a skeletal survey. Consulting a textbook of radiologic identification of syndromes is very helpful in interpreting the radiographs.

F. Children with corneal opacities and short forearms have a short list of possible syndromes. Consult the syndrome identification books to help in establishing a diagnosis.

G. The combination of corneal opacities and coarse facies should immediately make one think of the lysosomal storage disorders. Screening for these problems begins with urine tests for mucopolysaccharides (MPS) and oligosaccharides. By identifying the abnormal substances in the urine screening, one can determine which specific assays to order for definitive diagnosis.

H. The last group of patients to consider are those with corneal opacity and a problem in one other body system. By following the decision tree, you should be able to place the patient in the appropriate category. Remember that not every patient fits into a clear-cut diagnostic category. Some children remain with a diagnosis of corneal opacity with or without other clinical findings.

References

Aase JM. Diagnostic dysmorphology. New York: Plenum, 1990.

Gorlin RJ, Cohen MM, Levin LS. Syndromes of the head and neck. New York: Oxford University Press, 1990.

Jones KL. Smith's recognizable patterns of human malformation. Philadelphia: WB Saunders, 1988.

Taybi H, Lachman RS. Radiology of syndromes, metabolic disorders and skeletal dysplasias. Chicago: Year Book, 1990.

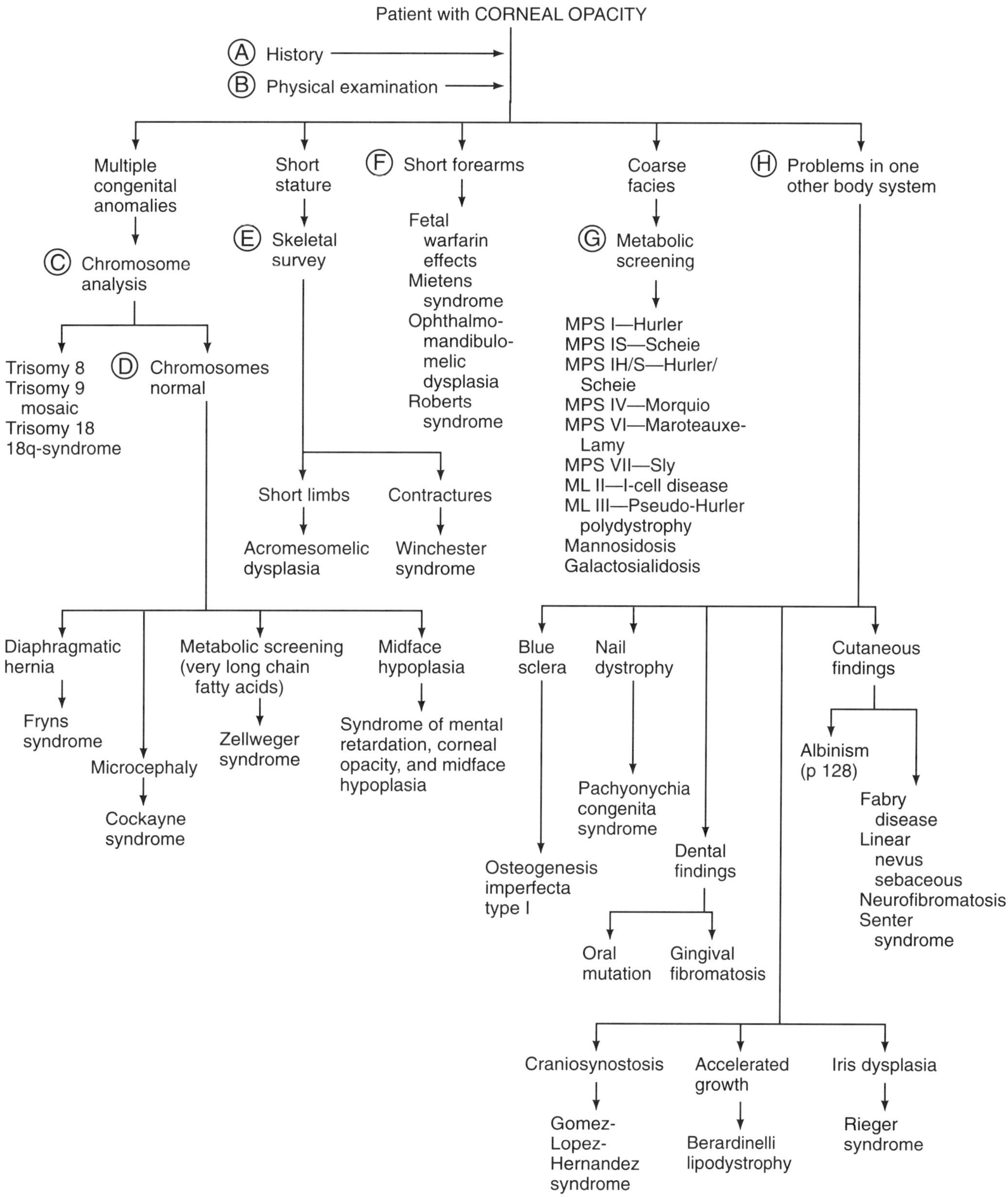
Patient with CORNEAL OPACITY
(A) History
(B) Physical examination
Multiple congenital anomalies
(C) Chromosome analysis
Trisomy 8
Trisomy 9 mosaic
Trisomy 18
18q-syndrome
(D) Chromosomes normal
Diaphragmatic hernia
Fryns syndrome
Microcephaly
Cockayne syndrome
Metabolic screening (very long chain fatty acids)
Zellweger syndrome
Midface hypoplasia
Syndrome of mental retardation, corneal opacity, and midface hypoplasia
Short stature
(E) Skeletal survey
Short limbs
Acromesomelic dysplasia
Contractures
Winchester syndrome
(F) Short forearms
Fetal warfarin effects
Mietens syndrome
Ophthalmo-mandibulo-melic dysplasia
Roberts syndrome
Coarse facies
(G) Metabolic screening
MPS I—Hurler
MPS IS—Scheie
MPS IH/S—Hurler/Scheie
MPS IV—Morquio
MPS VI—Maroteauxe-Lamy
MPS VII—Sly
ML II—I-cell disease
ML III—Pseudo-Hurler polydystrophy
Mannosidosis
Galactosialidosis
(H) Problems in one other body system
Blue sclera
Osteogenesis imperfecta type I
Nail dystrophy
Pachyonychia congenita syndrome
Dental findings
Oral mutation
Gingival fibromatosis
Cutaneous findings
Albinism (p 128)
Fabry disease
Linear nevus sebaceous
Neurofibromatosis
Senter syndrome
Craniosynostosis
Gomez-Lopez-Hernandez syndrome
Accelerated growth
Berardinelli lipodystrophy
Iris dysplasia
Rieger syndrome

GLAUCOMA AND DYSMORPHOLOGY

Jill Cellars Rogers, M.S.
David J. Harris, M.D.

A. The patient's medical and developmental history can help distinguish whether the glaucoma is isolated or is associated with other abnormalities. Included in the interview should be a pregnancy, labor, and developmental history. Also, dietary habits of the individual should be addressed. Isolated glaucoma can be inherited, so a good genetic history should be taken.

B. The individual's anthropomorphics, including head circumference, should be plotted on a growth chart. If available, previous measurements should also be plotted. A thorough physical examination should be performed, looking carefully for other major and minor malformations. Specific measurements such as canthal distances and ear length may help quantify dysmorphic features.

C. Glaucoma with no other apparent anomalies may be isolated or an indication of an inborn error of metabolism. Amino acid screening should be performed.

D. The diagnosis of homocystinuria or Lowe's syndrome is an indication for referral to a genetics center for management and follow-up.

E. Isolated glaucoma can be inherited in an autosomal dominant or autosomal recessive fashion. The ages of onset also vary. Genetic counseling may be appropriate for the affected individual's family.

F. The individual with glaucoma and involvement in other systems should always have a high-resolution chromosome analysis to rule out any chromosome abnormalities. If previous chromosome analysis was performed (i.e., amniocentesis, chorionic villus sampling) and high-resolution studies were not done, the analysis should be repeated.

G. The presence of abnormal chromosomes is an indication for referral to a genetics center. Also, the child should be referred to the appropriate pediatric specialists to treat his or her specific anomalies.

H. A child with multisystem abnormalities and normal chromosomes presents a diagnostic dilemma. Therefore, it is important to examine the child carefully and identify specific abnormalities. The list presented here includes the many syndromes that can include glaucoma. After consulting a syndrome identification book, a diagnosis may seem clear. Alternatively, the child may not fit into a diagnostic category. Nevertheless, the family should be referred for genetic counseling.

I. If the child has numerous defects of the eye, the Rieger eye malformation sequence should be considered. If the child has dental anomalies, he may have the Rieger syndrome. Both the sequence and syndrome can be inherited, and affected individuals and family members should be referred for genetic counseling.

References

Gorlin RJ, Cohen MM, Levin LS. Syndromes of the head and neck. New York: Oxford University Press, 1990.

Jones KL. Smith's recognizable patterns of human malformation. Philadelphia: WB Saunders, 1988.

McKusick VA. Mendelian inheritance in man. Baltimore: The Johns Hopkins University Press, 1990.

GLAUCOMA AND DYSMORPHOLOGY

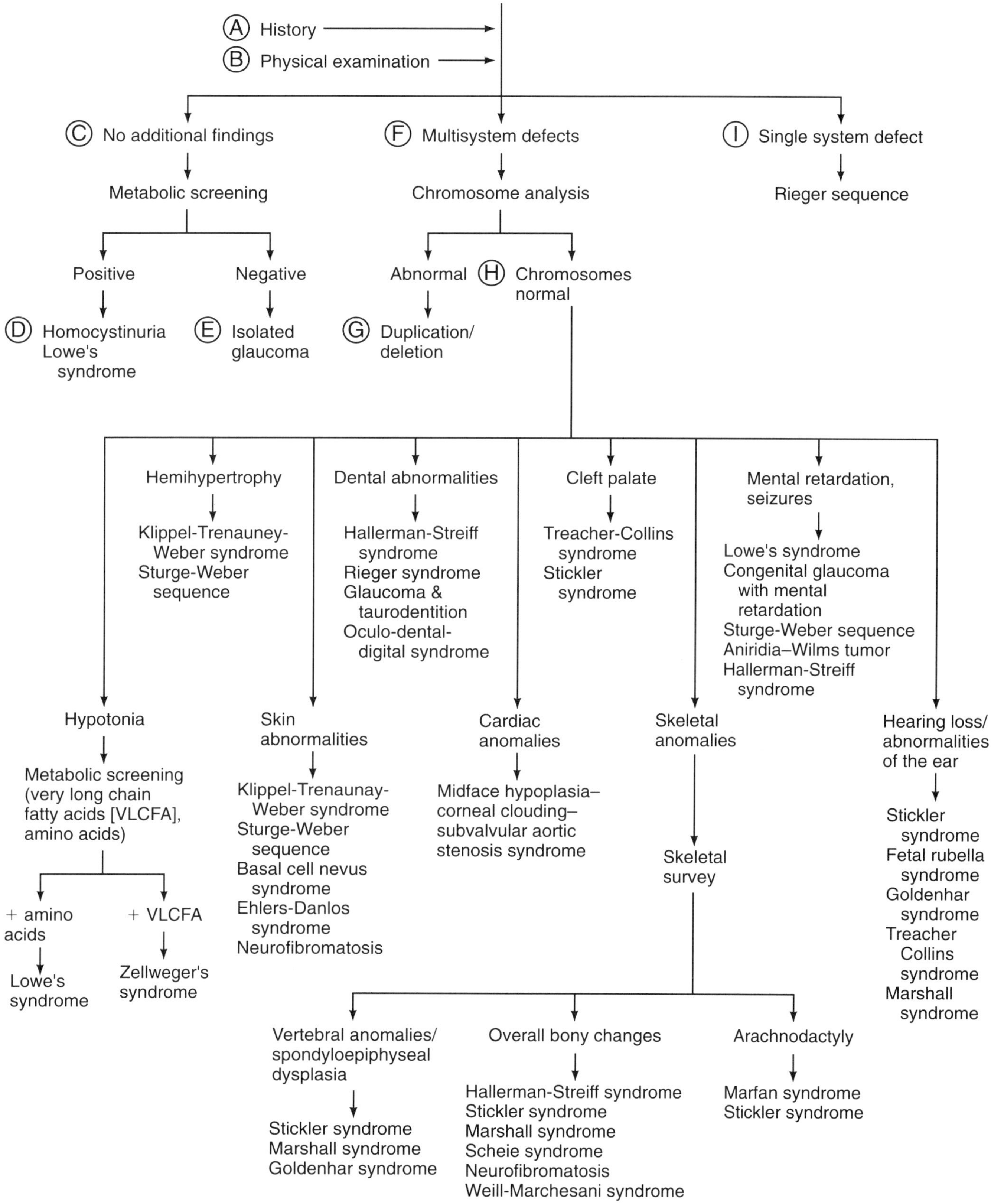

COLOBOMA AND DYSMORPHOLOGY

Jill Cellars Rogers, M.S.
David J. Harris, M.D.

A. A history of the patient's medical and developmental progress helps distinguish whether the coloboma is associated with other system defects or is an isolated finding. A prenatal and perinatal history should be included as well as a family history. Specific questions regarding each family member are useful to help the family recall particular individuals.

B. The anthropomorphics, including head circumference, of the affected individual should be plotted on growth charts along with previous measurements (if available). The presence of a coloboma should always raise the suspicion of other defects. A thorough physical examination should be performed to look carefully for other minor or major malformations. Dysmorphic features can often be quantified by taking measurements of, for example, canthal distances, ear length, and limb length.

C. If no abnormalities are noted from a medical or developmental standpoint, the coloboma is most likely isolated. Isolated colobomata can be inherited but usually are not. The family may wish genetic counseling. If no other specific anomalies are recognized but the child seems developmentally delayed or has nondescript dysmorphia, he should be referred for genetic evaluation.

D. A chromosome analysis should be performed on any child with multisystem defects, dysmorphia, or developmental delay. A high-resolution study should be specifically requested to look for smaller deletions that may not be recognizable on standard analysis. Therefore, if the child had normal chromosomes previously (i.e., amniocentesis, chorionic villus sampling), an additional high-resolution study is still indicated.

E. If a chromosome abnormality is identified, the child should be referred to a genetic service for further evaluation. Additionally, if the child has other system defects, he should be referred to the appropriate pediatric specialist.

F. If the chromosome evaluation is normal but the child has other system defects, the differential diagnosis is extensive. Echocardiography may be appropriate to rule out congenital heart defects. Specific physical characteristics may help to classify the child's anomalies. After reviewing the list provided and consulting syndrome identification books, the child may or may not be fit into a specific syndrome. In either case, it is important to refer the family for genetic consultation.

G. The Rieger eye malformation sequence involves iris dysplasia, abnormal pupils, and occasionally coloboma. If the child has abnormalities in dentition as well, he most likely has the Rieger syndrome. Both the sequence and syndrome can be inherited. Affected individuals and family members should be referred for genetic counseling.

References

Gorlin RJ, Cohen MM, Levin LS. Syndromes of the head and neck. New York: Oxford University Press, 1990.

Jones KL. Smith's recognizable patterns of human malformation. Philadelphia: WB Saunders, 1988.

McKusick VA. Mendelian inheritance in man. Baltimore: The Johns Hopkins University Press, 1990.

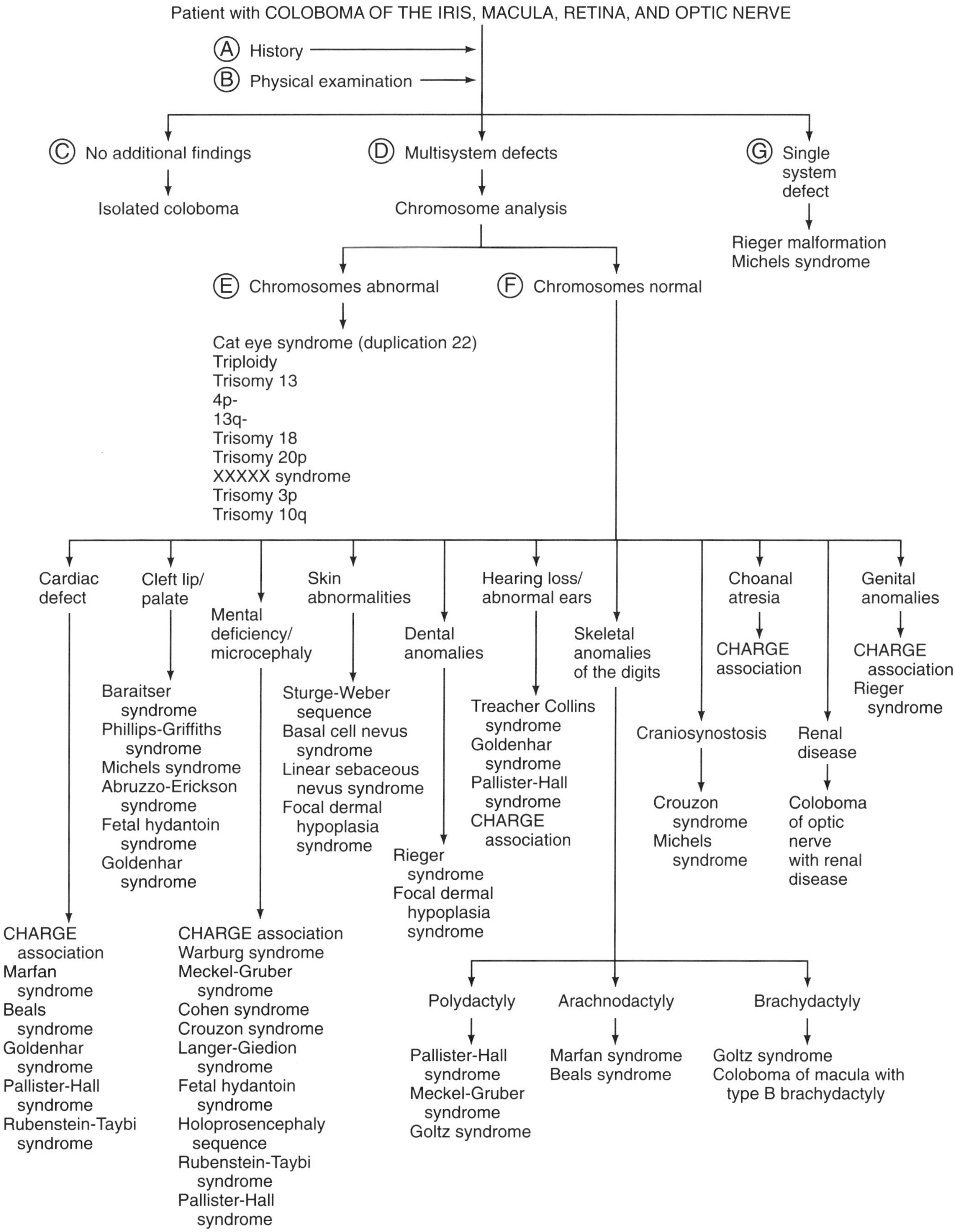
Patient with COLOBOMA OF THE IRIS, MACULA, RETINA, AND OPTIC NERVE
(A) History
(B) Physical examination
(C) No additional findings
Isolated coloboma
(D) Multisystem defects
Chromosome analysis
(G) Single system defect
Rieger malformation
Michels syndrome
(E) Chromosomes abnormal
Cat eye syndrome (duplication 22)
Triploidy
Trisomy 13
4p-
13q-
Trisomy 18
Trisomy 20p
XXXXX syndrome
Trisomy 3p
Trisomy 10q
(F) Chromosomes normal
Cardiac defect
CHARGE association
Marfan syndrome
Beals syndrome
Goldenhar syndrome
Pallister-Hall syndrome
Rubenstein-Taybi syndrome
Cleft lip/ palate
Baraitser syndrome
Phillips-Griffiths syndrome
Michels syndrome
Abruzzo-Erickson syndrome
Fetal hydantoin syndrome
Goldenhar syndrome
Mental deficiency/ microcephaly
CHARGE association
Warburg syndrome
Meckel-Gruber syndrome
Cohen syndrome
Crouzon syndrome
Langer-Giedion syndrome
Fetal hydantoin syndrome
Holoprosencephaly sequence
Rubenstein-Taybi syndrome
Pallister-Hall syndrome
Skin abnormalities
Sturge-Weber sequence
Basal cell nevus syndrome
Linear sebaceous nevus syndrome
Focal dermal hypoplasia syndrome
Dental anomalies
Rieger syndrome
Focal dermal hypoplasia syndrome
Hearing loss/ abnormal ears
Treacher Collins syndrome
Goldenhar syndrome
Pallister-Hall syndrome
CHARGE association
Skeletal anomalies of the digits
Polydactyly
Pallister-Hall syndrome
Meckel-Gruber syndrome
Goltz syndrome
Arachnodactyly
Marfan syndrome
Beals syndrome
Brachydactyly
Goltz syndrome
Coloboma of macula with type B brachydactyly
Craniosynostosis
Crouzon syndrome
Michels syndrome
Choanal atresia
CHARGE association
Renal disease
Coloboma of optic nerve with renal disease
Genital anomalies
CHARGE association
Rieger syndrome

CYTOGENETICS

Barbara K. Hecht, Ph.D.
Frederick Hecht, M.D.

This chapter relates to the laboratory science of cytogenetics, in which chromosomes are visually examined through the microscope. This is a key area in genetics, particularly as it pertains to dysmorphology and mental retardation.

A. The general medical history and physical examination are essential to evaluating the patient and should be provided by the referring pediatrician or family physician to the ophthalmologist.

B. The family history (p 2) is the ubiquitous tool in clinical genetics. This history should be recorded in pedigree form using the international code of squares (for males), circles (for females), and diamonds (sex unspecified), and should minimally contain three generations (children, parents, and grandparents).

C. The history and examination of the eyes, face, and head can be done by the ophthalmologist. The ophthalmologist is in a unique position to evaluate the face and head. Pertinent areas include the forehead, eyebrows, eyelashes, nose, midface, philtrum (between the nose and upper lip), lips, chin, ears, and head shape and size.

D. No notable findings may be present. Parents of such children still need the reassurance and continuing concern of their child's primary doctor and ophthalmologist.

E. An isolated defect may be found such as strabismus or a refractive error in the absence of abnormalities beyond these treatable entities. Parents should be effectively educated and reassured.

F. Multisystem defects require further evaluation. This should include consideration of chromosome studies.

G. A lymphocyte chromosome study should be ordered in children with multisystem defects and/or a personal or family history of developmental delay or mental retardation. This test is the entry-level chromosome study and requires a small sample of blood. The test can be ordered from a qualified chromosome laboratory. The chromosomes should always be banded at least at the 400-band stage.

H. A positive lymphocyte chromosome study can, for example, confirm trisomy 21 (Down syndrome) or establish the diagnosis of more severe conditions such as the trisomy 18 or 13 syndromes.

I. A family chromosome study is triggered by abnormal chromosome findings in the patient. Ideally, at least the parents and/or siblings should have chromosome

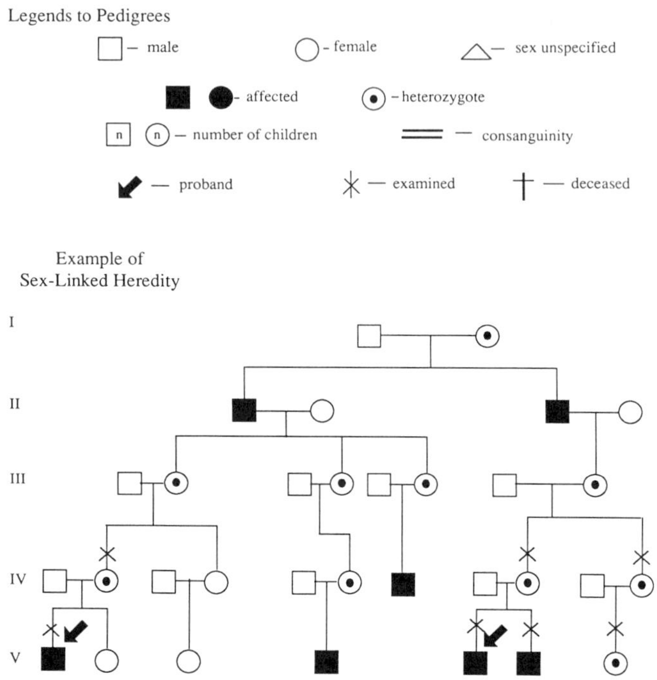

Figure 1 Pedigree chart for sex-linked hereditary condition.

TABLE 1 Examples of Autosomal Chromosome Abnormalities

Trisomies
- Trisomy 21 (Down syndrome)
- Trisomy 18 (Edwards syndrome)
- Trisomy 13 (Patau syndrome)

Deletions
- Deletion 4p (Wolf-Hirschorn syndrome)
- Deletion 5p (cat cry syndrome)
- Deletion 11p (aniridia–Wilms' tumor syndrome)
- Deletion 13q (retinoblastoma–mental retardation syndrome, p 132)

Duplications
- Duplication (or mosaic trisomy) 8
- Duplication (or mosaic trisomy) 9
- Duplication 22q (cat eye syndrome)

Sex chromosome anomalies
- 45,X (Turner syndrome)
- 47,XXX (triple-X syndrome)
- 47,XXY (Klinefelter syndrome)

Fragile X chromosome syndrome (p 130)

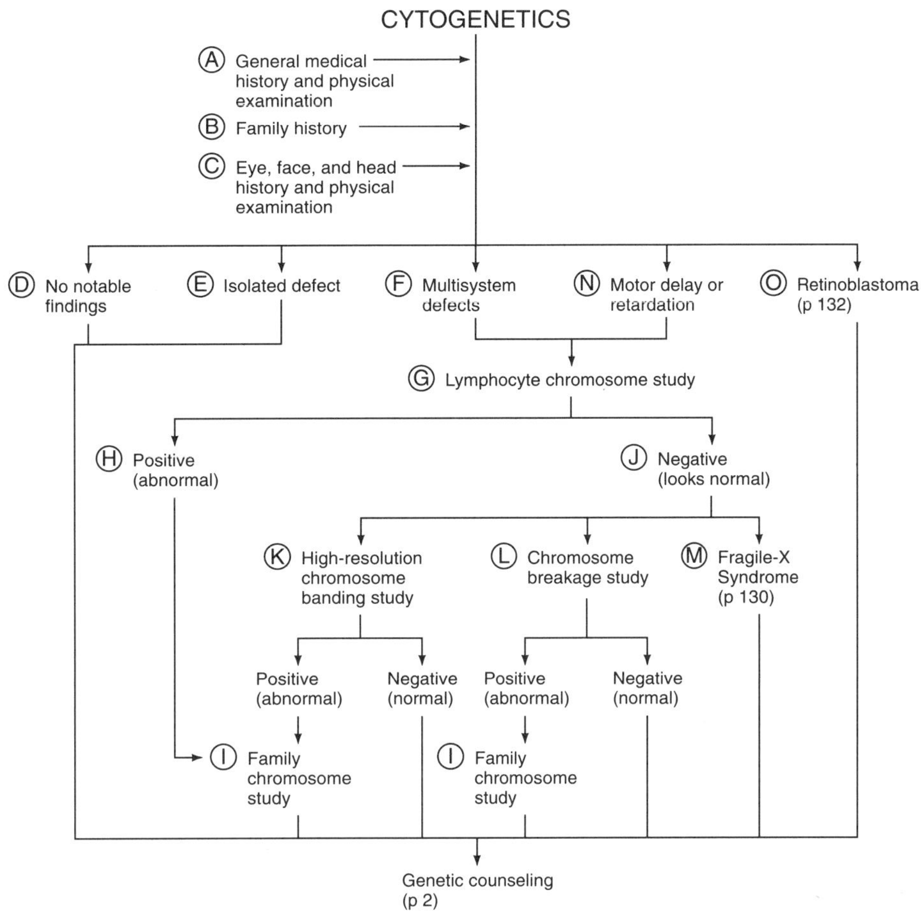

studies, but whether the costs will be borne by third-party medical insurers or the family may influence the decision. Genetic counseling (p 2) should be done to inform the family of the laboratory findings and to explain their consequences.

J. A negative lymphocyte chromosome result can reflect a truly normal karyotype or simply look, but not be, normal. If one seriously suspects a chromosome abnormality, further testing must be done. These additional cytogenetic tests are high-resolution chromosome banding, chromosome breakage studies, and special fragile-X chromosome assays.

K. A high-resolution chromosome banding study involves focused analysis of chromosomes in anaphase and prometaphase (i.e., at early, less condensed stages) to analyze the karyotype at approximately the 800 to 850 band level. Providing the laboratory with a list of the specific clinical findings permits the laboratory to focus on specific areas of the karyotype, the aim being to detect very small deletions, duplications, and other rearrangements.

L. A chromosome breakage study should be ordered if a chromosome instability syndrome such as ataxia-telangiectasia, Bloom syndrome, Fanconi anemia syndrome, or xeroderma pigmentosum is suspected.

M. The fragile X syndrome is the most common heritable cause of developmental delay and mental retardation. It requires special chromosome and/or molecular genetic testing (p 126).

N. Motor delay or mental retardation calls for additional evaluation of the child, including chromosome studies. It is essential that the referring physician and ophthalmologist be alert to developmental delay in infants and, later in childhood, to mental retardation.

O. Retinoblastoma should initiate a special work-up.

References

Gardner RJM, Sutherland GR. Chromosome abnormalities and genetic counseling. New York: Oxford University Press, 1989.

Jones KL. Smith's recognizable patterns of human malformation. Philadelphia: WB Saunders, 1988.

Sutherland, GR, Hecht F. Fragile sites on human chromosomes. New York: Oxford University Press, 1985.

MOLECULAR GENETICS

Barbara K. Hecht, Ph.D.
Frederick Hecht, M.D.

Molecular genetics is the basis for molecular medicine: the detection and diagnosis of diseases at the level of DNA and RNA. This discussion concentrates on DNA.

A. DNA can be isolated from any nucleated cell. Once it has been extracted from the cell, DNA is relatively stable. If DNA is stored under appropriate conditions, it can be banked for an indefinite length of time.

B. Traditional chromosome disorders are due to gross abnormalities easily detected under the ordinary light microscope (p 124). The parental origin of these chromosome anomalies can be determined by chromosome differences called chromosome polymorphisms or by molecular analysis using DNA polymorphisms.

C. Contiguous gene syndromes are intermediate between the traditional chromosome disorders and submicroscopic mutations and are due to deletion (loss), duplication (gain), or other rearrangements of DNA containing two or more contiguous genes. Contiguous gene syndromes are difficult or impossible to detect at the level of the microscope. Molecular analysis can confirm the existence of the contiguous gene syndrome and determine the extent of the DNA lesion. This is done by using direct DNA probes (DNA sequences that detect complementary sequences by molecular hybridization) aimed right at the suspect chromosome region. Among the contiguous gene syndromes is that described by Langer and Giedion. It is the trichorhinophalangeal syndrome with multiple bony exostoses and is associated with bushy eyebrows and deep-set eyes. The Langer-Giedion syndrome is due to a deletion in band 8q24. Cytogenetics and molecular genetics laboratories should focus on this region with high-resolution analysis and DNA probes. The Prader-Willi syndrome involves chromosome 15, as does the Angelman syndrome. The different clinical outcome may be due to imprinting, the differential expression of genetic material transmitted by the father versus the mother. If the deleted chromosome 15 is from the father, the patient has the Prader-Willi syndrome with almond-shaped, upslanting palpebral fissures and obesity due to binge eating. Even before the obesity is evident, the baby is hypotonic and has small hands and feet. Conversely, if the deleted chromosome 15 is from the mother, the child presents with Angelman "happy puppet" syndrome characterized by severe developmental delay, puppet-like gait, paroxysmal laughter, and hypopigmentation of the iris and choroid.

D. All information from molecular genetic testing should be conveyed to the patient and, in the case of a child, to his or her family.

E. Genetic disorders include autosomal dominant disorders (e.g., Marfan syndrome), autosomal recessive disorders (e.g., homocystinuria), X-linked conditions (e.g., choroideremia), and multifactorial disorders (e.g., myopia). Multifactorial disorders are not yet amenable to molecular analysis.

F. Linkage analysis is done to calculate the probability that a person carries a specific disease gene. Linkage studies for diagnosis are usually done when the disease gene has not been identified, different mutations are not yet known, and molecular probes directed to the gene itself are not yet available.

G. Because disease genes can follow different patterns of inheritance, a precise pedigree of the patient's family which identifies all affected individuals must be prepared. The patient's clinical findings must be well documented and an accurate diagnosis made. The general chromosomal location of the disease gene must also be known. Restriction fragment length polymorphisms (RFLPs) are normal heritable variations in DNA sequences detectable by restriction endonuclease enzymes that recognize specific sequences within the DNA and then cut (restrict) the DNA at these sites. Everyone has RFLPs within their genome, some between genes and some within genes. To be useful for linkage studies, an RFLP must be polymorphic (producing pieces of DNA of different sizes in different people), and it must be close to or actually within the disease gene (see below).

Family studies are the essence of linkage analysis. To do linkage studies, there must be at least one individual with the disease who carries the corresponding disease gene. Several generations of the patient's family must be tested. All family relationships, including parentage, must be established.

Probabilities are the result of linkage studies. If a disease gene is segregating in a family and the gene is close to a particular RFLP, so that they travel together as a package 95% of the time, from family linkage studies it can be stated that a given person has (or does not have) the disease gene with a probability of 95%. Linkage studies never yield an unequivocal answer but provide a probability estimate helpful in genetic diagnosis and counseling.

H. Direct molecular analysis is possible if a specific gene has been localized and the base sequence of at least part of the gene is known. Probes directed to a particular DNA sequence are then used to decide whether the gene is "normal" or contains a mutation that corresponds to a specific genetic disease. Direct diagnosis can also involve the sequencing of the DNA within the gene. Testing with direct molecular diagnosis may be restricted to a single individual, unlike the family studies required for linkage analysis. The polymerase chain reaction (PCR) has facilitated direct diagnosis. A short DNA sequence can be replicated and amplified a million times with PCR, permitting analysis of a short DNA sequence from very small quantities of DNA. DNA can now be analyzed from a

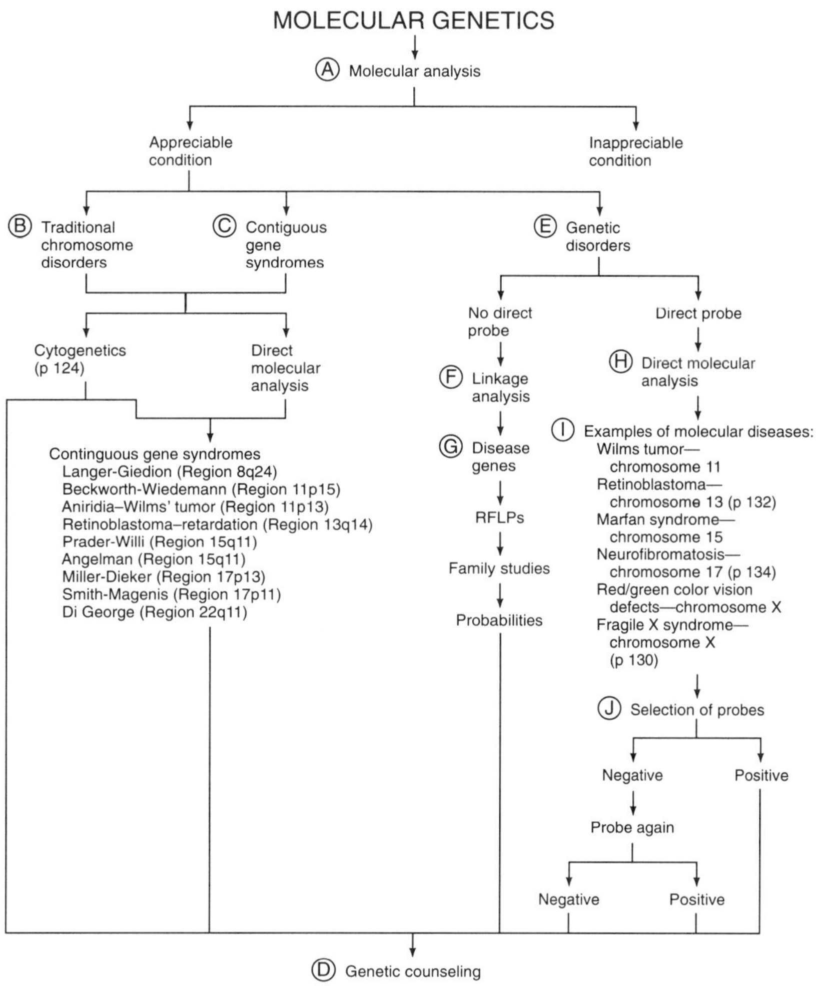

single cell, irrespective of whether that cell is a single egg or sperm or an ordinary somatic cell.

I. The number of genetic disorders amenable to direct DNA diagnosis increases every day, so one should contact a genetic clinic or laboratory for the current status of a specific diagnostic test.

J. Direct DNA testing can be positive or negative. A positive result indicates that the patient is carrying a specific mutation. A negative result can mean that a mutation is absent or that no mutation was identified with the probes used. A decision has to be made as to which probes and how many to use in testing for each genetic disorder. A single mutation can account for all or a high proportion of cases of a particular disorder so that use of a single probe is informative. However, for many single-gene disorders there are different mutations that cause the same clinical disease, and these different mutations can occur at different frequencies within different ethnic groups. In the search for the mutation, the laboratory may have to employ a number of probes, first using the most informative probes, then decreasingly informative probes. Issues of cost effectiveness become relevant. If the laboratory test results are negative, the final report should include a list of mutations analyzed, the percentage of individuals estimated to carry these mutations within different populations, and the probability that the patient is, in fact, a mutation carrier who was simply not detected by the testing performed. Additional molecular testing can be undertaken by a different laboratory which uses other probes specific for rarer mutations. As methods for sequencing become more efficient and cost effective, it may be possible to sequence each and every disease gene in order to identify any and all mutations. With the difficulty of sequencing and producing probes for larger genes, indirect or linkage analysis may still be appropriate for diagnosis if the direct DNA results are uninformative. The patient can be retested at a later date when more is known about the gene in question and when new probes are available.

References

Goodman RM, Gorlin RJ. The malformed infant and child. An illustrated guide. New York: Oxford University Press, 1983.

Jones KL. Smith's recognizable patterns of human malformation. Philadelphia: WB Saunders, 1988.

McKusick VA. Mendelian inheritance in man. Catalog of autosomal dominant, autosomal recessive and X-linked phenotypes. 9th ed. Baltimore: The Johns Hopkins University Press, 1990.

Weatherall DJ. The new genetics and clinical practice. New York: Oxford University Press, 1991.

ALBINISM

Karen S. Shimshak, M.D.

A. Albinism is a group of genetic disorders with congenital hypopigmentation of skin, hair, and eyes (oculocutaneous albinism) or eyes only (ocular albinism). Reduced vision, nystagmus, photophobia, iris transillumination with foveal hypoplasia, and hypopigmentation are present. This results from an absence or deficiency of melanin production due to an abnormality of the enzyme tyrosinase. Optic nerve fibers decussate abnormally at the chiasm, this is reflected in their visual evoked response (VER). Abnormalities of the lateral geniculate body and geniculocortical tracts are present. Binocular stereoscopic vision and electrophysiologic tests of the eye are abnormal (pp 294, 296, 298). Strabismus and high refractive errors occur frequently (90%).

B. Oculocutaneous albinism (OCA) has autosomal recessive transmission. Pigmentation of skin, hair, and eyes is absent to poor. Certain forms of OCA may have systemic abnormalities with important clinical implications. OCA is subdivided into 10 forms based upon clinical findings and the hairbulb incubation test for tyrosinase activity.

C. Autosomal-dominant OCA is rare. Patients have blond hair, hazel eyes, typical findings of ocular albinism, and reduced acuity of 20/60.

D. In tyrosinase-negative OCA (TNOCA), one of the most common forms, melanin formation is absent. Patients have white hair and skin throughout life. The iris is translucent, giving a pink red reflex to the eye. Patients develop nystagmus in the first few months of life, which may lessen with age. Photophobia is severe. Visual acuity is 20/200 or less.

E. Yellow mutant OCA (YMOCA), an allele of the TNOCA locus, is seen in Amish, blacks, Ceylonese, and British whites. Skin biopsy shows premelanosomes. Hair and skin are white at birth. Skin pigmentation develops early with yellowing of the hair. Nystagmus, photophobia, and poor vision may be severe and may improve with age.

F. Tyrosinase-positive OCA (TPOCA), the second most common form, is the most common form seen in blacks. Skin biopsy shows dense premelanosome and melanosome complexes within the melanocyte. Skin pigmentation varies with ethnic origin. Clinical expression varies as indistinguishable from TNOCA to those with blue to brown eyes, blond hair, and ability to tan. Typical patients have yellow hair, lightly pigmented skin, mild photophobia, and nystagmus.

G. Chediak-Higashi syndrome has variable pigmentation, bleeding diathesis, increased incidence of pyogenic infection, and early death. Skin biopsy shows macromelanosomes, giant melanosomes, and polyphagosomes. Patients may be mentally retarded with generalized lymphadenopathy. Skin pigmentation is patchy with light brown hair and hazel to brown irides. Vision is poor with the stigmata of OCA. The diagnosis is confirmed by the presence of giant cytoplasmic granules within the leukocytes (the Chediak anomaly).

H. Hermansky-Pudlak syndrome is a triad of OCA, a bleeding diathesis, and ceroid-like accumulation in the body causing interstitial pulmonary fibrosis, inflammatory bowel disease, renal failure, or cardiomyopathy. Bleeding time is prolonged owing to decreased platelet aggregation. Tyrosinase activity is weak, with giant melanosomes on skin biopsy. The bleeding tendency can be fatal after minor surgery, trauma, or aspirin ingestion.

I. Minimal pigment OCA, rare and clinically similar to YMOCA, may be an allelic form of the TNOCA gene. Skin biopsy shows normal melanocytes with variable premelanosome pigmentation. Patients are born with snow white hair and blue irides.

J. Brown OCA, described in Nigerian blacks, manifests light-brown skin and hair with blue or light brown irides. Vision ranges from 20/60 to 20/100.

K. Cross syndrome is seen in the Amish. They have blond hair, white skin, mental retardation, and microphthalmos with corneal clouding.

L. Red OCA occurs in the "red-skinned natives" of Papua New Guinea with brown-red skin and hair. Irides and fundi have a reddish brown discoloration. Mild nystagmus and photophobia are present with minimally reduced vision.

M. The black locks, OCA, and sensorineural deafness syndrome (BADS) patients have patchy pigmentation of the skin and hair (black and white), heterochromic irides with severe sensorineural hearing loss, and nystagmus with poor vision. Skin biopsy shows amelanotic areas interspersed with normally pigmented zones.

N. Clinical findings in ocular albinism (OA) are predominantly ocular with normal-appearing skin. However, skin biopsy of both affected and carrier females shows abnormal pigment ultrastructure in the form of macromelanosomes. In blacks there may be no iris transillumination. The VER is an excellent way to decide clearly whether a questionable case is or is not albinotic.

O. Ocular albinism (Nettleship-Falls, XLOA) is X-linked recessive. Skin biopsy shows macromelanosomes. Eyes have translucent blue irides, pale fundi, foveal hypoplasia, nystagmus, photophobia, and poor vision. Strabismus and high refractive errors are common. Patients may develop brown irides and good vision. Female carriers have iris transillumination with patchy (mosaic) fundus pigmentation. Some female carriers appear to be heterozygotes with nystagmus, poor vision, and iris and fundus findings.

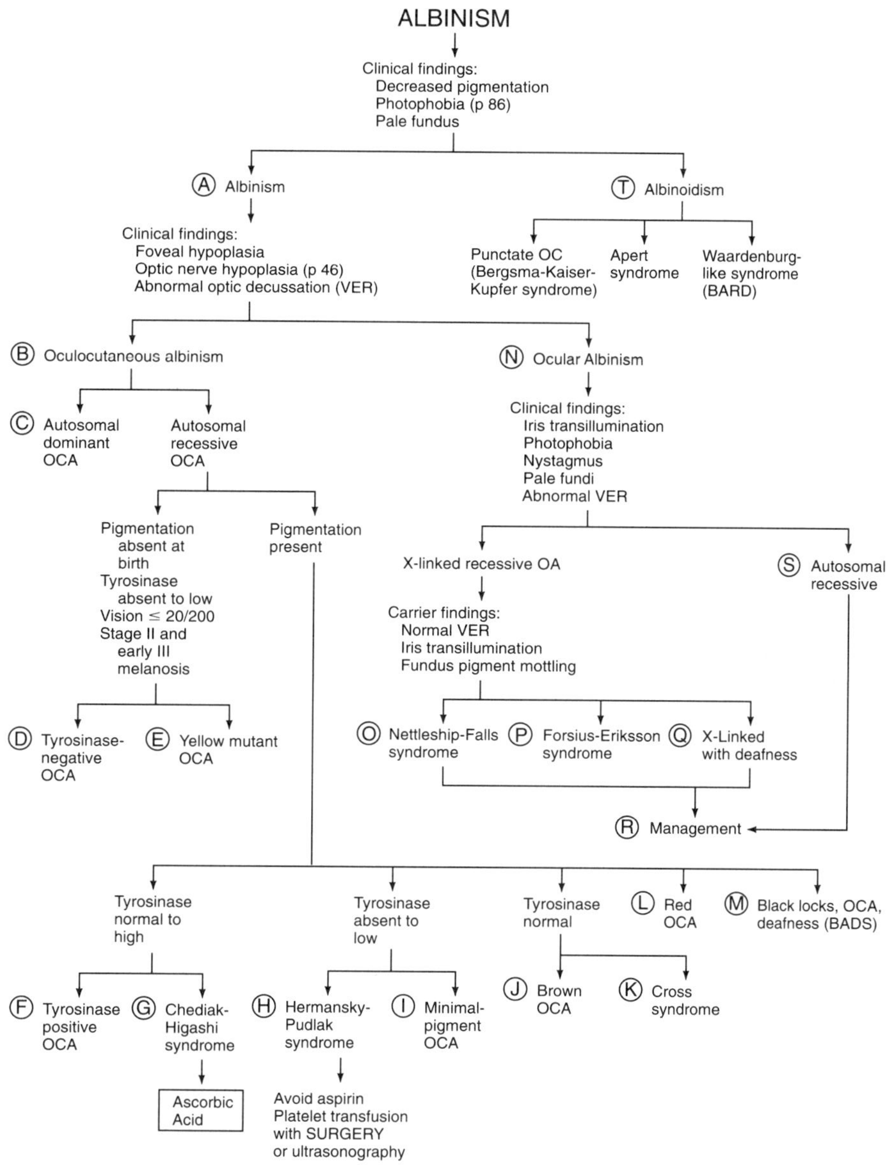

P. Forsius-Eriksson OA has findings of XLOA. Tyrosinase test is positive with regular melanosomes and normal optic pathways. Female carriers are normal.

Q. XLOA with late-onset sensorineural deafness is described in a white South African family with hearing loss in the fifth decade.

R. Patients with albinism are best managed with tinted amber (10% transmission) and dark amber (2% transmission) sunglasses, surgery for strabismus or head turn, protection from sun exposure, and genetic counseling. When young, albinos inevitably are able to hold things close enough that they prefer not to use low vision aids. With time this changes and magnifiers for reading are practical, along with hand-held telescopes for distance vision. The head bob and nystagmus make use of magnifying devices difficult. When myopic, patients prefer to go uncorrected, as the glasses make little difference for distance and they lose the built-in magnifying effect of their myopia for near. Maximum plus (+5 diopters) bifocals are useful.

S. Patients with autosomal recessive ocular albinism have the features of ocular albinism. Skin biopsy shows normal melanosomes.

T. Albinoidism is hypopigmentation of the skin, hair, and eyes in the absence of nystagmus, photophobia, and foveal hypoplasia. Vision is normal. Autosomal dominant transmission is described.

References

Ai E, Coonan P. Disorders of amino acid metabolism. In: Gold DH, Weingeist TA, ed. The eye in systemic disease. Philadelphia: JB Lippincott, 1990:311.

Broodbakker JTW, Westerhof W, Van Dorp DB. Ultrastructure of the skin of human albinos. Ophthalmic Paediatr Genet 1983; 2:95.

Creel DJ, Summers GC, King RA. Visual anomalies associated with albinism. Ophthalmic Paediatr Genet 1990; 11:193.

Jimenez-Sierra JM. Inherited retinal diseases: A diagnostic guide. St. Louis: CV Mosby, 1989:100.

Merlin S. Inherited eye diseases: Diagnosis and clinical management. New York: Marcel Dekker, 1991:480.

THE FRAGILE-X SYNDROME: UNSTABLE DNA

Barbara K. Hecht, Ph.D.
Frederick Hecht, M.D.

The fragile-X syndrome has emerged as the most common heritable cause of mental retardation. It affects approximately 1 in 1000 boys and fewer girls. (Down syndrome is more common but it is usually sporadic.)

A. The clinical picture is, at first glance, nonspecific developmental delay in infancy and mental retardation later in childhood. Boys are rather severely retarded, whereas girls are more mildly delayed. The child may present to the ophthalmologist (and audiologist) with the parents questioning whether the child can see (and hear) normally. The answer generally is yes.

The head circumference tends to be large, and the child on the big side. Seizure disorders are a known complication. It has been argued, perhaps rightly, that the irides may be lighter in color than usual. The ears are definitely large, with a tendency to be longer than normal. In later childhood the face is long with a moderately prominent jaw. There also tends in time to be a connective tissue disturbance with mitral valve prolapse, long digits, hyperflexible joints, and flat feet. Macro-orchidism (large testes) occurs in about one-quarter of preadolescent and a much higher proportion of postadolescent boys. The behavior is characteristically very troublesome, with hyperactivity and schizoid outbursts, and presents endless problems for the parents, teachers, and doctors.

B. The family history should be taken with care (p 2). The pattern of inheritance one is looking for is X-linked, with males affected by retardation and females acting as carriers. Female carriers can be normal or mildly mentally retarded. (Phenotypically normal male carriers are known but are distinctly in the minority.)

One may find a positive family history, with the fragile X segregating much as would hemophilia or Duchenne muscular dystrophy. Or one may encounter a seemingly negative family history.

C. Laboratory tests are required if any suspicion of the fragile-X syndrome arises based on clinical acumen or family history. There are a number of ways to proceed with laboratory tests;
   1. Cytogenetics only—the traditional way
   2. Cytogenetics + linkage—the next approach
   3. Cytogenetics + linkage + DNA probes—the newest triad
   4. Cytogenetics + DNA probes—currently in vogue
   5. DNA probes only—assuredly the future

D. Cytogenetics (p 124) is still prerequisite at the time of this writing. The fragile site is on the X chromosome in band q27.3, where it manifests most often by gaps in the continuity of the chromosome, less often by frank breaks in the chromosome, and least commonly by so-called polyradial formations. These cytogenetic manifestations are visible through the light microscope in lymphocytes (and other cells) grown in the laboratory in culture media deficient in folic acid and thymidine or to which methotrexate or 5-fluorodeoxyuridine has been added.

E. Molecular genetics studies (p 126) are the wave of the present and future with the fragile X. Linkage analysis relies on nearby DNA markers, usually restriction fragment length polymorphisms (pp 124, 126), and provides a probability estimate of fragile X versus nonfragile X. Direct DNA analysis of the fragile-X gene has yielded startling information:
   1. The fragile-X gene consists of unstable DNA.
   2. This unstable DNA involves a repeating sequence.
   3. This repeat is cytidine cytidine guanosine (CCG).
   4. This repeat can get longer with each succeeding generation in a family.
   5. The length of the repeating CCG can vary between siblings and even within different cell populations in a person.
   6. The longer the CCG repeating sequence, the more severe the clinical phenotype.
   7. The elongation of the CCG repeating sequence provides a biologic basis for anticipation—progressively earlier appearance and greater severity of a genetic disease in successive generations.

A similar molecular mechanism appears to account for myotonic dystrophy, X-linked spinal and bulbar atrophy, and, in all likelihood, a number of other genetic disorders. Unstable DNA is a dramatic new molecular genetic phenomenon, not new in nature but new in understanding its behavior.

F. Genetic counseling for the fragile-X syndrome is crucial, can be complex, and should be done in consultation with a genetics center.

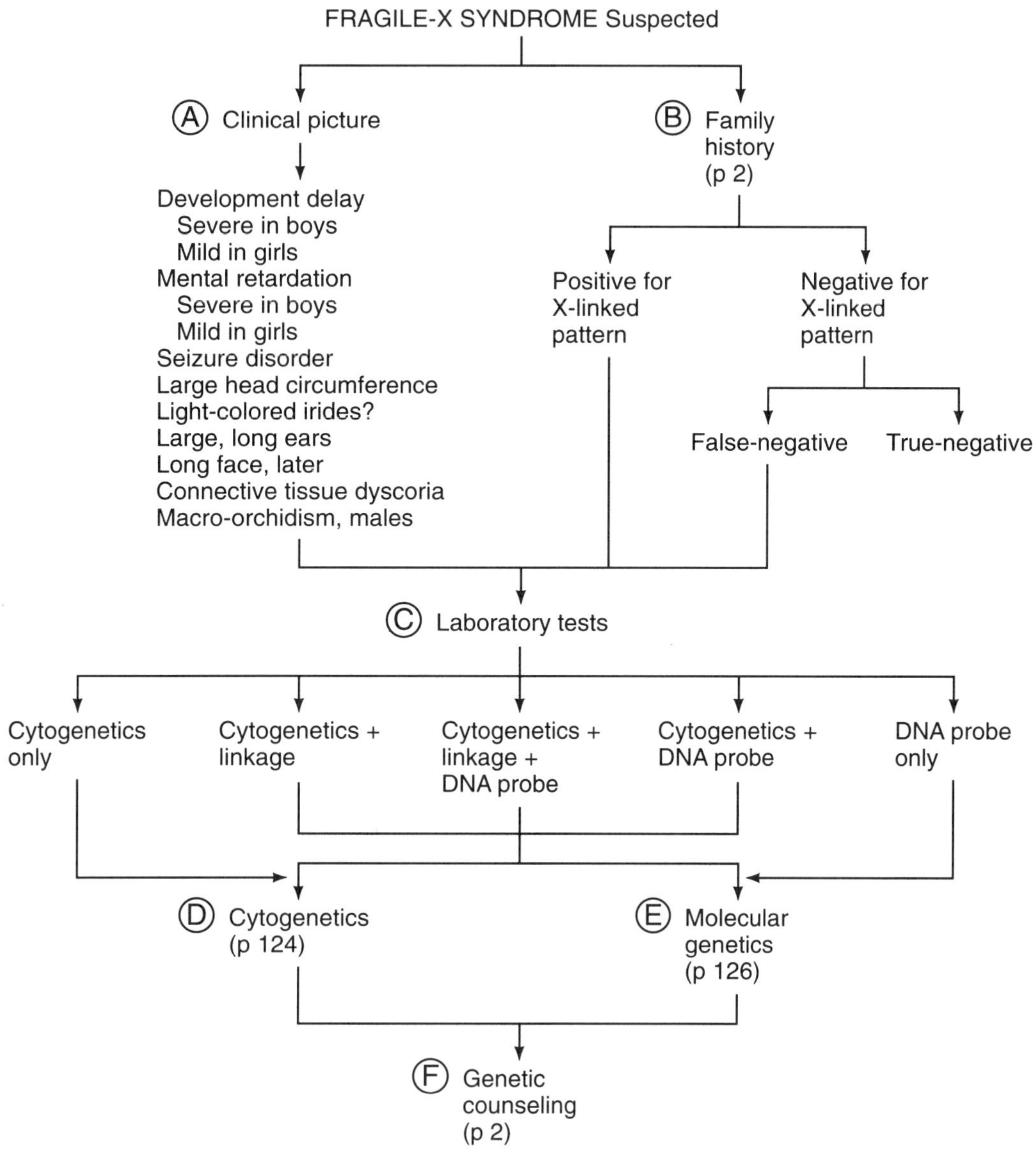

References

Pergolizzi RG, Erster SH, Goonewardena P, Brown WT. Detection of full fragile X mutation. Lancet 1992; 339:271.

Rousseau F, Heitz D, Biancalana V, et al. Direct diagnosis by DNA analysis of the fragile X syndrome of mental retardation. N Engl J Med 1991; 325:1673.

Sutherland GR, Gedeon A, Kornman L, et al. Prenatal diagnosis of fragile X syndrome by direct detection of the unstable DNA sequence. N Engl J Med 1991, 325:1720.

Sutherland GR, Hecht F. Fragile sites on human chromosomes. New York: Oxford University Press, 1985.

Sutherland GR, Hecht F. Unstable DNA. The fragile X chromosome and myotonic dystrophy (tentative title). New York: Oxford University Press, 1993.

RETINOBLASTOMA

A. Linn Murphree, M.D.
Gerhard W. Cibis, M.D.

A. Leukocoria is the most common clinical finding bringing retinoblastoma (RB) patients to ophthalmologists. Other clinical findings are less common as the presenting sign. Strabismus occurs with decreased vision from tumor. RB may mimic other presenting disorders such as posterior uveitis, preseptal or orbital cellulitis, spontaneous hyphema, or vitreous hemorrhage.

B. Inquire about family history of RB. If no specific RB history is found, did any family member have an eye enucleated as a child?

C. Childhood retinal detachment without trauma is rare and underlying exophytic RB is suspect. Funduscopy alone may rule out RB. If a question remains, diagnostic tests are encouraged. Fluid drainage to look for suspected RB cells is not advisable, as this may spread tumor into the orbit.

D. Other intraocular masses should be differentiated from RB (see E). Typical RB has a white fish flesh appearance with surface and deep blood vessels visible in the mass lesion. Calcium may not be clinically discernible. Vitreous seeds or satellite lesions are classic for RB. RB cells can remain alive in the vitreous and form balls. The center of these often necrose, as they are furthest from the vitreous nutrients.

E. RB can mimic vitreous hemorrhage, spontaneous hyphema, or posterior uveitis and appear simply as media opacities. Systemic corticosteroids for 3 days can reduce inflammation, providing a better look for classic RB signs or, if it clears the opacification, ruling out RB.

F. CT imaging is most helpful to look for calcium. Ten percent of tumors show no calcium (calcifications need to be at least 2 mm for CT detection). Almost no other intraocular lesion has calcification. *Toxocara* granulomata may calcify. *Toxocara* lesions are hyperintense in T_1 and T_2 images, unlike RB, which is moderately hyperintense on T_1 and hypointense on T_2. CT and MRI can aid in finding extraocular extension of tumor prior to enucleation. MRI gives better resolution of optic nerve involvement and recurrence, both extracranial and intracranial.

G. More problematic are tumors not containing calcium. Other differentials need careful consideration. Usually they are sufficiently characteristic in retinoscopic appearance that lack of calcification confirms a non-RB nature. Persistent hyperplastic primary vitreous is the most common RB-mimicking lesion. Choroidal melanomas are extremely rare in childhood. Leiomyoma and medulloepithelioma occur but arise outside of the retina and are not usually posterior pole lesions. *Toxocara* and astrocytic hamartoma are the most common differential tumors to consider. ELISA (enzyme-linked immunosorbent assay), eosinophil counts, and MRI may assist identification. Brain imaging, genetic consultation, search for appropriate skin lesions, and subungual hamartomas can help establish tuberous sclerosis as the underlying disease with retinal hamartoma.

H. If there is no intraocular mass or calcification and the clinical appearance could be posterior uveitis, consider Coats' disease, endophthalmitis, sarcoidosis, and amyloidosis, which can all mimic an infiltrating flat RB. Strong suspicion for RB, especially if the clinical presentation is atypical, is needed to avoid draining subretinal fluid, doing anterior chamber or vitreous taps, or injecting antibiotics without realizing the underlying RB. These techniques may release tumor cells outside the eye.

I. Enucleate in unilateral cases if there is no hope for vision in the affected eye. External beam radiation (EBR) or radioactive plaque should be considered if vision is preserved in unilateral and bilateral RB. In bilateral cases, the eye with the worse visual prognosis should be enucleated and the remaining eye treated conservatively. With poor bilateral visual potential, external beam radiation or radioactive plaques may preserve some vision. When vision is good, an attempt to save the eye is reasonable. Photocoagulation of small posterior pole lesions and cryotherapy of small peripheral tumors may also be considered. Chemotherapy is used when the tumor has extended outside the eye. Radioactive plaques deliver large doses of radiation to vitreous seeds or very anterior lesions that EBR may not properly reach. Plaques are also useful when maximum EBR has been given and the tumor is still viable. Whenever nonenucleative therapy is used, monitor meticulously and enucleate if the tumor spreads and threatens extraocular invasion. Only if orbital tumor recurs would radiation be done to an anophthalmic socket.

J. Tumor genetics is of great importance. Many cases of RB are associated with a defective RB gene in the consitutional DNA. Most of these present bilaterally. There is a 10% nonpenetrance rate for people having the gene defect with no manifestation of tumor or with spontaneous regression, leaving behind a lesion called a retinoma. A distinction must be made between inherited RB (gene defect inherited from parent) and a new mutation potentially heritable in future generations. For this reason, parents of all children with unilateral and especially bilateral RB need dilated fundus examinations. All bilateral cases automatically are known to be genetic, but some unilateral cases are actually genetic, having the RB gene defect in all somatic cells of the body but manifesting tumor only in one eye.

If the eye is removed, Southern blot DNA analysis can identify and characterize the gene defect in 10% of cases. It is then relatively easy to check for a similar

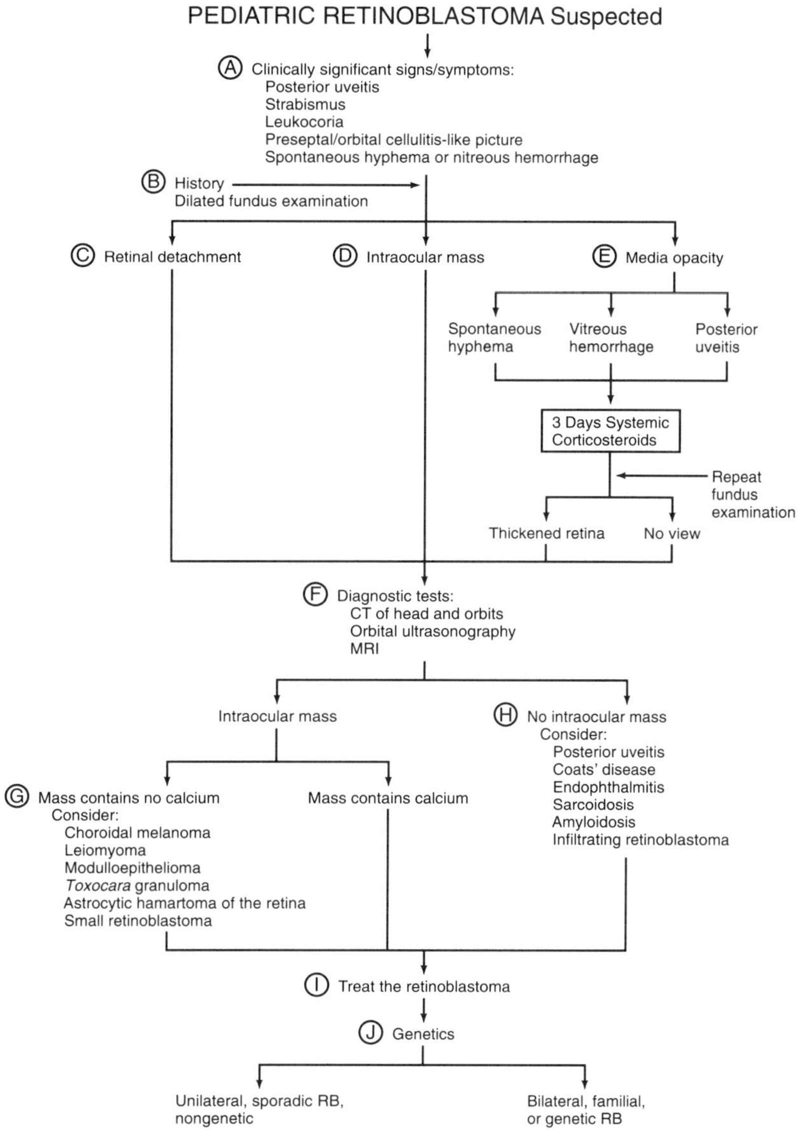

defect in somatic cells (white blood cells are used). It is more difficult to locate and characterize gene defects in all cases. That can be done using nucleotide sequencing but is more resource intensive. All enucleated specimens therefore should be considered for DNA analysis to identify the gene defect, which can then be looked for in white blood cell DNA. If present, parents and other relatives can be similarly screened and properly counseled. If the tumor defect is absent in peripheral blood DNA, the patient's family can be reassured.

Enucleated adults planning to have children need to know genetic risks. Gene defects can be looked for in their systemic cells, but it is often easier to work with the tumor DNA, first establishing the defect and then studying constitutional DNA. This is beginning to be done even on old, fixed specimens on slides or in wax. Defects can also be detected in amniocentesis and chorionic villus specimens. In addition to direct detection, linkage analysis can be used in some cases for prenatal diagnosis and carrier status evaluation.

If a unilateral RB infant does not have the gene defect systemically, clinicians have leeway in scheduling evaluation under anesthesia (EUA). With a systemic defect, there is an 80% likelihood that tumor will develop in the other eye. In enucleated unilateral cases with no knowledge of genetic status, we do an EUA every 3 months up to 3 years old, every 6 months until 5 years old, and annual office examinations thereafter. Patients with unilateral RB, in whom the defect is known not to be systemic can be examined under anesthesia less often, and office visits may suffice.

References

Dryja TP, Mukai S, Petersen R, et al. Parental origin of mutation of the retinoblastoma gene. Nature 1989; 339:556.

Goodrich DW, Lee WH. The molecular genetics of retinoblastoma. Cancer Surveys 1990; 3:529.

Greger V, Passarge E, Hopping W, et al. Epigenetic changes may contribute to the formation and spontaneous regression of retinoblastoma. Hum Genet 1989; 83:155.

NEUROFIBROMATOSES

Stefan-Matthias Pulst, M.D., Dr. med.

The neurofibromatoses (NF) now include at least two genetically and clinically distinct phenotypes. NF1, previously called von Recklinghausen disease, is caused by a mutation on human chromosome 17. NF2, previously called bilateral acoustic neurofibromatosis, is caused by a mutation on chromosome 22. When patients present with typical clinical findings, little overlap exists between the two diseases. The greatest diagnostic difficulty is encountered when a patient presents with multiple cutaneous or CNS tumors. In these patients, at least one tumor should be examined histologically. Neurofibromas and gliomas are typically seen in NF1, whereas schwanomas, meningiomas, and ependymomas typically occur in NF2.

A. Lisch nodules are iris hamartomas. They are clear to brown-colored dome-shaped elevations from the iris. A slit-lamp examination is usually necessary to distinguish them from iris nevi. More than two Lisch nodules are found in more than 90% of individuals over 6 years of age with NF1 and in less than 1% of normal individuals. The incidence is age dependent.

B. The diagnostic criteria for NF1 are met in an individual if two or more of the following are found (some may develop over time):
   1. Six or more café-au-lait spots more than 5 mm in diameter in prepubertal individuals and more than 15 mm in diameter in postpubertal individuals.
   2. Two or more neurofibromas of any type or one plexiform neurofibroma.
   3. Axillary or inguinal freckling.
   4. Optic glioma.
   5. Two or more Lisch nodules (iris hamartomas).
   6. A distinctive osseous lesion such as sphenoid dysplasia or thinning of the long bone cortex with or without pseudarthrosis.
   7. A first-degree relative with NF1 by the above criteria.

C. Posterior subcapsular cataracts are found in more than 40% of patients with NF2. They can be found in individuals as young as 4 years of age and may even be present at birth. Although posterior subcapsular cataracts are the most common type of lens opacity found in NF2, cortical or nuclear cataracts have also been described.

D. NF1 is an autosomal dominant disease with age-dependent penetrance that reaches 100% in adulthood. About 50% of NF1 cases are new mutations. When a patient with NF1 is identified, first-degree relatives should be examined. For NF1 this can usually be accomplished by a physical examination. At times a slit-lamp examination may be necessary.

E. Genetic counseling and regular follow-up visits are important aspects of the care of patients with NF1 and NF2. Prenatal and presymptomatic DNA-based diagnosis is possible in familial cases of NF1 and NF2. Treatment is symptomatic.

F. Involvement of the angle can sometimes be seen in NF1 and is associated with glaucoma. Uveal schwanomas of the retina and glial hamartomas like those in tuberous sclerosis can also be seen. Neurofibromas may be found in the eyelid. Prominent or thickened cranial nerves may be seen.

G. The criteria for NF2 are met by an individual who has:
   1. Bilateral eighth nerve masses seen with the appropriate imaging techniques (CT or MRI), or
   2. A first-degree relative with NF2 and either (a) unilateral eighth nerve mass or (b) two of the following: neurofibroma of any type, meningioma, glioma, schwanoma, juvenile posterior subcapsular lenticular opacity.

H. NF2 is an autosomal dominant disease. The percentage of new mutations causing NF2 is unknown. For the diagnosis of NF2, imaging studies are necessary. MRI with gadolinium enhancement is the most sensitive technique to detect small schwannomas. The spine should be imaged as well because asymptomatic spinal tumors are very common in NF2.

I. The phenotypic spectrum of NF2 may be more varied than the definition in G. NF2 should be considered in cases of multiple CNS tumors, acoustic schwanomas or meningiomas at a young age, or the presence of brain or spinal tumors accompanied by juvenile lens opacities.

References

Kaiser-Kupfer MI, Kupfer C, Pulst SM, et al. The association of posterior capsular lens opacities with bilateral acoustic neurofibromas in patients with neurofibromatosis type 2. Arch Ophthal 1989; 107:541.

Lubs MLE, Bauer M, Formas ME, Djokic B. Iris hamartomas in the diagnosis of neurofibromatosis-1. Pediatr 1990; 5:261.

National Institutes of Health Consensus Development Conference Statement on Neurofibromatosis. Arch Neurol 1988; 45:575.

Pulst SM. Prenatal diagnosis of the neurofibromatoses. In: Clinics in Perinatology. Philadelphia: WB Saunders, 1990:829.

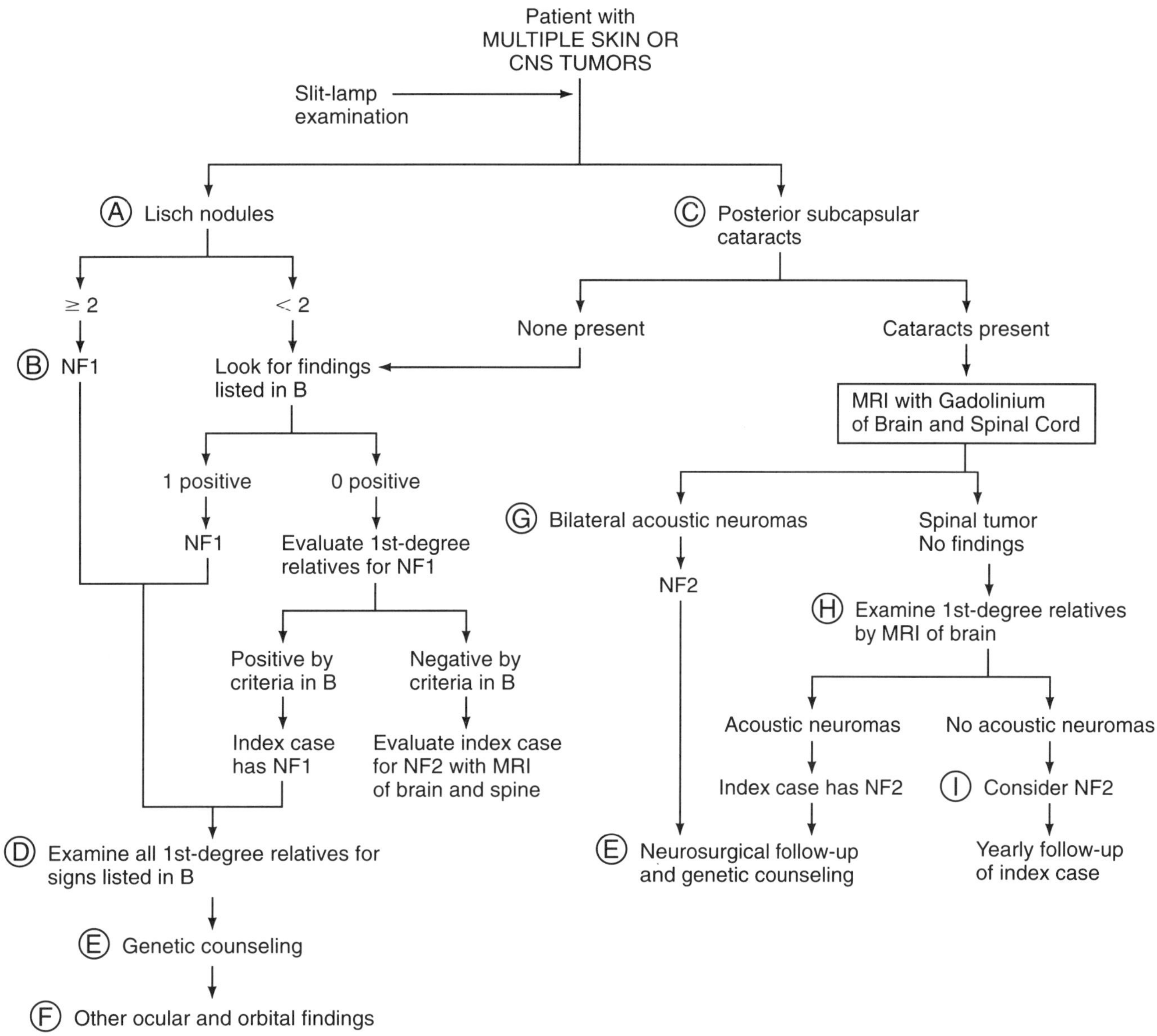
Patient with
MULTIPLE SKIN OR
CNS TUMORS
Slit-lamp
examination
(A) Lisch nodules
≥ 2
< 2
(B) NF1
Look for findings
listed in B
1 positive
0 positive
NF1
Evaluate 1st-degree
relatives for NF1
Positive by
criteria in B
Negative by
criteria in B
Index case
has NF1
Evaluate index case
for NF2 with MRI
of brain and spine
(D) Examine all 1st-degree relatives for
signs listed in B
(E) Genetic counseling
(F) Other ocular and orbital findings
(C) Posterior subcapsular
cataracts
None present
Cataracts present
MRI with Gadolinium
of Brain and Spinal Cord
(G) Bilateral acoustic neuromas
NF2
Spinal tumor
No findings
(H) Examine 1st-degree relatives
by MRI of brain
Acoustic neuromas
No acoustic neuromas
Index case has NF2
(I) Consider NF2
(E) Neurosurgical follow-up
and genetic counseling
Yearly follow-up
of index case

VITREORETINOPATHIES

David M. Brown, M.D.
Thomas A. Weingeist, M.D., Ph.D.

A. Many vitreoretinopathies and some forms of simple myopia are heritable. Family history of retinal detachments, joint pains, cleft palate, and cataracts suggest Stickler syndrome. A family history of early retinal detachments is also common in patients with familial exudative vitreoretinopathy (FEVR). X-linked disorders such as X-linked juvenile retinoschisis, congenital stationary night blindness, and Nettleship-Falls ocular albinism often have positive family histories, particularly when questioned about brothers and maternal uncles. A history of prematurity or neonatal oxygen exposure should be ascertained because of the high incidence of myopia in premature births.

B. Myopia, photophobia, or tearing may be the presenting sign of congenital glaucoma. Progressive enlargement of the globe from high intraocular pressure must be excluded in all infants and children found by retinoscopy to have myopia. Anterior segment examination should exclude corneal enlargement, corneal edema, breaks in Descemet's membrane, and buphthalmos. Retroillumination should exclude transillumination defects in children with myopia, particularly if nystagmus is present. Both Nettleship-Falls X-linked ocular albinism and Äland Island disease may demonstrate moderate to high myopia and diffuse transillumination defects.

C. Poor visual acuity or poor fixation in one or both eyes has important diagnostic and management implications. Unless complicated by retinal detachment or concomitant amblyopia, patients with Stickler syndrome, FEVR, and simple myopia may have relatively good corrected visual acuity. Congenital stationary night blindness, X-linked retinoschisis, and Goldmann-Favre disease may present with decreased central visual acuity. Amblyopia should be considered and treated appropriately with corrective lenses and patching therapy. Myopic anisometropia of 3 diopters or more may be amblyogenic, and corrective lenses should be considered. To prevent ametropic amblyopia, myopic correction should also be considered in children less than 6 months of age with greater than 6 diopters of myopia and in children more than 6 months old who have more than 3 diopters of myopia.

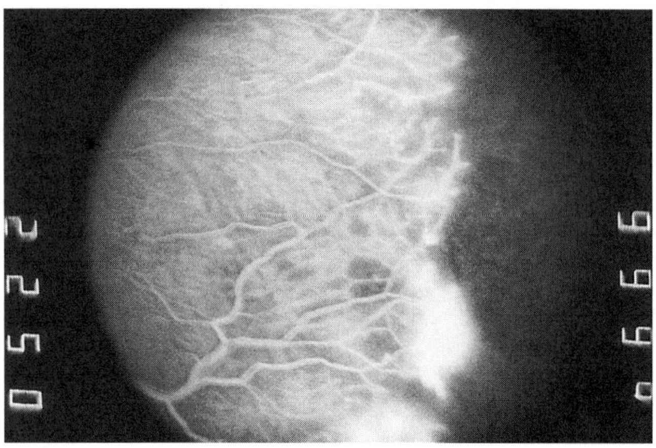

Figure 1 Fluorescein angiogram in familial exudative vitreoretinopathy (FEVR), showing vascular ridge and avascular retina resembling retinopathy of prematurity.

D. Ocular features of Stickler syndrome include high myopia (−8 to −18 diopters) and frequent retinal detachments in the first decade of life. The vitreous appears optically clear with syneretic vitreous strands, vitreous membranes, and veils. Vitreous degeneration can present in the first several months of life, or the vitreous can appear normal into the second decade. The retina often has perivascular pigmentary changes, but bone spicule–like formation is not seen. Chorioretinal degeneration and retinal holes and breaks are prevalent, and complicated retinal detachments occur in up to 50% of affected eyes. Primary open-angle glaucoma and premature cataracts are commonly seen in Stickler syndrome. Systemic manifestations include degenerative changes of the weight-bearing joints and generalized epiphyseal dysplasia. Bone survey radiographs reveal generalized epiphyseal dysplasia of the long bones. Orofacial anomalies such as submucous clefting of the palate and bifid uvula are noted in up to 75% of patients.

E. FEVR resembles retinopathy of prematurity (ROP), but patients have no history of premature birth or antenatal oxygen administration. It is inherited in an autosomal dominant pattern, and the most constant ocular finding is an abrupt cessation of retinal vessels in a scalloped edge at the equator. The avascular area can be quite extensive or confined to only several clock hours. Often an elevated fibrovascular scar in the temporal periphery is present, very similar to the cicatricial stage of ROP. Peripheral neovascularization can be present adjacent to this area, and maturation and organization of the fibrovascular scar produces the striking signs of retinal traction ("dragged disc" and macular heterotopia). Retinal detachments are predominantly tractional in the first decade of life and rhegmatogenous in the second decade. The overall incidence of retinal detachment varies from 4 to 30%. Macular ectopia is present in up to one-half of patients, and resultant positive angle kappa and strabismus are common.

F. Foveal changes and peripheral retinoschisis are seen in both X-linked juvenile retinoschisis (p 300) and Goldmann-Favre syndrome, a very rare autosomal recessive degenerative condition consisting of progressive loss of vision and night blindness due to retinoschisis, progressive cataract, and pigmentary

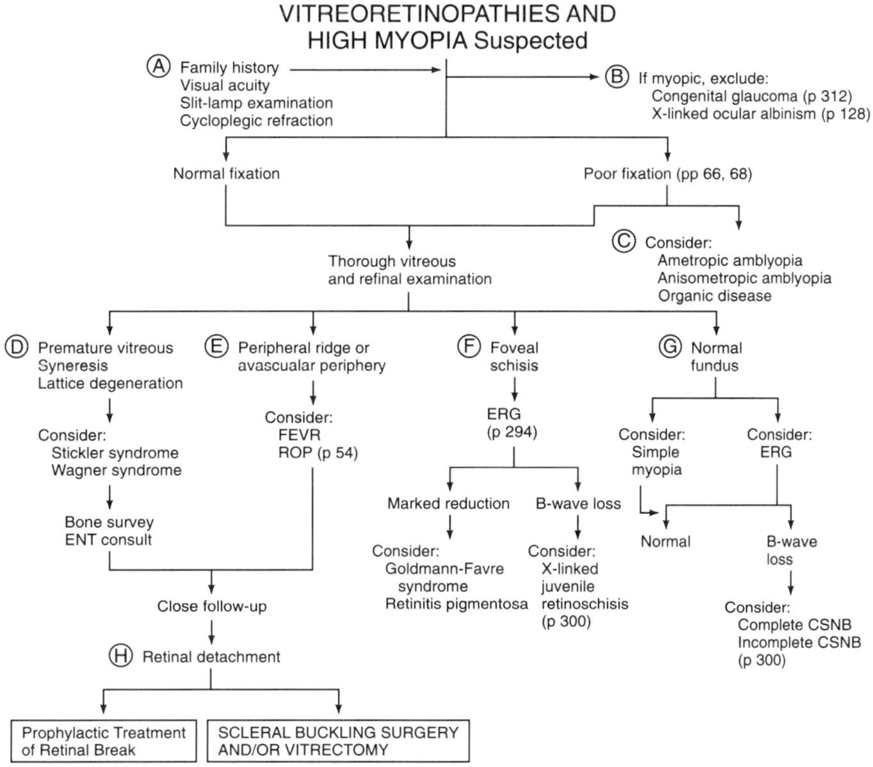

chorioretinal degeneration with bone spicule–like formation. Generally, the central macula has microcystic changes and a "beaten-copper" appearance. Patients with Goldmann-Favre syndrome have nondetectable or strikingly abnormal electroretinographic (ERG) responses. Juvenile X-linked retinoschisis, although relatively rare worldwide, is common in boys of Finnish decent. It is transmitted as an X-linked recessive trait, occurring almost exclusively in males, and is invariably bilateral. The most constant ocular finding is a cystic, stellate maculopathy or foveal schisis, which is present in almost every case and may be the only feature in approximately one-half of cases. Although bilateral inferotemporal retinoschisis has been considered the classic presentation of this disorder, only 40% of patients have peripheral retinoschisis in addition to the macular findings The natural history of the macular changes is rapid progression during the first 5 years of life and then very slow progression until the sixth or seventh decade. Visual loss is generally related to macular involvement, although retinal detachment or vitreous hemorrhage may cause sudden visual loss. ERG in patients with juvenile X-linked retinoschisis typically reveals selective reduction of the B-wave amplitudes. Visual fields are constricted corresponding to areas of involved retina, with absolute scotomas in areas of peripheral retinoschisis. As juvenile X-linked retinoschisis progresses slowly, prophylactic treatment of retinoschisis and holes in schisis cavities is not recommended. Management includes treatment of retinal detachments and vitreous hemorrhages.

G. Normal fundus examinations in the presence of moderate to high myopia may be seen in simple myopia, early Stickler syndrome, and congenital stationary night blindness (CSNB) (p 300). A normal fundus examination and decreased visual acuity are also seen in patients with Leber's congenital amaurosis and achromatopsia, but myopia is infrequent in these entities.

Patients with CSNB generally have normal funduscopic examinations and present with decreased visual acuity and night blindness. CSNB is generally X-linked recessive, although females with autosomal recessive inheritance are reported. Average myopia in complete CSNB is −7.9 diopters, and ERG reveals nonrecordable rod function with a "negative ERG" (amplitude of the A wave is less than that of the B wave.) Dark adaptation shows absent rod adaptation and elevated cone thresholds. Twenty percent of affected patients have nystagmus, and exotropia is present in up to 17%.

H. Patients with Stickler syndrome and familial exudative vitreoretinopathy are at higher risk of developing retinal detachments and should be followed at least semiannually. Peripheral breaks should be treated prophylactically because retinal detachments are common and are often complicated and difficult to repair.

References

Fishman GA, Jampol LM, Goldberg MF. Diagnostic features of the Favre-Goldmann syndrome. Br J Ophthalmol 1976; 60:345.

Forsius H, Krausc U, Helve J, et al. Visual acuity in 183 cases of X-chromosomal retinoschisis. Can J Ophthalmol 1973; 8:385.

van Nouhuys CE. Dominant exudative vitreoretinopathy and other vascular developmental disorders of the peripheral retina. Documenta Ophthalmol 1982; 54:1.

Weingeist TA, Hermsen V, Hanson JW, et al. Ocular and systemic manifestations of Stickler's syndrome: A preliminary report. Birth Defects 1982; 18:539.

STURGE-WEBER SYNDROME

Ramesh C. Tripathi, M.D., Ph.D., F.A.C.S.
Susmitha P. Kolli, B.A.
Brenda J. Tripathi, Ph.D.

A. Sturge-Weber syndrome is a congenital, nonfamilial disease characterized by nevus flammeus that is usually unilateral and limited to the sensory distribution of the trigeminal nerve. Thirty percent of the eyes with the nevus develop glaucoma. Choroidal hemangioma occurs in 40% of the patients and gives the fundus a tomato catsup appearance. Other ocular manifestations of Sturge-Weber syndrome include discoloration of the iris, vascular dilation of the episclera, chamber angle defect, optic disc cupping, and retinal detachment.

Sturge-Weber syndrome manifests as an abnormality of the vasculature of the face, choroid, and meninges. Vascular endothelium is derived from mesodermal mesenchyme. Neural crest cells form the facial dermal connective tissue, choroid of the eye, pia mater, as well as pericytes and smooth muscle cells of the vasculature. A morphogenic error arising in a limited region of the cephalic neural crest and its interaction with mesodermal mesenchyme could partially explain the clinical findings. Glaucoma results from two main factors: anomalous angle development in early-onset cases, and blockage of trabecular meshwork–Schlemm's canal system in late-onset cases. The rise in intraocular pressure (IOP) could result from (1) increased vascularity of the iris, (2) occlusion of angle with anterior synechiae, (3) elevated episcleral pressure, and/or (4) increased permeability of thin-walled vessels in choroidal hemangioma.

Variants of Sturge-Weber syndrome include Jahnke syndrome (nevus flammeus) without glaucoma, Schirmer syndrome with buphthalmos, Lawford syndrome with late-onset glaucoma but without buphthalmos, and Mille syndrome with choroidal hemangioma in the absence of glaucoma.

B. Corneal clouding and buphthalmos are the most common signs in children under the age of 2 years with glaucoma. Elevated IOP leads to enlargement of the cornea as well as the posterior portion of the globe, which in turn causes breaks in Descemet's membrane and a compromise in the corneal endothelial barrier that results in clouding of the cornea. Among patients with congenital glaucoma, 60% manifest it early enough (prior to 2 years of age) to develop unilateral hydrophthalmos. The congenital glaucoma is often associated with the nevus that involves the upper eye lid. The glaucoma may be bilateral if the nevus crosses the midline. Bilateral nevus flammeus with bilateral hydrophthalmos is rare but is reported in cases of Klippel-Trenaunay syndrome, a variant of Sturge-Weber syndrome.

Bilateral hydrophthalmos is more common in certain syndromes and unilateral hydrophthalmos in others, but there are exceptions. Syndromes that result in bilateral congenital glaucoma include aniridia, anomalous superficial iris vessels, Axenfeld anomaly, Rieger anomaly, Peters anomaly, Rubenstein-Taybi syndrome, and retinopathy of prematurity. The incidence of unilateral versus bilateral glaucoma in each of the congenital glaucoma syndromes is discussed on p 316.

C. In a young patient, IOP and corneal diameters should be measured and angle structures examined under sedation. Intraocular pressure greater than 23 mm Hg and corneal diameter greater than 12 mm indicate congenital glaucoma. Gonioscopically, patients with Sturge-Weber syndrome may have prominent iris processes that adhere to the trabecular meshwork or Schwalbe's line; this finding indicates a primary congenital defect in the development of the angle.

D. Primary congenital glaucoma is differentiated from Sturge-Weber syndrome by the absence of systemic findings in the former. The gonioscopic findings are indistinguishable.

E. In older children, medical therapy is the initial treatment. Beta-adrenergic blocking agents, although not approved for use in children, can be effective. Topical pilocarpine is effective in children with normal-looking angles, but the miotic and myopic effects limit its use. Pilocarpine gel at bedtime is tolerated better than drops because maintenance of miosis reduces the irritation. Synthetic anticholinesterases such as isofluorophate are tolerated well in adolescents. The side effects of these agents include development of cataracts and iris cysts. Once the ciliary spasm is established, vision may be corrected with appropriate glasses. Topical 1% epinephrine is effective in juvenile patients. When young patients do not respond to topical agents, oral carbonic anhydrase inhibitors may be used at a daily dose of 15 to 30 mg/kg body weight, although one should be aware of bone marrow depression and aplastic anemia. Methazolamide has fewer side effects than acetazolamide except for cerebral depression. However, medical treatment has limited long-term success and often is used before primary or secondary surgical treatment can be instituted.

F. Because of problems with compliance, administration, and side effects of the drugs in younger children, surgical treatment is preferred. For most cases of congenital glaucoma, goniotomy is the procedure of choice because of its low incidence of complications. However, because the failure rate for goniotomy is high in Sturge-Weber glaucoma, trabeculotomy is the preferred surgical approach. Several precautions have to be taken prior to this procedure: induction of low IOP preoperatively with beta-blocking agents, car-

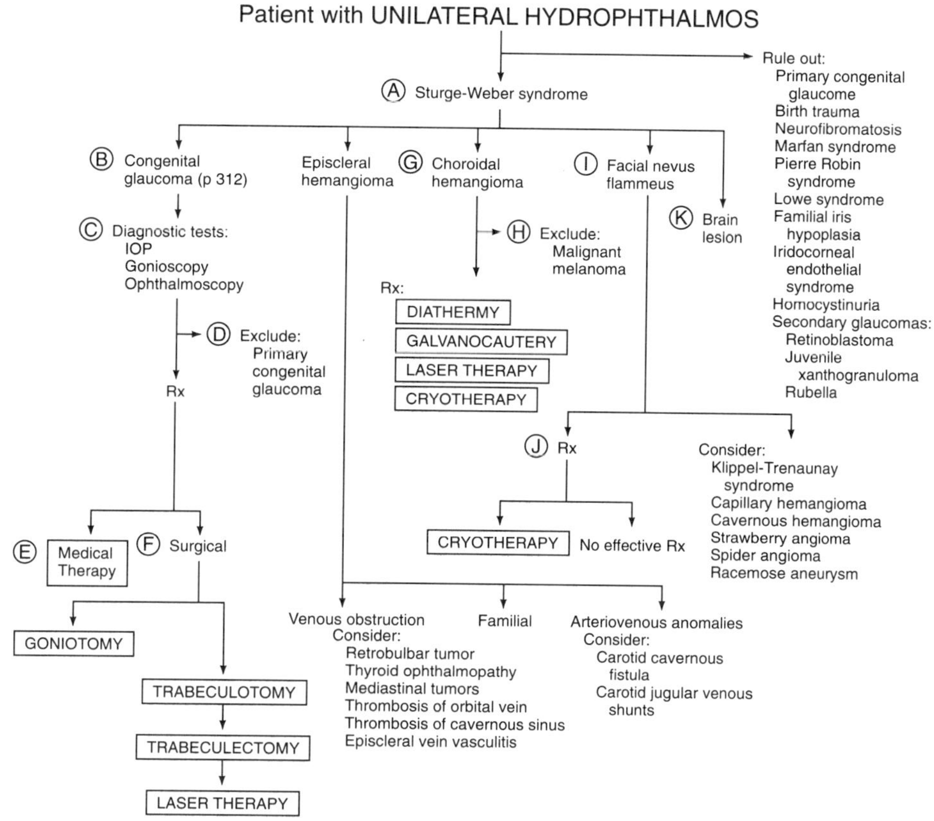

bonic anhydrase inhibitors or osmotic agents, and cauterization of dilated subconjunctival, episcleral, and scleral vessels to avoid hemorrhage and prolapse of intraocular contents. Trabeculectomy carries risk of surgical complications that include expulsive hemorrhage, choroidal effusion, prolapse of the ciliary process into the trabeculectomy wound, scleral ectasia, and prolonged persistence of flat anterior chambers. Trabeculectomy is indicated in patients with failed trabeculotomy or glaucoma that manifests in adolescence. In some patients a repeat trabeculectomy may be required. Cryotherapy, transcleral YAG photocoagulation, setons, and valves are final resorts in failed cases (see pp 312, 314).

G. Choroidal hemangioma is often situated temporal to the optic disc, with its greatest height in the macular region, and it is surrounded by dilated choroidal and retinal vessels. The hemangiomas induce prominent cystoid degeneration of the overlying sensory retina, which eventually results in exudative retinal detachment and intractable secondary glaucoma. The treatment for choroidal hemangiomas is often disappointing, but large leaking lesions may be coagulated.

H. It is often difficult to differentiate choroidal hemangiomas from malignant melanomas and may lead to accidental enucleation of globe.

I. The nevus may be flat, nodular, or verrucous. It is present at birth and generally darkens and becomes nodular with age.

J. The nevus usually does not regress but in some cases may respond to sclerosing agents, topical corticosteroids, laser photocoagulation, and cryotherapy.

K. The neurologic manifestations of the syndrome include angiomatosis of the ipsilateral meninges, secondary degeneration and subsequent calcification of the underlying cortex, contralateral jacksonian seizures in 80% of the patients (in 50% before age 1 year), mental retardation in 54% as well as contralateral hemiplegia, hemianopia, and facial hemihypertrophy.

References

Cibis GW, Tripathi RC, Tripathi BJ. Glaucoma in Sturge-Weber syndrome. Ophthalmology 1982; 91:1061.

Hoskins HD Jr, Kass M. Developmental and childhood glaucoma. In: Becker-Shaffer's diagnosis and therapy of the glaucomas. 6th ed. St. Louis: CV Mosby, 1989: 355.

Lever WF, Shaumberger-Lever G. Tumors of vascular tissue. In: Histopathology of the skin. 6th ed. Philadelphia: JB Lippincott, 1983:623.

Richards RD. Hemangioma. In: Fraunfelder FT, Roy FH, eds. Current ocular therapy. 3rd ed. Philadelphia: WB Saunders, 1990:268.

Tripathi BJ, Tripathi RC, Cibis GW. Sturge-Weber syndrome. In: Gold DH, Weingeist TA, eds. Eye in systemic disease. Philadelphia: JB Lippincott, 1990:443.

Welch RB. Retinal disease. Ocular fundus: Its relation to central nervous system and systemic disease. In: Walsh TJ, ed. Neuro-Ophthalmology: clinical signs and symptoms. 2nd ed. Philadelphia: Lea & Febiger, 1985:127.

NEUROCRISTOPATHY

Gerhard W. Cibis, M.D.

A. Neurocristopathies are disorders resulting from pathology of structures embryologically derived from the neural crest. Knowledge of neural crest cell derivations and interaction with tissues of other derivation is helpful in understanding otherwise seemingly inexplicable syndrome relationships.

Cranial neural crest cells contribute most of the mesenchyme of the face and give rise to all the embryonic facial processes (medial and lateral, nasal and maxillary). Neural crest cells arise at the summit of the neural folds as the neural tube closes. Neural crest cells from the anterior mesencephalic and diencephalic regions begin to migrate anteriorly along the dorsum of the embryo. The neural crest cells, migrating in specific waves, quickly envelop most of the optic cup, following dorsal to ventral and medial to lateral pathways. The crest cells in their early migrations are pluripotent. Local factors affect final differentiation considerably.

The neural crest cells contribute most of the connective tissue components of the eye and orbit. These include the corneal stroma and endothelium, most of the sclera, the sheath of the optic nerve, all the uveal melanocytes, the choroidal stroma, the ciliary body including the muscle, the iris stroma, orbital bones, fat, trochlear cartilage, neural sheath, muscle sheaths, and connective tissues of the orbit (Tenon's capsule). The major exceptions are the striated fibers of the extraocular muscles and the endothelial cells of all the vessels of the eye and orbit.

The extrinsic ocular muscles, including the orbicularis oculi, arise from mesoderm, but the satellite and connective tissue cells of the muscles are of crest origin. In the orbital region, including the eye, all the endothelium of the blood vessels arises from mesoderm, but the components of the vessel walls, including the smooth muscle coats of the vessels, arise from neural crest cells. Generally, connective tissues superiorly and temporally in the orbit are mesodermal in origin. The nasal, inferior, and medial components are formed by neural crest cells. The orbital bones of the floor, medial wall (including the upper median facial bones), and most of the roof develop from the cranial neural crest cells.

B. Pathology is possible with a disturbance in induction, migration, proliferation, or regression of neural crest cells and their derivatives. The exact disturbance determines the clinical picture. Defects may be general or very localized.

C. Iris stroma and melanocytes are derived from neural crest cells. Although aniridia may not be a primary neurocristopathy, the failure of iris stromal development makes it one. The chamber angle and trabecular meshwork are formed by regression of neural crest–derived tissues. Failure to do this is the origin of goniodysgenesis and is supported by the step-ladder classification of anterior segment disorders (see F). The iris-lens pupillary membrane with goniodysgenesis (Fig 1) is a disorder of regression of neural crest–derived tissue. Muscular coats of the great vessels are neural crest derived, providing the linkage of cardiac anomalies and colobomata in CHARGE.

D. Melanocytes are of neural crest origin. The Waardenburg condition with heterochromia and white forelock is a localized failure of melanocyte expression (Fig.2). Iris transillumination in the Prader-Willie syndrome has a similar origin. Albinism qualifies because of the inborn error of metabolism in the melanocytes.

E. The posterior corneal stroma and corneal endothelium are derived from neural crest. Hereditary endothelial dystrophies such as posterior polymorphous and con-

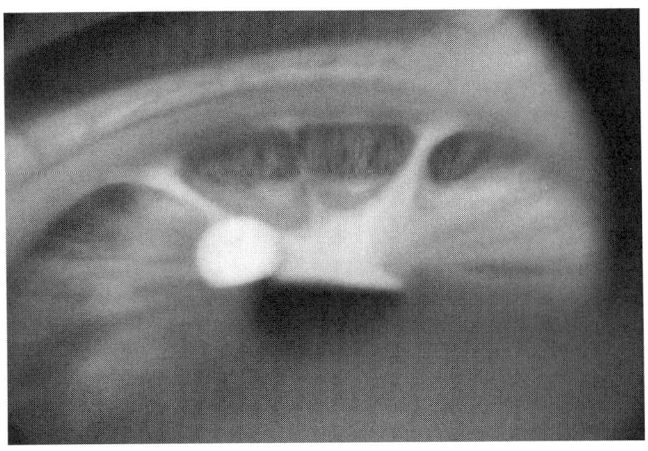

Figure 1 Iris-lens membrane with goniodysgenesis.

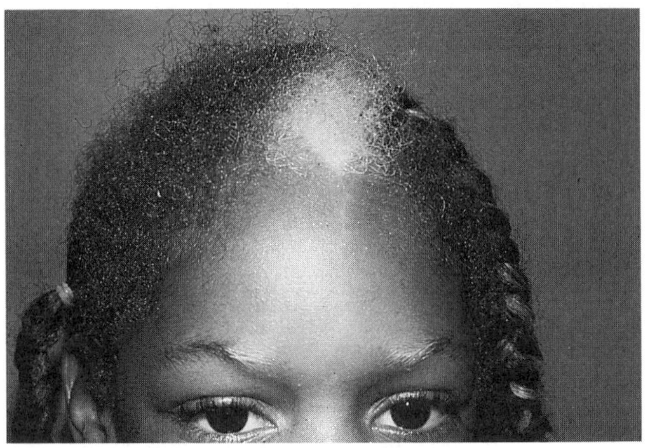

Figure 2 Waardenburg syndrome with white forelock and telecanthus.

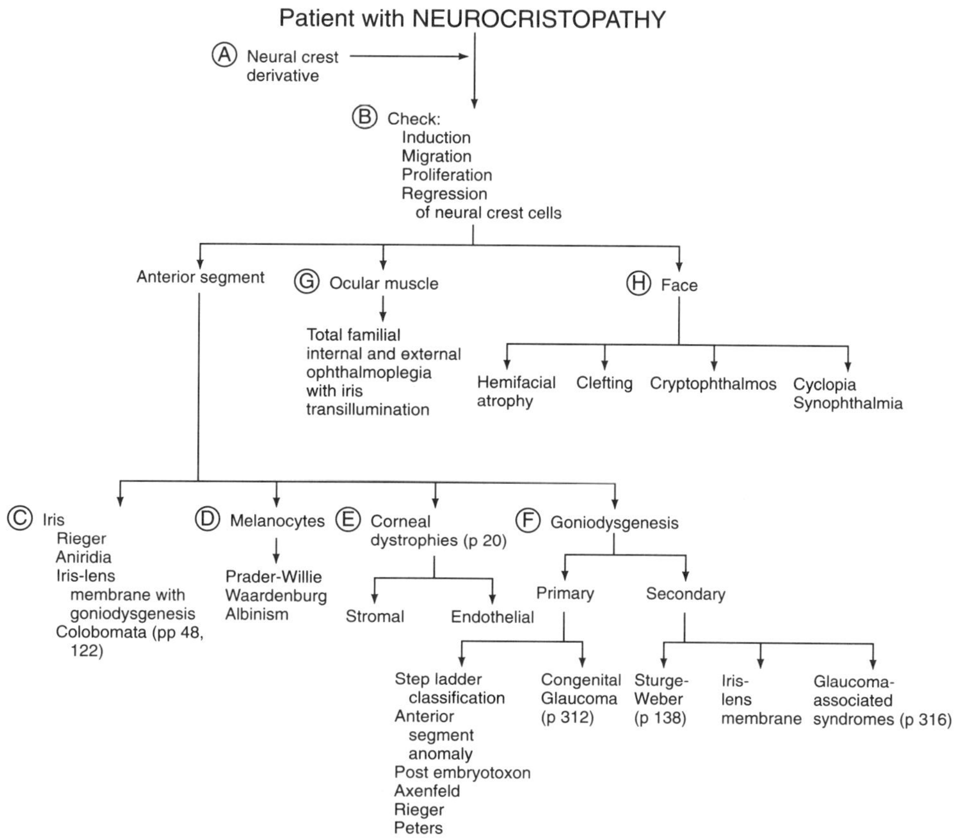

genital hereditary dystrophy are neurocristopathies. Stromal dystrophies such as cornea verticillata also qualify.

F. All primary (congenital glaucoma) and secondary (Sturge-Weber syndrome) goniodysgeneses are neurocristopathies.

G. Total familial internal and external ophthalmoplegia with iris transillumination in all clinical aspects can be explained on the basis of neural crest cell involvement, the lack of stromal melanocytes giving iris transillumination, and lack of internal and external muscles. The ciliary muscles are neural crest cell derived.

TABLE 1 Neural Crest Cell–Derived Ocular Structures

Corneal stroma and endothelium
Sclera
Trabecular meshwork
Sheaths and tendons of extraocular muscles
Connective tissues of iris
Ciliary muscles
Choroidal stroma
Melanocytes (all uveal and epithelial)
Meningeal sheaths of the optic nerve
Schwann cells of ciliary nerves
Ciliary ganglion
Orbital bones (all midline) and inferior orbital, as well as parts of orbital roof and lateral rim
Cartilage
Connective tissue of orbit
Muscular layer and connective tissue sheaths of all ocular and orbital vessels

H. Facial defects result from a deficiency in the number of neural crest cells or from failure of fusion of the processes, either laterally or in the midline. Primary cleft palate can be produced by extirpation of the neural fold prior to crest cell migration. The median face malformation (severe orbital hypertelorism) is thought to result from a failure of the midline coalescence of the frontonasal process. With cryptophthalmos there is also lack of iris and ciliary body development that is neural crest related.

Disturbances of midline structures disrupt neural crest cell–derived migration. Cyclopia with a proboscis above the single or synophthalmic eye is explainable as a failure of the neural crest to migrate between the two eye placodes to form the nose.

References

Cibis GW, Tripathi RC, Tripathi BJ, Seidel G. Familial total internal and external ophthalmoplegia with iris transillumination (a neurocristopathy). Am J Ophthalmol 1992; 113:443.

Cibis GW, Waeltermann JM, Hurst E, et al. Congenital pupillary-iris-lens membrane with goniodysgenesis (a new entity). Ophthalmology 1986; 93:847.

Johnston MC, Sulik KK. Embryology of the head and neck. In: Serafin D, Georgiade N, eds. Pediatric plastic surgery. St. Louis: CV Mosby, 1984.

Tripathi BJ, Tripathi RC. Embryology of the anterior segment of the human eye. In: Ritch R, Shields MB, Krupin T, eds. The glaucomas. St Louis: CV Mosby, 1989:3.

Tripathi BJ, Tripathi RC. Neural crest origin of human trabecular meshwork and its implications for the pathogenesis of glaucoma. Am J Ophthalmol 1989; 107:583.

DECREASED VISION FROM INTRACRANIAL TUMOR

Michael X. Repka, M.D.

A. Decreased visual acuity in childhood is usually due to amblyopia. However, a thorough examination of each patient including determination of visual acuity, presence or absence of an afferent pupillary defect, assessment of color vision, visual field determination, and inspection of the optic nerve and nerve fiber layer is necessary to make an accurate diagnosis. Evidence of an optic neuropathy includes optic atrophy, nerve fiber layer loss, afferent pupillary defect, or dyschromatopsia. Confirmatory evidence of amblyopia includes the absence of the previously described findings with strabismus, monofixation syndrome, or anisometropia.

B. An optic neuropathy in childhood may occur from tumor, infiltration, compression, inflammation, or heredity.

C. There are several hereditary optic neuropathies: dominant optic atrophy, autosomal recessive optic atrophy, and Leber hereditary optic neuropathy (LHON). Each of these may present insidiously in late childhood or early teenage years. Examination of the patient's parents or other affected siblings is useful. Wedge-shaped temporal optic nerve pallor associated with blue-yellow dyschromatopsia is seen with dominant optic atrophy. Peripapillary telangiectasias may be seen in relatives and in the other eye of patients with LHON. Analysis of mitochondrial DNA can establish the diagnosis in 50% of cases of LHON by demonstrating the 11,778 deletion or four other recently reported mutations of the mitochondrial DNA.

D. Optic gliomas are juvenile pilocytic astrocytomas of the optic nerve, the optic chiasm, or both. These tumors may occur sporadically or in patients with neurofibromatosis type 1 (see p 134). They generally have a benign histology and clinical course but occasionally are associated with aggressive behavior. They are readily diagnosed with MRI.

E. The management of optic nerve glioma is careful follow-up until there is profound visual loss. If there is continuing growth, particularly growth that is progressing toward the intracranial space or severe proptosis, resection is warranted. This is generally performed via a combined orbitalcraniotomy approach. MRI with gadolinium is better for glioma management than CT scanning.

F. Optic chiasm gliomas are treated with biopsy if it is difficult to confirm the diagnosis with neuroimaging. Increasingly the diagnosis can be made solely on the basis of neuroimaging and evidence of unilateral visual loss. If the tumor is small and intrinsic, no therapy is initiated. If there is mass effect with compression of the third ventricle, the hypothalamus, or the contralateral optic nerve or optic tract or a large exophytic component, subtotal resection is recommended. Such tumors are readily resected without a deleterious effect on visual acuity. Following initial therapy, patients are generally examined every 3 months and undergo neuroimaging every 3 to 6 months.

G. If there is a decline in visual function or enlargement in tumor volume, the patient is considered a candidate for treatment. Patients over the age of 4 years receive radiation therapy. Patients under the age of 4 years receive chemotherapy, usually a combination of vinblastine and carboplatin. The goal of chemotherapy is to delay the need for radiation therapy until the patient is over the age of 4 years, when the brain is less susceptible to radiation toxicity.

H. Four other suprasellar tumors may present with visual loss. These tumors—craniopharyngioma, germinoma, arachnoid cyst, and hypothalamic glioma—produce visual loss by optic nerve compression. Craniopharyngioma is treated by surgical resection and adjuvant radiation therapy, usually external beam. Germinoma is typically treated with biopsy and radiation therapy. Symptomatic arachnoid cysts are drained and the capsule is partially resected. They rarely recur. Hypothalamic gliomas present with failure to thrive, poor nutrition, poor temperature control, and reduced vision. The visual acuity is usually only mildly to moderately affected, unlike the patients with primary optic glioma, who have profound visual loss. Therapy is partial resection followed by chemotherapy or radiation therapy.

I. Tumors of the cerebrum, particularly astrocytomas, may involve the thalamus, producing evidence of optic tract disease with a contralateral afferent pupillary defect and homonymous hemianopsia. They may also involve the geniculocalcarine radiations or striate cortex.

References

Miller NR. Walsh and Hoyt's clinical neuro-ophthalmology, Vol. 3. Baltimore: Williams & Wilkins, 1988.

Repka MX, Miller NR. Optic atrophy in childhood. Am J Ophthalmol 1988; 106:191.

Wallace DC, Singh G, Lott MT, et al. Mitochondrial DNA mutation associated with Leber's hereditary optic neuropathy. Science 1988; 242:1427.

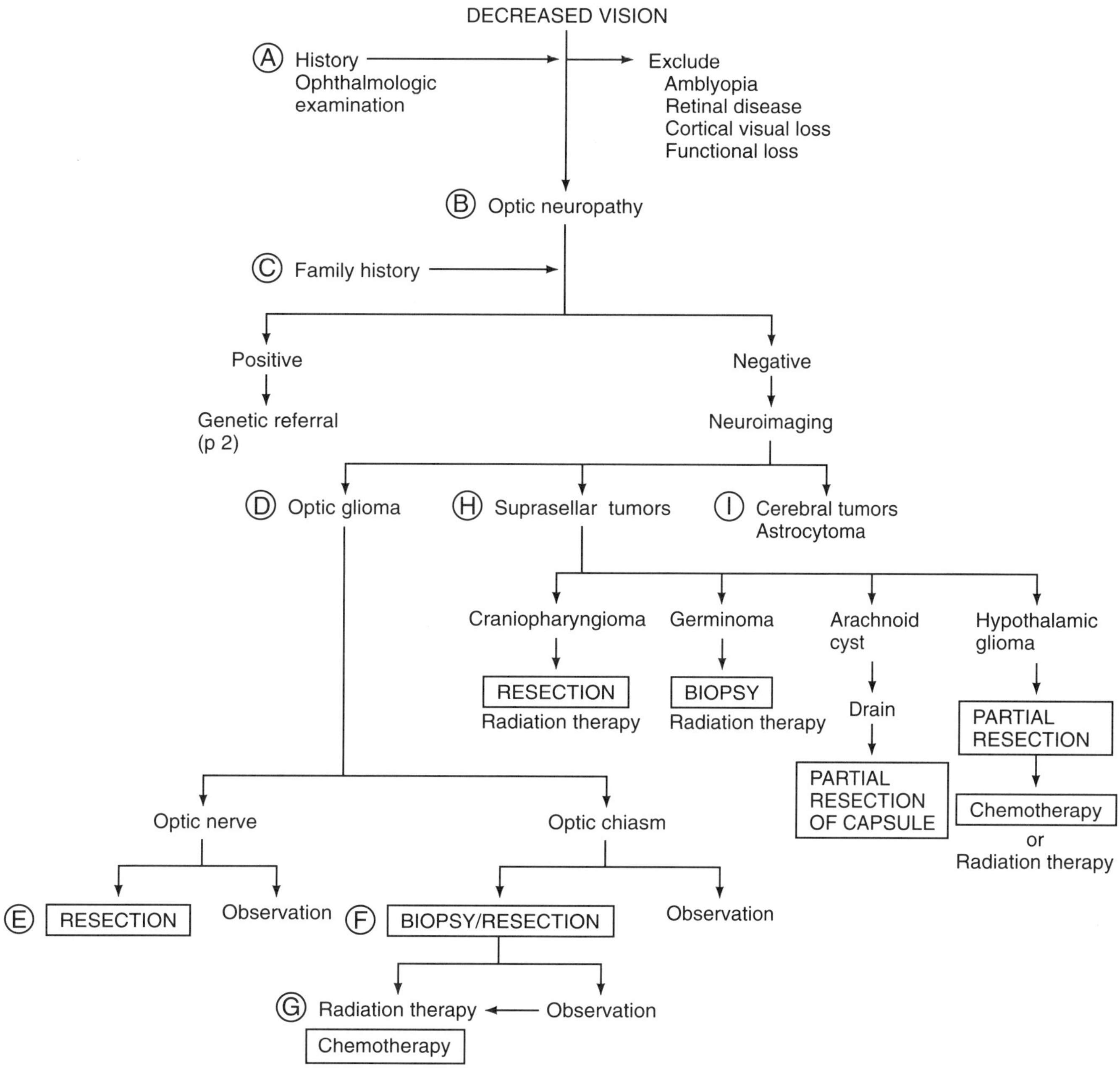
DECREASED VISION
Ⓐ History
Ophthalmologic examination
Exclude
Amblyopia
Retinal disease
Cortical visual loss
Functional loss
Ⓑ Optic neuropathy
Ⓒ Family history
Positive
Genetic referral (p 2)
Negative
Neuroimaging
Ⓓ Optic glioma
Ⓗ Suprasellar tumors
Ⓘ Cerebral tumors
Astrocytoma
Craniopharyngioma
RESECTION
Radiation therapy
Germinoma
BIOPSY
Radiation therapy
Arachnoid cyst
Drain
PARTIAL RESECTION OF CAPSULE
Hypothalamic glioma
PARTIAL RESECTION
Chemotherapy
or
Radiation therapy
Optic nerve
Ⓔ RESECTION
Observation
Optic chiasm
Ⓕ BIOPSY/RESECTION
Observation
Ⓖ Radiation therapy
Chemotherapy
Observation

THE PRESCHOOL AND SCHOOL-AGE CHILD

ACQUIRED MYOGENIC PTOSIS IN THE CHILD

Holly L. Barbour, M.D.
Jonathan J. Dutton, M.D., Ph.D.

Ptosis is an abnormally low position of the upper eyelid margin caused by a dysfunction of either the levator palpebrae superioris muscle or Muller's sympathetic tarsal muscle. The condition has a diversity of causes that may or may not be associated with other ocular or systemic abnormalities. The general pathophysiologic categories are myogenic, aponeurogenic, mechanical, or neurogenic. Trauma, which in the past was considered a distinct etiologic classification, may actually involve any of the above causes. Although the surgical choices for ptosis repair are limited and usually depend upon levator muscle function (Table 1), a knowledge of the underlying pathology is imperative to guide the surgeon in the overall care of the patient.

A. A complete ophthalmic and medical history is an essential first step in evaluating the ptosis patient. A determination should be made of the time of onset, rate of progression, any associated signs or symptoms, and previous illnesses or ophthalmic surgeries. A list of current medication use, allergies, or exposure to toxins should also be obtained.

B. A thorough ophthalmic examination is mandatory, including visual acuity and a current refraction, or retinoscopy in a young child. Evidence of ptosis-related amblyopia should be recorded. The size, symmetry, and reactivity of the pupils are noted. External examination includes observation of any head tilt or turn, associated neuromuscular or structural anomalies, the presence or absence of spontaneous eye and lid movements, anomalous synkinetic movements, or evidence of trauma. Symmetry and contour of the lids and orbit should be noted. The anterior orbit should be palpated for the presence of masses. Versions and ductions are evaluated, as is the presence of an adequate Bell's phenomenon. Specific measurements are taken, including interpalpebral fissure height, distance from the upper eyelid margin to the mid-pupillary reflex (MRD), total levator muscle excursion, and height of the upper eyelid crease. In most cases, the history and physical examination clarify the cause of the ptosis.

C. Pseudoptosis is a narrowing of the interpalpebral fissure not associated with a levator or Muller's muscle dysfunction. Causes of pseudoptosis include hypotropia, contralateral eyelid retraction, enophthalmos (retraction syndrome or orbital volume loss), microphthalmos, phthisis bulbi, blepharospasm (secondary to ocular surface irritation or encephalitis), and hemifacial spasm.

D. Myogenic ptosis involves a primary disorder of the striated levator muscle, resulting in diminished function on examination. Although other extraocular muscles may also be affected, the hallmarks of third nerve palsy such as anisocoria and superior rectus muscle weakness are not seen unless neurogenic involvement also exists.

E. Chronic progressive external ophthalmoplegia (CPEO) is characterized by gradual paralysis of all extraocular muscles. Both idiopathic and familial forms are known. The onset is usually before 20 years of age, and ptosis is typically an early sign. Diplopia is notably absent. There may be a neurogenic form of CPEO, but it is clinically indistinguishable from the myopathic form. CPEO may exist as part of a syndrome, such as Werdnig-Hoffman syndrome and Bassen-Kornzweig syndrome, which are associated with other neurodegenerative disorders. Ocular pharyngeal dystrophy is a rare form of CPEO, and myotonic dystrophy may mimic CPEO. Both tend to occur later in life.

TABLE 1 Surgical Choices for Ptosis

Procedure	*Indications*	*Relative Contraindications*
Fasanella-Servat	Minimal ptosis (1–2 mm) Good levator function (8–15 mm)	More than 2 mm ptosis Poor to fair function Tarsal deformities
Aponeurotic advancement	Mild to severe ptosis Fair to good function (5–15 mm)	Absent to very poor function
Levator resection	Moderate to severe ptosis Poor to fair function (3–8 mm)	Absent to very poor function Weak to absent Bell's phenomenon
Frontalis suspension	Moderate to severe ptosis Absent to very poor function (0–2 mm)	Fair to good function Weak to absent Bell's phenomenon

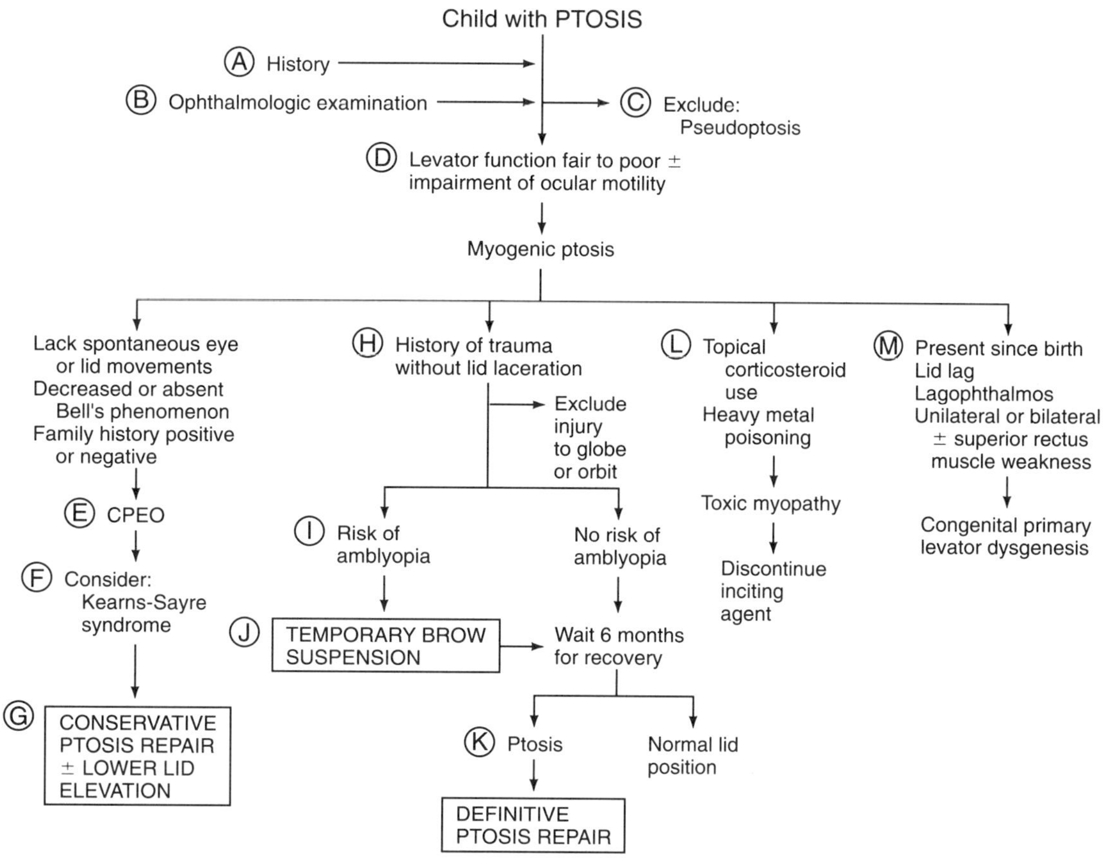

F. All patients with CPEO must have a cardiac evaluation for evidence of Kearns-Sayre syndrome, a triad of CPEO, heart block, and pigmentary retinopathy.

G. The poor ocular motility and Bell's phenomenon in these patients mandate a conservative approach to ptosis repair. The aim of surgery is to allow a functional visual field without risking corneal exposure. Simultaneous surgical elevation of the lower eyelid may offer additional corneal protection. The specific surgical procedure is based upon levator muscle function.

H. Blunt trauma to the anterior orbit and eyelid often results in a temporary ptosis, usually resulting from hematoma or contusion of the levator muscle. Pain or iritis-induced photophobia may cause a pseudoptosis. A foreign body or orbital fracture must be ruled out by appropriate clinical and radiographic studies. Surgical trauma to the eyelids and orbit may also cause a myopathic ptosis that is typically temporary.

I. Any child under the age of 8 years is at risk for deprivation amblyopia when the upper eyelid obscures the pupillary axis. The younger the child, the more rapidly amblyopia may develop.

J. For children at risk for amblyopia, a temporary brow suspension can be performed. The lid is suspended from the frontalis muscle with a submuscular sling of silicone tubing, synthetic suture, or fascia lata. Eyelid elevation is achieved with contraction of the frontalis muscle. Liberal topical lubrication of the globe is mandatory in the postoperative period because of the inevitable lagophthalmos following this operation. The sling can be removed after recovery of levator muscle function.

K. If ptosis remains at 6 months, definitive repair is indicated. The choice of procedure depends upon the amount of levator muscle function.

L. The chronic use of topical corticosteroids or heavy metal exposure, such as with the ingestion of lead, has been associated with ptosis. The ptosis is believed to be due to a localized toxic myopathy and is potentially reversible with discontinuance of the toxic agent.

M. The majority of myogenic ptoses in children are congenital in origin and involve a primary dysgenesis of the levator muscle. The most characteristic sign is an increase in ptosis on upgaze and an apparent decrease in ptosis or even frank retraction on downgaze. This results from the partially fibrotic levator muscle and its inability to contract or stretch normally.

References

Anderson RL, Baumgartner SA. Amblyopia in ptosis. Arch Ophthalmol 1980; 98:1068.

Dutton JJ. A color atlas of ptosis—a practical guide to evaluation and management. Singapore: PG Publishing, 1989.

Kemp EG, James CR, Collin JR. Brow suspension in the management of ptosis: An analysis of over 100 cases. Trans Ophthal Soc UK 1986; 105(Pt 1):84.

ACQUIRED APONEUROGENIC AND NEUROGENIC PTOSIS IN THE CHILD

Holly L. Barbour, M.D.
Jonathan J. Dutton, M.D., Ph. D.

A. History, physical examination, and exclusion of pseudoptosis are requisite first steps (p 2).

B. Aponeurogenic ptosis, the most common form of acquired ptosis in the adult, can also be seen in children as a congenital or an acquired disorder. In the former case it usually results from birth trauma. The mechanism is a thinning or stretching of the levator aponeurosis or actual disinsertion of the tendon from the tarsus. This causes a loss of transmission of levator muscle force to the upper eyelid. The high or attenuated eyelid crease and excellent levator muscle function support the clinical diagnosis.

C. Ptosis in the setting of an eyelid laceration should always prompt exploration for additional injury to the globe and anterior orbit. A penetrating foreign body should be ruled out, and the levator aponeurosis must be carefully evaluated for transection.

D. A levator aponeurosis laceration should be repaired primarily. Whenever possible in older children, the procedure should be performed under local anesthesia to allow voluntary cooperation for more accurate placement of lid position. The orbital septum should not be repaired because this carries the risk of lid retraction and lagophthalmos. The orbicularis muscle and skin are closed in layers.

E. In the absence of an eyelid laceration, redundancy, dehiscence, or frank disinsertion of the aponeurosis can result from patching, traumatic edema, allergic angioneurotic reactions, or blepharochalasis.

TABLE 1 Causes of Mechanical Ptosis

Mass effect
Lid abscess
Lid tumor
Conjunctival tumor
Orbital mass lesion
Dacryoadentitis
Traumatic bony abnormalities
Cellulitis
Lid edema
Cicatricial changes
Stevens-Johnson syndrome
Chemical burns
Trauma or surgery

F. Repair is achieved by tucking or reinserting the aponeurosis to the tarsal plate through an upper eyelid incision at the site of the desired supratarsal skin crease.

G. Mechanical ptosis can result from a number of causes (Table 1). These result in a mass effect that depresses the eyelid downward or in a cicatricial restriction of eyelid movement. Treatment is directed toward the underlying pathology.

H. Often, removing the inciting mass or scar tissue corrects the ptosis without the need for further repair. Any residual ptosis can usually be corrected with aponeurotic advancement.

I. Ptosis of neurogenic origin almost invariably coexists with other signs of neurologic dysfunction that distinguish it from other causes of droopy eyelid.

J. Unexplained third nerve or sympathetic paresis requires appropriate radiographic evaluation for central or orbital apex lesions.

K. Once the underlying condition has been treated, it is advisable to wait 6 to 12 months for spontaneous recovery of levator function before repair. The exception is in young children at risk for amblyopia. For

TABLE 2 Lesions Affecting the Third Cranial Nerve

Third nerve nuclear or fascicular lesions:
Ischemic infarction
Demyelination
Metastases
Interpeduncular lesions:
Trauma
Meningitis
Vascular anomalies
Cavernous sinus lesions:
Inflammatory or infectious processes
Metastatic and pituitary tumors
Meningiomas and gliomas
Vascular fistulas and aneurysms
Orbital apex or superior orbital fissure lesions:
Inflammatory processes
Trauma

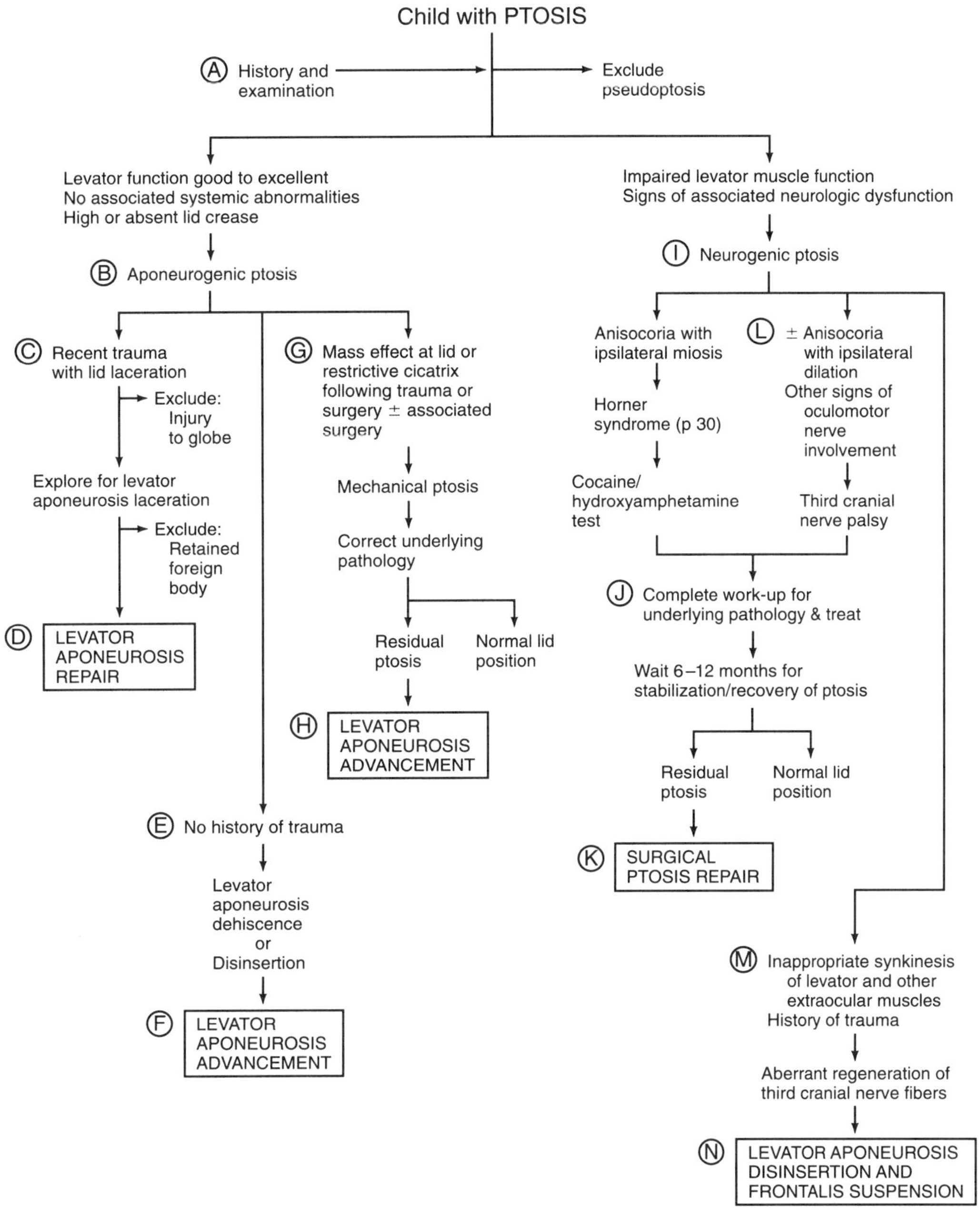

persistent ptosis after 6 to 12 months, the choice of operative procedure must be carefully tailored to the individual patient and depends largely upon the residual levator muscle function, if any.

L. The third cranial nerve runs a long intracranial course, and oculomotor nerve dysfunction can result from a variety of insults. Dilation of the involved pupil is common, and multiple other signs of extraocular muscle dysfunction are typically present. Table 2 lists some of the more common causes by location.

M. Aberrant peripheral regeneration of third nerve fibers is a sequela of compression or trauma. Nerve fibers intended for the levator muscle redirect to other extraocular muscles. This is distinct from the congenital Marcus-Gunn phenomenon, in which there is a central misdirection of nerve fibers between the third nerve and muscles served by the fifth cranial nerve.

N. Inappropriate synkinetic ptosis is corrected surgically by aponeurosis shortening if ptosis is the major clinical symptom. For children in whom the synkinetic component is of primary concern, the levator muscle is disinserted and the eyelid repaired by frontalis muscle suspension.

References

Anderson RL, Baumgartner SA. Amblyopia in ptosis. Arch Ophthalmol 1980; 98:1068.

Berlin AJ, Vestal KP. Levator aponeurosis surgery: A retrospective review. Ophthalmology 1989; 96:1033.

Dutton JJ. A color atlas of ptosis—a practical guide to evaluation and management. PG Publishing, 1989.

Kemp EG, James CR, Collin JR. Brow suspension in the management of ptosis: An analysis of over 100 cases. Trans Ophthal Soc UK 1986; 105(Pt 1):84.

ACQUIRED PROPTOSIS

Barrett G. Haik, M.D.,
Zeynel A. Karcioglu, M.D.

A. Presence of pain at the time of detection of proptosis and rate of progression are important diagnostic clues. Hamartoma, choristoma, teratoma, microphthalmia with cyst, and meningoencephaloceles are congenital but may not be detected until significant growth has occurred. Rhabdomyosarcoma, metastatic tumors, teratoma, and capillary hemangioma can grow rapidly over days or weeks. Explosive growth over hours or days is usually a result of hemorrhage from trauma, bleeding diatheses, blood cyst formation in lymphangioma, or infectious disorders such as orbital cellulitis. Thyroid ophthalmopathy does occur in children.

B. Physical examination should include systemic, dermatologic, and ocular examination. Dermatologic examination may yield valuable information in patients with phakomatosis, hamartomas, and metastatic disease. Ocular examinations are performed to detect intraocular tumors, pathology of the optic nerve, extraocular muscles, and globe compression. Palpation is important to detect abnormal resistance to retropulsion, bony orbital abnormalities, or palpable masses. Pulsation abnormalities may be detected in patients with vascular anomalies, neurofibromatosis, and meningoencephaloceles; bruits and/or crepitation may be detected on auscultation.

C. Diagnostic imaging is critical to the evaluation of pediatric patients with proptosis. Ultrasonographic examination enables one to detect neoplastic mass lesions and distinguish them, with a high degree of reliability, from inflammatory and vascular causes of proptosis. Ultrasonography is of limited value in evaluating deep orbital tumors and lesions involving the bones. High-resolution CT detects well over 95% of all orbital tumors as well as depicting intracranial extension. The technique is somewhat limited by beam-hardening and volume-averaging artifacts in the orbital apex, optic canal, and chiasmal region. MRI with surface coils and gadolinium-DTPA is also extremely valuable for providing anatomic and biochemical information concerning orbital disease (pp 278, 284). It is especially well suited for visualizing intracranial extension of orbital tumors. MRI is limited in its ability to detect calcific orbital abnormalities. Plain films are valuable in evaluating bony abnormalities, and angiography is indicated in selected vascular disorders.

D. Pseudoproptosis may be seen with unilateral high myopia or contralateral microphthalmia. It may occur when contralateral enophthalmia results from prior orbital blowout fracture. It may result from buphthalmos and orbital asymmetry, as occurs in craniofacial disorders.

E. In orbital trauma with proptosis, the detection of orbital fractures, foreign bodies, and hemorrhage are critical to appropriate therapy. If hemorrhage, bone fragments, or foreign bodies are mechanically threatening the nerve or globe, surgical intervention is indicated. Nonreactive foreign bodies do not require extraction, whereas organic and copper foreign bodies should be removed. MRI should be used judiciously in cases of metallic foreign bodies. Use of CT is preferable.

F. Proptosis secondary to sinus infection usually represents bacterial orbital cellulitis. Broad-spectrum intravenous antibiotic therapy and otolaryngologic examination are usually indicated. When an orbital or subperiosteal abscess is detected on imaging studies, surgical drainage is indicated if there is not a rapid response to antibiotic therapy or rapid visual impairment.

G. Diversity of orbital tumors reflects the numerous embryologic derivations of tissues throughout the orbit. Fortunately, the great majority (>75%) are benign. Clinical and imaging characteristics are valuable in the differential diagnosis of these masses. Well-circumscribed cystic masses include microphthalmia with cyst, meningoencephalocele, choristomas, and teratomas. In microphthalmia with cyst, an extreme form of ocular coloboma, a bluish orbital mass displaces a microphthalmic eye superiorly.

H. Encephaloceles and meningoceles are associated with a focal cranial defect at the base of the nasal cavity, telecanthus, and optic nerve anomalies. Aspiration of cerebrospinal fluid may be evaluated chemically, or a communication between the orbital mass and CNS may be detected with CT following the intrathecal administration of nonionic contrast.

I. Epidermoid and dermoid cysts are among the most common pediatric lesions. These choristomatous lesions may be detected at birth or later in life after significant growth has occurred. They are typically firm, immobile, painless, and located adjacent to bony suture lines. On CT and MRI a spherical circumscribed mass is seen, commonly an adjacent focal bony defect. Fat density material is often present in dermoids and is detected as negative Hounsfield density tissue on CT, and hyperintense on T1- and hypointense on T2-weighted MRI. Surgical excision is employed in symptomatic patients and to avoid traumatic rupture. Orbital cystic teratomas are rare but dramatic. They may result in hideous proptosis as fluid accumulates within the cysts and/or glandular tissues proliferate. Teratomas are managed by excision, although exenteration may be required.

J. Enhancing infiltrative lesions may be associated with intraocular tumors such as retinoblastoma and medulloepithelioma. These may be diagnosed with the assistance of indirect ophthalmoscopy. Confirmation by incisional biopsy is followed by radiation and chemotherapy in extraocular retinoblastoma and medulloepithelioma. Enhancing infiltrative tumors associated with enlarged orbit include capillary hemangioma, lymphangioma, and neurofibroma. Capillary hemangiomas occur within the first 6 months of life. They may grow rapidly and are commonly associated with amblyopia from pupillary occlusion and/or ani-

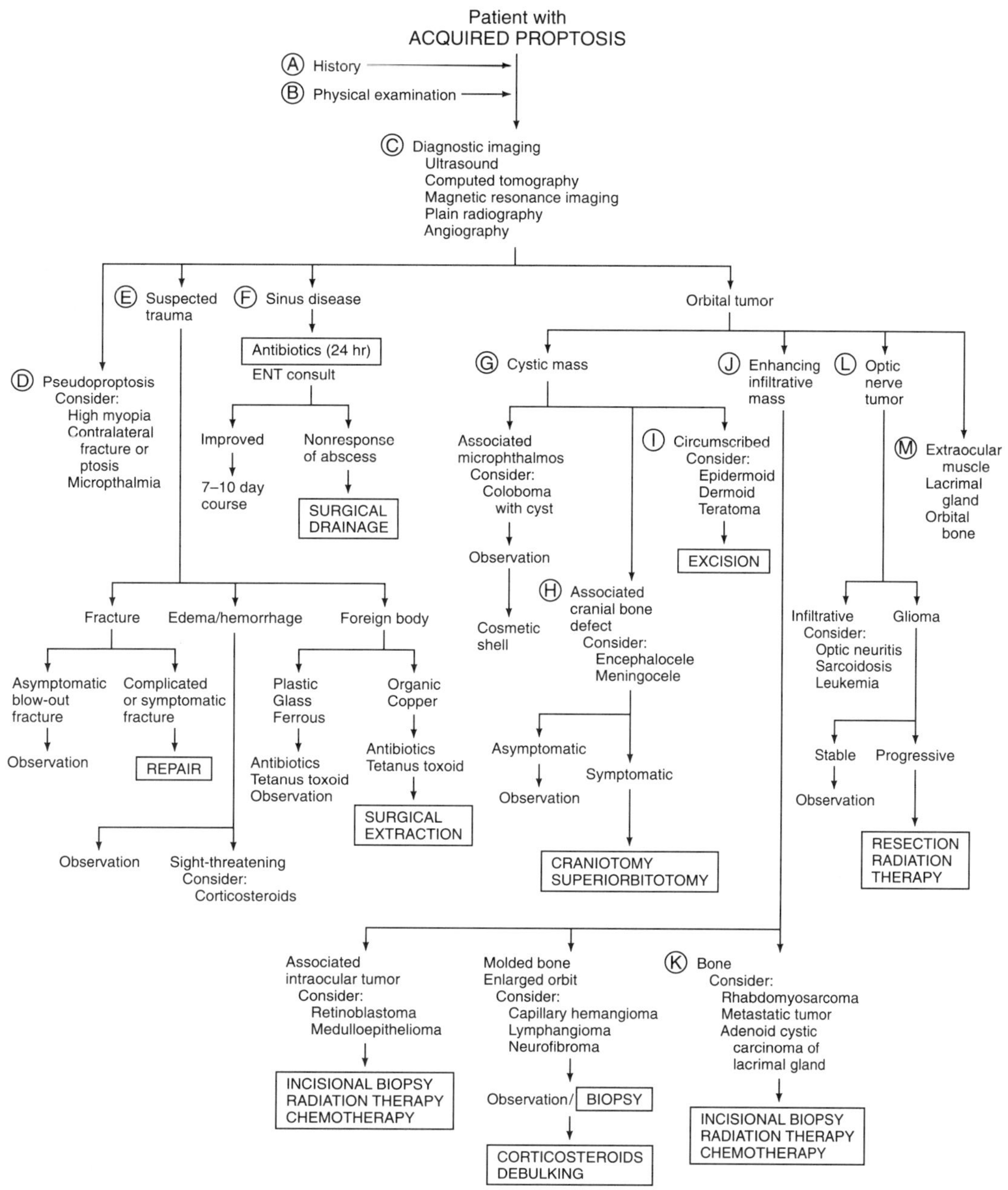

sometropia. Therapy for vision-threatening lesions is usually corticosteroid injections. Orbital lymphangioma usually develops in the first decade. These typically grow at the same rate as the child, unless rapid enlargement occurs following blood cyst formation or systemic bleeding disorders. Examination of the palate may reveal extraorbital focus of a vascular lesion, particularly lymphangioma. Orbital lymphangioma and neurofibroma are nonresponsive to medical and radiation therapy; therefore, surgical debulking is a mainstay of management.

K. Infiltrating, enhancing masses with bone destruction include rhabdomyosarcoma and metastatic neuroblastoma. Once diagnosis is secured with incisional biopsy, a combination of regimens including debulking surgery, radiation, and chemotherapy are undertaken.

L. Optic nerve enlargement may be secondary to infiltrative lesions or optic nerve glioma. Optic nerve glioma is diagnosed radiographically, and MRI may demonstrate chiasmal or intraocular extension in more than 50%. A great deal of controversy exists over the most effective mode of therapy.

M. Primary and secondary diseases of the extraocular muscles, lacrimal gland, and bony orbit must be considered and appropriately evaluated.

References

Haik BG. Advanced imaging techniques in ophthalmology. In: Haik BG, ed. International ophthalmology clinics, Vol. 26, No. 3. Boston: Little, Brown & Company, 1986.

Karcioglu ZA. Tissue diagnosis: Orbit. In: Karcioglu ZA, ed. Laboratory diagnosis in ophthalmology. New York: Macmillan Publishing Company, 1987.

Rootman J, ed. Diseases of the orbit: A multidisciplinary approach. Philadelphia: JB Lippincott, 1988.

Shields JA, ed. Diagnosis and management of orbital tumors. Philadelphia: WB Saunders, 1989.

PRESEPTAL CELLULITIS IN CHILDREN

Don Liu, M.D.

A. Preseptal and orbital cellulitis begin with inflammatory signs in the eyelid. In children, preseptal cellulitis is more common than orbital cellulitis. The presence or absence of inflammation of the orbital tissues is the most important clinical findings that distinguishes these two entities. Children with preseptal diagnosis can be hospitalized or managed as outpatients.

B. If orbital inflammatory signs are absent, the patient has a preseptal cellulitis. The presence or absence of skin trauma or infection determines whether this is a suppurative or nonsuppurative preseptal cellulitis. A relatively common cause of pediatric preseptal cellulitis is impetigo, which is seen most often in children under the age of 6 with poor hygiene. The dermatopathy begins with small, red macules that progress rapidly to vesicles. When these vesicles rupture, a characteristic thick golden yellow crust forms. Laboratory investigations should include Gram's stain of a smear, the vesicle fluid, as well as culture and sensitivity studies. Usually organisms typical of *Staphylococcus aureus* or *S. pyogenes* (group A) are identified. Treatment includes intravenous nafcillin; topical antibiotic ointment; hot, wet compresses; and good hygiene.

C. A rare form of suppurative preseptal cellulitis caused by *S. pyogenes,* group A, is erysipelas. This begins typically as an elevated erythematous plaque on the skin of the eyelid and progresses to an edematous, painful eyelid with a sharply demarcated area of deep red discoloration. Unlike other forms of preseptal cellulitis, orbital inflammatory signs such as chemosis, proptosis, and mild limitation of ocular motility are present. Vision usually remains normal. The patient tends to have a high temperature, chills, and malaise. A CT scan of the orbit should be obtained. Treatment consists of intravenous penicillin G, followed by oral penicillin once clinical improvement occurs.

D. Despite a history and other clinical evidence of trauma, it may not always be possible to identify an entry site. When purulent material is present, it should be aspirated for Gram's stain, culture, and sensitivity studies. A CT scan should be performed if there is a suspicion of injury to the globe or other orbital structures, or if there is a possibility of a retained foreign body. Organisms most commonly recovered are *S. aureus* and *S. pyogenes,* but anaerobes are found frequently following animal or human bites. Treatment includes incision and drainage of the purulent material, removal of the foreign body, topical

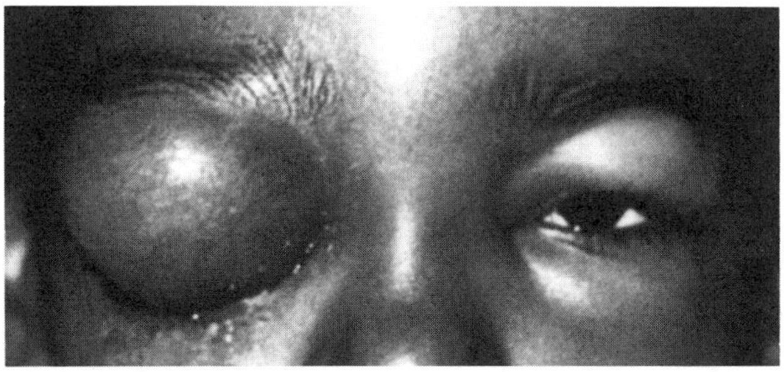

Figure 1 Although this child has marked swelling of the eyelids, he does not have proptosis or limitation of eye movement. The disease process is limited to the preseptal compartment.

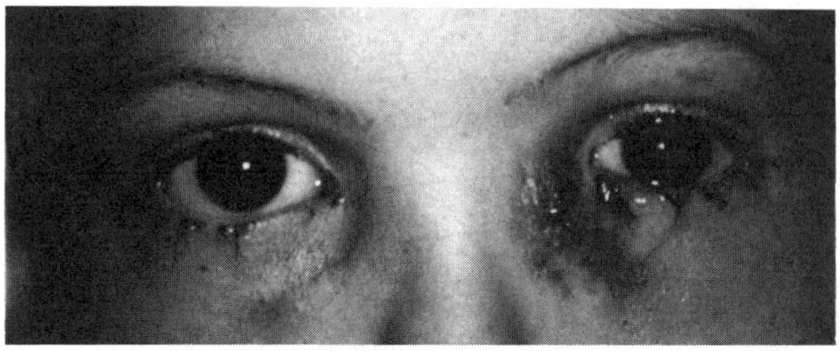

Figure 2 This child has impetigo secondary to an infectious process in the nasolacrimal system. The skin lesion is a wet process with red macules that begin to form vesicles.

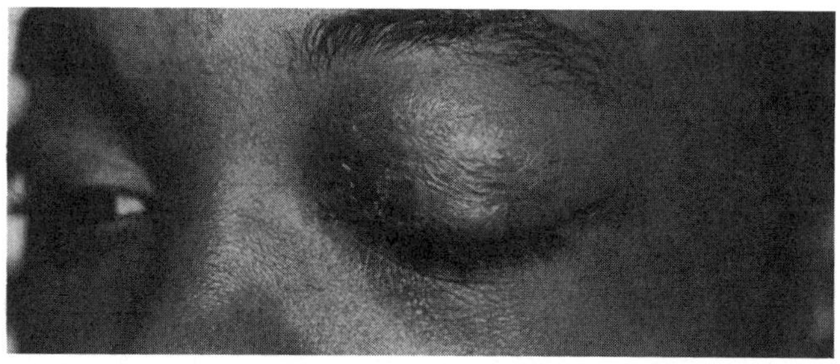

Figure 3 This child has preseptal cellulitis secondary to skin trauma. However, evidence of trauma is not always so obvious.

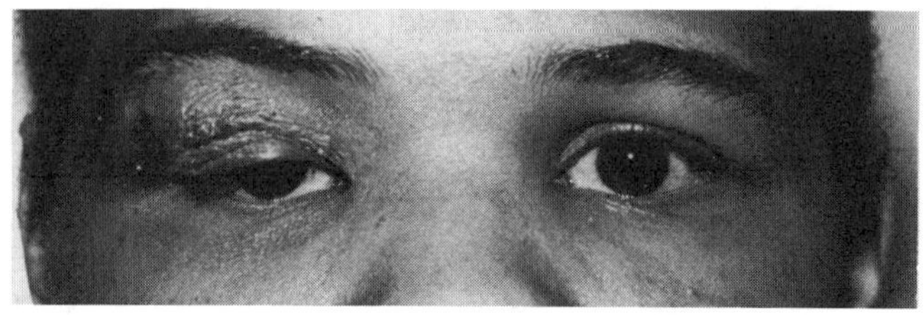

Figure 4 A large, protruding piece of wood penetrating the orbital septum was removed from this child's right upper eyelid laterally. With intravenous antibiotic treatment, the patient never developed any orbital inflammatory signs but the disease process is still evident in the preseptal compartment.

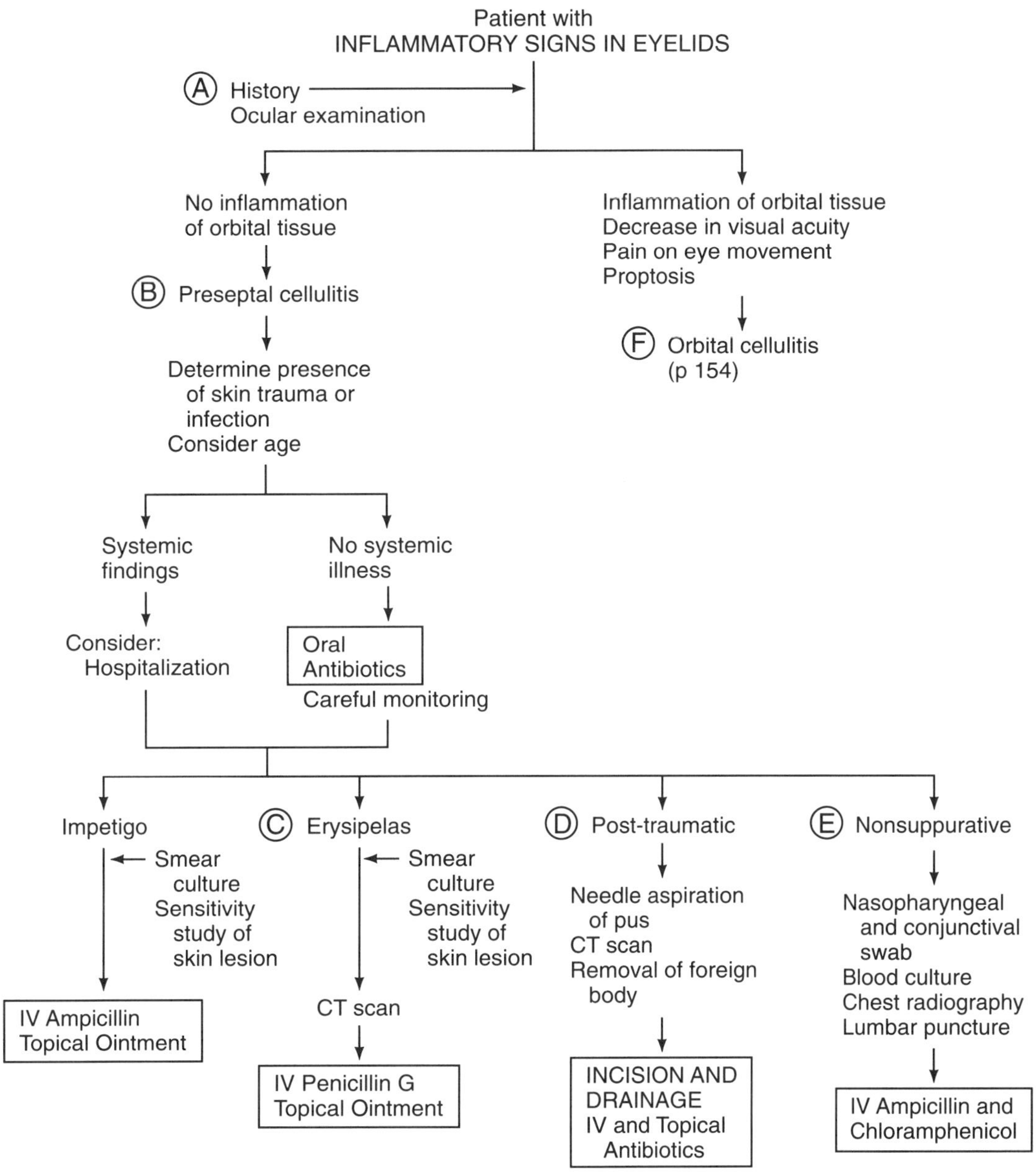

antibiotic ointment, and hot compresses. Appropriate antibiotics are given intravenously based on the Gram's stain and culture and sensitivity studies.

E. A nonsuppurative preseptal cellulitis in children less than 6 years of age is caused almost exclusively by *Haemophilus influenzae* type B or by *Streptococcus pneumoniae*. Work-up of these children should include chest radiography, nasopharyngeal and conjunctival swabs for culture and sensitivity studies, and a blood culture. If the child presents with a high fever and irritability, lumbar puncture should be performed to rule out meningitis. The treatment of nonsuppurative preseptal cellulitis is intravenous ampicillin and chloramphenicol.

F. Orbital cellulitis is covered on p 154.

References

Jones DB, Steinkuller PG. Strategies for the initial management of acute preseptal and orbital cellulitis. Trans Am Ophthalmol Soc 1988; 86:94.

Molarte AB, Isenberg SJ. Periorbital cellulitis in infancy. J Pediatr Ophthalmol Strabismus 1989; 26:232.

Powell KR, Kaplan SB, Hall CB, et al. Periorbital cellulitis: Clinical and laboratory findings in 146 episodes, including tear countercurrent immunoelectrophoresis in 89 episodes. Am J Dis Child 1988; 142:853.

ORBITAL CELLULITIS IN CHILDREN

Don Liu, M.D.

A. Orbital cellulitis begins with inflammatory signs in the eyelid and/or orbit. In children, preseptal cellulitis is more common than orbital cellulitis. The presence or absence of inflammation of the orbital tissues is the most important clinical finding that distinguishes these two entities. When the orbital tissues are involved, there is an accompanying decrease in visual acuity, pain on eye movement, proptosis, and conjunctival chemosis. Children with orbital cellulitis should be hospitalized for intravenous antibiotic management.

B. In a child with orbital cellulitis, CT scans of the orbits and the paranasal sinuses are essential for diagnosis and management. History often reveals a predisposing factor such as trauma, surgery, sinusitis, dental work, diabetes mellitus, immunosuppression, or upper respiratory infection. Orbital cellulitis is frequently accompanied by other constitutional symptoms and signs such as malaise, fever, chills, and rhinorrhea.

C. If there is a history or suspicion of trauma, echography studies in addition to the CT scans may be helpful in localizing an orbital foreign body or orbital fracture. A large or protruding foreign body should be removed promptly, whereas conservative management is advisable for small objects that are deeply embedded in the orbit. Concurrent suppuration in the preseptal compartment should be drained and the material submitted for Gram's stain and culture and sensitivity studies. Blood cultures should also be obtained. *Staphylococcus aureus* is most commonly identified, although mixed organisms and anaerobes are also seen. The preferred initial treatment is intravenous nafcillin and Tobramycin; using the Gram's stain and culture sensitivity studies as a guide, other antibiotics may be added.

D. When orbital cellulitis is the result of recent intraorbital surgery, the management is essentially the same as that for post-traumatic cellulitis. Infected or extruding implants should be removed promptly. Purulent material should be collected for Gram's stain and cultures, and blood culture should be performed. The choice of intravenous antibiotics is based initially on clinical judgment and is guided by the results of culture and sensitivity studies.

E. When there is radiographic evidence of sinusitis, the orbital cellulitis is, in general, an extension of that process. These patients may also have a high fever, headache, rhinorrhea, irritability, and general malaise. Blood cultures and nasopharyngeal and conjunctival swabs should be obtained, although these studies tend to be inconclusive. Pathogens identified are almost invariably in the nasopharyngeal secretions. Intravenous nafcillin and chloramphenicol are drugs of choice initially. Based upon results of culture and sensitive studies, other antibiotics may be added.

F. If there is clear-cut evidence by CT scan of a subperiosteal abscess, and if fever fails to abate with intravenous antibiotics, if vision is threatened, or if other orbital inflammatory signs worsen, surgical drainage of the subperiosteal material and of the involved paranasal sinuses is indicated. Rarely, orbital cellulitis may be a complication of infections in other parts of the face. The management of these patients is essentially the same as for those with sinusitis.

G. When the child is a severe diabetic or is immunosuppressed, mucormycosis must be considered. Typically, the patient has a severe metabolic acidosis, and initial symptoms include headache, orbital pain, high fever, and rhinorrhea. The patient's condition may rapidly worsen to include altered consciousness, neurologic deficit, and development of orbital apex syndrome. Typically, a dark, gangrenous lesion is found in the mucosa of the nasal portion of the hard palate. The nasal septum may be perforated. Blood cultures and lumbar punctures are usually not helpful. A tissue biopsy and smear and culture of the necrotic tissue are necessary. The tissue scrapings should be examined under the microscope using 20% potassium hydroxide (KOH) to make the diagnosis. The material should be inoculated onto blood agar, Sabouraud's agar, and an anaerobic medium and incubated at 25° C and 37° C for at least 2 weeks before being considered negative. To confirm the presence of organisms, tissue should be fixed in 10% formalin, embedded in paraffin, and stained with hematoxylin and eosin, periodic acid–Schiff, and Grocott's methenamine stains. Correction of the metabolic acidosis, restoration of electrolyte balance, and rehydration are of the utmost importance in the management of these patients. In addition, wide debridement of necrotic tissues should be performed and intravenous amphotericin B treatment should be initiated prior to laboratory confirmation of the organism.

(Continued on page 156)

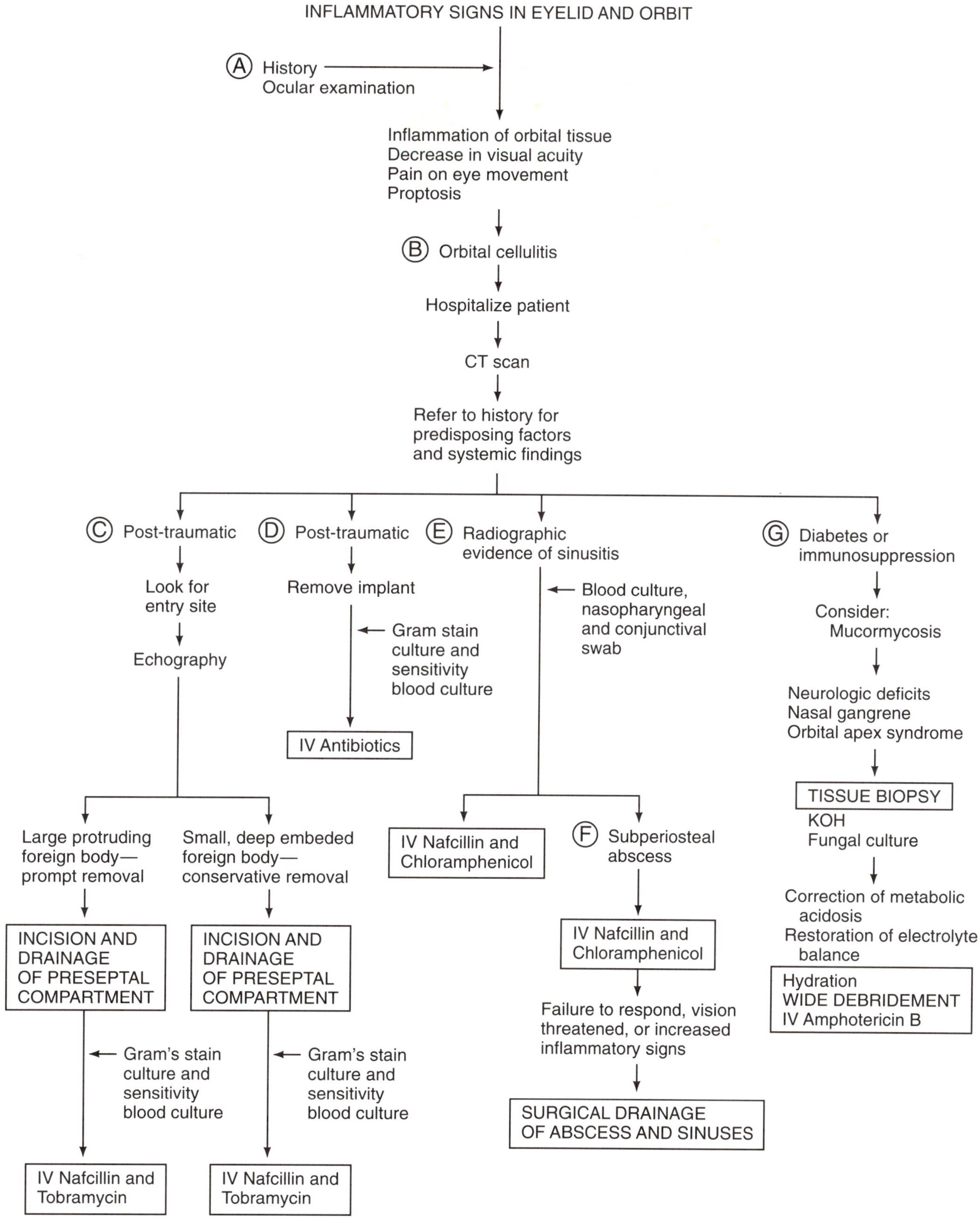
INFLAMMATORY SIGNS IN EYELID AND ORBIT
(A) History
Ocular examination
Inflammation of orbital tissue
Decrease in visual acuity
Pain on eye movement
Proptosis
(B) Orbital cellulitis
Hospitalize patient
CT scan
Refer to history for predisposing factors and systemic findings
(C) Post-traumatic
Look for entry site
Echography
Large protruding foreign body—prompt removal
INCISION AND DRAINAGE OF PRESEPTAL COMPARTMENT
Gram's stain culture and sensitivity blood culture
IV Nafcillin and Tobramycin
Small, deep embeded foreign body—conservative removal
INCISION AND DRAINAGE OF PRESEPTAL COMPARTMENT
Gram's stain culture and sensitivity blood culture
IV Nafcillin and Tobramycin
(D) Post-traumatic
Remove implant
Gram stain culture and sensitivity blood culture
IV Antibiotics
(E) Radiographic evidence of sinusitis
Blood culture, nasopharyngeal and conjunctival swab
IV Nafcillin and Chloramphenicol
(F) Subperiosteal abscess
IV Nafcillin and Chloramphenicol
Failure to respond, vision threatened, or increased inflammatory signs
SURGICAL DRAINAGE OF ABSCESS AND SINUSES
(G) Diabetes or immunosuppression
Consider: Mucormycosis
Neurologic deficits
Nasal gangrene
Orbital apex syndrome
TISSUE BIOPSY
KOH
Fungal culture
Correction of metabolic acidosis
Restoration of electrolyte balance
Hydration
WIDE DEBRIDEMENT
IV Amphotericin B

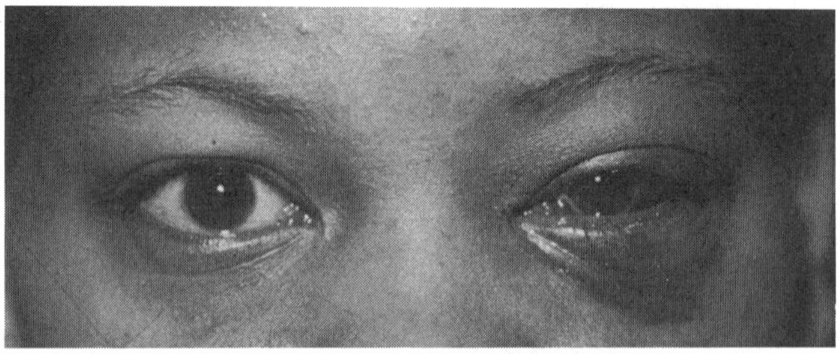

Figure 1 This child has erysipelas. In addition to the red, edematous, painful eyelid, there is mild proptosis, subconjunctival hemorrhage, and limitation of ocular motility.

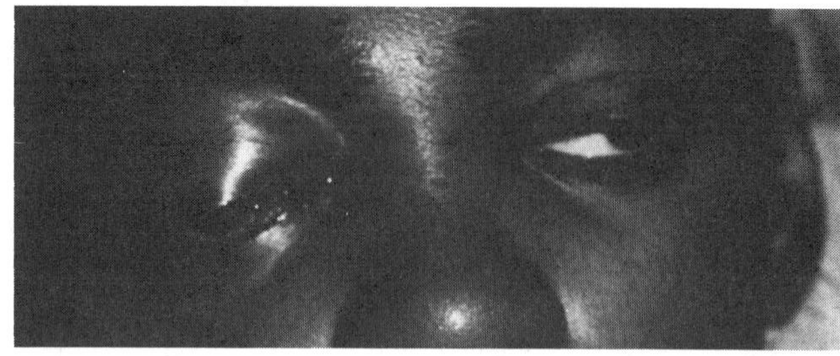

Figure 3 This child presented with a high fever and general malaise and looked toxic. His vision in the involved eye was hand motion and the globe was frozen. A STAT CT scan revealed subperiostal abscess. Immediate surgical drainage of the orbit and ethmoidal cells restored his vision and motility to normal.

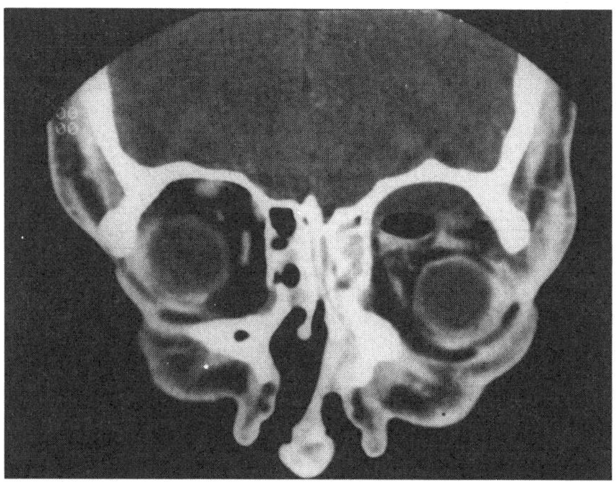

Figure 2 A typical CT scan of orbital cellulitis secondary to sinusitis. Note the air in the orbit and the opacification of the ethmoidal cells.

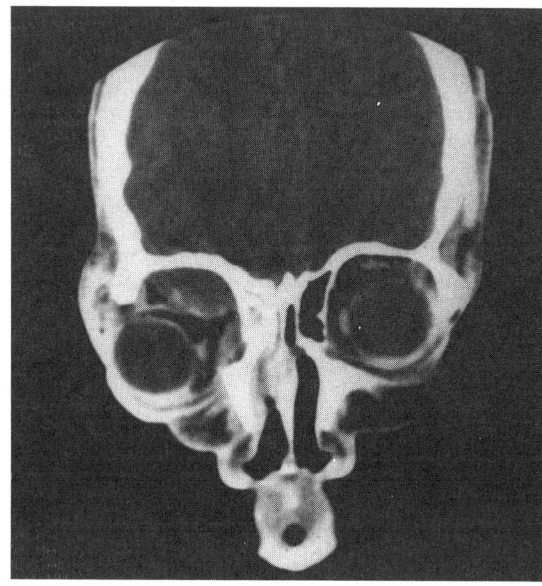

Figure 4 CT scan shows a subperiosteal collection of pus both superiorly and medially. Ethmoidal cells are also involved.

References

Noel LP, Clark WN, MacDonald N. Clinical management of orbital cellulitis in children. Can J Ophthalmol 1990; 25:11.

Rubin SE, Rubin LG, Zito J, et al. Medical management of orbital subperiosteal abscess in children. J Pediatr Ophthalmol Strabismus 1989; 26:21.

Williams BJ, Harrison HC. Subperiosteal abscesses of the orbit due to sinusitis in childhood. Aust NZ J Ophthalmol 1991; 19:299.

PIGMENTED LESIONS OF THE EYELIDS, PERIOCULAR SKIN, AND CONJUNCTIVA

Curtis E. Margo, M.D.

A. Pigmented lesions of the eyelid and periocular skin consist of a heterogeneous collection of conditions characterized by their color (i.e., nonflesh). The vast majority of all periocular skin lesions in the pediatric age group are benign tumors or hamartomatous malformations. Most of these have a vascular or melanocytic origin. The distinction between these two groups is relatively easy based on color. A complete analysis of the lesion's clinical features (size, shape, topography, texture, and color) and its behavior establishes the diagnosis. In some situations a biopsy may be needed.

B. The two most commonly encountered congenital vascular lesions are the capillary hemangioma of infancy and the nevus flammeus, or port wine stain. The predominantly macular port wine stain is often found in the distribution of the trigeminal nerve and rarely enlarges after birth, although lesions may become darker and focally nodular. Capillary hemangioma of infancy (strawberry nevus) is a vascular malformation present at birth or appearing shortly thereafter. These red bosselated tumors have a smooth surface and rubbery texture. The spider angioma is a rare vascular malformation characterized by its central feeding vessel and peripheral radiating arms. Pyogenic granuloma is a polypoid growth of granulation tissue. The rich vascular supply of these lesions gives the pyogenic granuloma the appearance of a primary vascular tumor.

C. The spectrum of congenital melanocytic lesions may be subdivided into two broad categories: nevus of Ota and congenital melanocytic nevi. The nevus of Ota is a large cutaneous macule associated with ocular melanosis. The macule has no palpable edge and can be delineated by its color (light tan, grey, or blue-grey color). Some macules do not become clinically evident for months or years after birth. Patients need periodic life-long follow-up because of the propensity for ocular melanosis to spawn a uveal melanoma. There is virtually no risk of melanoma developing in the cutaneous macule, however. By convention, all other congenital melanocytic malformations are referred to collectively as congenital melanocytic nevi. Most congenital nevi appear as elevated lesions with irregular topographic features. Their size, heavy pigmentation, and hair make them cosmetic problems. Most are considerably larger than acquired nevi, which rarely exceed 6 mm in diameter. Some congenital melanocytic nevi can involve as much as one-third of all facial skin. These lesions may have a propensity for malignant transformation, based on anecdotal experiences with large congenital nevi located elsewhere. Unfortunately, there is no clinically practical method of estimating the magnitude of this risk. Onset of ominous changes in color or contour, signs of ulceration, and bleeding require a biopsy to exclude the possibility of malignant transformation.

D. The diagnosis of acquired melanocytic lesions in infants and children is based on their clinical features and course. One must determine if the lesion is flush with the skin surface (macule) or elevated (nodule). Small tan to brown macules include ephelides (freckles), lentigines, and junctional nevi. These lesions are all benign and rarely exceed 7 mm in diameter. Facial freckles are common and easily recognized by their orange-brown color and distribution on sun-exposed skin. A solitary childhood lentigo is clinically indistinguishable from a junctional nevus without biopsy, but this distinction rarely needs to be made. Multiple lentigines are often associated with systemic disorders such as the Peutz-Jegher syndrome, the LAMB syndrome, the LEOPARD syndrome, and xeroderma pigmentosum. Café-au-lait spots are considerably larger than junctional nevi and childhood lentigines and have a more irregular shape.

E. There are a variety of benign acquired melanocytic nodules. Differentiating these nodules clinically often requires biopsy, but because most are benign there are few clinical indications for surgical excision. As junctional nevi mature into compound nevi, they become elevated. The acquired melanocytic nevus carries a very small risk of malignant transformation. Biopsy is indicated when a stable lesion changes in size or color (although this is not an uncommon phenomenon during adolescence) or if a lesion has atypical clinical features (e.g., dysplastic nevus). The blue nevus, combined nevus, halo nevus, and spindle/epithelioid nevus are other benign pigmented nodules whose diagnoses often require biopsy. Surgical excision is usually not required because these nodules appear clinically benign and pose minimal life-long risk of malignant transformation.

F. Malignant melanoma of the eyelid and periocular skin is exceptionally rare in infants and children. A malignant melanoma needs to be considered in the differential diagnosis of any progressively enlarging tan, brown, black, maroon, or dark blue nodule. Other signs of malignancy include the presence of irregular margins, an ulcerated surface, and mottled coloration. The histopathologic evaluation of melanocytic tumors in infants and children is challenging because a certain degree of cellular atypia is normally found in benign melanocytic nevi during the first decade of life. Because large congenital melanocytic nevi are considered precursors to melanoma, they

(Continued on page 160.)

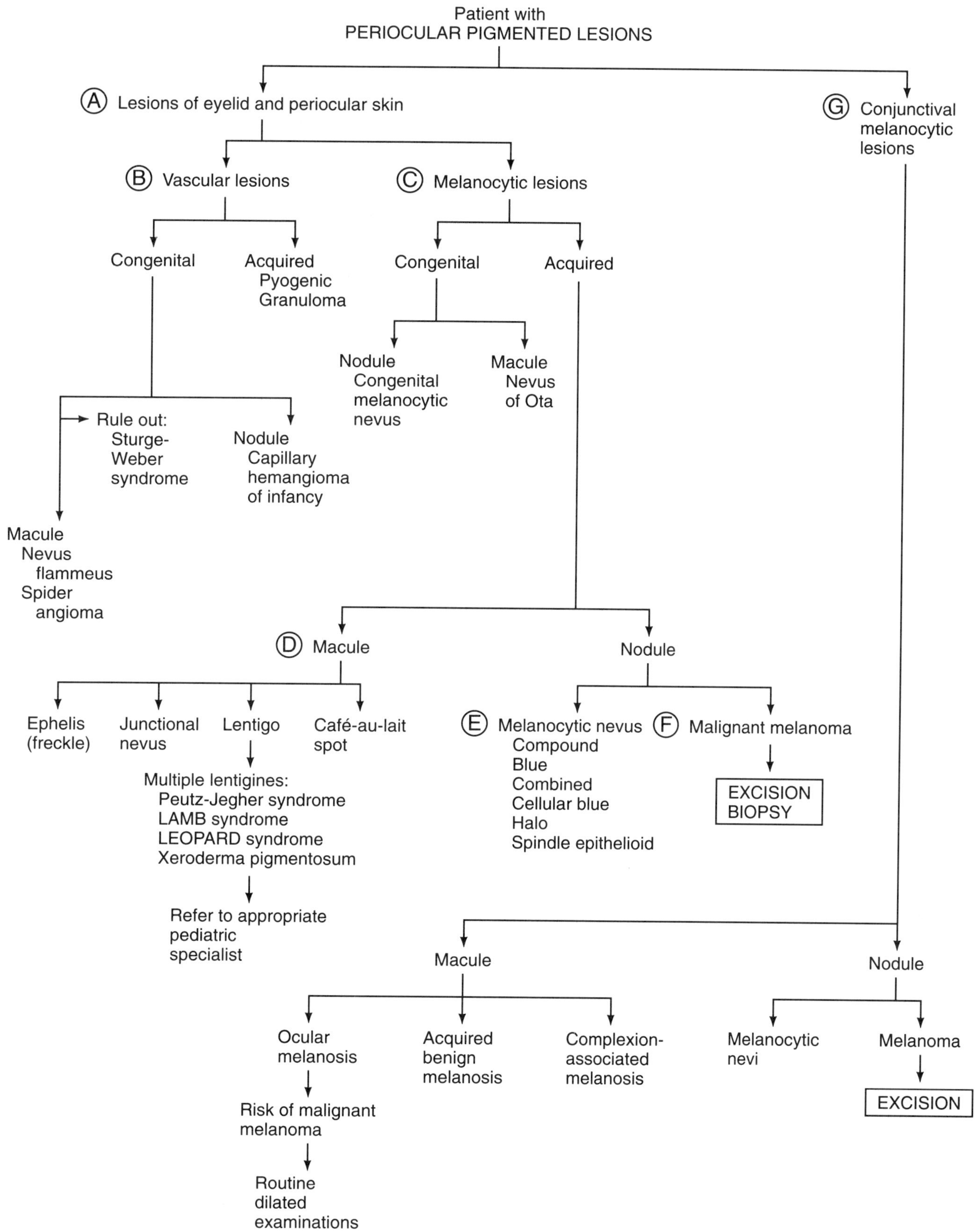
Patient with
PERIOCULAR PIGMENTED LESIONS
Ⓐ Lesions of eyelid and periocular skin
Ⓑ Vascular lesions
Congenital
Acquired
Pyogenic
Granuloma
Rule out:
Sturge-
Weber
syndrome
Nodule
Capillary
hemangioma
of infancy
Macule
Nevus
flammeus
Spider
angioma
Ⓒ Melanocytic lesions
Congenital
Acquired
Nodule
Congenital
melanocytic
nevus
Macule
Nevus
of Ota
Ⓓ Macule
Ephelis
(freckle)
Junctional
nevus
Lentigo
Café-au-lait
spot
Multiple lentigines:
Peutz-Jegher syndrome
LAMB syndrome
LEOPARD syndrome
Xeroderma pigmentosum
Refer to appropriate
pediatric
specialist
Nodule
Ⓔ Melanocytic nevus
Compound
Blue
Combined
Cellular blue
Halo
Spindle epithelioid
Ⓕ Malignant melanoma
EXCISION
BIOPSY
Ⓖ Conjunctival
melanocytic
lesions
Macule
Ocular
melanosis
Risk of malignant
melanoma
Routine
dilated
examinations
Acquired
benign
melanosis
Complexion-
associated
melanosis
Nodule
Melanocytic
nevi
Melanoma
EXCISION

should be observed periodically and biopsied if focal changes are noted.

Not all melanocytic lesions are pigmented. The small nodule of the spindle/epithelioid nevus, for example, often has a flesh-orange color. In addition, not all tan-colored lesions are due to primary melanocytic malformations or proliferations. Secondary melanocytic hyperplasia occurs with inflammatory dermatoses, cutaneous scar formation, and in a variety of nonmelanocytic tumors such as the dermatofibroma. In infants and children, the low incidence of malignant melanoma makes it unlikely that any small pigmented nodule is a melanoma. A specific diagnosis for most benign-appearing skin nodules rarely needs to be made because their management is the same: observation and family reassurance.

G. Pigmented lesions of the conjunctiva share many of the clinical and biologic features of their cutaneous counterparts. The diagnostic approach is similar. Congenital ocular melanosis (with or without cutaneous involvement) is the most common pigmented macule found in infants and young children. Small acquired, pigmented macules can be found in patients with Peutz-Jegher syndrome and von Reckinhausen disease. Some degree of complexion-associated melanosis (so-called racial melanosis) usually becomes evident near puberty. The vast majority of all conjunctival melanocytic nevi are benign and begin to appear in late childhood or during puberty. Histologically, these small nodular lesions can be classified into a variety of subtypes (e.g., compound nevus, epithelioid nevus, pigmented limbal spindle cell tumor, melanocytoma, blue nevus). Biopsy, however, is seldom required because the incidence of malignant melanoma of the conjunctiva is exceptionally low in the pediatric age group. Conjunctival nevi may grow during adolescence and usually raise concern over the possibility of malignant transformation. Because benign nevi of the forniceal or palpebral conjunctiva are rare, they should be biopsied when found. Conjunctival nevi are freely movable over the sclera and often contain clear microcysts. Benign limbal nevi may overlap the cornea. Signs of corneal stromal invasion are worrisome and warrant biopsy. Inflammation and cellular atypia in benign conjunctival nevi in children may make the objective evaluation of a biopsy difficult.

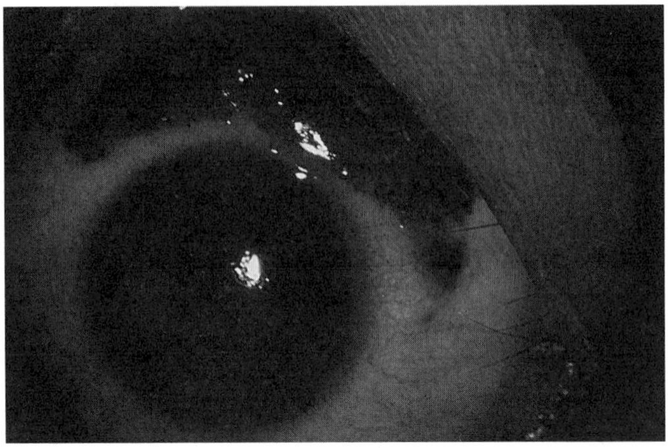

Figure 1 Conjunctival nevus growing at puberty.

References

Folberg R, Jakobiec FA, Bernardino AB, Iwamoto T. Benign conjunctival melanocytic lesions. Clinicopathologic features. Ophthalmology 1989; 96:436.

Margo CE, Rober DLJ, Hadayat AA. Borderline melanocytic tumor of the conjunctiva: Diagnostic and therapeutic considerations. J Pediatr Ophthalmol Strabismus 1991; 28:268.

Margo CE. Pigmented lesions of the eyelid. In: Albert DM, Jakobiec FA, eds. Principles and practice of ophthalmology. Philadelphia: WB Saunders (in press).

Margo CE, Habal MB. Large congenital melanocytic nevus. Light and electron microscopic findings. Ophthalmology 1987; 94:960.

McDonnell JM, Carpenter JD, Jacobs P, et al. Conjunctival melanocytic lesions in children. Ophthalmology 1989; 96:986.

Trozak DJ, Rowland WD, Funan H. Metastatic malignant melanoma in prepubertal children. Pediatrics 1975; 55:191.

CHILDHOOD BLEPHARITIS

William D. Mathers, M.D.

A. Blepharitis in childhood can be caused by a number of processes, including bacterial infection, allergy, parasitic infestation, and meibomian gland dysfunction. Differentiating these processes by their symptoms is difficult because most produce a similar chronic irritation, itching, burning, and erythema of the eyelid margin. Careful biomicroscopy of the eyelid margin, conjunctival surface, and cornea with meibomian gland expression is essential in making the correct diagnosis.

B. Three species of lice parasitize humans: *Pediculus humanus corporis* (human body louse), *Pediculus humanus capitis* (head louse), and *Phthirus pubis* (crab louse). All of these can cause infestation of the lid margin and lashes. Adult females lay eggs that are glued to the lashes and are easily seen by biomicroscopy. Transmission is through close contact, particularly bedding and clothing. Lice may also cause follicular conjunctivitis, marginal keratitis, and madarosis. Treatment consists of mercuric oxide ointment, physostigmine, or tetraethyl pyrophosphate applied to the lid margins for the entire life cycle (14 days). Ilotycin ointment may also be used. Child abuse can be considered when infestations involve young children.

C. Granulomatous inflammation and destruction of individual meibomian glands occurs in childhood, often in association with chronic blepharitis. Meibomian gland dysfunction, however, is not always evident by meibomian gland expression. Firm and somewhat tender nodules may be quite inflamed during the acute stage. Treatment for acute chalazia is palliative and includes warm compresses. If infection and preseptal cellulitis are suspected, systemic oral antibiotics may be indicated. Chalazia that persist longer than 3 months may be incised in the same way as chalazia in adults are treated. Low-dose oral tetracycline* or erythromycin may be justified if the problem is particularly unresponsive and severe. However, tetracycline may permanently stain newly formed teeth if given during the time of dental calcification (approximately 5 months' gestation to 8 years of age).

D. Blepharitis is often accompanied by conjunctivitis. With careful biomicroscopy, it is usually possible to discriminate between a follicular and papillary response in the conjunctiva, although follicles are usually present in the normal child. Acute follicular conjunctivitis is frequently associated with viral infection. Chlamydial infection and molluscum contagiosum should also be considered.

E. A papillary response in the conjunctiva is usually associated with an allergic process. The most severe example occurs in vernal conjunctivitis. Giant papillary conjunctivitis is associated with contact lens use and may present a similar picture. Environmental allergies often associated with hay fever produce symptoms that range from extremely mild and occasional to severe and protracted. Treatment consists of antihistaminic and sympathomimetic medications; topical steroid use should be avoided.

F. Bacterial conjunctivitis with blepharitis may produce injection and thickening of the conjunctiva and may or may not be associated with a papillary response. Other signs of bacterial conjunctivitis include loss of lashes and crusting of the lid margin. A short course of topical antibiotics can be used when acute bacterial infection is suspected. Chronic treatment with topical antibiotics is counterproductive and should be avoided.

G. Perilimbal inflammation is often associated with chronic blepharitis and probably represents an immune response to resident bacteria rather than a bacterial infection. Marginal infiltrates with perilimbal inflammation represent antigen-antibody deposition and respond quickly to short-term topical antibiotic and steroid combinations. A cellular immune response creates phlyctenular disease, which responds more slowly to topical antibiotics and steroids. Chronic treatment of the blepharitis with systemic tetracycline* may be indicated if the phlyctenular disease is resistant to local treatment.

H. Meibomian gland dysfunction (MGD) with alteration of meibomian gland excreta may begin in later childhood and adolescence, although it is more common in adults. Meibomian gland drop-out from obstructive meibomian gland dysfunction can be seen with meibography and is associated with markedly thickened excreta and decreased excreta volume. Seborrheic meibomian gland dysfunction is associated with increased meibomian excreta volume that is only slightly thickened. Both may produce similar blepharitis symptoms. Seborrheic meibomian gland dysfunction does usually not require treatment except local measures, including lid scrubs with baby shampoo. Obstructive meibomian gland dysfunction may also be treated with lid scrubs and in severe cases with low-dose long-term oral tetracycline* or erythromycin. Chronic application of topical antibiotics is not generally effective.

*Because of age-related tooth deposition do not use in children younger than 8 to 10 years of age.

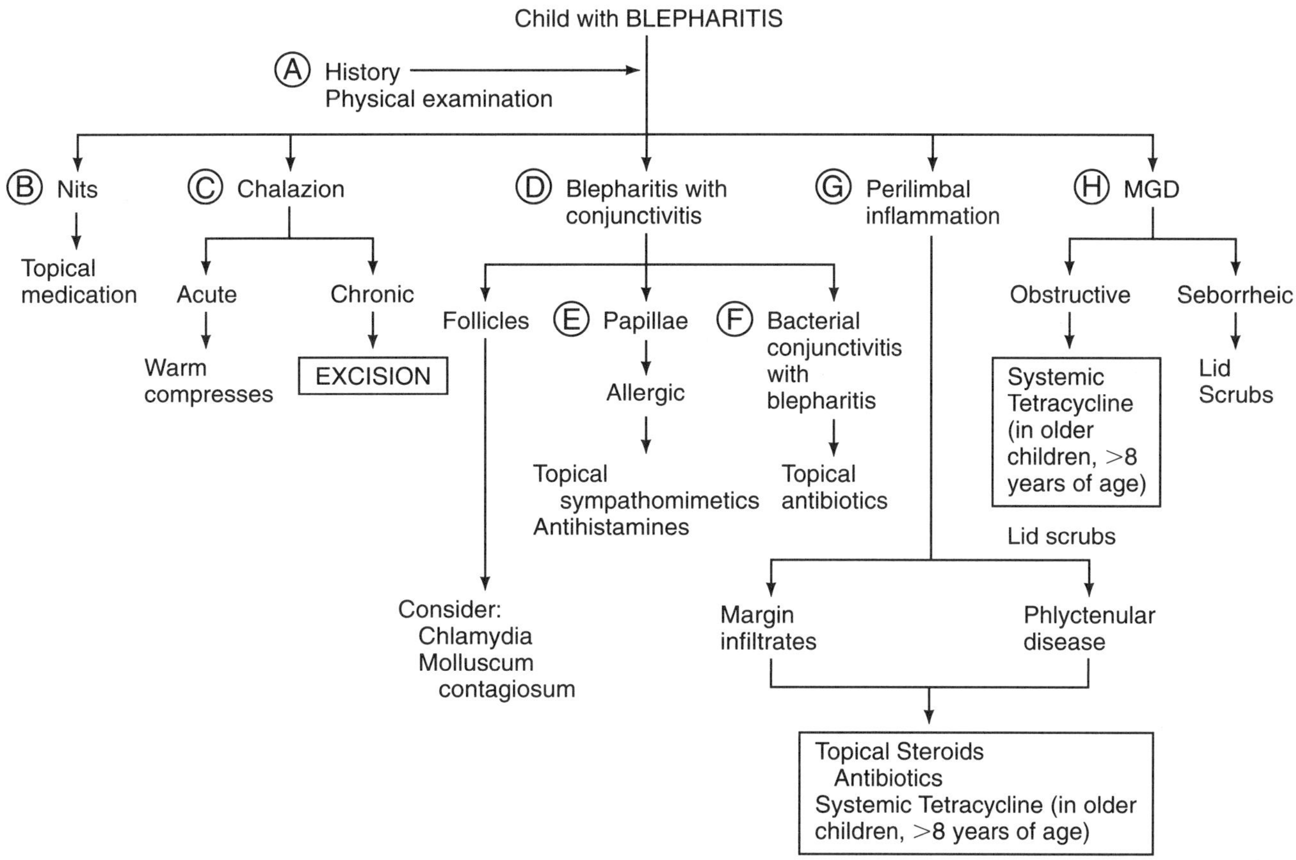

References

Couch SM, Green WR, Hirst LW, De La Cruz ZC. Diagnosing and treating *Phthirus pubis* palbebrarum. Surv Ophthalmol 1982; 26:219.

Dougherty JM, McCulley JP. Comparative bacteriology of chronic blepharitis. Br J Ophthalmol 1981; 68:524.

Mathers WD, et al. Meibomian gland dysfunction in chronic blepharitis. Cornea 1991; 10:277.

ACUTE CONJUNCTIVITIS IN CHILDHOOD

Avery H. Weiss, M.D.

A. Acute conjunctivitis, defined as conjunctival redness with discharge of less than 14 days' duration, is a common problem in preschool and school-age children. Most cases are due to bacterial rather than viral infections, but both can spread to family members and other close contacts. It may be associated with the seasonal appearance of ocular itching, hay fever, and atopic skin disease. Exposure to noxious agents (including topical medications) and airborne irritants should be considered as possible causes of conjunctival injection.

B. Although the various causes of conjunctivitis are not reliably distinguished on the basis of examination alone, certain findings are suggestive of bacterial, viral, or allergic conjunctivitis and serve to exclude nonconjunctival disorders. Both bacterial and viral infections occur bilaterally and cause eyelid swelling with conjunctival erythema. However, the conjunctival discharge tends to be serous in viral infections and purulent in bacterial infections. The presence of preauricular adenopathy and pharyngitis is more indicative of viral infections and otitis media of bacterial infections. The conjunctival response is follicular in viral infections, mixed or nonspecific in bacterial infection, and papillary in allergic conditions. Because papillary hypertrophy shows a predilection for the palpebral conjunctiva of the upper eyelid, it is best demonstrated by eversion of the lid. In infants, the presence of purulent discharge with conjunctival injection might suggest lacrimal duct obstruction, which can be confirmed by showing delayed clearance of 5% fluorescein applied topically. Care should be taken to inspect the eyelids and globe for abnormalities that can be mistaken for conjunctivitis, such as conjunctival foreign bodies, keratitis, scleritis, and uveitis.

C. Bacterial cultures are not done routinely. They are obtained in cases of neonatal conjunctivitis, when there is an associated preseptal cellulitis, and in cases that have been recalcitrant to standard therapy. To maximize their yield, the culture media should be inoculated directly or the sample taken immediately to the microbiology laboratory in transport media. Culture media should include blood and chocolate agar, both of which are enriched with blood or other growth factors. Selective media such as mannitol salts, agar, and eosin methylene blue agar are used to enhance the growth and to facilitate the identification of staphylococcal and gram-negative organisms, respectively. Viral cultures (except in herpes infections) are not useful because there is little clinical efficacy and no therapeutic benefit (p 288).

D. Once again, routine conjunctival scrapings are not obtained except for cases delineated in paragraph C. After topical anesthetic drops are instilled in each eye, the palpebral conjunctiva is scraped gently with a Kimura spatula. The material is placed onto labeled glass slides and prepared with Gram and Giemsa stains. The Gram stain results help to predict the presence and type of bacterial pathogens and guide the selection of initial antibiotic treatment. Giemsa stains provide information about the conjunctival inflammatory response showing neutrophilia in bacterial infections, lymphocytosis in viral infections, eosinophils or eosinophilic granules in allergic conditions, and degenerative changes of the epithelial nucleus and cytoplasm in toxic reactions (p 292).

E. The most common bacterial pathogens are *Haemophilus influenzae, Streptococcus pneumoniae* and other streptococcal isolates, and *Branhamella catarrhalis*. Other gram-negative organisms can be recovered in individual patients. Recovery of staphylococci has questionable significance because they are part of the normal eyelid flora. Staphylococcal blepharitis is reliably diagnosed when there are clinical signs of blepharitis, heavy growth of *Staphylococcus aureus* from the lids, and evidence of conjunctival inflammation. Persistent staphylococcal blepharitis may be indicative of an underlying allergic disease or immunodeficiency state.

F. Although acute bacterial conjunctivitis tends to be a self-limited disease lasting 7 to 14 days, antibiotic treatment is recommended because it shortens the duration of clinical disease. There are numerous antibiotic choices. Sulfacetamide drops are inexpensive, but they have a bacteriostatic mechanism of action and sting upon instillation. Both erythromycin and polysporin (combination of bacitracin and polymyxin) have activity against the most common bacterial pathogens, but the ointment vehicle causes visual blurring that makes them undesirable in school-age children. Polytrim (combination of trimethoprim and polymyxin B) is a good first-line antibiotic because it has broad-spectrum coverage and comes in solution form. Topical aminoglycosides should be reserved specifically for gram-negative infections and Ciloxin (ciprofloxacin) for serious or recalcitrant infections.

G. Adenoviruses are important causes of pediatric conjunctivitis. The hallmark of pharyngoconjunctival fever (associated with adenovirus types 3, 4, 7, and occasionally 5) is fever and pharyngitis. Epidemic keratoconjunctivitis (due to adenovirus types 8 and 19) is probably the most common viral pathogen in children older than 10 years. It can be associated with the appearance of subepithelial corneal infiltrates 10 to 14 days after its onset. These immune-mediated opacities may elicit a foreign body sensation and disturb vision. Herpes simplex presents as a follicular

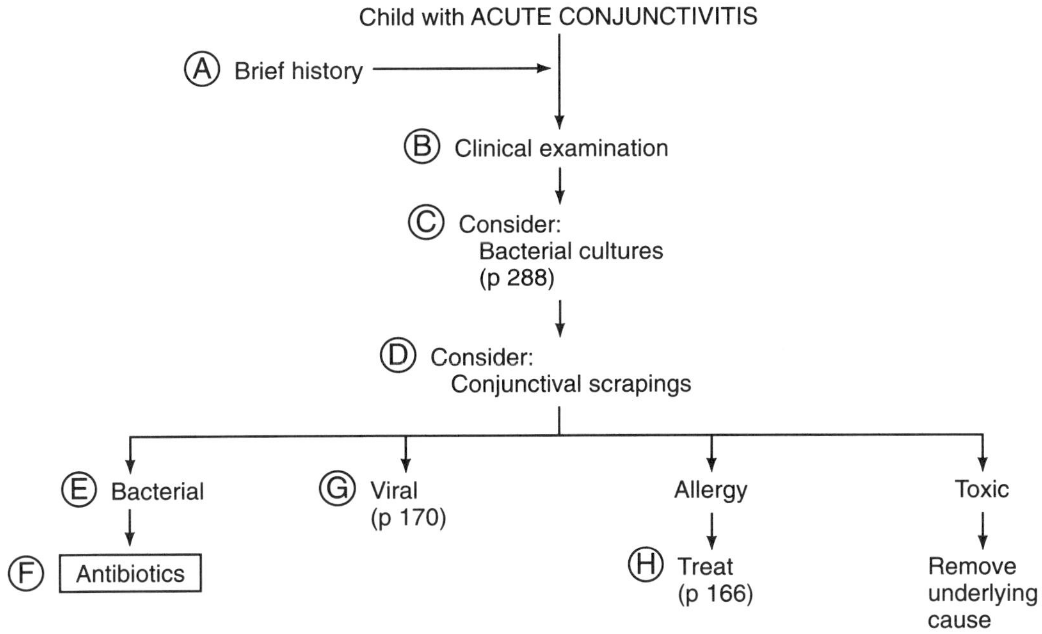

conjunctivitis that can be distinguished on the basis of associated ocular involvement, particularly eyelid vesicles and corneal dendrites. Varicella-zoster, measles, and vaccinia can invade the ocular surface and are easily recognized by their accompanying systemic involvement, particularly skin exanthema (p 170).

H. Treatment is symptomatic using topical and, less frequently, systemic decongestants and antihistamines. Cromolyn sodium drops and other agents that prevent mast cell degranulation are sometimes very helpful. Topical corticosteroids are indicated for unusually severe and intractable symptoms (p 166).

References

Brinser JH, Weiss A. Laboratory diagnosis in ocular disease. In: Tasman W, Jaeger EA, eds. Duane's clinical ophthalmology. Philadelphia: JB Lippincott, 1990:1.

Gigliotti F, Hendly JO, Morgan J, et al. Efficacy of topical antibiotic therapy in acute conjunctivitis in children. J Pediatr 1984; 104:623.

Gigliotti F, Williams WT, Hayden FG, Hendley JO. Etiology of acute conjunctivitis in children. J Pediatr 1981; 98:531.

Lohr JA, Austin RD, Grossman M, et al. Comparison of three topical antimicrobials for acute bacterial conjunctivitis. Pediatr Infect Dis J 1988; 7:626.

ALLERGIC CONJUNCTIVITIS

Andrea Cibis Tongue, M.D.

A. Presenting symptoms of allergic conjunctivitis frequently give a clue to the etiology. Acute symptoms occur upon contact with allergens, usually associated with hay fever—pollen, mold, and animal hairs, especially cat hair. The conjunctivitis is usually bilateral. Unilateral acute allergic conjunctivitis occurs with insect bites and localized contact with particle allergens such as an insect part, plant seed, and so forth. The most common symptoms are itching and/or irritation and tearing; the most common signs are watery, red eyes with boggy conjunctival chemosis and sometimes lid chemosis. Onset is hours to days before the patient seeks help. Patients with hay fever usually have associated rhinorrhea; their symptoms are often seasonal and recurrent.

Patients who come in contact with a chemical allergen may present with unilateral or bilateral conjunctivitis depending on the site of exposure. Acute chemical allergic conjunctivitis develops in sensitized patients with prior exposure to the allergen. Often the lids are involved with pale, boggy, or occasionally hyperemic chemosis. Neomycin, atropine, sulfur, and merthiolate are some of the more common chemical allergens used in ophthalmology. However, any ophthalmic drops, ointments, or solutions may contain ingredients to which a patient is allergic.

Treatment of acute allergic conjunctivitis is withdrawal of suspected or known contact allergens. Topical and/or systemic antihistamines and the use of cold compresses usually provide sufficient symptom relief. Patients with recurrent hay fever symptoms may benefit from desensitization to the allergen. Cromolyn sodium ophthalmic solution* has been useful in preventing eye symptoms of hay fever as well.

B. Onset is more gradual in atopic conjunctivitis, vernal conjunctivitis, giant papillary conjunctivitis, staphylococcal keratoconjunctivitis, phlyctenular conjunctivitis, and chronic chemical allergen exposure. Patients may have had irritation, itching, or conjunctival hyperemia for weeks, even months, before seeking definitive care. Corneal involvement may be found with associated photophobia, tearing, and discomfort.

C. Atopic conjunctivitis is characterized by itching, burning, watery eyes and mucoid discharge. The eyelids may be red, thickened, and crusty with associated staphylococcal blepharitis or eczema. Conjunctival papilla are most prominent in the lower fornix. Conjunctival hyperemia, when present, is mild. The cornea may be involved with punctate epithelial staining. A familial history of atopic disease is relatively common. Treatment consists of lid hygiene and use of antibiotic ointment if staphylococcal disease is present. Antihistamine eye drops and artificial tears or ointment are helpful in some patients, as is cromolyn sodium ophthalmic solution.* Topical steroids should be used judiciously for short-term treatment only. Some patients with severe atopy may develop keratoconus and cataracts as part of their disease.

D. Allergic conjunctivitis secondary to chronic chemical allergen exposure is most usually seen in contact lens wearers. It may develop insidiously over a period of weeks before becoming sufficiently bothersome to cause the patient to seek care. Hyperemia, irritation, and discomfort upon insertion of the contact lenses are often the initial symptoms; itching is usually a mild or minor symptom. A bulbar follicular reaction, mild tarsal follicular and papillary reactions, or corneal epithelial keratitis may be seen. The most common causative agent is the contact lens solution preservative merthiolate (thimerosal). There may be early stages of giant papillary conjunctivitis. Treatment is removal of the suspected allergen and use of astringent or lubricating eye drops. Cromolyn* or topical antihistamine eye drops are helpful for itching and conjunctival chemosis. Other chronic exposure to topical eye medications or solutions, foreign substances such as particles of eye make-up, viral particles of molluscum contagiosum at the eyelid margin, eye sutures, and artificial eyes may cause a chronic follicular conjunctivitis. It is thought that the reaction may be toxic rather than allergic, but the treatment is essentially the same.

E. Vernal conjunctivitis is a seasonally recurring disease lasting 4 to 10 years. Symptoms, which commonly appear in the spring with warm weather, include watery red eyes with a ropy thick discharge and photophobia. Pseudoptosis may occur. The primary symptom is itching, although patients on systemic antihistamine drops may have amelioration of this. A family or personal history of atopic disease is not uncommon. Examination reveals papillary hypertrophy of the superior tarsal conjunctiva. In the palpebral variety of vernal conjunctivitis, the papillary hypertrophy is marked, with large, flat, pale or hyperemic papilla, resembling a cobblestone pattern. Vessels originate from a central core in the papilla and then branch in an arcade over the tops of the papillae. Histologically, papillae consist of collections of inflammatory cells (lymphocytes, plasma cells, eosinophils, basophils) supported by newly proliferated collagen and blood vessels. The surface of the tarsus is often coated with a whitish stringy exudate, and a similar thick and stringy accumulation may be present

(Continued on page 168)

*Cromolyn sodium ophthalmic solution is no longer available at the time of the writing of this chapter.

Patient with ALLERGIC CONJUNCTIVITIS

- **(A) Acute**
  - Itching
  - Conjunctival discharge
  - Boggy lid swelling
  - Hyperemia
  - Tearing
  - → Unilateral
    - Chemical allergen
    - Insect bite
  - → Bilateral
    - Hay fever
    - Chemical allergen
  - → Removal of allergen
    - Cold compresses
    - Artificial tears or astringents
    - Antihistamines, topical/systemic
    - Short course of topical steroids
    - Cromolyn sodium ophthalmic solution
    - Desensitization to allergen

- **(B) Subacute chronic:**
  - Itching
  - Hyperemia
  - Tearing
  - Irritation
  - Photophobia

  - Plus: Mucoid discharge; Erythematous lids; History of eczema or atopy; Follicular/papillary reaction
    - → **(C) Consider:** Atopic conjunctivitis
    - → Artificial tears; Astringents; Lid hygiene; Antibiotics for concomitant staplyloccal infection; Antihistamine ophthalmic drops; Cold compresses; Steroids, only short term for severe symptoms; Cromolyn sodium ophthalmic drops

  - Plus: History of contact with eye solutions, ointments, contact lenses; Punctate keratitis
    - → **(D) Consider:** Chemical conjunctivitis
    - → Removal of allergen; Artificial tears; Astringents; Antihistamine drops; Steroids, short term for severe symptoms

  - Plus: Pseudoptosis; Stringy thick discharge; Giant superior tarsal papillary reaction; Limbal papillary reaction; Horner-Trantas dots; Superficial keratitis; Oval grey corneal ulcers
    - → **(E) Consider:** Vernal conjunctivitis
    - → **Antihistamines, systemic**
    - Antihistamines, topical; Astringents; Cromolyn sodium ophthalmic drops; Cold compresses; Topical steroids (short-term use); Climate change

  - Plus: Giant superior tarsal papillae; History of contact lens or prosthesis wear; Keratitis
    - → **(F) Consider:** Giant papillary conjunctivitis
    - → Remove contact lenses; Topical antihistamines; Topical short-term steroid use; Switch to different type of contact lens; Avoid merthiolate-preserved solutions

  - Plus: Limbal follicles; Marginal infiltrates; Punctate keratitis; Blepharitis
    - → **(G) Consider:** Staphylococcal keratoconjunctivitis
    - → Antibiotic/steroid drops or ointment; Lid hygiene; Long-term low-dose antibiotic drops or ointment

  - Plus: Isolated nodule with leash of vessels; Severe photophobia
    - → **(H) Consider:** Phlyctenular keratoconjunctivitis
    - → Treat underlying microbial disease if present (staphylococcal most common); Topical steroid drops or ointment

in the lower fornix. Histologically the distinguishing feature is the presence of many eosinophils and eosinophilic granules. If the patient has limbal involvement, raised nodules, either isolated or confluent, are seen primarily along the upper limbus. The nodules have central vascular cores of papillae, unlike limbal follicles, which have vessels that come up around the sides of the follicles from the base of the follicle, not from the center. Superiorly the nodules may be confluent and appear gelatinous, overhanging the cornea. White/yellow calcific-appearing dots or concretions may appear within the mounds around the limbus and much more rarely on the bulbar conjunctiva. These concretions, composed of collections of eosinophils, are referred to as Horner-Trantas dots, pathognomonic of vernal conjunctivitis. Superficial corneal epithelial keratitis or more extensive epithelial involvement may be seen. Rarely patients develop oval shallow gray-white ulcers, usually located superiorly under the lid. Photophobia and tearing are symptoms of corneal involvement.

Vernal conjunctivitis is treated with systemic and topical antihistamine drops or Cromolyn.* Artificial tears, astringent eye drops, and cold compresses often help. Steroids are reserved for severe cases and should not be used long term. Patients need to be followed carefully while receiving topical steroid therapy. Use of antihistamine eye drops and systemic antihistamines often allows the steroid dosage to be decreased rapidly. Patients and parents need to be advised that the disease cannot be cured or eliminated. Changing climatic conditions, eliminating known allergens, and desensitization can be helpful. However, specific allergens usually do not seem to trigger vernal conjunctivitis. Concomitant lid or conjunctival bacterial infections should be treated.

F. Giant papillary conjunctivitis (GPC) has many similarities to vernal conjunctivitis. Papillary hypertrophy, usually of the superior tarsal conjunctiva, occurs. Patients may develop superficial punctate epithelial keratitis, often of the superior cornea. Itching, hyperemia, irritation, mucous discharge, photophobia, and tearing are prominent symptoms. GPC is most often a result of contact lens wear, soft contacts more often to blame than hard or gas-permeable contact lenses. Patients may develop GPC as a response to contact lens-care products. Symptoms at first are mild, and the onset of more severe disease is generally insidious. The diagnosis of GPC may be missed in a contact lens wearer unless the upper lid is everted and the tarsal conjunctiva inspected. Treatment is removal of contact lenses, use of topical antihistamine eye drops, or a short-term course of topical steroid eye drops if the symptoms are severe. Cromolyn* should not be used while soft contact lens wear is continued. Patients often can resume contact lens wear with a different type of lens. Disposable lens systems with frequent lens replacement (i.e., every 2 weeks) may work for some patients. Contact lens solutions containing merthiolate should be avoided, and rinsing the lenses well before insertion with nonpreserved sterile saline may also be helpful. Giant papillary conjunctivitis may also result from prosthesis wear.

G. Staphylococcal keratoconjunctivitis is a relatively common cause of chronic red eyes. Patients complain of irritation, photophobia, and tearing. Some may have been treated for conjunctivitis with antibiotics with little or no relief. Symptoms appear to be secondary to an antibody reaction to bacterial allergens. Examination may reveal associated blepharitis, superficial punctate epithelial keratitis, and limbal follicular reaction. Marginal corneal infiltrates, separated from the limbus by a clear zone, are at first subepithelial but may later ulcerate. Patients respond rapidly to a combination of antibiotic steroid eye drops. Lid hygiene should be continued long term if signs of blepharitis exist. If the disease recurs frequently, use of longer-term low-dose prophylactic antibiotic ointment or eye drops may be helpful in decreasing the bacteria that lead to the allergic reaction.

H. Phlyctenular conjunctivitis is postulated to be a delayed hypersensitivity reaction to bacterial or fungal infections, the most commonly implicated microbes being *Staphylococcus,* tuberculosis bacillus, *Candida albicans,* and *Coccidioides.* The phlyctenules are localized and may occur at the limbus or bulbar conjunctiva. The lesions are isolated elevated gelatinous nodules with a *leash* of vessels extending from the nodule like a tail. If phlyctenules involve the cornea, severe debilitating photophobia results. Most lesions last 2 weeks but may recur in other sites. Treatment is directed toward the underlying disease, and topical steroids are helpful in eliminating symptomatic phlyctenular lesions.

*Cromolyn sodium ophthalmic solution is no longer available at the time of this writing.

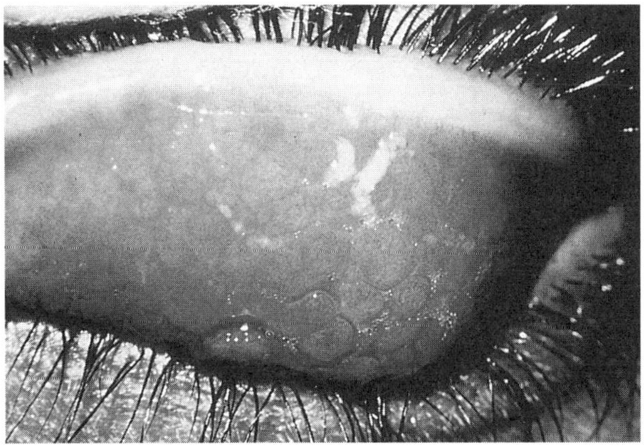

Figure 1 Giant papillae.

References

Allansmith MR. Vernal conjunctivitis. In: Wilson L, ed. External diseases of the eye. Hagerstown: Harper & Row, 1979:83.

Friedlaender MH. Allergy and immunology of the eye. Hagerstown: Harper & Row, 1979.

Ocular allergy. In: Int Ophthalmol Clin 1988; 28:261.

Rodriguez RD, Smith LM, George M, Abelson M. Recent advances in the therapy of ocular allergy. Ophthalmol Clin North Am 1990; 3.

VIRAL CONJUNCTIVITIS

Merril L. Stass-Isern, M.D.

By far the most common form of viral conjunctivitis seen in children is adenovirus. There are other types, but they are associated with systemic diseases. Their diagnosis is easily made because the systemic findings usually precede the ocular disease. A few other conjunctivitides are associated with viruses affecting another organ system. Often their diagnosis may be obscure because the ocular findings can precede those of the other organ system affected.

A. When taking a history of a red eye, inquire into the following:
   1. If any other family members, close contacts, or fellow classmates (including children at daycare or nurseries, preschool, or elsewhere) have had any similar problems. Epidemic keratoconjunctivitis is highly contagious and typically is present within a given city in epidemic form (thus its name).
   2. If there has been any diagnosis of systemic illnesses (e.g., varicella, mumps, rubella).
   3. If there has been no specific diagnosis but systemic findings are present (e.g., fever, sore throat), consider pharyngoconjunctival fever (adenovirus types 3 and 7). If systemic findings include skin lesions and flulike symptoms, consider Lyme disease.
   4. If there has been a periocular skin eruption only, consider herpes simplex, herpes zoster, and molluscum contagiosum.

B. Epidemic keratoconjunctivitis (EKC) is most frequently caused by adenoviruses 3, 8, and 19. It is highly communicable. The patient usually presents with an acute onset of unilateral, then bilateral conjunctival reaction. Chemosis and punctate hemorrhages may be present. Preauricular and submandibular adenopathy are typical. Lids may swell. Discharge is usually watery. In severe cases a pseudomembrane may occur, causing marked lid swelling that mimics a preseptal or orbital cellulitis. Subepithelial infiltrates may occur, usually 11 to 15 days after onset. The usual course is resolution in 1 week, but if pseudomembranes or subepithelial infiltrates occur, the course is protracted.

C. Supportive measures include ice packs, artificial tears, and topical decongestants. Secondary infection is treated with topical antibiotic drops. Frequent hand washing and the use of individual bed linens, bath towels, and other personal items to avoid spread to close contacts should be emphasized. School and work (if in close contact with others) should be curtailed until recovery.

D. If subepithelial infiltrates occur, they may obscure the visual axis or be associated with an iritis. If an iritis is present, topical Pred Forte should be used. If there is no iritis but subepithelial infiltrates only, FML/FML forte should be considered, but this is controversial. Some believe that topical steroids may relieve symptoms but that final visual outcome is unchanged, with actually a delay of resolution.

E. Pseudomembranes need to be stripped and topical Pred Forte or FML/FML forte applied. It is important that they be treated because they are uncomfortable and can cause residual conjunctival scarring.

F. Primary herpes simplex infection of the eye is characterized by vesicles on the skin of the lids, follicular conjunctivitis, and sometimes punctate keratitis. Recurrent attacks are usually in the form of dendritic ulceration of the cornea. Most cases are type I. Type II (genital) occurs in newborns. Treatment of primary disease consists of corneal debridement and/or topical antivirals (trifluorothymidine, vidarabine, or idoxuridine). Ointments are used five times a day and drops every hour while awake. A cycloplegic may be used to

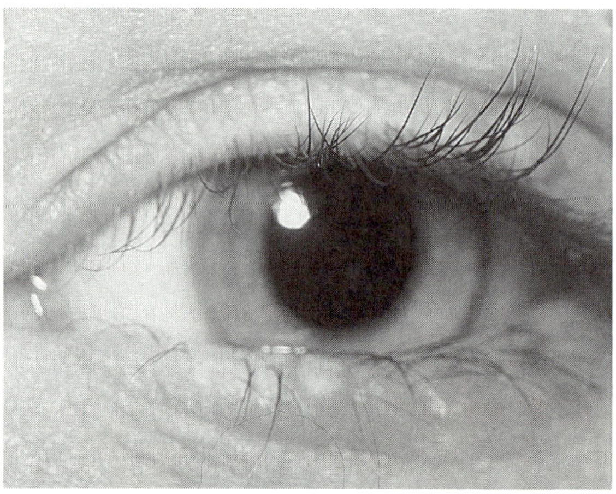

Figure 1 Molluscum contagiosum.

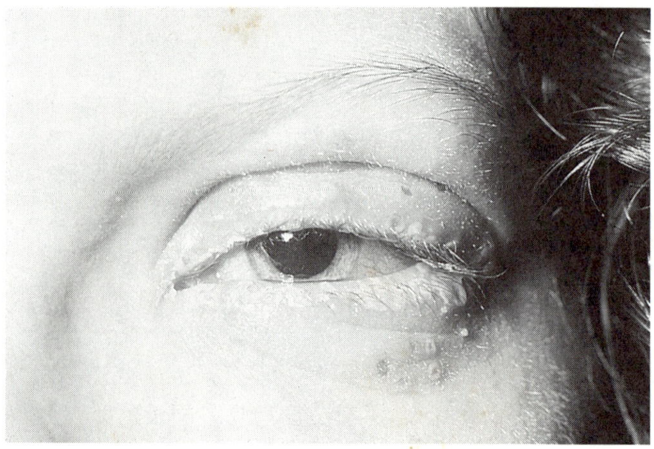

Figure 2 Primary herpes simplex infection of skin, conjunctiva, and cornea.

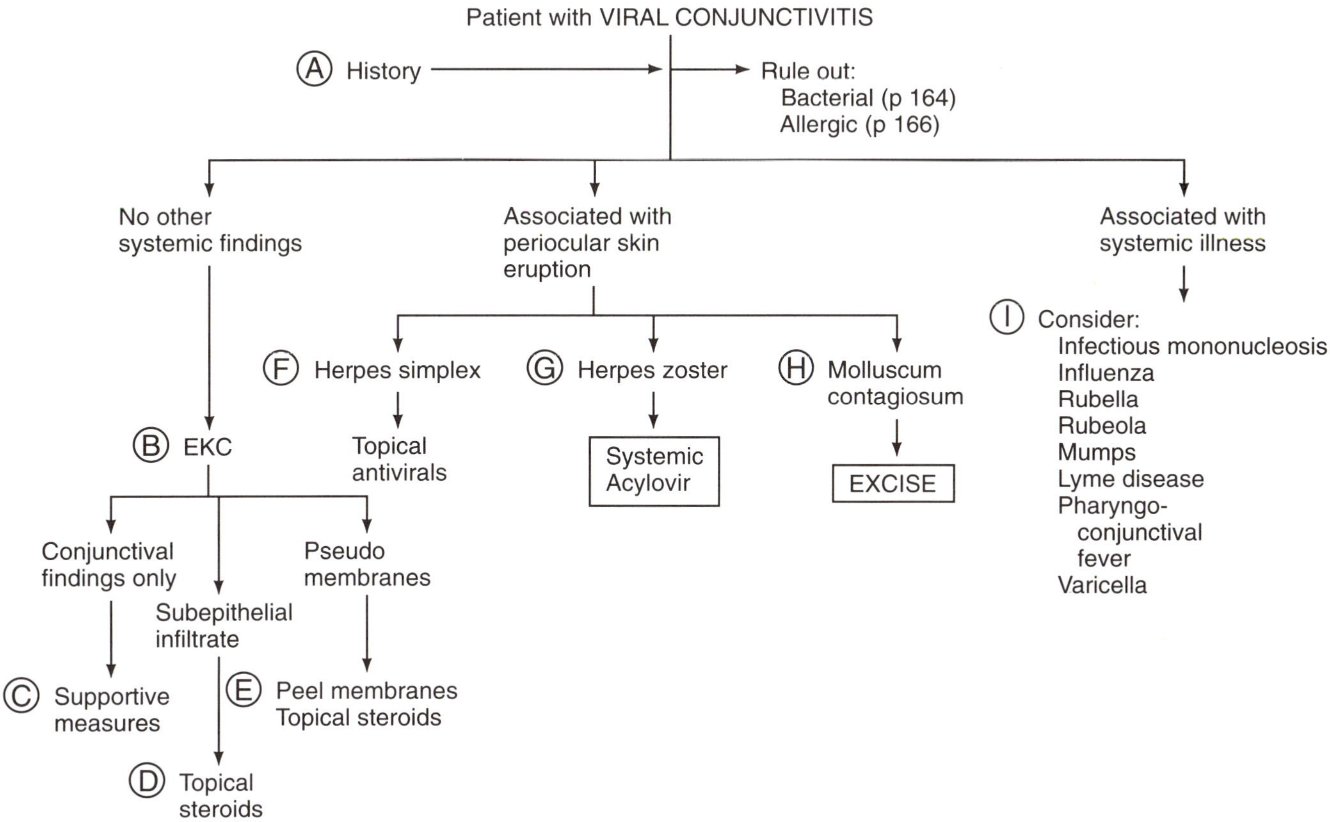

reduce ciliary spasm and photophobia. Close follow-up is necessary.

G. Herpes zoster seldom affects the healthy child but may be seen more commonly in the immunosuppressed child (e.g., chemotherapy for cancer, HIV infection, diabetes). It is caused by the varicella-zoster virus. A periorbital vesicular eruption occurs. Ocular involvement may be heralded by vesicles on the tip of the nose (Hutchinson's sign). Ocular involvement may be as simple as a conjunctivitis or may progress to a keratitis, uveitis, episcleritis, optic neuritis, or paralysis of cranial nerves III, IV, or VI. Intravenous acyclovir is used for immunosuppressed patients. The role of oral acyclovir is controversial in otherwise healthy patients (800 mg/day for 7 days). During the phase when lid vesicles are discharging and forming crusts, an antibiotic-steroid solution may be applied to the eye and continued for 3 weeks. Tetracycline ointment may be applied to inflamed lid lesions. Steroids are used topically for episcleritis, sclerokeratitis, iritis, or vasculitis.

H. Molluscum contagiosum is a mildly contagious disease caused by a poxvirus. Lesions are small, dome-shaped, umbilicated, shiny, skin-colored papules. A follicular conjunctivitis may occur when the virus is shed into the conjunctiva. Molluscum is best treated by simple excision of the lesion by scissors, blades, electrocautery, curretage, or cryosurgery.

I. The conjunctivitis caused by infectious mononucleosis, influenza, rubella, rubeola, and mumps is self limited and treated supportively with cool compresses and topical decongestants. Lyme disease conjunctivitis may be treated with tetracycline ointment. Pharyngoconjunctival fever is most commonly caused by adenovirus type 3. There is usually a fever, follicular conjunctivitis with serofibrinous exudate, and pharyngitis. Chemosis and punctate hemorrhages may be present. Preauricular and submandibular adenopathy complete the picture. Treatment is the same as for EKC.

Varicella ophthalmic involvement consists primarily of unilateral small papular, phlyctenular eruptions along the lid margin, on the similunar fold of the conjunctiva and the limbus. Virus shed into the conjunctiva can cause a conjunctivitis. Treatment is supportive. Antibiotic ointments may be used for lid lesions that are crusting and possibly becoming secondarily infected. Topical antibiotic drops may be used if a secondary bacterial conjunctivitis is suspected. Iritis is not uncommon.

References

Aaberg TM. The expanding ophthalmic spectrum of Lyme disease. Am J Ophthalmol 1989; 107:77.

Dawson CR, Hanna L, Wood TR, et al. Adenovirus type 8 keratoconjunctivitis in the United States. III. Epidemiologic, clinical and microbiologic features. Am J Ophthalmol 1970; 69:473.

Fraunfelder FT, Hamptomroy F. Current ocular therapy. 3rd ed. Philadelphia: WB Saunders, 1990:72.

ACQUIRED CORNEAL CLOUDING

Gerhard W. Cibis, M.D.

A. Most corneal dystrophies are autosomal dominant in inheritance. Penetrance and therefore clinical onset and manifestation can vary enormously. When dystrophies are suspected, examination of parents and other family members can be helpful. We have encountered situations in which findings in individuals were vague, but compiling all the findings in different family members allowed the diagnosis to be made. Nearly all hereditary corneal dystrophies manifest in childhood. Most are not clinically evident until the second decade of life (Table 1).

B. The cornea is able to enlarge secondary to glaucoma up to 3 years of age. After that time, elevated intraocular pressure causes edema and optic nerve damage but does not increase corneal diameter or cause myopia from globe enlargement.

C. In the syndromes of Rieger and Lowe, aniridia, and post–cataract surgery, glaucoma commonly develops late in childhood without corneal enlargement. These conditions need routine intraocular tensions either in the office, when possible, or by evaluation under anesthesia (EUA) (see p 154). We try to do that at least annually. Optic nerve drawings or photos can be helpful.

D. Inborn errors of metabolism that cause corneal clouding typically do so after birth. Lipidoses, mucopolysaccharidoses, mucolipidoses, and sphingolipidoses are all storage diseases associated with corneal clouding. Diagnosis is made by clinical suspicion confirmed by a metabolic work-up (see pp 61, 150) and/or conjunctival, or, rarely, corneal biopsy. Therapy when available is drug or dietary. Transplantation surgery may be needed.

E. Band keratopathy (see Table 2 for a list of causes) occurs with degeneration of the globe after trauma, including surgical (phthisis) or severe disease such as long-standing retinal detachment, Coats disease, uveitis, and radiation for retinoblastoma. It also occurs with systemic illnesses, particularly renal, involving calcium and parathyroid metabolism. Chelation therapy is only temporary. With corneal transplantation, unless the underlying cause is treated, the transplant develops band keratopathy.

F. Pannus occurs with allergic conjunctivitis (p 166). Shield-shaped corneal scarring keratopathy occurs with vernal conjunctivitis.

G. Appropriate cultures and antibiotics or antifungal and antiviral agents need to be chosen based on clinical presentation.

H. Noninfectious keratitis includes neurotropic disorders. Corneal hypesthesia occurs with many causes, including familial dysautonomia (Riley-Day syndrome). Bell palsy and various types of trauma result in keratitis sicca. Artificial tears are the treatment of choice.

I. Post-traumatic hyphema with pressure elevation leads to blood staining of the cornea.

J. The cornea is partially ectodermally derived and therefore is afflicted in a number of conditions that affect the skin. The most common of these is deep cornea farinata associated with ichthyosis, usually sex-linked recessive in heredity. Richner-Hanhart syndrome can be controlled by diet. Other conditions may require medical therapy or antibiotic ointments and lubricants.

TABLE 1 Corneal Dystrophies with Onset in the First Decade of Life

Meesman	Recurrent erosions
Reis-Bueckler	Granular
Schnyder crystalline	Lattice
Posterior polymorphous corneal dystrophy	Macular
Congenital hereditary endothelial dystrophy	Map dot fingerprint

TABLE 2 Conditions with Band Keratopathy

Fanconi's syndrome	Uremia
Vitamin D toxicity	Hypophosphatasia
Juvenile rheumatoid arthritis	Milk-alkali syndrome
Autoimmune diseases such as lupus erythematosus	Sarcoidosis
Hyperphosphatemia	Renal failure
Hypercalcemia	
Ocular Disease	
Degeneration of globe	Traumatic degeneration
Corneal dystrophies secondary to long-standing corneal edema	Glaucoma

References

Cibis GW, Krachmer JH, Phelps CD, Weingeist TA. The clinical spectrum of posterior polymorphous dystrophy, Arch Ophthalmol 1977; 95:1529.

Good W, Hoyt C. Corneal abnormalities in childhood. In: Taylor D, ed. Pediatric ophthalmology. Boston: Blackwell Scientific, 1990:178.

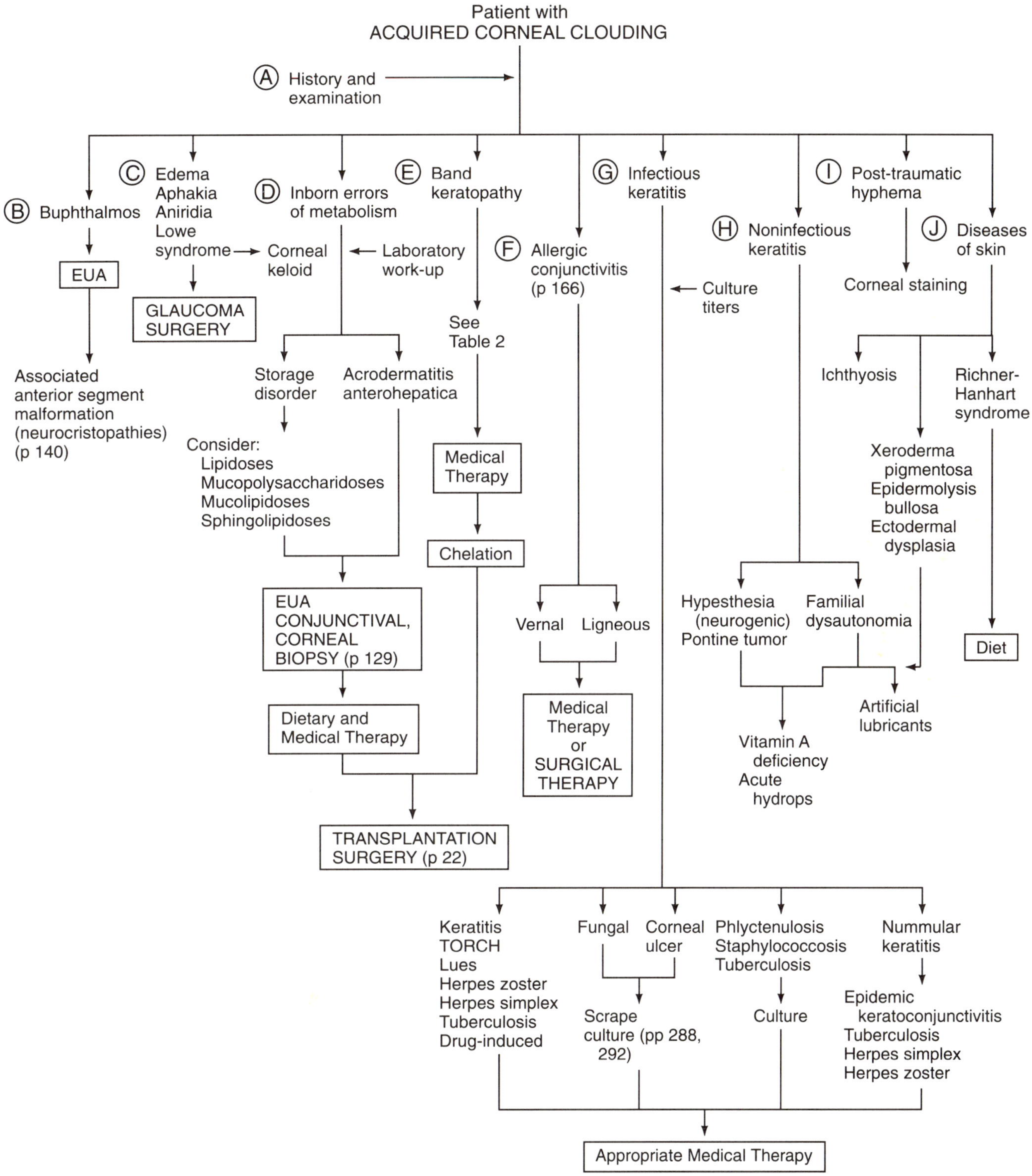
Patient with
ACQUIRED CORNEAL CLOUDING
Ⓐ History and examination
Ⓑ Buphthalmos
EUA
Associated anterior segment malformation (neurocristopathies) (p 140)
Ⓒ Edema
Aphakia
Aniridia
Lowe syndrome
GLAUCOMA SURGERY
Corneal keloid
Ⓓ Inborn errors of metabolism
Laboratory work-up
Storage disorder
Acrodermatitis anterohepatica
Consider:
Lipidoses
Mucopolysaccharidoses
Mucolipidoses
Sphingolipidoses
EUA CONJUNCTIVAL, CORNEAL BIOPSY (p 129)
Dietary and Medical Therapy
Ⓔ Band keratopathy
See Table 2
Medical Therapy
Chelation
TRANSPLANTATION SURGERY (p 22)
Ⓕ Allergic conjunctivitis (p 166)
Vernal
Ligneous
Medical Therapy or SURGICAL THERAPY
Ⓖ Infectious keratitis
Culture titers
Keratitis
TORCH
Lues
Herpes zoster
Herpes simplex
Tuberculosis
Drug-induced
Fungal
Corneal ulcer
Scrape culture (pp 288, 292)
Phlyctenulosis
Staphylococcosis
Tuberculosis
Culture
Nummular keratitis
Epidemic keratoconjunctivitis
Tuberculosis
Herpes simplex
Herpes zoster
Appropriate Medical Therapy
Ⓗ Noninfectious keratitis
Hypesthesia (neurogenic)
Pontine tumor
Familial dysautonomia
Vitamin A deficiency
Acute hydrops
Artificial lubricants
Ⓘ Post-traumatic hyphema
Corneal staining
Ⓙ Diseases of skin
Ichthyosis
Richner-Hanhart syndrome
Xeroderma pigmentosa
Epidermolysis bullosa
Ectodermal dysplasia
Diet

ABNORMALITIES OF THE RETINA WITHOUT DIAGNOSTIC ELECTRORETINOGRAPHY

King Y. Lee, M.D.
Gerhard W. Cibis, M.D.

A. Although electroretinography (ERG) may be reduced, it is not diagnostic. ERG reduction is based on retinal disruption from the disease process. The examination and clinical appearance provide the major diagnostic information.

B. Retinal angiomata first discovered by an ophthalmologist should lead to a search for tumors of the CNS and kidneys. A thorough family study must be undertaken to identify other affected family members. Therapy is localized destruction of the tumors.

C. Tuberous sclerosis is associated with retinal, brain, skin, and subungual hamartomas. Those in the retina are usually benign, not disturbing vision. Neurologic implications of the diagnosis mandate that proper referrals be made. Although uncommon, retinal hamartomas may appear at birth. Incidence of appearance increases each year in the first decade of life.

D. Telangiectasias may be minimal (miliary aneurysms of Leber) or significant (Coats disease). Cryotherapy is the treatment of choice for Coats disease. Laser therapy may be valid for miliary aneurysm if it is associated with localized pathology such as lipid exudates or recurrent hemorrhages.

E. Pseudoglioma is a scarring and detachment process similar to retinopathy of prematurity but occurs in older children with incontinentia pigmenti. Skin lesions are verrucous at birth but become pigmented with time. It is autosomal dominant, mothers usually having skin findings. Nearly always fatal to male concepti, which are aborted, it appears almost exclusively in females. Alopecia and dental malformations are associated. Fortunately, the blinding process tends to be unilateral. Because of this complication, all incontinentia pigmenti patients should be followed at regular intervals with dilated fundus examinations. Cryotherapy or laser therapy in the early stages should abort the pseudoglioma development.

F. Trauma and its sequelae as well as its therapy are self-explanatory. The proper way to follow children at risk for toxicity while on therapeutic drugs such as juvenile rheumatoid arthritis (JRA) medications is more controversial. Retinal sensitivity visual fields and color vision (Farnsworth 100, not plates or Farnsworth 15) should be done at regular intervals. We also do baseline ERG and electro-oculography (EOG) prior to instituting therapy and annually thereafter and fundus examinations at least every 6 months. Mellaril toxicity is a retinitis pigmentosa–like change best diagnosed early with ERG and EOG. Baseline tests are very important, especially in the JRA group, because they are often on steroids. Steroids give a supernormal ERG. Knowledge of the baseline ERG/EOG with no drugs and with the steroids is helpful. A significant decrease of a supernormal ERG/EOG toward normal in a patient on both chloroquine and steroids is an indication of toxicity.

G. Blindness in one eye from dog worm is common. We see it almost as often as blindness from trauma. Fundus findings are characteristically those of inflammation, differentiating them from hamartomas or congenital problems. The worm has a predilection for the macula, either because that is a watershed region of choroidal circulation or because arterioles at that point are less than 20 μ in diameter, trapping the worm in a vascular dead end. Subretinal "tracks" of previous worm migration prior to dying and setting off a granulomatous reaction can aid in the differential diagnosis. In the acute phase, a blood eosinophil count may be helpful. Enzyme-linked immunosorbant assay (ELISA) testing for *Toxocara canis* should be done in all suspected cases.

H. *Toxoplasma gondii* is an intracellular protozoan parasite that can cause congenital toxoplasmosis in utero by placental transfer when the mother acquires the disease during the first 90 days of pregnancy. The acute ocular lesion is a yellow-white retinal inflammation with vitreous cells and haziness. These may heal within 3 weeks to 6 months. Most children appear normal and healthy, and the healed chorioretinal scars are usually discovered later on a routine examination. If the infection occurs early in the pregnancy, there may be much more systemic involvement of the fetus, with hepatosplenomegaly, jaundice, petechiae, cerebral calcification, and hydrocephalus. Ocular findings in these patients are usually bilateral and posterior. The diagnosis can frequently be made in the acute stage by its appearance as described above. In the inactive stage the typical scar is one-fourth to several disc diameters in size with a dry atrophic retinochoroidal scar surrounded by dark pigmentation. Usually recurrences manifest between ages 10 and 35 years. Diagnostic tests include the Fabin-Feldman dye test, indirect fluorescent antibody (FA) test, hemagglutination test, and ELISA. The organisms can also be identified from placental tissue or cord blood. Medical treatment includes pyrimethamine (Daraprim), folinic acid, sulfonamides, clindamycin, corticosteroids, tetracycline, and spiramycin. Because of the toxicity of the drugs, treatment is recommended only for active lesions that threaten the macula or optic nerve and when the vitreous inflammation seriously impairs vision. Photo-

(Continued on page 176)

ABNORMALITIES OF THE RETINA WITHOUT DIAGNOSTIC ELECTRORETINOGRAPHY

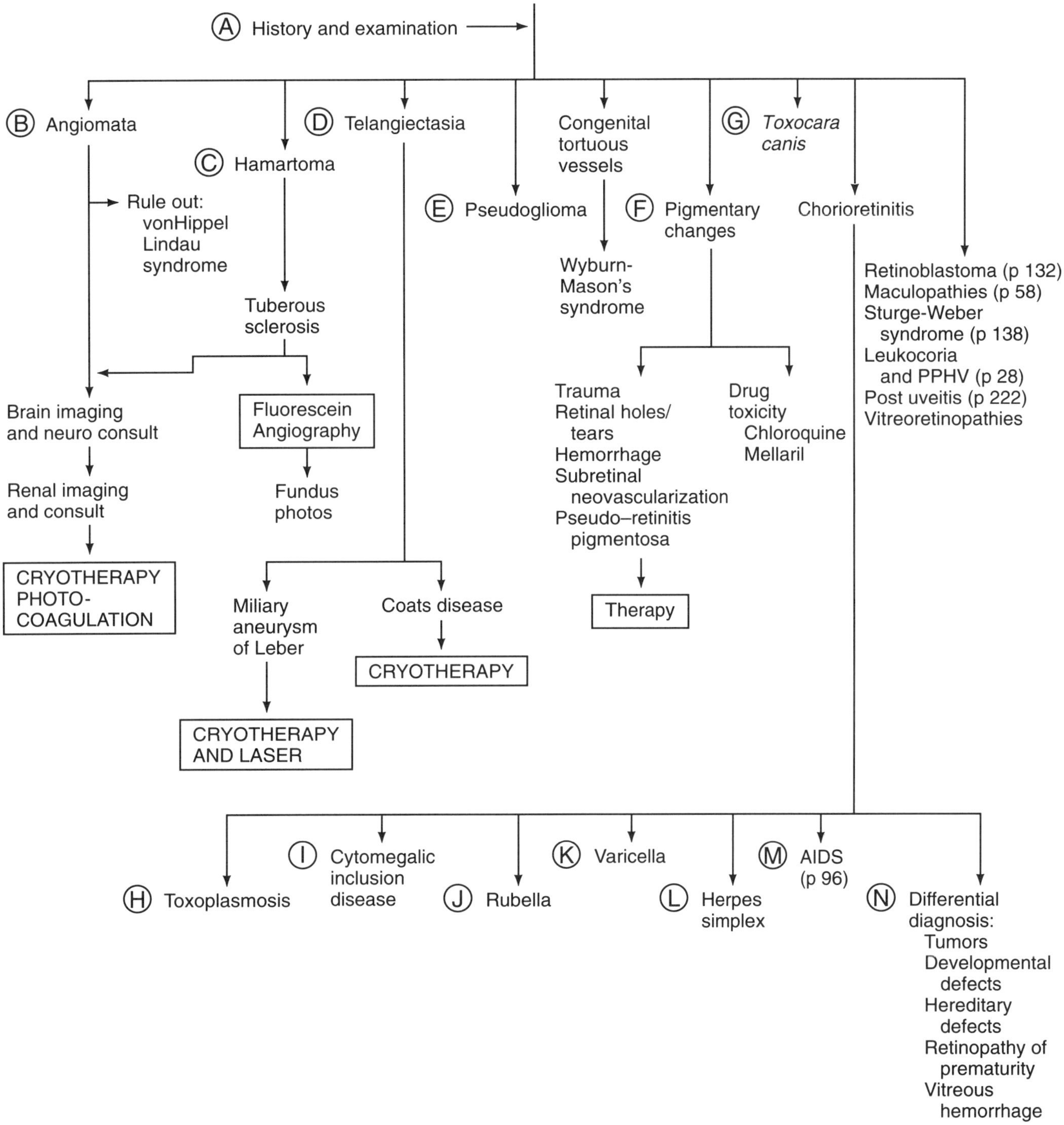

coagulation and cryopexy have been used, but experience is limited.

I. Cytomegalovirus (CMV), part of the herpesvirus group, can cause fetal infection by transplacental transfer from an asymptomatic mother. Most infections are subclinical. Severe cases may show jaundice, hepatosplenomegaly, anemia, thrombocytopenia, microcephaly, deafness, seizures, and pneumonitis. Like toxoplasmosis, it produces retinochoroiditis and can cause intracranial calcification. Other ocular features are coloboma, optic atrophy, cataract, microphthalmos, and uveitis. Appearance of CMV retinitis in immunocompetent neonates is different from that in adults with acquired immunodeficiency syndrome (AIDS). Laboratory tests include blood and urine cultures. Examination of urine can show epithelial cells with large basophilic inclusion bodies in the nuclei and cytoplasm. Ganciclovir has been found to be beneficial in treatment but when used systemically can be very toxic and recurrences are frequent. Some success has been obtained with intravitreal injections.

J. Rubella (German measles) is a virus that can affect the fetus when the mother is infected during the first trimester. The newborn may display congenital heart disease, deafness, and retardation.

K. The varicella-zoster virus is neurotropic and can cause chorioretinitis in utero. Ocular findings include hypoplasia and optic disc atrophy, congenital cataract, and Horner's syndrome. Chorioretinal scars may occur in the posterior pole and may be confused with the scars caused by toxoplasmosis. Systemic involvement includes cicatricial skin lesions, hemiparesis, bulbar palsy, psychomotor retardation, seizures, and neurotropic bladder. Diagnosis can be made by culture studies, but serologic testing is also helpful.

L. Herpes simplex virus infects infants during birth passage through the uterine cervix and vagina of an affected mother. The retinitis is characterized by subretinal and retinal hemorrhage, perivascular sheathing, and yellowish white punctate lesions. Systemic manifestations include encephalitis and hepatosplenomegaly.

M. AIDS in pediatric patients differs from that found in the adult population (p 96).

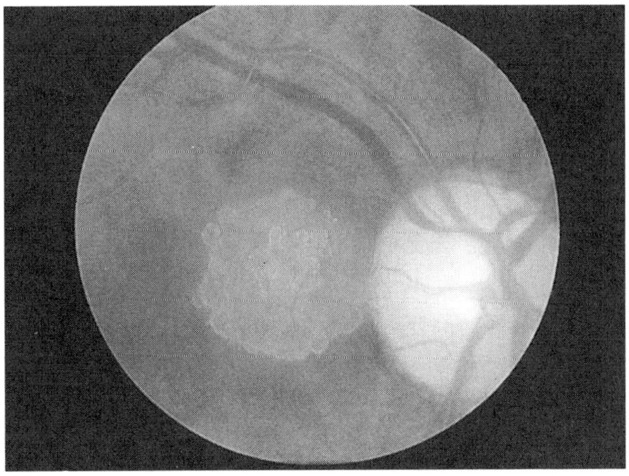

Figure 1 Glioma of retina.

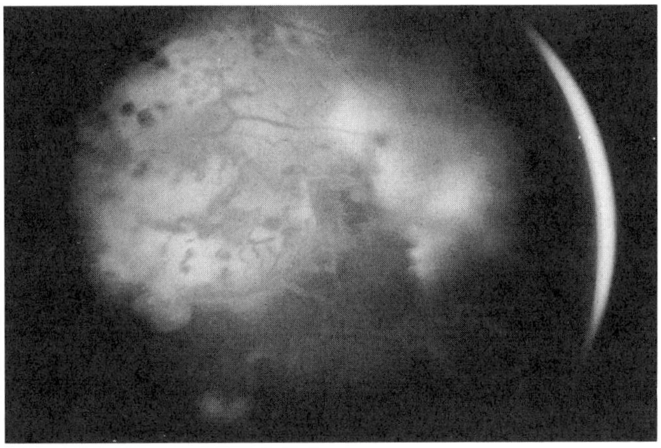

Figure 2 Telangiectasias.

N. Differential diagnosis should include tumors, developmental defects, hereditary defects, retinopathy of prematurity, and vitreous hemorrhage. In these conditions the culture and serologic tests are negative and the clinical history is usually different.

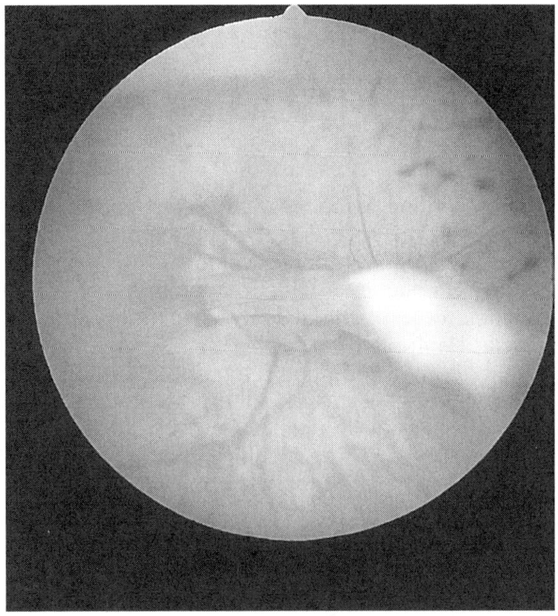

Figure 3 *Toxocara canis.*

References

Boger III WP. Late ocular complications in congenital rubella syndrome. Ophthalmology 1980; 87:1244.

Cibis GW, Flynn JT, Davis EB. Herpes simplex retinitis. Arch Ophthalmol 1978; 96:299.

Cochereau-Massin I, Lehoang P, Lautier-Frau M, et al. Efficacy and tolerance of intravitreal ganciclovir in cytomegalovirus retinitis in acquired immune deficiency syndrome. Ophthalmology 1991; 98:1348.

Lambert S, Hoyt C. Ocular manifestations of intrauterine infection In: Taylor D, ed. Pediatric ophthalmology. Boston: Blackwell Scientific, 1990:91.

Lewis RA, Crowder WE, Eierman LA, et al. The Gardner syndrome. Ophthalmology 1984; 91:916.

POOR VISION IN CHILDHOOD

Kevin M. Miller, M.D.

A. The presenting complaint that a child "sits too close to the television set" is heard frequently in pediatric ophthalmology. In most instances no pathology is found. The same systematic approach that is used to evaluate other complaints involving the visual system should be applied to this problem, with emphasis on visual acuity testing and refraction. Normally sighted children may sit close to the television set because they are hearing impaired. One should question the parents about hearing problems, and refer the child to an otologist or audiologist if appropriate.

B. Many normal children sit within a few feet of the television set. Just as the infant's visual world is within arm's reach, the young child's visual preference is for near objects. Unless the television set was manufactured in the 1950s, sitting close is not harmful to the eyes. Most children outgrow this behavior with time.

C. If auditory testing reveals a hearing defect, further otologic testing should be conducted to determine whether the loss is conductive or sensorineural. A hearing aid may help.

D. The visual acuity test that is selected should be appropriate for the developmental age of the child (see p 304). If the child is less than 3 years of age, it may be impossible to measure optotype acuity. Monocular fixation reflexes can be observed (the notation "CSM" refers to a corneal light reflex that is *centered* in the pupil, *steady,* and *maintained*). In some centers, preferential looking acuity can be measured using grating targets. Beyond 6 years of age, most children can read the Snellen eye chart. Between the ages of 3 and 6 years, it may be feasible to test visual acuity with individual Snellen E's, numbers, Landolt C's, or Allen object recognition figures. Grating targets, Snellen E's, and Landolt C's are resolution rather than recognition acuity targets and may overestimate the acuity of eyes with amblyopia. Acuity measurements should be compared with those of the other eye and of age-matched controls.

E. A prescription for optical correction should be written if it substantially improves visual acuity. It is usually unnecessary to correct low to moderate hyperopia unless it is accompanied by esotropia or anisometropic amblyopia. It also is unnecessary, in most cases, to correct low amounts of myopia and astigmatism. The reader is encouraged to consult the referenced textbooks for an expanded discussion of the indications for prescribing glasses and contact lenses (see p 186).

F. Anterior segment pathology may account for poor vision. Such pathology is usually detected early in life because it is obvious to the parents. Specific conditions should be excluded at each anatomic location: *conjunctiva* (conjunctivitis); *cornea* (band keratopathy, congenital hereditary endothelial dystrophy, congenital hereditary stromal dystrophy, cystinosis, interstitial keratitis, irregular astigmatism, keratoconus, keratoglobus, microcornea, mucolipidoses, mucopolysaccharidoses, Peters anomaly, Rieger anomaly, and scars); *iris* (corectopia, iritis); *lens* (anterior lenticonus, aphakia, cataract, coloboma, posterior lenticonus, spherophakia, subluxation); and *muscles* (amblyopia, nystagmus, strabismus).

G. Posterior segment pathology may not be detected until later in childhood because of its concealed location. The following conditions, grouped according to anatomic location, can cause poor vision: *vitreous* (endophthalmitis, persistent hyperplastic primary vitreous); *retina* (achromatopsia, albinism, Best vitelliform dystrophy, Coats' disease, juvenile retinoschisis, Leber's congenital amaurosis, leukemia, retinal detach ment, retinitis pigmentosa, retinoblastoma, retinopa thy of prematurity, Stargardt disease, Stickler syndrome, toxocariasis, and toxoplasmosis); *choroid* (hemangioma, histoplasmosis, pars planitis, sympathetic ophthalmia, Vogt-Koyanagi-Harada syndrome); *optic nerve* (atrophy, coloboma, glaucoma, glioma, hypoplasia, meningioma, and optic neuritis); and *orbit* (dermoid and epidermoid cyst, hemangioma, metastatic tumor, microphthalmos with cyst, pseudotumor, rhabdomyosarcoma, and varices).

H. In some cases, poor vision is one aspect of a multisystem disorder. Some conditions manifest at birth, whereas others become apparent with time. Full evaluation may require the coordinated efforts of the ophthalmologist, pediatrician, geneticist, neurologist, and other subspecialists. A partial list of multisystem disorders that should be considered includes *neonatal infections* (toxoplasmosis, rubella, cytomegalovirus, herpes simplex, and syphilis); *phakomatoses* (Bourneville disease, Louis-Bar syndrome, Sturge-Weber syndrome, von Hippel-Lindau disease, von Recklinghausen disease, and Wyburn-Mason's syndrome); *developmental defects of the eye and brain* (see p 140) (chromosomal abnormalities, colobomata (see pp 48, 122), cortical blindness, craniofacial syndromes, hydrocephalus, meningoencephalocele, microencephaly (see p 110), microphthalmia, neonatal anoxia, neurodegenerative diseases, toxic encephalopathies, trauma, and tumors); and *storage diseases* (gangliosidoses, lipidoses, mucopolysaccharidoses, mucolipidoses, and others). Consider developmental delay (see p 66) or delayed maturation of the visual system if visual acuity is inappropriately low for age but the ophthalmic and neurologic examinations are otherwise normal.

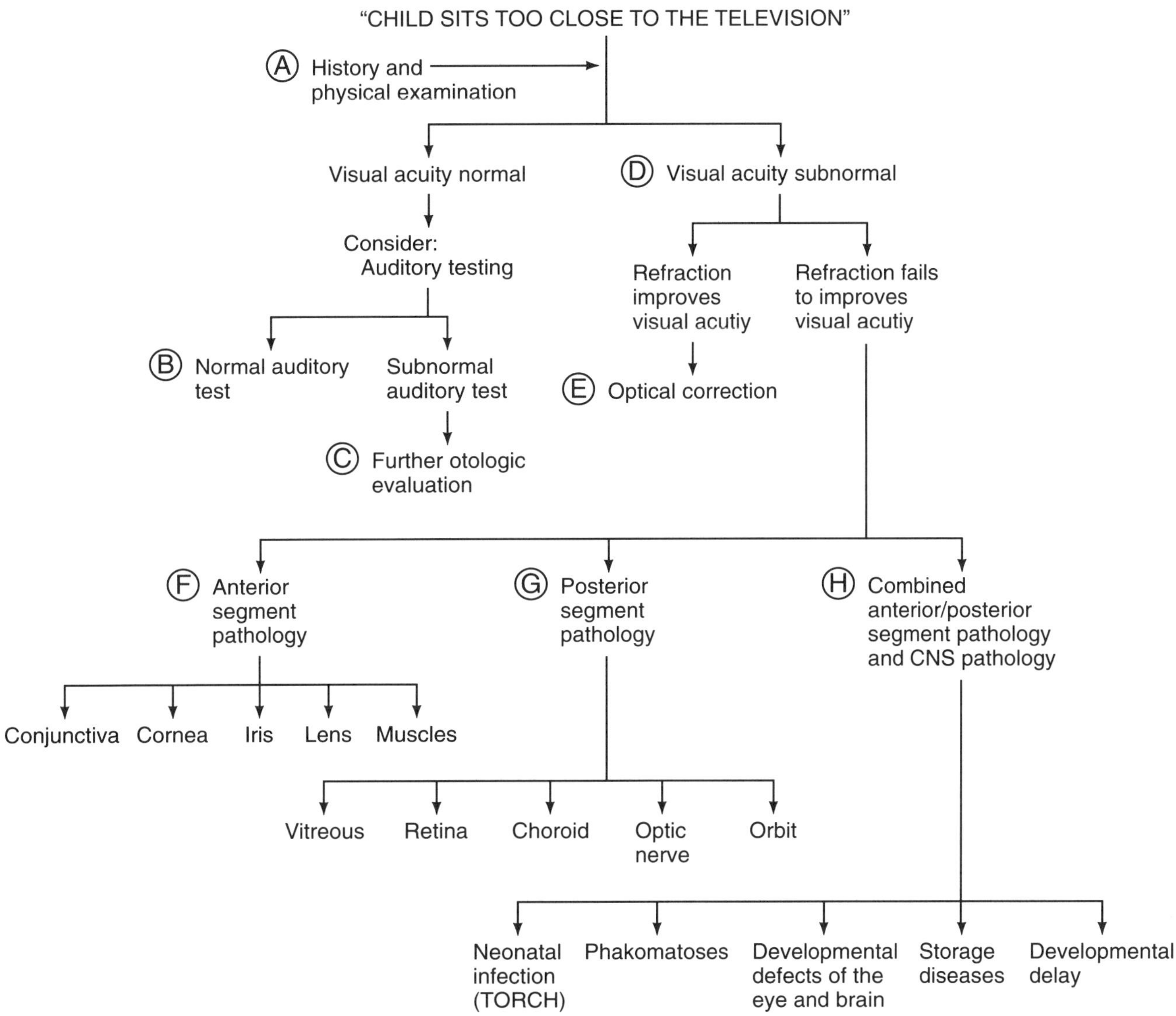

References

Fern KD, Manny RE. Visual acuity of the preschool child: A review. Am J Optom Physiol Opt 1986; 63:319.

Michaels DD. Visual optics and refraction. 3rd ed. St. Louis: CV Mosby, 1985.

Milder B, Rubin ML. The fine art of prescribing glasses without making a spectacle of yourself. 2nd ed. Gainesville, Fl. Triad Publishing, 1991.

Simons K. Visual acuity norms in young children. Surv Ophthalmol 1983; 28:84.

FUNCTIONAL VISUAL LOSS

Andrew W. Lawton, M.D.

By definition, a patient with a visual complaint but no identifiable organic cause has functional visual loss. This problem may present at any age but has a frequency peak between 8 and 15 years of age. Girls outnumber boys about 3 to 1. Inclusion of this possibility in the differential diagnosis of visual change can save the child and parents considerable anxiety and expense. You must prove normal visual acuity in order to make the diagnosis of functional visual loss. Examination needs to be particularly directed at picking up any organic disease by means of careful evaluation of pupils, macula, and optic nerve. Color vision should be evaluated if visual acuity is subnormal. Dry retinoscopy is valuable to determine if a significant refractive error is a possible cause of poor vision. Preliminary fundus examination should rule out optic nerve anomaly or maculopathy. Then all the tests and tricks listed should be directed at trying to elicit a normal acuity before cycloplegia is used (Table 1).

A. If functional visual loss is suspected, parents and patients should be questioned about school performance and any changes in social or family situations. Casual questioning about who else wears glasses in school and if any friends have recently gotten glasses may give a clue as to why the child is experiencing problems with vision in spite of a normal examination. Many times no unusual circumstances or concerns are vocalized by child or parent, and frequently the child's school performance is good in spite of professed visual difficulties. Characteristically, patients with functional visual loss relate their symptoms with a remarkably indifferent affect, in spite of professed severe visual dysfunction.

B. The physician's task may be very difficult if a patient complains of poor vision in both eyes. All "tricks" are fair game in establishing true visual acuity, and it is totally appropriate to "lead" the patient to the proper response. For example, the suggestion that dilating drops can make visual fields expand is implausible to the trained physician but may result in just such a response in a child. Observe patient function; If you hold out your hand for shaking or an object for testing, is this taken despite claims of poor vision and a tunnel field? Can the child maneuver around the examination room or find a parent across a wide waiting area despite poor performance on Snellen testing? "Inverting" the eye chart by starting with 20/10 rather than 20/400 letters may elicit better visual acuity. Fogging and then unfogging an eye may yield the same result. The presence of good stereopsis despite claims of bad vision suggests functional disease.

C. More tests become available with monocular complaints. A 4Δ base-out (BO) prism over the "bad" eye produces refixation when the child looks at small letters. A 4Δ base-down (BD) prism over the "good" eye should produce vertical diplopia. Are both letters equally clear? Does a 7Δ base-down prism over the "bad" eye make it harder for the child to read? Occult occlusion or a 40Δ base-out prism over the "good" eye may trick the child into reading better with the "bad" eye. Red-green glasses and the Worth four-dot flashlight can help. Another test is to put the red lens over the "good" eye and ask the child to read text written with red pencil on white paper.

D. Although most children do not initially complain of visual field alterations, perimetry almost universally elicits an abnormality. The classic change is a tunnel field of between 5 and 10 degrees, which paradoxically constricts the farther the patient sits from the fixation target. This is related to the size of the frame of reference; confrontation at 1 meter using the examiner's face as a background produces a smaller perimeter than the same target on the larger tangent screen at the same distance. Less frequently, a hemianopia or quadrant loss may be mimicked. The presence of a central scotoma is uncharacteristic of functional disease and should prompt further evaluation for organic disease.

E. Visual evoked response, especially sweep testing (p 304), can establish a diagnosis when objective waveform acuity does not correlate with claimed decrease in vision. Contrast sensitivity can also be objectively determined. If visual acuity is not normal but the ophthalmologic examination is normal, one should re-evaluate within 1 to 2 months. If it is still not normal, electrophysiologic testing should be instituted

TABLE 1 Tricks That Often Elicit a Normal Visual Response

1. Visual field testing
2. Inverting the eye chart
3. Polaroid glasses, red-green glasses for acuity testing
4. Teller preferential looking test, electroretinography, sweep visual evoked potential (p 304)
5. Use plano lenses, suggesting that they are magnifiers and that acuity will be better.
6. Tell child to draw rather than name the letter.
7. Stereo testing
8. Tumbling E and C to check acuity
9. Use a phorometer, starting with high plus or high cylinder and work down to plano.
10. Use a (+) and a (−) lens of equal power to neutralize each other and suggest improvement.
11. Use (−) lenses for near acuity testing and see if visual acuity improves.

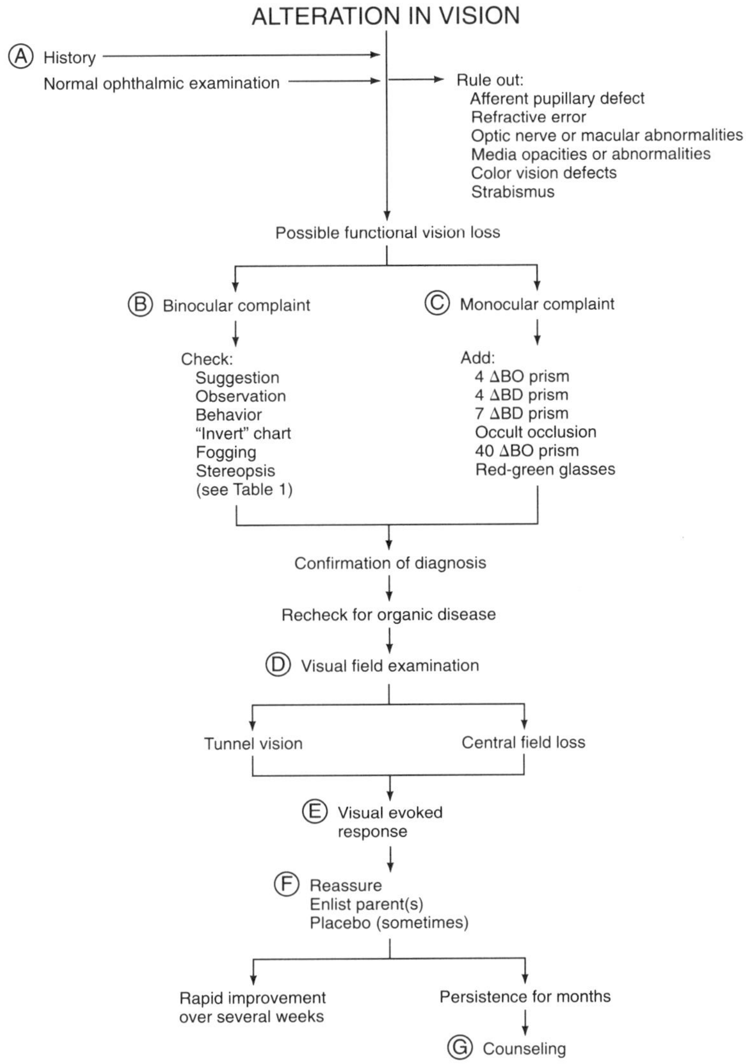

and neurologic consultation considered. Some ophthalmologists go straight to the electrophysiologic tests. Admittedly, that is expensive and the technology is not readily available to all practitioners.

F. Simple reassurance that the child's eyes are healthy and vision is normal should be directed at both parent and child. This reassurance, however, can be given only if visual acuity has been proven to be normal during the examination. If functional visual loss is suspected but visual acuity is not proven to be normal, further evaluation and follow-up are indicated. Many parents are surprised when they are told that nothing is wrong with their child's eyes or vision. They should be reassured that this type of complaint is not uncommon, that it is at times secondary to stress or tension or other underlying problems the child may have discussed, or may be due to attention another child has received from wearing new glasses or having eye problems. If complaints continue despite reassurance that vision is normal, psychological counseling is indicated. The patient's pediatrician should be informed about the patient's complaints and the examination findings at the time of the first ophthalmic visit.

G. Some children may not respond to reassurance and persist in visual complaints past 2 months. Professional psychological counseling is necessary to allow them to deal with their precipitating stress.

References

Bangash IH, Worley G, Kandt RS. Hysterical conversion reactions mimicking neurological disease. Am J Dis Child 1988; 142:1203.

Gratton-Smith P, Farley M, Procopis P. Clinical features of conversion disorder. Arch Dis Child 1988; 63:408.

Slavin ML: The prism dissociation test in detecting unilateral functional visual loss. J Clin Neuro-ophthalmol 1990; 10:127.

Sletteberg O, Bertelstein T, Høvding G. The prognosis of patients with hysterical visual impairment. Acta Ophthalmol 1989; 67:159.

Smith TJ, Baker RS. Perimetric findings in functional disorders using automated techniques. Ophthalmology 1987; 94:1562.

AMBLYOPIA

Oscar A. Cruz, M.D.
John T. Flynn, M.D.

Amblyopia (from the Greek "blunt vision") is a developmental defect in spatial vision of one or both eyes. It is associated with conditions occurring early in life during the critical period of visual development (0 to 4 years of age). Amblyopia is a leading cause of monocular visual loss in the United States up to the eighth decade of life. Clinical findings in addition to the decreased vision include the inability to discriminate optotypes that are crowded closely together ("crowding phenomena"). Most amblyopic eyes have better "single E" acuity. Also, neutral density filters characteristically reduce the acuity of eyes with amblyopia much less than eyes with poor vision secondary to organic disease. Currently, amblyopia is classified according to the condition with which it is associated, that is, strabismus, anisometropia, deprivation (cataract), occlusion (ptosis), and so forth. Evidence is accumulating that all amblyopia may have a common cause and differs only in the severity of its manifestations.

A. History and ophthalmologic examination should include pupillary testing for an afferent pupillary defect, cycloplegic retinoscopy, ocular alignment, and indirect ophthalmoscopy of optic nerve and macula. One must exclude any disease processes that disrupt the cellular structure of the retina or visual pathways.

B. In preverbal children, amblyopia is detected by observing the fixation behavior. The key is comparison of the infant's behavior with one eye versus the other occluded. Newer techniques, such as the gradient filter test, photorefraction screening, preferential looking, and visual evoked potential testing, may help in the assessment of preverbal children. Modified Allen pictures with "crowding" bars induces contour interaction similar to that of line letter tests and may be a more sensitive test of amblyopia in the preschool child. The usual clinical criterion for defining unilateral amblyopia quantitatively is a two-line difference in best-corrected Snellen visual acuity between the two eyes.

C. Strabismus is the most common cause of amblyopia. Esotropia is more commonly associated, but it does occur with all other forms of strabismus. Strabismus surgery should be delayed until the vision in the two eyes is equal or maximum vision has been obtained in the amblyopic eye. Exceptions to this rule may be justified, as when fixed deviations complicate patching.

D. Anisometropic amblyopia usually occurs in the more hyperopic eye when the degree of anisometropia is small and in the more ametropic eye when the difference between the two is large. A difference of + 1.00 or greater than −3.00 diopters is thought to be amblyogenic.

E. Isometropic amblyopia is bilateral amblyopia associated with large, approximately equal refractive errors. Therapy in this condition, as well as in anisometropic amblyopia, is directed at early optical correction. It may take months, even years, of glasses wear for vision to maximize.

F. Idiopathic amblyopia is a very infrequent form of amblyopia, presumably secondary to exposure to a transient amblyogenic factor early in life.

G. Visual deprivation amblyopia includes all conditions that prevent foveal form vision, including iatrogenic (after prolonged patching of the previous fixating eye) causes.

H. Ocular media opacities of the cornea, lens, or anterior segment or persistent hyperplastic primary vitreous requires clearing of the visual axis by surgery.

I. Eighty percent of capillary hemangiomas regress spontaneously. Amblyopia secondary to periorbital and orbital hemangioma may be due to anisometropia, occlusion of visual axis, and strabismus. If vision is jeopardized and cannot be expected to respond to amblyopia treatment alone, treatment with intralesional or systemic steroids may be indicated. Medical treatment is usually reserved for lesions that occlude. The development of high astigmatic refractive errors in the involved eye may also be an indication for treatment if glasses cannot be worn successfully.

J. Congenital ptosis is often associated with strabismus and high refractive errors that often contribute to the occlusion amblyopia. Definitive lid surgery depends on levator function.

K. Occlusion therapy is best accomplished with adhesive patches. Patching should be instituted as soon as the amblyopia is detected, preferably in the first years of life. In general, full-time occlusion should not be prescribed in excess of 1 week of occlusion for each year of age. Patching should be continued until visual acuity in the amblyopic eye reaches and maintains a plateau for 3 to 6 months. Maintenance patching may be required until approximately 9 years of age.

L. Although patching can safely be discontinued when equal vision is achieved, maintenance patching is usually required when there is persistent unequal acuity. It must be remembered that amblyopia can recur until approximately 9 years of age.

M. Penalization therapy is usually reserved for patching failure or difficulties with the patching therapy. This pharmacologic therapy usually consists of 1% atropine placed in the good eye to blur the better eye at near. Optical penalization degrades the image in the

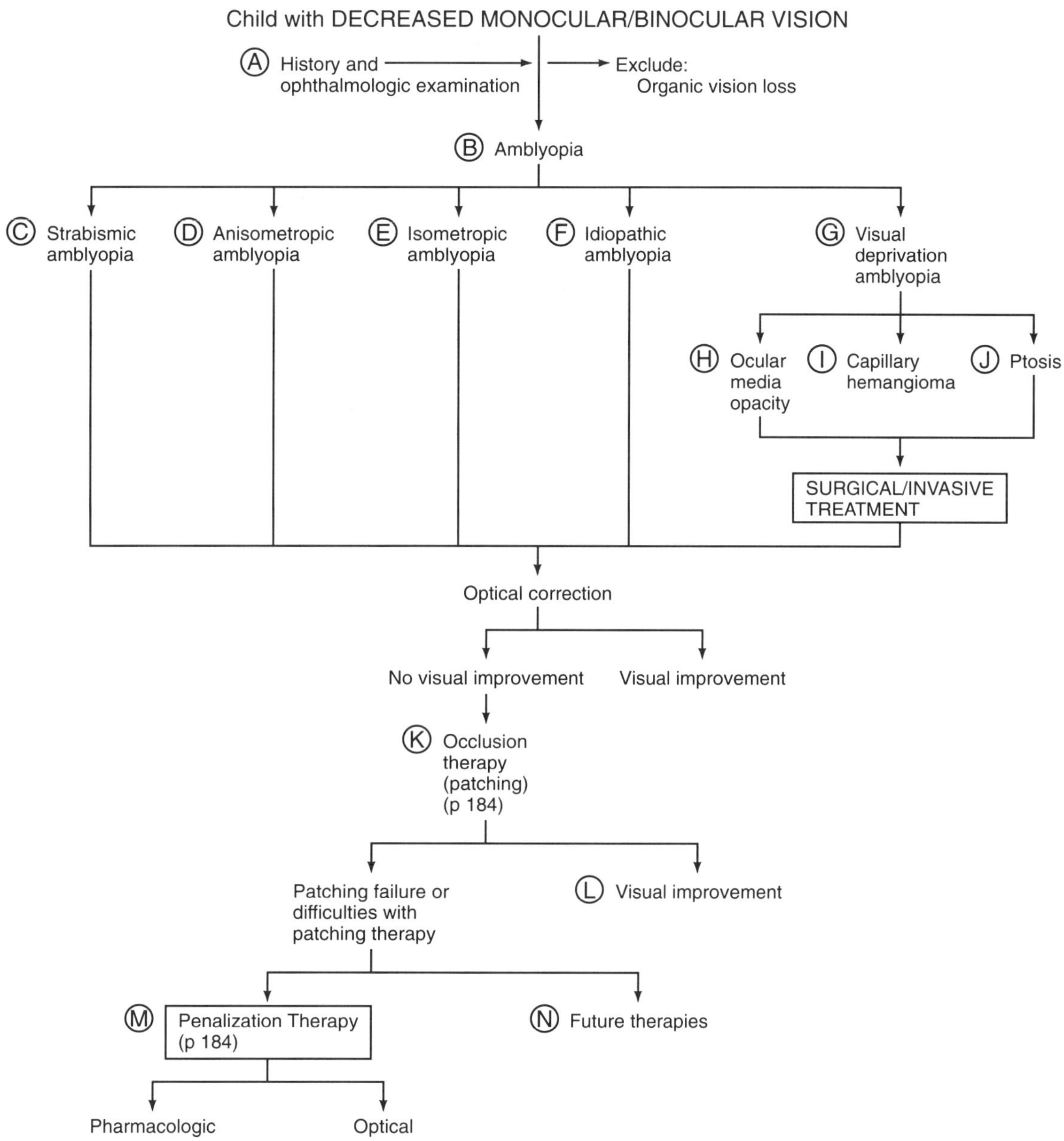

better eye to such a degree that the amblyopic eye has a competitive advantage at a given fixation distance.

N. Basic amblyogenic mechanisms may be the same: an interference with the developing synaptic neuron substrate with subsequent compromised binocular interaction. In animals with monocular deprivation, shrinkage of cortical dominance columns from the deprived eye, in addition to expansion by the sprouting of axonal terminals from the deprived eye, can be demonstrated. Biomolecular mechanisms such as neurotransmitters (dopamine) or synaptic facilitators hold the most promise as potential pharmacologic agents in the treatment of amblyopia. Amblyopia prevention must be aimed at screening nonverbal or barely verbal children. Successful treatment modalities must not obviate a primary objective—amblyopia prevention.

References

Flynn JT. Amblyopia revisited. (17th Annual Frank Costenbader Lecture). J Pediatr Ophthalmol Strabismus 1991; 28:183.

Gottlob I, Stangler-Zuschrott E. Effect of levodopa on contrast sensitivity and scotomas in human amblyopia. Invest Ophthalmol Vis Sci 1990; 31:776.

Keech RV, Kutschke PJ. The gradient filter test to assess amblyopia. Am J Ophthalmol 1990; 110:57.

Mayer DL, Gross RD. Modified Allen pictures to asses amblyopia in young children. Ophthalmology 1990; 97:827.

von Noorden GK. Binocular vision and ocular motility. 4th ed. St. Louis: C.V. Mosby, 1990.

OPTIONS IN AMBLYOPIA THERAPY

Gerhard W. Cibis, M.D.

A. Various types of amblyopia respond differently to therapy, some types being more recalcitrant than others. Congenital cataracts and other forms of early occlusion such as ptosis are very difficult to correct if not caught early. The later the onset of the amblyopia and the earlier its diagnosis, the more successful treatment is. Therefore, age of onset and age of diagnosis are important. Response to therapy also varies with cause. With anisometropic amblyopia, high hyperopic differences are more difficult to treat than astigmatic anisometropia or modest myopic anisometropia. A difference of 1 diopter hyperopia or 3 diopters myopia is considered to be amblyogenic. The greater the dioptric difference, the more likely amblyopia is to develop.

High unilateral myopia is often associated with organic problems and can be very difficult to correct. The "rabbit eye syndrome" of high myopia with myelinated nerve fibers of the retina is an example, as are staphyloma. Electroretinography may be helpful in such cases in documenting the presence or absence of an associated organic problem (see p 296). Large afferent pupillary defects may be seen with significant amblyopia.

B. The clinical impression of the depth of amblyopia determines the need for full-time versus part-time occlusion or inverse occlusion.

C. Reserve inverse occlusion for older, school-aged, socially conscious children with a deep and difficult-to-treat amblyopia. Patch the amblyopic eye full time for 6 weeks. This serves two purposes. The first is to acclimate parents and child to patching without the acute vision loss. Secondly, it has clinically and experimentally been shown to hasten full-time good eye patching. Reverse occlusion of the amblyopic eye stops active brain inhibition to that eye.

D. If the amblyopia is deep and severe, full-time occlusion is used. Also, if part-time occlusion fails to make progress, full-time occlusion is the only way to clearly determine if progress is possible. The rule for observing the patient for occlusion amblyopia is 1 week of patching per year of age. By this is meant it is safe to follow a 4 year old every 4 weeks, a 2 year old every 2 weeks, and so forth.

E. If no progress is made for 3 consecutive months, patching is considered a failure. When vision is maximized (either normal or no more progress with full-time patching for 3 months), move to part-time maintenance patching.

F. Maintenance patching can take many forms, mechanical and optical, varying in time periods. From full-time patching one may usually go to half-time for some months, then to several hours per day. Always follow up to ensure that vision remains stable. Ultimately go to half an hour per day of maintenance patching and stop after 9 years of age. A decline in vision on any part-time regimen is a sign to increase patching time.

G. Half-time patching is used until 9 years of age in unilateral aphakes from congenital cataracts. After the age of 9 years, the visual system is thought to be mature. Half time has been shown to be adequate to treat and prevent amblyopia regression yet gives an adequate amount of time for binocularity to develop. If binocularity does develop with contact lenses, less than half-time patching can be done.

H. Optical occlusion can take the form of eye drops to blur the better eye. This is called penalization. Atropine 1% is instilled daily. The distance refraction is worn and the eye used at distance. At near range, the amblyopic eye has the advantage and is used. An examination 1 week after starting is needed to ensure that the amblyopic eye is actually being used at near range. Often, despite the atropine, the good eye continues to be used. If penalization does not work, another method is needed. Penalization, in our experience, works only if vision is better than 20/100. Bangarter filters are graded neutral-density filters that reduce normal vision in a graded way. They can be used for primary full-time occlusion or to give the amblyopic eye a one or two line advantage over the good eye for maintenance patching. An unscientific but useful way to simulate filters is to degrade vision by applying layers of nail polish to the spectacle lens of the good eye.

I. Although it is not my preference, some practitioners do no maintenance patching. They restart patching whenever vision drops on follow-up visits.

J. Unproven alternatives to patching are constantly surfacing. At one time, Cambridge Amblyopia Meridional (CAM) therapy, consisting of short periods of looking at rotating stripes of varying size, was popular. This has been shown to be ineffective. Currently, no drug therapy is clinically done, although several agents have been shown to improve vision in amblyopia. None is practical at this time, although this is an area of great future promise.

K. Different philosophies of part-time patching exist. Some practitioners advocate one day off per week with full-time patching. Others reverse eyes for one day or patch full time every other day. My choice is to patch a varying number of hours every day. The amount is based on clinical experience and trial and error. The end point is maximum vision, which often

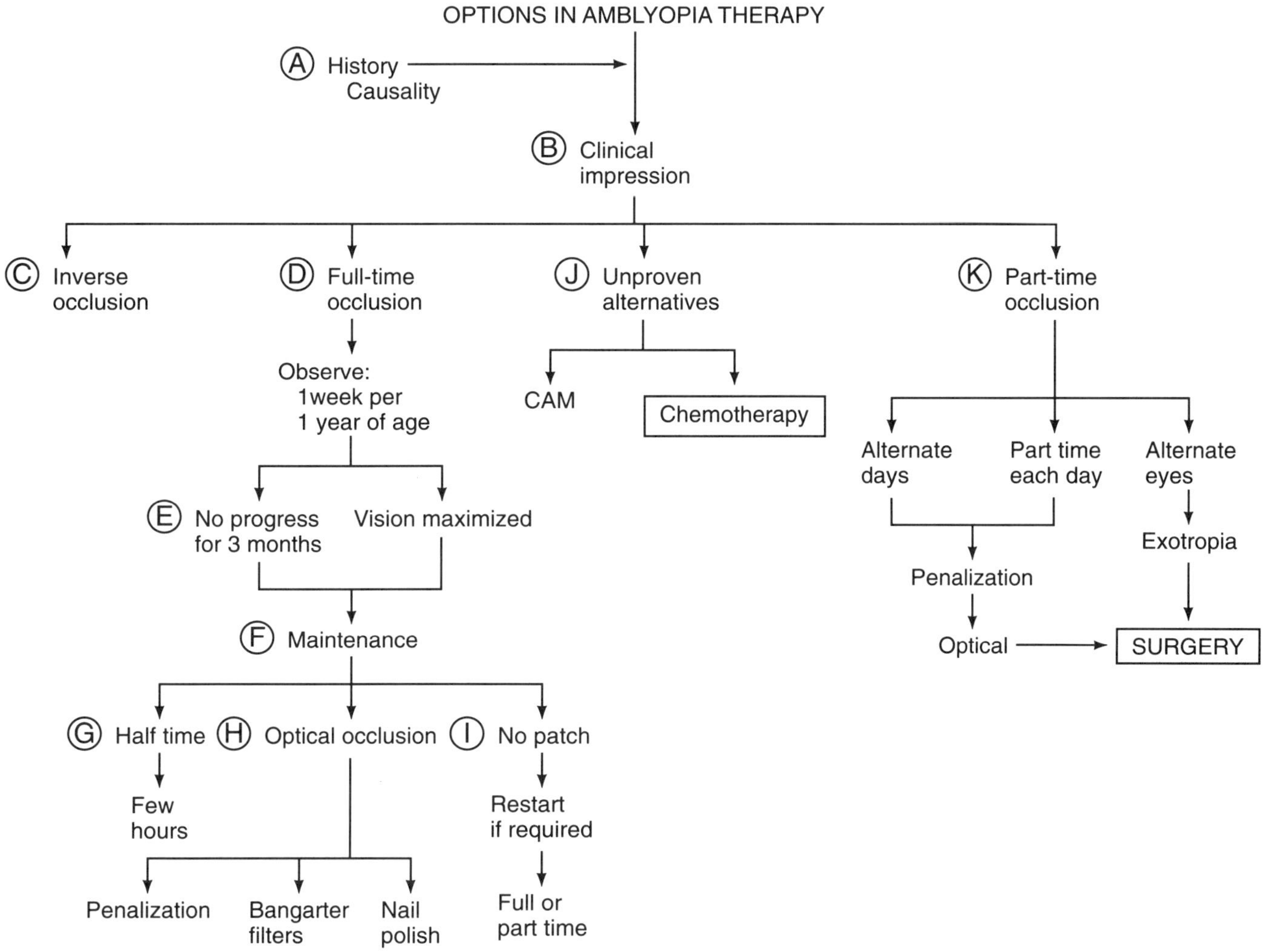

is one or two lines less than the better eye. Alternate patching of eyes with exotropia in anticipation of surgery is based on the concept of breaking down active suppression to allow a better result for the surgery. This is done for 6 weeks before surgery. Once vision is maximized, surgery, if needed, is done. Part-time maintenance patching continues after surgery.

References

Burian GM, von Noorden GK. Binocular vision and ocular motility: theory and management of strabismus. 3rd ed. St. Louis: CV Mosby, 1985.

Cibis GW. Strabismus. Trans. by J Lang. Thorofare, NJ: Slack Publishing, 1983.

Parks MM. Atlas of strabismus surgery. Philadelphia: Harper & Row, 1983.

REFRACTIVE ERRORS AND GLASSES FOR CHILDREN

Andrea Cibis Tongue, M.D.
Trudi R. Grin, M.D.

The refractive state of a child's eye is a dynamic one. The factors that contribute to the overall refractive error—axial length, corneal curvature, and lens power—undergo significant changes from birth through adolescence, accounting for the ever-changing refractive error. Glasses are prescribed for children for four reasons: (1) to achieve normal visual development (see chapter on "Amblyopia, pp 182, 184), (2) to see better, (3) to manipulate accommodative convergence (p 238), and (4) for safety or protection of an eye.

Unlike adults, who have different visual needs, infants and young children can function quite normally with uncorrected mild to moderate myopia or astigmatism. Infants and young children also have the ability through accommodation to overcome a fairly large amount of hyperopia. Hyperopic refractive errors unassociated with esophoria or esotropia of less than +4.00 to +5.00 diopters often do not need to be corrected in the infant or toddler. The same refractive error would most likely need to be corrected in the older child or teenager and clearly would need to be corrected in the adult.

A. Infants and young children are at risk for developing permanent visual loss, i.e., amblyopia, if they have anisometropia or high ametropic refractive errors that are not corrected early in life. Individuals appear to vary in their susceptibility to developing amblyopia. Refractive correction should be provided for patients in the amblyogenic age group (infancy to age 7 to 9 years) who have refractive errors equivalent to or greater than those noted in Table 1.

   Symmetric astigmatic refractive errors of up to +2.50 diopters are not uncommon in infancy. Usually the astigmatism decreases in magnitude by the time the infant is 2 years old. Glasses do not necessarily need to be prescribed for astigmatism in the infant if all other visual parameters appear to be normal. Follow-up is necessary. In children over 2 years of age, astigmatism of +2.50 diopters or more is unusual and in general should be corrected to avoid astigmatic amblyopia. Anisometropic astigmatism of +1.00 to + 1.50 diopters or greater should be corrected at any age. There are unfortunately no definitive guidelines for the correction of refractive errors for the purpose of preventing amblyopia. Clinical judgment is exercised by the individual practitioner.

TABLE 1 Amblyogenic Refractive Errors (Infancy to 7 to 9 Years)*

Myopia	−2.00 – −3.00
Hyperopia	+4.00 – +5.00
Anisometropia	
Hyperopic	+1.00 – 1.50
Myopic	−2.00 – −3.00
Astigmatism	+1.00 – +2.50

*Minimum refractive errors believed to be amblyogenic. Individual variations and sensitivity to development of amblyopia exist.

B. Correction of refractive errors because of visual impairment is a less complicated issue. One needs to look at how the refractive error and the decreased vision impact the patient's life. If there is no impact and the refractive error is not amblyogenic, there is no need to make the patient wear glasses. Follow-up is recommended. Prescribing glasses when the child begins school may be appropriate. Most preschool children are hyperopic and live comfortably with a hyperopia of up to +3.00 to +4.00 diopters. Glasses do not need to be prescribed just because hyperopia is discovered on an examination. If the visual acuity is normal at distance and near and the patient has no evidence of esophoria or esotropia and no visual complaints, glasses are not necessary. Unfortunately "stress-relieving glasses" are prescribed all too frequently just because an asymptomatic hyperopic refractive error is discovered on an examination. Older children and teens most likely have symptoms of asthenopia if their high hyperopia persists and is uncorrected. However, some teens who are asymptomatic choose not to wear a +4.00 or +5.00 diopter correction.

C. If the visual acuity cannot be corrected to a normal level in the office, glasses should be prescribed, even if the visual impairment is not causing the patient any problems or concerns. For example, if a 6-year-old child has an uncorrected acuity of 20/50 and with correction in the office is 20/40 at best, glasses should be prescribed because of concern about bilateral refractive amblyopia. The criteria used for prescribing bilateral correction can be essentially the same as for prescribing an anisometropic correction. If one can correct the vision to 20/20 and the patient demonstrates no sensorimotor or fusion problems, glasses are most likely not necessary in an asymptomatic child. If glasses are not prescribed, follow-up while the child is in the amblyogenic age is essential.

D. The use of spectacle correction in pediatric aphakia is reserved for bilateral aphakia. Unilateral aphakia is best corrected by a contact lens (p 42). The aphakic refractive error changes dramatically in most infants during the first 2 years of life. The refraction may decrease by more than 10 diopters. Single-vision lenses are usually prescribed for the first 2 years of life and bifocals for the preschool and school-age years. Unilateral aphakes who are unable to wear a contact lens can use spectacles while they are patched and

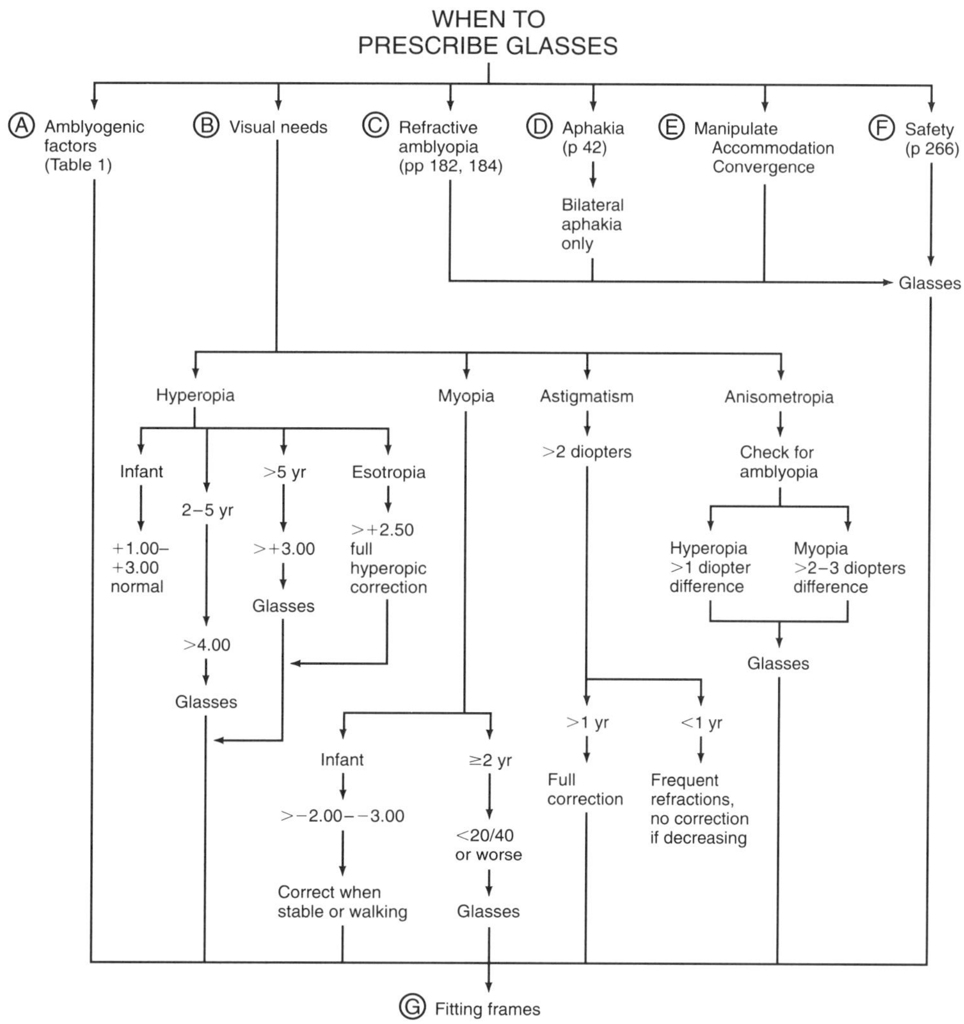

undergo amblyopia treatment. However, other modalities such as epikeratophakia and intraocular lenses should be considered in children over 1 year of age.

E. Glasses to manipulate accommodation are used in accommodative esotropia and in patients with strabismus and high accommodative convergence ratios. The latter group may be esotropic or exotropic. In the case of esotropia one aims to reduce accommodative effort by prescribing plus lenses; in the case of exotropia one wants to induce accommodative effort by prescribing minus lenses. Patients with high hyperopia may have normal accommodative convergence, and simply by correcting their hyperopia one is able to eliminate the esotropia. Patients with high accommodative convergence have a greater esotropic deviation at near and frequently require bifocals to control the deviation. These patients may be hyperopic, emmetropic, or myopic. Bifocals are prescribed if fusion is present or presumed achievable and if the distance deviation is controlled but near esotropia is present secondary to accommodative effort.

F. Safety glasses should be prescribed for all children who have permanent visual loss of one eye and whose life style and activities would be adversely affected if they lost vision in their good eye. Safety frames and 3-mm polycarbonate lenses are recommended. Sports safety goggles should be used for athletic activities that carry a risk of trauma to the head or eye (p 266).

G. Correcting refractive errors should not end with writing the prescription for glasses. Children deserve glasses that fit well and serve their purpose. In young children flexible cable temples usually provide a superior solution to bands and help prevent the glasses from sliding off the child's nose. Nose pads, particularly rocking pads, may be required if the child has a flat nasal bridge. Bifocals should be placed high enough (usually the top of the segment should bisect the pupil) for the child to use them easily but not so high that they interfere with distance vision or sports activities. High myopic lenses have thick edges that need to be beveled to prevent the lens from cutting into the child's skin (particularly in case of falls or blows to the glasses). The new plastics (high refractive index) that allow for thinner lenses are advantageous for cases of high refractive error.

References

Isenberg SJ. Physical and refractive characteristics of the eye at birth and during infancy. In: Isenberg SJ. The eye in infancy. Chicago: Year Book, 1989:31.

Safir A, Merker C. Refraction in children. In: Harley RD. Pediatric ophthalmology. 2nd ed. Philadelphia: WB Saunders, 1983:276.

DIAGNOSTIC USE OF PRISMS IN STRABISMUS

John P. Burke, M.D., FRCS
William E. Scott, M.D.

Acquired comitant esotropia accounts for approximately 25% of all strabismus cases. Many have a residual esotropia despite wearing their full cycloplegic refraction or may develop an esotropia while wearing the full hyperopic correction. Many of these patients experience a functional improvement in their binocularity following surgery, provided that their eyes are aligned (within 8Δ of orthophoria). Patients may have an esotropia that is equal at near and distance, an esotropia equal at near and distance but with an associated small comitant vertical deviation, or an acquired comitant esotropia with a distance-near disparity (i.e., near deviation greater than distance deviation by ≥10Δ).

A. Conventional surgery may produce variable results, even among patients with similar versions and measurements. Preoperative prism adaptation has been shown to determine the angle of deviation and the patient's capacity for fusion in nonaccommodative, deteriorated accommodative, and partially accommodative esotropia. It identifies a group of patients who can safely receive larger amounts of surgery without increasing their risk of overcorrection. It has the disadvantage of requiring more time, effort, and expense preoperatively than conventional management.

B. The amount of esotropia measured in the distance by alternate cover and prism testing (ACPT) is neutralized by Fresnel Press-On prisms. The patient's motor and sensory response to prism wear is assessed weekly, and he or she is classified as a prism adaptation responder when the deviation stabilizes at 8Δ or less on simultaneous prism cover testing (SPCT) at 6 meters, with evidence of peripheral fusion. These patients remain in their temporary prisms until surgery and undergo surgery for an angle of deviation equalling the total amount of prism worn at response (prism-adapted angle). A recent multicenter study of patients with acquired esotropia operated on for their prism-adapted angle showed that 89% were within 8Δ of orthotropia by SPCT at 6 months postoperatively.

C. A prism adaptation nonresponder may develop one of three possible situations during prism adaptation: (1) The patient develops an exotropic shift through the prisms on the SPCT at distance and near, with a suppression response on sensory testing. (2) The deviation on SPCT remains between 0 and 8Δ of esotropia at distance and near for 30 days but without fusion development. (3) The deviation continues to build through the course of the adaptation process until it exceeds 60Δ (the maximum amount of Fresnel prism available). Prism therapy is discontinued in this group and surgery is based on their initial distance deviation measured by the ACPT. These patients have a significantly worse prognosis at 6 months than the prism-adapted responders. Only 73% were within 8Δ of SPCT 6 months postoperatively.

D. Patients with a horizontal deviation may have a coexisting small comitant vertical deviation. Prisms can be used to offset the horizontal deviation. The vertical deviation can be considered insignificant if it disappears when the horizontal deviation is neutralized with prisms, and its postoperative disappearance can then be predicted if horizontal alignment is accomplished. If the vertical deviation does not disappear after neutralizing the horizontal deviation, it is considered significant and requires surgical or permanent prismatic correction.

E. Patients with a distance-near disparity can be treated with prism adaptation for their near angle. Base-out Fresnel prisms are mounted over the entire lens. The prism prescription is based on the ACPT measurements, with the patient fixating on an accommodative target at one-third meter. Through the prisms, patients may initially demonstrate a distance exotropia that is quickly controlled by their fusional convergence amplitudes. Sensory status is evaluated through the prisms using the Worth four-dot test at distance and near and the Titmus stereotest. If, on weekly follow-up, the deviation measures more than 8Δ of esotropia on SPCT at near, then prism power is increased to neutralize the angle. The patient's motor and sensory responses are evaluated weekly until stability is achieved and the prism response determined.

F. A patient is a prism adaptation responder if there is a fusional response on sensory testing and a deviation of 8Δ or less of esotropia measured by SPCT at distance and near through prisms. A responder wears his prisms until surgical correction, at which time he is operated on for his prism-adapted near angle. A recent study showed that 68% of patients with a distance-near disparity were prism responders and 94% of these had fusion postoperatively. None was overcorrected, and their need for bifocals was obviated.

G. Prism adaptation nonresponders developed either (1) an exotropic shift through prisms at distance or near or (2) an esotropic shift of 8Δ or less without fusion, or (3) their deviation built to an angle >60Δ with prisms. Prism wear can be discontinued in these patients and surgery performed to correct the esodeviation found originally at distance, followed by use of bifocals to correct the residual near esodeviation.

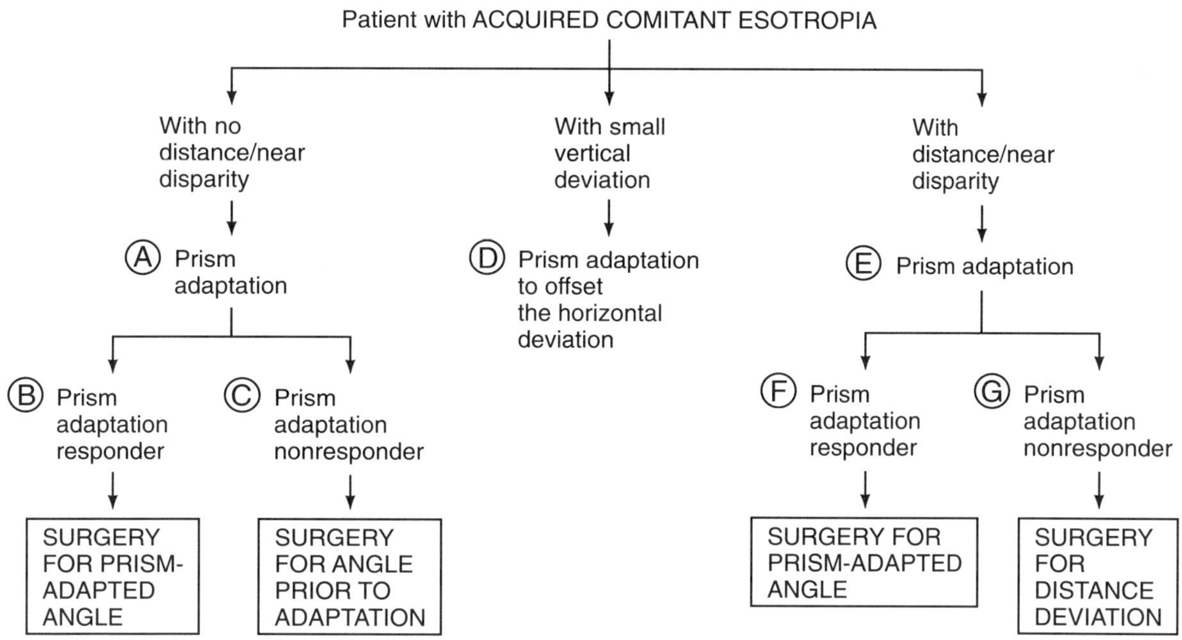

References

Kutschke PJ, Scott WE, Stewart SA. Prism adaptation for esotropia with a distance-near disparity. J Ped Ophthalmol Strab (in press).

Prism Adaptation Study Research Group. Efficacy of prism adaptation in the surgical management of acquired esotropia. Arch Ophthalmol 1990; 108:1248.

THERAPEUTIC USE OF PRISMS

John P. Burke, M.D.
William E. Scott, M.D.

Prism therapy may be considered in patients to restore or maintain binocular single vision or to relieve asthenopic symptoms in heterophoria. Prism power is determined by the purpose for which it is to be used and generally is the amount necessary to neutralize the deviation to permit fusion or until no shift is seen on the alternate cover and prism test (ACPT).

A. Horizontal and/or vertical tropias that develop in visually mature patients cause diplopia. If the horizontal deviation is less than 10Δ and is comitant, prisms can be a comfortable way to permanently control the deviation. If fusion is restored with temporary Fresnel Press-On prisms, glasses can be ordered with ground-in prisms. Concomitant vertical deviations measuring less than 10Δ often respond well to prismatic correction. If a small vertical and horizontal deviation coexist, correction of the vertical component alone may enable horizontal fusional vergences to maintain binocularity. If this is not the case, the prism axis should be rotated so that both components of the deviation can be neutralized.

B. Prisms can relieve asthenopic symptoms in patients with heterophorias in whom fusional amplitudes are poor. However, they should be used with caution because these patients frequently require periodic increases in their power owing to increasing dependence. Base-in prisms can provide comfort in patients with exophoria in whom orthoptic exercises are not helpful and surgery is not indicated. Small base-up or base-down prisms may give relief to patients with hyperphorias, and base-out prisms may be used in patients with esophoria.

C. Surgical therapy to alleviate moderate to large abnormal head positions is preferred for congenital nystagmus, but prisms could be used when the abnormal head position is small, as the null zone is close to the primary position. The prisms are introduced so that the eyes are maintained in an eccentric position that corresponds to the null position, thereby eliminating the abnormal head position. One achieves this by placing the prisms over each eye with their bases toward the direction of the head turn. However, this may cause a cosmetic problem because the patient appears to look away from the object of visual regard. Prisms may also be used to "fine tune" the results of surgery by shifting the gaze position to the null position when the procedure is insufficient. Occasionally, if the nystagmus is damped by convergence and the patient possesses fusion, bilateral base-out prisms can encourage convergence and improve acuity.

D. Generally the treatment of overcorrected esotropia is one of watchful waiting except for cases of large overcorrections with severe restriction of motility in which early reoperation should be considered. The initial management is reduction of the hyperopic correction in patients with hypermetropia. Base-in prisms position the eyes in orthotropic or slightly esotropic positions and prevent suppression. Hardesty found that 50% of his patients did not require further surgery after wearing decreasing amounts of prism for 6 months to 1 year. Small residual postoperative esodeviations respond less well to prism therapy. The residual esodeviation can be compensated for by giving the least amount of base-out prism that produces fusion. If the amount of prism required is small, then time and/or orthoptics can be helpful, with the gradual reduction and discontinuation of the prisms.

E. Most patients with undercorrection of exotropia require additional surgery. Base-in prisms at least 10Δ greater than the residual exotropia should be initially tried to simulate esotropia and produce diplopia, which the patient seeks to alleviate by adapting to a more convergent position. This convergent motor adaptation is actually a lessening of the exodeviation. Prism wear is tapered on average over 6 months and may occasionally result in resolution of the exotropia. In general, observation is advocated in the first month after small degrees of overcorrection of exotropia. This may be followed by miotic therapy and/or a period of full-time occlusion. Thereafter, base-out prisms can be introduced to neutralize the deviation if the esotropia is not lessening. As long as the patient fuses constantly, surgery can be postponed indefinitely. Hardesty reported that secondary esotropias of 15Δ or slightly greater could be cured after some months of tapering prism therapy. For large deviations, base-out prisms may be used to prevent diplopia until the time of second surgery, usually 6 months after the first surgery. Operations for overcorrected exotropia often result in a recurrence of exotropia.

F. Small postoperative hyperdeviations, when comitant, can respond to prism use. If prisms are "eaten up," surgery is needed. Often the hyperdeviations are incomitant and prisms are of little help.

References

Bagolini B. Therapeutic uses of prisms. Ocular motility. Int Ophthalmol Clin 1971; 11:272.

Hardesty HH. Treatment of undercorrected and overcorrected intermittent exotropia with prism glasses. Am Orthop J 1969; 19:110.

Reinecke RD, Simonsz K, Moss A, et al. An improved method of fitting resultant prism in treatment of two-axis strabismus. Arch Ophthalmol 1977; 95:1255.

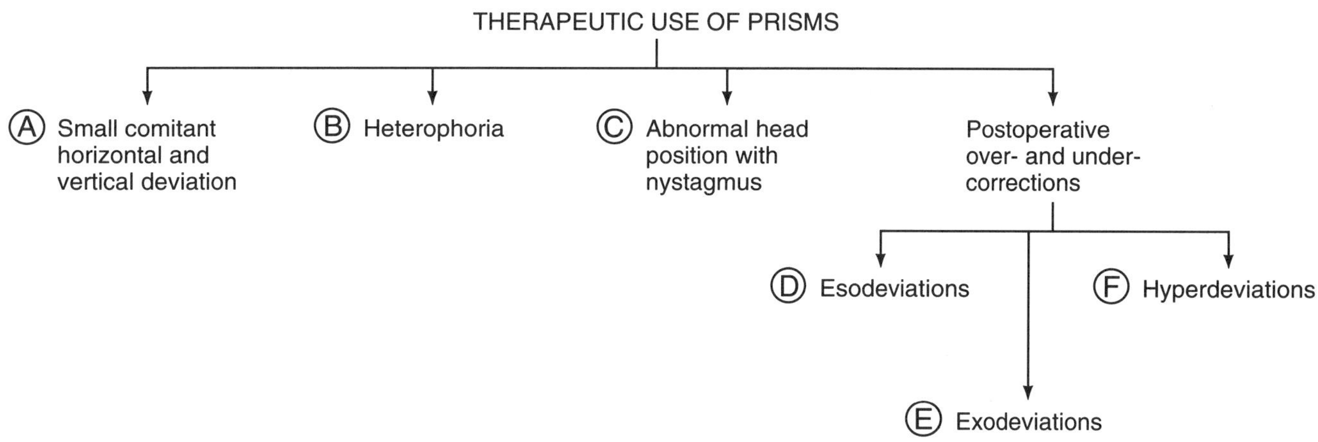
THERAPEUTIC USE OF PRISMS
(A) Small comitant horizontal and vertical deviation
(B) Heterophoria
(C) Abnormal head position with nystagmus
Postoperative over- and under-corrections
(D) Esodeviations
(E) Exodeviations
(F) Hyperdeviations

LEARNING DISABILITY SUSPECTED

Marilyn Newman Metzl, Ph.D.
Marva K. Newberry, M.S.

Learning disability (LD) is impaired ability to store, process, or produce information. This disability is due to a known or presumed CNS dysfunction rather than to psychological or social factors or inappropriate academic instruction. "Minimal brain damage," "minimal brain dysfunction," "dyslexia" (inability to read), "dysgraphia" (writing problems), and "dyscalculia" (difficulty with mathematics) are terms used to describe LD patients. "Attention deficit disorder (ADD)" and "attention deficit hyperactivity disorder (ADHD)," although not actually a part of LD, occur frequently with LD and are often considered together. Between 10 and 20% of all school-aged children have LD. LD can affect various aspects of life. Problems with self-esteem, frustration, anxiety, disruptive behavior, immaturity, and difficulty understanding social situations hinder achievement.

A. School personnel are often the first to notice learning problems. Difficulties in physical activity level, ability to attend, and peer relationships as well as academic achievement may be noted by teachers and counselors. The family medical specialist is frequently the first professional from whom the family seeks help. Concerns about a child's schoolwork may be voiced to the pediatrician. Ophthalmologic and audiologic assessments are frequently sought, hoping that the learning problem resides in the sensory organs and may be corrected. Advice from neurologists and other medical specialists may also be sought. The frequent overlay of social and emotional problems in the LD patient and the family often requires intervention of psychiatrists, psychologists, social workers, and counselors.

B. LD symptoms, unique to each individual, fall into four general categories: physical symptoms, academic difficulties, behavioral concerns, and emotional problems. These cannot be easily separated, and individuals rarely possess only one type of symptom. Overt physical symptoms may need neuropsychological evaluation. These range from weak or distorted sensory (visual, auditory, and tactile) acuity to perceptual difficulties, including weaknesses in visual and auditory discrimination, "figure-ground" differentiation, and processing speed. Weak or delayed gross or fine motor skills and writing ability, as well as hyper- or hypoactivity levels, are also frequently observed.

C. Difficulty in the development of a specific academic skill area often leads to referral for testing for LD. Difficulties range from broad to specific, from mild to severe.

D. Inappropriate behavioral manifestations observed by school teachers include maturational delays, ability to attend to task and follow through with work completion, impulse control, organizational skills, and problem-solving ability.

E. Emotional concerns frequently come from parents, who identify poor self-esteem in a child who exhibits anxiety, depression, and difficulty acquiring and maintaining satisfactory peer and family relationships.

F. LD evaluation must determine which symptoms actually exist and what the primary underlying causal condition is. The formal intake interview must explore the feelings of the referred client and parents. The person performing this evaluation must be qualified and aware of individual differences in approaches to task. Formal testing should consist of physical/neurologic assessment, standardized cognitive testing, psychological/projective techniques, and review of information acquired from other professionals working with the individual.

G. Physical/neurologic testing should begin with determination of visual and auditory acuity. This screening should be completed prior to other testing, with referral made to medical specialists and acuity corrections made. Visual and auditory perceptual skills are carefully assessed. Perception refers to a neurologic process rather than the physical condition of the sensory organ. An individual with excellent visual or auditory acuity may confuse this input, causing visual reversals, omissions, difficulty distinguishing a figure from its background, inability to "hear" someone speak to him when engrossed in listening to another source, or difficulty distinguishing subtle differences in sounds. Perceptual information may be processed correctly but at so slow a rate that a child misses part of the input unless it is presented slowly.

H. Detailed coverage here of the balance of the psychologist's LD evaluation is so complex as to be prohibitive. Comprehensive understanding of cognitive, psychological, and physical/neurologic testing not presented here may be gained from the references at the end of the chapter. Only mention of the evaluative testing an ophthalmologist might do has been made.

I. Only after the complete assessment by a qualified professional can a specific, individualized set of remediation strategies be developed. Parents and professionals should be wary of any standardized treatment program that professes to help all children. Eye, hearing, and neurologic problems should be addressed by appropriate specialists before LD therapy is begun. One must always be sure that treatment tasks are within the physical capabilities of the LD child.

J. Treatment modifications in the school environment include changing seat assignments, altering the nature of assigned tasks (extra time for task completion, shorter or less complex tasks, recorded instructions, notes or color-coded cues, word processor/computer) and aid with specific organizational techniques. Speech, language, and physical and/or occupational therapy within the school setting should also be investigated. Remediation of deficit skill areas should be attempted before placement in special classes for individual instruction.

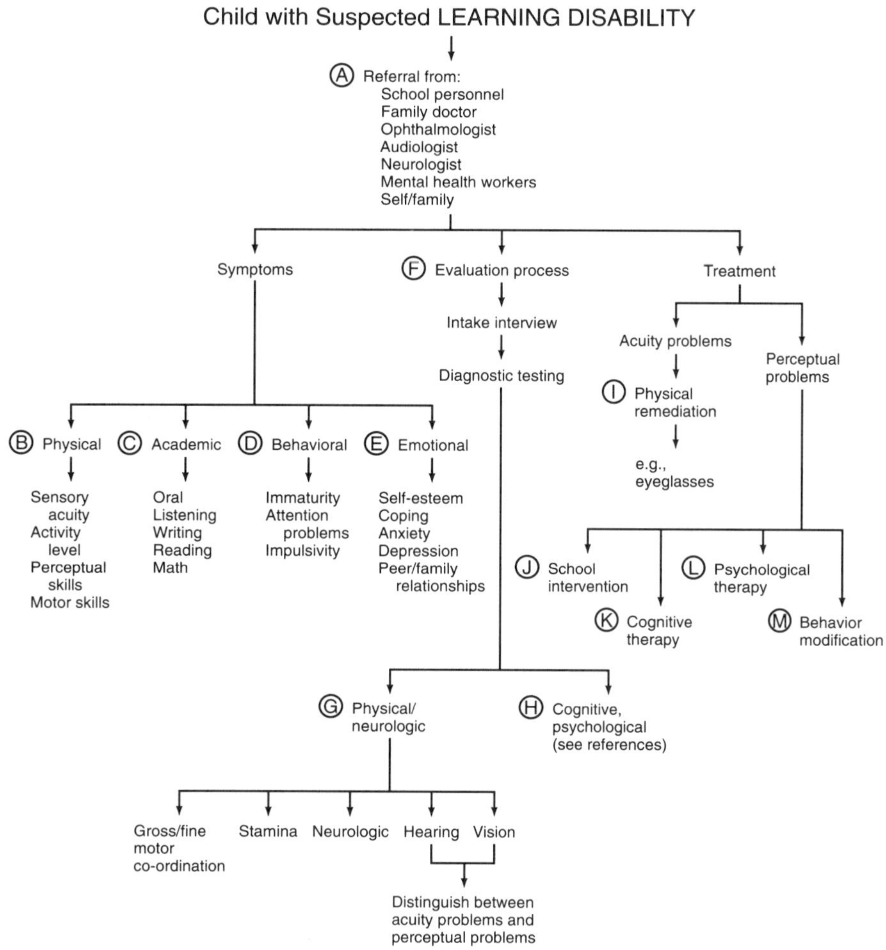

K. Cognitive therapy techniques help LD individuals improve self-awareness. In "demystification," one learns about his own disability and how it affects his performance. Issues discussed include neurologic factors, the fact that his disability is physiologically based, and that he can expect to improve with remediation. The difference between his intellectual ability and achievement levels is explained, as are his strengths and weaknesses.

L. Psychological therapy may be required to alleviate negative self-perceptions, the result of trying to function despite the presence of LD. Treatment for situational self-esteem issues involves developing techniques to overcome difficulties in that specific area, using strengths from the functioning areas of a person's life. Characterologic low self-esteem is more pervasive, derived from a feeling of being a bad person, and requires more intensive psychotherapy. Depressed children have severely restricted interpersonal relationships and often benefit from social skill training. Children with anxiety disorder, in which excessive worrying and fearful behavior is not focused on a specific situation or person, respond to medication and to psychotherapy. Often parental dysfunction interacts with the child's problem, and family therapy and direct treatment of parents may be needed. Stress management training, including systematic desensitization for phobic and assertiveness training for socially withdrawn behavior, has proven effective. Children with learning and attention problems often have difficulty in relationships and activities requiring verbal and nonverbal communication. Individual and group therapy consisting of specific skill training in communication, anger control, reasoning, problem solving, and stress management is beneficial.

M. Behavior modification techniques can help an individual deal with the effects of his LD. These may decrease environmental distractions, improve goal setting, prioritize assignments, provide cues for appropriate behaviors and refocus of attention to task, encourage social interactions, and reward close approximations of desired behaviors.

References

Copeland ED. Attention please! A comprehensive guide for successfully parenting children with attention disorders and hyper-activity (ADHD/ADD). Atlanta: Southeastern Psychological Institute, 1991.

Levine MD, Busch B, Aufesser C. The dimension of inattention in children with school problems. Pediatrics 1982; 70:387.

Levine MD. The pediatric assessment system for learning disorders. Cambridge, MA: Educators Publishing Service, 1986.

Levine MD, Brooks R, Shonkoff J. A pediatric approach to learning disorders. New York: John Wiley and Sons, 1980.

Silver LB. The misunderstood child, a guide for parents of learning disabled children. New York: McGraw-Hill, 1984.

VISUAL PHENOMENA

Andrea Cibis Tongue, M.D.

Children commonly present with a chief complaint of "seeing things." Often they describe seeing shapes colored "purple, silver, or shiny." These type of visual experiences are referred to as hallucinations. Other children complain of micropsia, with selective parts of the visual image described as being smaller, i.e., a small head or entire person, with the rest of the environment appearing normal. Less frequently, children complain of macropsia. Visual phenomena that alter the size or shape of real objects in space are referred to as visual illusions. Children may complain of seeing a cloud or spot in their vision or describe near-total loss of vision.

A. Complaints of visual phenomena require a careful history to ascertain specifically what it is the child notices. Onset, frequency, duration of each episode, unilaterality or bilaterality, and at what time of day it occurs need to be charted. If old enough, the child should be asked to draw the shapes and describe the usual colors of the shapes. It is important to establish whether these visual phenomena are ever associated with headaches and whether the child has had or there is a family history of headaches or migraine equivalents. Question parents as to how they first became aware of these visual phenomena and whether they have ever observed the child experiencing an episode. Does the child stop other activities, appear distressed or nonresponsive, or complain of a headache? Do episodes occur at school? If so, are teachers aware of them? The child's medical background and general health status may contribute important information. It is important to ask whether the initial symptoms were associated with a febrile illness or the use of medication.

B. Children with complaints of visual phenomena should have a comprehensive eye examination and ideally a screening neurologic examination (may be performed by pediatrician) if cortical origin is suspected. If the complaint is unilateral, optic nerve or eye pathology should be suspected; if bilateral, central or cortical pathology is implicated.

C. Rarely is ocular pathology responsible for a child's complaints of visual phenomena. Retinal and optic nerve disease may cause distortion of vision, blurriness, scotomas, and photopsias. However, these are usually unilateral and ocular pathology is detected on examination.

Children infrequently complain of monocular illusions or hallucinations. This may be because of the rapid onset of suppression in early childhood and the relatively rare occurrence of acute macular, retinal, or optic nerve disease. Monocular illusions and hallucinations may be due to refractive problems, maculopathy, optic neuropathy, acquired retinal lesions (inflammations or retinal tears), migraine, and, most commonly, physiologic phenomena seen with photoreceptor deformation such as phosphenes and Moore's lightning flashes or vitreous floaters. Retinal tears need to be considered if there is a history of trauma or high myopia or retinal detachments in the family. Optic nerve disease may be associated with seeing light or light flashes.

D. Visual phenomena lasting more than a few seconds, recurring sporadically, and causing the child to stop current activity may be migraine equivalents or acephalgic migraines. Visual phenomena may be prodromal symptoms of typical migraines; more often they are isolated occurrences unassociated with headaches. In 25% to 50%, family members are known to suffer from migraines.

Visual hallucinations associated with migraine may be uniocular or binocular depending on the site of vascular dynamic change. Generally, visual symptoms of migraine last 5 to 30 minutes. They may progress in size and intensity and march across the visual field. However, almost every conceivable visual phenomenon has been attributed to migraines. The most commonly described childhood hallucinations are "seeing lights, flashes, sparklers, varicolored circles, points, dots, star-like shapes, triangles, wavy or zigzag lines." Scotomas and transient loss of vision are also visual phenomena seen with migraine.

E. Some very perceptive children note physiologic visual phenomena that adults ignore. A child may complain of seeing double. When questioned about the double vision, it becomes clear that they are talking about physiologic diplopia. The same can occur with vision. Objects at distance become smaller (and blurrier) when the child focuses on an object in the same line of vision at near. Children with uncorrected hyperopia who accommodate may note change in image size with accommodation. If glasses correct the hyperopia, image magnification is appreciated. Micropsia may be noted by myopes when first corrected or if the prescription is increased. Hyperopes who change from spectacles to contact lenses may complain of micropsia. Some individuals appear to be very sensitive to the size change induced by optical correction.

The first complaint of visual phenomena may follow observation of a normal physiologic phenomenon such as an afterimage from a camera flashbulb. Children may complain of afterimages from ordinary lights.

Phosphenes may also be noted. They are due to stimulation of the retina by rubbing the eye, pull of the vitreous on the retina from eye movement, or sudden change in position. Usually these are small, may have a streak appearance, and are silver or shiny. Children may observe entopic phenomena, complaining of seeing dots when looking at a blue sky or floaters, particularly when looking at a white ceiling or wall.

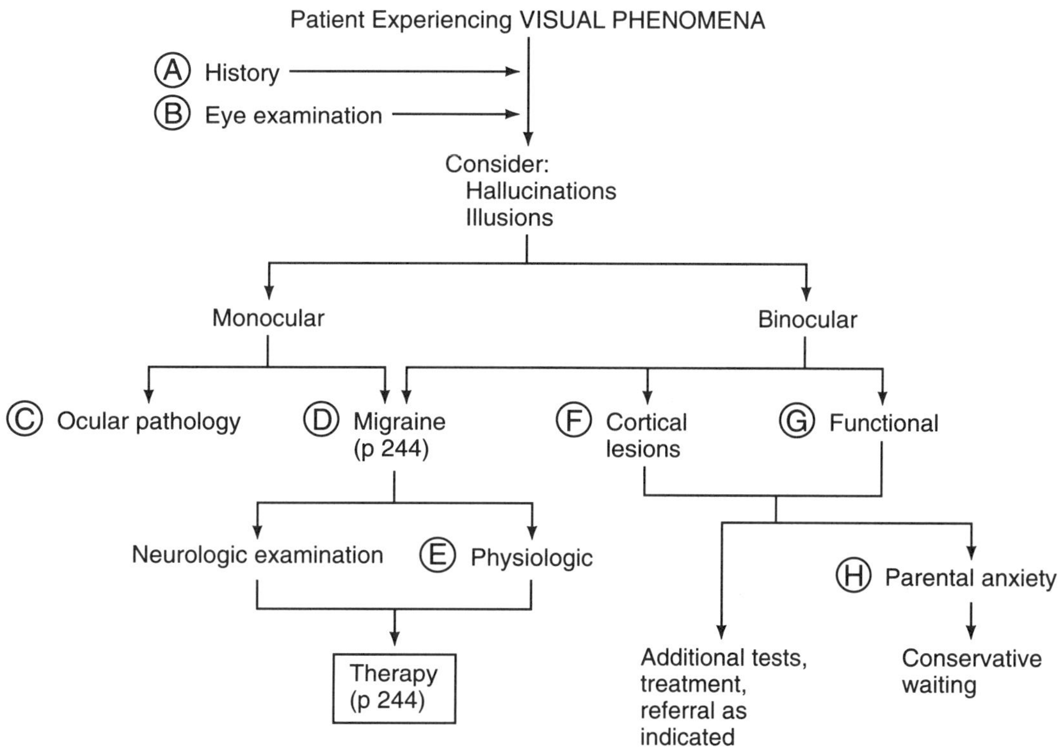

F. Cortical pathology is occasionally responsible for visual phenomena. The binocular visual aura of migraines is secondary to cortical changes due to transient abnormalities of cerebral vascular dynamics. However, tumors, vascular abnormalities, and seizures have been implicated in visual phenomena. These are extremely rare, and one would expect that the episodes would last more than a few seconds and be disturbing to the individual experiencing them. One would expect the visual images to be more reminiscent of migraine-type episodes or formed visual hallucinations. Clinical judgment is needed when evaluating a child's description of visual phenomena as to whether they seem to be due to underlying pathology that requires neurologic or neuroimaging studies or whether conservative management and reassurance is in order.

G. Most frequently, children complain of the visual hallucinations or illusions described for migraine, i.e., seeing lights, lines, dots, or shapes of different colors or noting micropsia, macropsia, or scotomas. The micropsia or macropsia is usually selective, affecting only part of the visual scene. However, children indicate that the visual phenomenon lasts only a few seconds. Parents and teachers are rarely aware of any abnormal visual symptoms until the child volunteers at a later time that he or she has been experiencing them. If the child is healthy, the ophthalmologic examination negative, and a pediatric examination negative (most parents see the pediatrician first and the ophthalmologist second), watchful waiting is indicated.

H. Children may note details in an object that parents are not aware of and overly concerned parental reaction to the child's observation may become the source of prolongation or embellishment of the initial observation.

References

Burde R, Savino P, Trobe J. Visual illusions and hallucinations. In: Clinical decisions in neuro-ophthalmology. 2nd ed. St. Louis: Mosby-Year Book, 1992:145.

Miller NR. Clinical neuro-ophthalmology. 4th ed. Baltimore: Williams & Wilkins, 1991:2515.

Taylor D. Peculiar visual images. In: Taylor D. Pediatric ophthalmology. Boston: Blackwell, 1990:708.

VISION SCREENING GUIDELINES

Earl R. Crouch, Jr., M.D.
Ross A. Kennedy, M.D.

Appropriate vision screening is one of the most important factors in pediatric health care. Because visual stimuli are critical to normal development, early detection and correction of problems can avoid serious vision impairment or blindness. The American Academy of Ophthalmology, the American Association of Pediatric Ophthalmology and Strabismus, and the American Academy of Pediatrics strongly support the goal of early detection and treatment of eye problems in children. In particular, vision screening is needed to detect and refer four major conditions: strabismus, amblyopia, ocular disease, and refractive errors.

A. For vision screening to be effective, it must be done in a uniform manner. Screening tests must be rapid, easy to use, and cost effective. An effective screening program uses the fewest procedures needed to identify children with vision problems. High sensitivity and specificity are important, thereby keeping over- and under-referrals to a minimum. Referrals should be prompt, and limitations of screening must always be kept in mind. Vision screening is not diagnostic and does not identify every child who has a vision difficulty. Screening rarely gives positive proof of the presence or absence of a defect. Some children with conditions needing treatment are not identified, regardless of the screening methods used. Only a professional examination can determine the presence of a defect, its nature and extent, and whether it requires treatment.

B. Unfortunately, no uniform program administered by a single agency exists, and thus screening may occur at a number of different times. Some children are screened in preschool settings, some in day-care centers. Some are not screened until first grade and others not at all. Children should be examined for eye problems in four stages.
   1. In the newborn nursery: Pediatricians or family physician should examine all infants; ophthalmologists should examine all high-risk infants, i.e., those at risk to develop retinopathy of prematurity and those with a family history of retinoblastoma, cataracts, or metabolic disease.
   2. By age 6 months: Pediatricians or family physicians should screen all infants.
   3. At age 3½ years: Pediatricians, family physicians, or ophthalmologists should examine all children.
   4. At age 5 years and older: Pediatricians or family physicians should screen children annually if this is not provided by school personnel or volunteer organizations.

C. Screening for medical conditions is most beneficial when the condition fulfills certain well-established criteria. Consider these criteria in the context of screening for amblyopia in the pediatric population:
   1. The condition sought should be an important health problem: Amblyopia is certainly an important health problem. It is the leading cause of blindness in one eye in the pediatric age group, affecting 2% to 5% of the population.
   2. There should be an efficacious treatment for the problem being screened: Amblyopia is a treatable

TABLE 1 Recommended Vision Screening by Pediatricians and Family Physicians

Age	*Examination*	*Referral Criteria*
Newborn	Penlight examination of cornea	Any ocular pathology
	Rule out nystagmus	Nystagmus
	Red reflexes	Abnormal red reflexes or white reflex
By 6 months	Fixation to light or small toys	Objection to occlusion
	Penlight examination	Nystagmus; any ocular pathology
	Corneal light reflex test, cover test	Strabismus
	Red reflexes	Abnormal red reflexes or white reflex
3.5 years	Visual acuity	Acuity of 20/40 or less in one or both eyes
	Corneal light reflex test, cover test	Strabismus
	Fundus examination	Any ocular pathology
5 years or older	Visual acuity	Acuity of 20/30 or less in one or both eyes
	Corneal light reflex test, cover test	Strabismus
	Fundus examination	Any ocular pathology

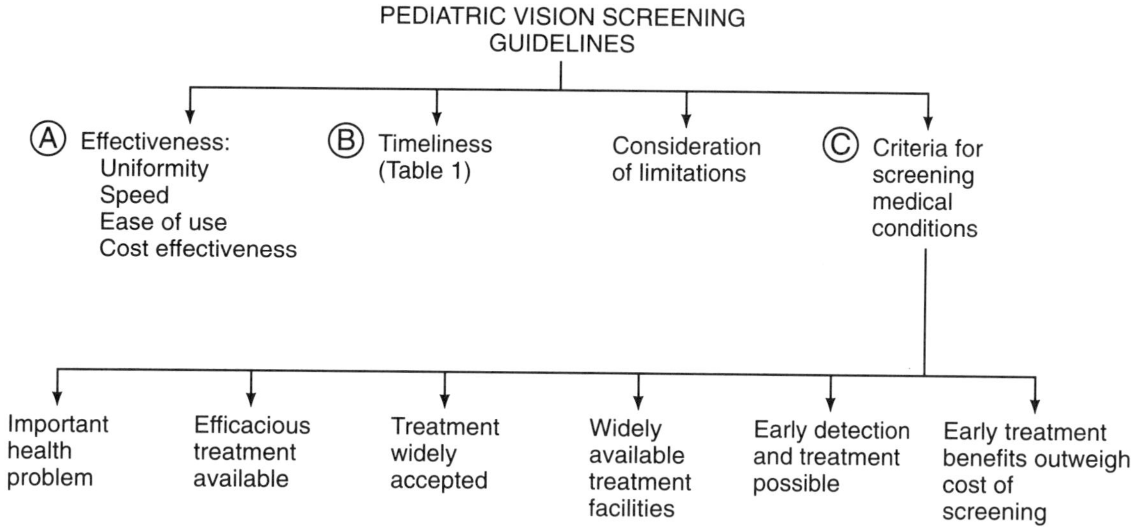

disorder with long-term effectiveness in the range of 80% to 90%.

3. There should be wide acceptance of the treatment for the condition: The treatment of amblyopia by patching is recognized and is not controversial.
4. Facilities for the diagnosis and treatment should be widely available: The present health care system in this country is well equipped with adequately trained personnel to deal with the total expected volume of amblyogenic problems.
5. There should be an early stage during which the disease is detectable and treatment is effective: Treatment for amblyopia is effective during the first 6 or so years of life. Research and clinical wisdom dictate that early treatment is most effective.
6. The cost of the screening should be offset by the health outcome of early treatment.

References

American of Academy of Ophthalmology. Infant and children's eye care—a position statement for the select panel on child health. Washington, DC: American Academy of Ophthalmology, 1980.

American Academy of Ophthalmology. The child's eye: strabismus and amblyopia. San Francisco: American Academy of Ophthalmology, 1982.

American Academy of Pediatrics Committee on Practice and Ambulatory Medicine. Vision screening and eye examination in children. Pediatrics 1986; 77:918.

American Optometric Association. The American Optometric Association guidelines on vision screening. Washington, DC: American Optometric Association, 1979.

Cadman D, Chamber L. Assessing the effectiveness of community screening program. JAMA 1984; 251:1580.

Crouch ER Jr, Goodrich KA. Practical aspects of pediatric vision screening. Am Orthop J 1988; 38:62.

PEDIATRIC VISION SCREENING TECHNIQUES

Earl R. Crouch, Jr., M.D.
Ross A. Kennedy, M.D.

A. Guidelines regarding who needs to be screened and when are covered in the previous chapter.

B. Specific screening tests may be more suited to certain ages and/or vision abnormalities. Each type of test has advantages and disadvantages (Tables 1 to 3).

C. Vision screening tests by primary care physicians include visual acuity assessment or fixation preference, motility examination, red reflex and fundus examination, stereoscopic tests, and photorefractive techniques. In infants and preverbal children, preferred tests include the corneal light reflex test and simultaneous examination of the red reflexes. In young children, a reliable subjective response is obtainable with methods such as forced choice preferential looking. However, the time and trained personnel required to do this test make it impractical as a mass screening tool.

D. In verbal preschoolers, distance visual acuity testing with Snellen tumbling "E" or letters is preferred. When letters or the "E" game cannot be used, picture tests such as the Allen cards or Lighthouse test can be used instead. At present, visual acuity is the most widely used vision screening test in the verbal child. Unfortunately, visual acuity may under-refer amblyopic children with strabismus in about 3% of patients.

E. Stereoscopic tests such as the random dot E stereogram are inexpensive, relatively accurate, and easy to use. Ehrlich, Reinecke, and Simons concluded that the use of random stereogram testing prevents under-referrals. Some studies indicate the test may miss patients with intermittent exotropia and anisometropia. Stereoacuity testing does not replace visual acuity testing as a screening method. The random dot stereograms may overlook a large amount of aniseikonia or amblyopia, but it appears to have the best performance of stereotests and is therefore the recommended test. It should be used in conjunction with visual acuity testing. Unfortunately, the random dot E stereogram has not been widely used by pediatricians, family physicians, and state and national volunteer agencies. As a screening test, the random dot stereogram depends on subjective responses. It is used along with the Snellen acuity test in school-aged children. Visual acuity charts that use letters of equal legibility with controlled spacing between letters and lines and those with logarithmic progression should be used.

F. As new tests are developed that are superior to the Snellen visual acuity test and that enable us to better perform vision screening in a more rapid, accurate, uniform manner, these tests must be incorporated into the vision screening process. Random adoption of vision screening tests by various city, state, and national organizations makes the entire process somewhat complicated. Most importantly, there must be uniform referral criteria.

G. Probably the best vision screeners are orthoptists, limited in number and specially trained. To use orthoptists, ophthalmologists, or optometrists as primary vision screeners underutilizes their skills and is not cost effective. At present, the American Optometric Association advocates a "modified clinical technique" of vision screening, including retinoscopy, ophthalmoscopy, cover/uncover test, and corneal light reflex test. In addition, testing of Snellen E visual acuity, color vision, and external observation is recommended. This is essentially a complete eye examination requiring eye care professionals and raising the cost of vision screening to a prohibitive level. Vision screening of preschool children falls to pediatricians, family physicians, school nurses, and volunteers trained by private groups, including the National Society to Prevent Blindness and similar state societies. Pediatricians and family doctors are able to access a great number of children through human resources already in place. They have the greatest ability to detect abnormalities at an early age. Essential elements of their vision screening examination include fixation preference or visual acuity, motility examination including corneal light reflex testing, the cover test, simultaneous red reflexes, and fundus examination. These procedures are cost effective and can be performed in a time-efficient manner. Education of pediatricians, family practitioners, and the public in vision screening is essential to the entire process.

H. Traditional tests of vision require a subjective response and are not fully adequate in preverbal and nonverbal children. Researchers, by comparing the qualities of the "red reflex" from the two eyes, have successfully identified the common precursors of amblyopia (strabismus, anisometropia, large refractive errors, and problems with ocular structure). Groups from several continents use various photographic and videographic techniques to capture the red reflex for study. The technologies differ mainly in the arrangement of the light source and the camera. Some photoscreeners are designed with the camera lens and the light source at the same theoretical axis, whereas others work with an off-axis arrangement. Off-axis photoscreening is preferred over on-axis photoscreening because of much lower cost and the limited assessment of media opacities and strabismus with the on-axis process. This technology provides accurate and reliable identification of the precursors of amblyopia in the preverbal infant when treatment is most effective. Compared with the "gold standard" assessment of a pediatric ophthalmologist, photoscreening produces sensitivity

(Continued on page 200)

VISION SCREENING TECHNIQUES

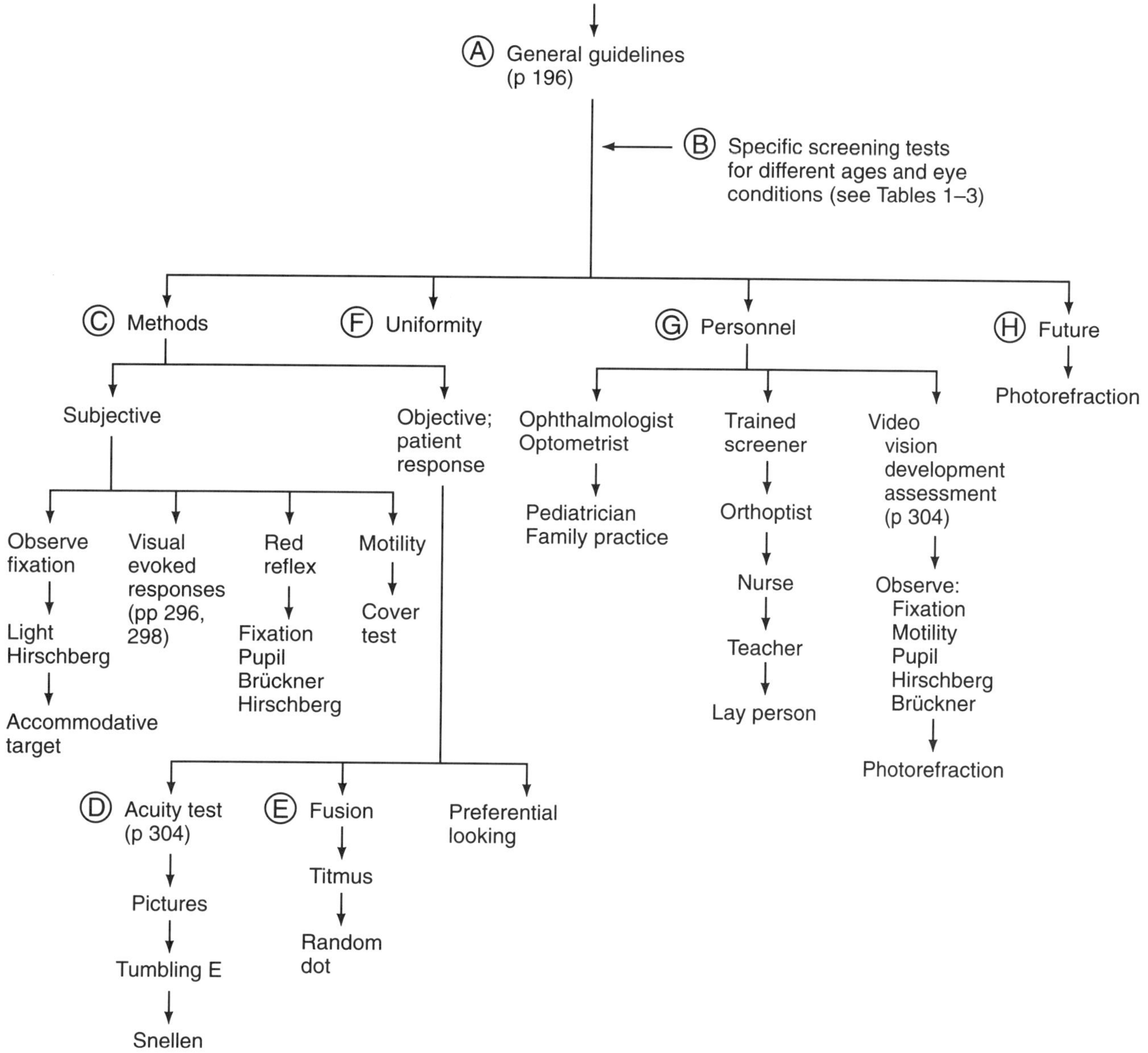

TABLE 1 Vision Screening Guidelines: Infants and Preverbal Children

Examination	*Abnormalities Identified*	*Advantages*	*Disadvantages*
Corneal light reflex test	Strabismus	Inexpensive Easy to perform	May yield false positive
Simultaneous red reflexes	Strabismus Media opacities Anisometropia High refractive errors	Inexpensive Easy to perform by physicians Excellent for media opacities, strabismus	May overlook refractive errors, especially anisometropia, amblyopia
Photoscreener Off-axis (para-axial) flash source with respect to optical axis of camera	Strabismus Anisometropia Media opacities High refractive errors	Can be performed by trained lay and allied health screeners Simultaneously records red reflexes, corneal light reflex, refractive errors; excellent to detect strabismus, media opacities Sensitivity—0.85 Specificity—0.87 Cycloplegia not required	Interpretation required by trained professionals or highly trained health care personnel Initial cost—approximately $4000 per unit Additional cost—$7.00 per student Refracts only one axis
On-axis (isotropic) flash source with respect to optical axis of camera	Anisometropia Refractive errors Some media opacities	Can be performed by trained lay or allied health screeners Sensitivity—0.94 Specificity—0.94, especially sensitive for astigmatism	Interpretation requires trained professionals or highly trained health care personnel Cost—approximately $10,000 to $15,000/unit Limited assessment for partial media opacities, strabismus Cycloplegia preferred to enhance sensitivity

TABLE 2 Vision Screening Guidelines: Preschoolers Ages 3 through 5 Years

Vision Function and Screening Method	*Abnormalities Identified*	*Referral Criteria*	*Advantages*	*Disadvantages*
Distance visual acuity				
Snellen acuity Tumbling E or ABCs	Refractive errors Amblyopia	Less than 4 of 6 correct on 20/40 line	Easy to perform	Over-referral of visually normal children
Picture test Allen pictures, lighthouse	Refractive errors Amblyopia	Incorrect response to 20/40 line	Easy to perform Can be used with children difficult to screen	
Ocular alignment—strabismus				
Unilateral cover test Distance (10 feet or 3 meters)	Strabismus	Any eye movement		Requires trained allied health professional, i.e., orthoptist or C.O.M.T., or primary care practitioner
Near (13 inches or 33 cm)	Strabismus	Any eye movement	Requires good accommodative target	
Random dot stereogram (16 inches or 40 cm)	Strabismus Amblyopia	Less than 4 of 6 correct	Can be administered by any trained screener Requires normally functioning optical, motor, and sensory systems	May overlook patients with anisometropic amblyopia and intermittent exotropia Must be used in conjunction with visual acuity testing
Photorefractive screener (see Table 1)				

TABLE 3 Vision Screening Guidelines: School-age Children 6 Years and Older

Vision Function and Screening Method	*Abnormalities Identified*	*Referral Criteria*	*Advantages*	*Disadvantages*
Distance visual acuity				
Snellen letters	Refractive errors Amblyopia	Less than 4 of 6 correct on 20/30 line, OR a two-line difference between the two eyes, i.e., 20/30 and 20/20	Can be administered by any trained screener	
Ocular alignment—strabismus				
Unilateral cover test Distance (20 feet or meters)	Strabismus	Any eye movement	Requires highly trained allied health professional, i.e., orthoptist, C.O.T., or C.O.M.T.	
Near (13 inches or 33 cm)	Strabismus	Any eye movement	Good accommodative target required	
Random dot stereogram (16 inches or 40 cm)	Strabismus Amblyopia	Less than 4 of 6 correct	Can be administered by any trained screener Requires normally functioning optical, motor, and sensory system	May overlook patients with anisometropic amblyopia and intermittent exotropia Does not replace visual acuity testing

and specificity in the range of 85% to 94%. Compared with a combination of illiterate E visual acuity and stereotest given by a lay health technician, photoscreening seems to recognize almost twice as many children with the disease in a study of a general population.

A photoscreener is operated by trained technicians. Refinement of the technology as these products are brought into service should reduce the cost and time of screening to a fraction of those of present "manual" techniques. Photoscreening of all children by 12 months of age could detect precursors of amblyopia with a high degree of sensitivity and specificity. These techniques can then become incorporated into vision screening and may well become the key elements in the early detection of amblyopia.

References

Avilla CW, von Noorden GK. Limitation of the TNO random dot stereo test for visual screening. Am Orthoptic J 1981; 31:87.

Day SH, Norcia AM. Photographic screening for factors leading to amblyopia. Am Orthoptic J 1988; 38:51.

Ehrlich MI, Reinecke RD, Simons K. Preschool vision screening for amblyopia and strabismus: programs, methods, guidelines. Surv Ophthalmol 1983; 28:145.

Hso-Winges C, Hammer RD, Norcia AM. Polaroid photorefractive screening of infants. J Pediatr Ophthalmol Strabismus 1989; 26:254.

Kennedy RA, Sheps SB. A comparison of photoscreening techniques for amblyopic factors in children. Can J Ophthalmol 1989; 24:259.

Molteno ACB, Hoare-Nairne J, Parr JC. The Otago photoscreener, a method of mass screening of infants to detect squint and refractive error. Trans Ophthalmic Soc NZ 1983; 35:43.

Ruttum MS. Vision screening with random dot stereograms. Am Orthoptic J 1988; 38:43.

Ruttum MS, Nelson DB. Stereoscopic testing to reduce over-referral in preschool vision screening. J Pediatr Ophthalmol Strabismus 1991; 28:131.

Tongue AC, Cibis GW. Bruckner test. Ophthalmology 1981; 88:1041.

Von Noorden GK. Stereoacuity testing does not replace visual acuity testing. Arch Ophthalmol 1986; 104:1112.

VIDEO VISION DEVELOPMENT ASSESSMENT

Gerhard W. Cibis, M.D.
Thomas P. Luke, B.S.

Video vision development assessment (VVDA) combines dynamic documentation of the Brueckner and Hirschberg reflexes with pupil movement assessment for fixation, with photo refraction. A Super VHS video camera with a specially modified light source (patent pending) captures the dynamic aspects of fixation, foveation, and accommodation. Individual video frames can be digitized for mathematical analysis. A video printer allows for documentation on hard copy to form a report to parents or referring physicians or to be placed in the medical record. Although usable as a screening tool, VVDA is actually a diagnostic assessment of fixation, foveation, accommodation, amblyogenic factors, and ocular alignment in real time (dynamic aspects) (Fig. 1).

A. A patient fixes a point light source situated within the plane of a video camera lens that records the Hirschberg and Brueckner reflexes from both eyes. When fixation on the light occurs, pupillary constriction, change in red fundus reflex (Brueckner), and shift in Hirschberg (first Purkinje) image are captured in real time and are available for analysis.

B. When both eyes are aligned and refractive errors nearly equal, the Brueckner reflex is equal and the Hirschberg reflex is appropriate. Hippus of the pupil can be monitored over time as fixation on the light is maintained. Often with accommodative or small angle intermittent esotropia, over time (a few seconds) a deviation manifests itself. Deviations are more readily seen with the video equipment than with a live observer, something we call the "lack of doctor" effect. Amblyogenic factors such as misalignment of the eyes, anisometropia, high refractive errors, and media opacities are apparent to the video viewer.

Although this test does not measure depth perception, fusion, or binocularity per se, the presence of symmetric Brueckner and Hirschberg reflexes allows the diagnosis of ocular alignment. When eyes are not aligned, lack of or interruption of binocular development can be assumed. Eccentric photorefraction allows determination of amblyogenic refractive errors. By decentering the fixation light, a crescent is created which can be used to monitor accommodation, testing it over time and under different conditions. Accommodation, convergence, and motility are recorded in real time. These factors can be assessed over time in normal conditions such as reading or working with video monitors.

C. VVDA can perform photorefraction and is much more accurate because of the ability to capture and analyze dynamic aspects. Most current photorefractors use still photographs. Our experience with VVDA shows that not only do patients not fixate as needed but that without the dynamic aspects it can be impossible to determine the difference between looking at the light and truly fixing (foveating) on it with proper accommodation and convergence.

Eccentric photorefraction works on the concept that with a sufficiently large refractive error, light reflected from the patient's fundus spills into the optical aperture of the viewing instrument, which can

A
B
C

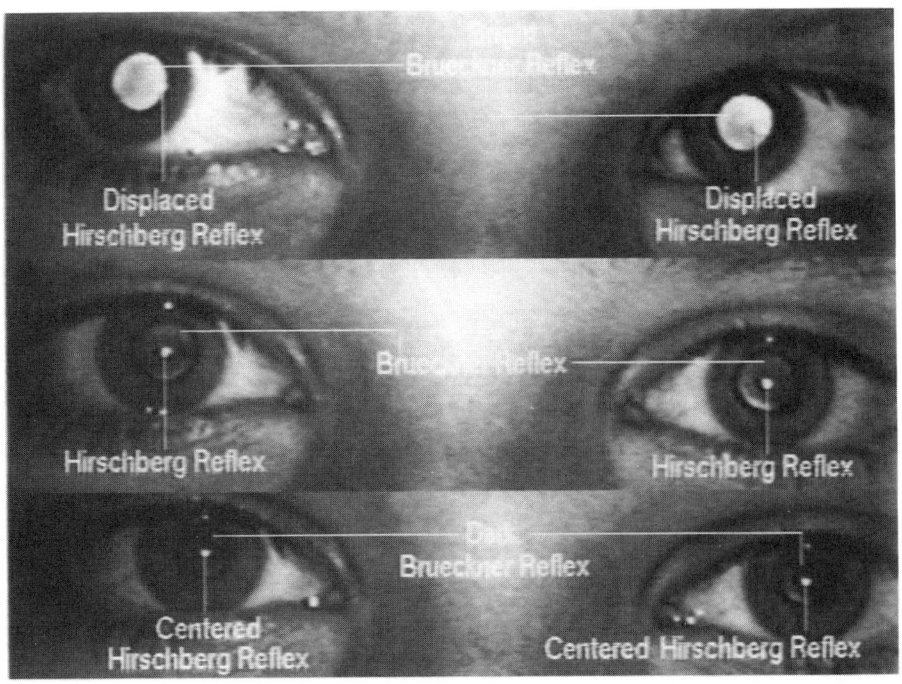

Figure 1 **A,** Patient not fixating light. Hirschberg reflexes are displaced. Bright Brueckner reflexes are unequal. **B,** Patient fixates light. Hirschberg reflexes are properly centered with small angle kappa, but patient is not foveating. **C,** Patient foveates light. Again, Hirschberg reflexes are appropriate for angle kappa but now pupil is constricted and Brueckner reflex is darker in both eyes than in **B,** indicating foveation and accommodation. The difference between fixating and foveating takes place in less than 1/30 of a second (one video frame).

VIDEO VISION DEVELOPMENT ASSESSMENT of
Nonverbal Children, 6 Months to 3 Years of Age

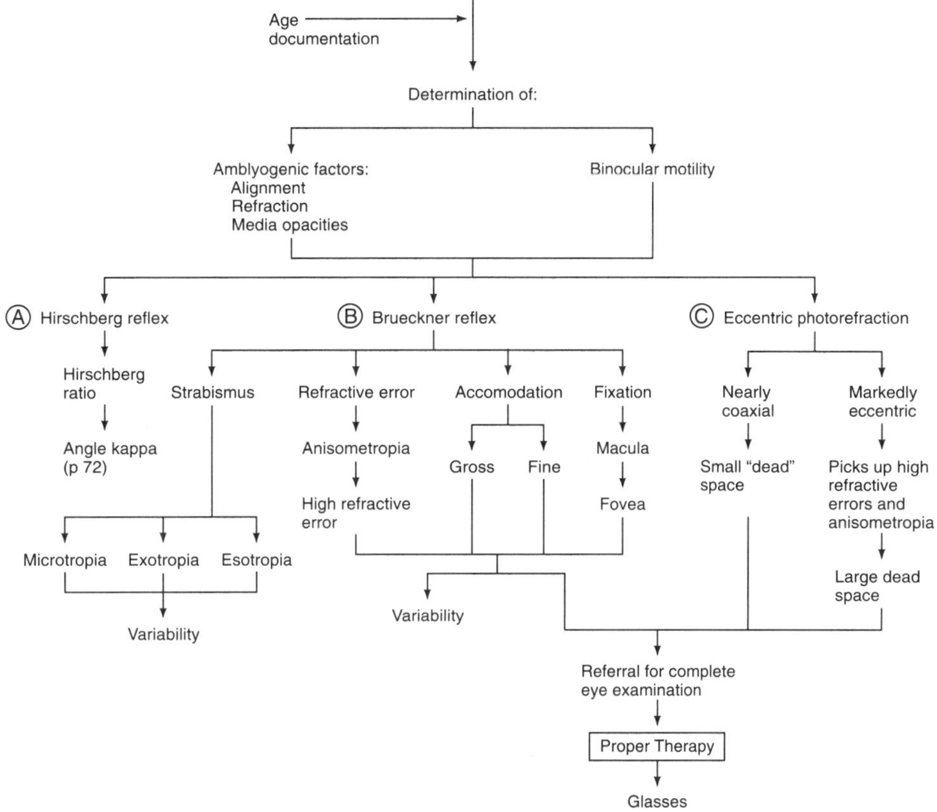

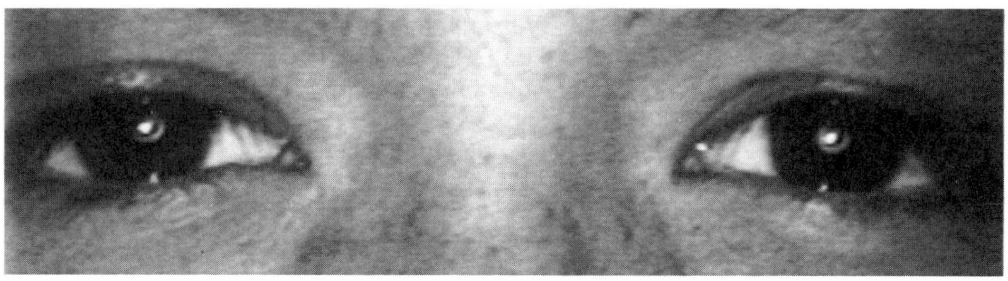

Figure 2 Photorefractive crescent measures 1 diopter of accommodation at 33-cm fixation target when 3 diopters are needed. Diagnosis: accommodative insufficiency.

be an ophthalmoscope. We use a video camera with light source in the plane of the camera lens. The more eccentric the light is from the center of the camera lens, the larger the refractive error needs to be for a crescent to be seen (dead space). Large decentration of the light therefore leaves a large refractive error that cannot be measured. Small decentrations with small dead space suffer from the crescent quickly reaching maximum; therefore, the range of errors that can be measured is limited to 3 to 4 diopters for any degree of eccentricity. Our test strategy therefore is to examine the patient with two settings of light eccentricity and to combine the information from both to determine refractive errors and amblyogenic potential. Crescent size is a factor of patient–to–light source distance, patient pupil size, and degree of light eccentricity. When all these are known, the refractive power of the eye can be calculated (eccentric photorefraction).

References

Bobier WR. Eccentric photorefraction: A method to measure accommodation of highly hypermetropic infants. Clin Vision Sci 1990; 5:45.

Cibis-Tongue AB, Cibis GW. Brueckner test. Ophthalmology 1981; 88:1041.

Day SH, Norcia AM. Photographic detection of amblyogenic factors. Ophthalmology 1986; 93:25.

Howell ER. The differential diagnosis of accommodation/convergence disorders. Behav Optometry Jan/Feb 1991; 20.

Kaakinen K. A simple method for screening of children with strabismus, anisometropia or ametropia by simultaneous photography of the corneal and the fundus reflexes. Acta Ophthalmol (Copenh) 1979; 57:161.

ABNORMAL AMPLITUDES OF ACCOMMODATION

Malcolm L. Mazow, M.D., F.A.C.S.

A. All people experience some nondescript symptoms associated with the use of the eyes at near. Significant symptoms causing complaints that need attention by an eye-care professional are labeled asthenopia. The change in visual acuity from distance to near requires a smooth transition of the disjunctive movements of the eyes. These include accommodation and convergence (proximal, fusional, accommodative, awareness of near). Abnormalities in these mechanisms may lead to difficulties with prolonged, or in some cases, any near effort visual task.

B. The following steps in the examination are needed:
   1. Visual acuity measured at distance and near, monocularly and binocularly.
   2. Fusional measurements to ensure that complaints originate from a binocular problem: 1) Divergence amplitudes—the amplitudes of fusional divergence should always be measured prior to convergence amplitudes. Amplitudes are passive and appear decreased or abnormal if the active (convergence) amplitudes of fusion and near are measured first. Near divergence should be two to three times distance, normal mean distance break and refuse points being 6/4. 2) Convergence fusional amplitudes are measured at distance and near, with the mean break/refuse for distance 18/14. The near convergence amplitude is two to three times distance.
   3. Near point of accommodation—measured from blurred to clear and clear to blurred, monocularly and binocularly.
   4. Near point of convergence measurement uses an accommodative target for *objective* and red glass for *subjective* testing. The normal for both should be less than 10 cm from the bridge of the nose.
   5. Pupillary evaluation is mandatory, including size at distance and near, reaction to light and to near, and consensual response. Adie's pupil, third cranial nerve palsy, and other clinical conditions cause asthenopia.
   6. A cyclomanifest refraction with the prescribing of the appropriate correction may alleviate asthenopic complaints.

C. In accommodative spasm the ciliary muscle tone is increased, and a constant accommodative effort is expended by the parasympathetic nervous system. This brings the far point and near point closer to one another, inducing a pseudomyopia. In milder cases, the spasm is intermittent, accentuated by near work. Distance vision is blurred. The individual becomes pseudomyopic. This worsens if an optical correction (minus) is given. Near vision is rarely impaired. In severe cases close work may be done at a very short distance. Symptoms are accentuated with close work. This results in brow pain, headache, and early fatigue with inability to maintain visual or mental concentration. Pain may induce nausea, vomiting, and abdominal discomfort. The accommodative disturbance is sometimes associated with spasm of the pupil. Excess convergence may also be seen, leading to an esotropia in some individuals. Conversely, convergence insufficiency may result in this condition. The diagnosis should be suspected when subjective and objective tests of refraction (dry manifest and cycloplegic refraction) vary and the range of accommodation is abnormal for the patient's age. Mild cycloplegic drops may not be sufficient, and total atropine cycloplegia may be required to unmask the pseudomyopia.

D. Organic accommodative spasm can result from irritative lesions of the brain stem and trunk of the third nerve, encephalitis, meningitis, trigeminal neuralgia, intraocular inflammation (when the ciliary body is involved), and systemic infections such as diphtheria. Morphine, the digitalis drugs, and sulfonamides can be causative. Closed head trauma may induce bilateral accommodative spasm, and local ocular trauma can cause unilateral spasm.

E. It is important to understand an individual's work habits requiring constant close work to help make the diagnosis of tonic accommodation. Diseases also associated with tonic accommodation include diabetes, alcoholism, ocular migraines, generalized migraines, and Graves' disease.

F. Total loss of accommodation results from paralysis of the parasympathetic component of accommodation. The near point of accommodation recedes until it approaches the far point. Pupils fail to contract. This accentuates the optical defect. Symptoms depend on the refractive state. Because the cause is often a lesion in the oculomotor nuclear complex or at the trunk of the third nerve, paralysis of accommodation rarely occurs alone. Fourth, sixth, and third cranial nerves are often affected. Iridoplegia with loss of accommodation occurs.

G. Accommodation palsy can be caused by topical or systemic anticholinergic cycloplegic drugs, especially atropine. Anti-Parkinson drugs such as trihexyphenidyl, benztropine, and L-dopa may also be causative. New drugs, including Anafranil (used in obsessive-compulsive disorders), may cause mild accommodative deficiencies but not total paralysis.

H. Closed head trauma affects accommodation. It may also disturb convergence, resulting in an internal ophthalmoplegia. Although rare, congenital defects in the ciliary muscle may produce the same phenomenon.

I. A variety of neurogenic conditions, including infec-

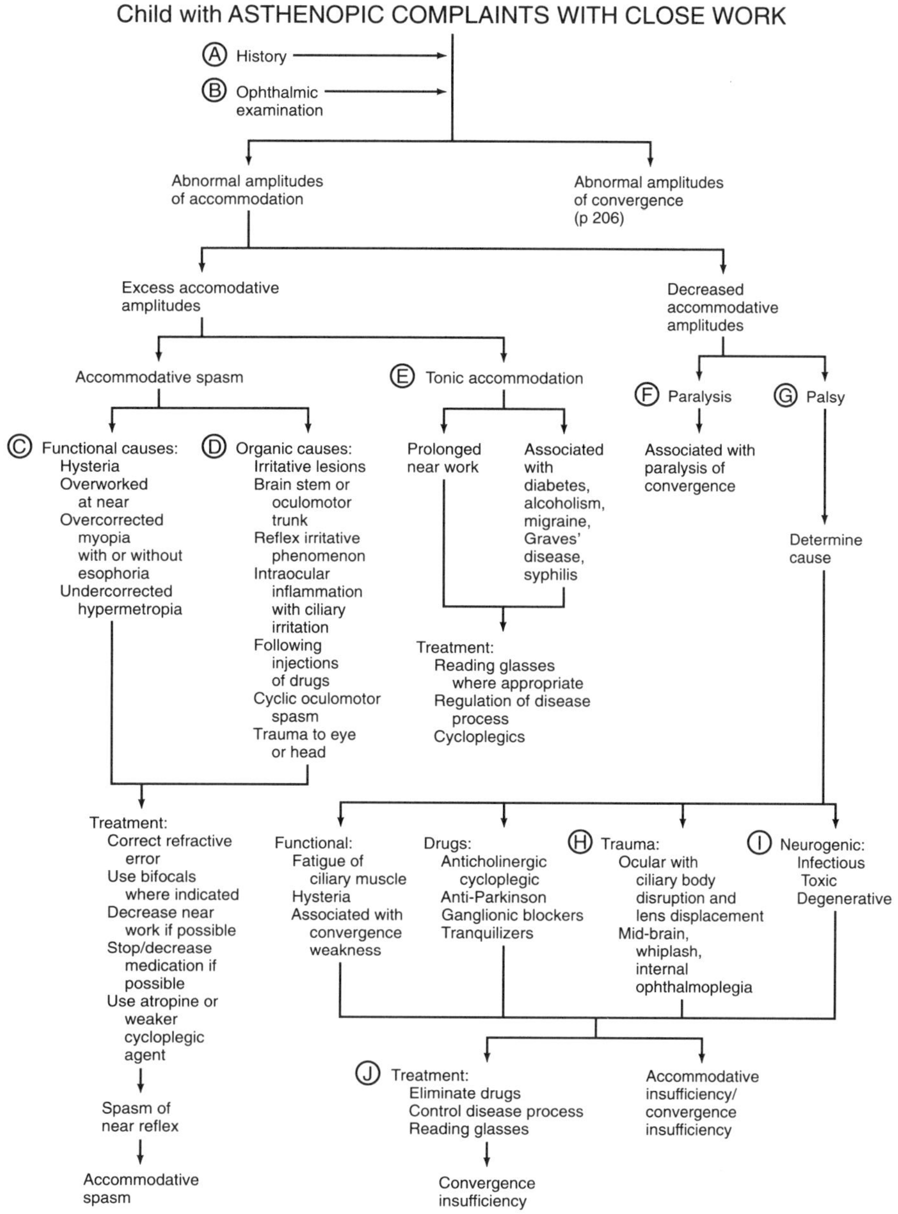

tions, toxins, degenerative diseases, and exogenous poisons, along with metabolic diseases (e.g., diabetes) should be considered in total paralysis. Infectious conditions including encephalitis, meningitis, herpes zoster, and syphilis may lead to total accommodation loss (paralysis) or weakness. The mechanism is not understood. It is possible that the toxin affects the nerve trunks or the nucleus. Postdiphtheric paralysis is attributable to a demyelinating toxin with special predilection for cranial nerves supplying the bulbar musculature of the palate, pharynx, larynx, and ciliary body. *Clostridium botulinum* causes dilated nonreactive pupils and weakness or paralysis of accommodation. Pupillary and ciliary musculature may be weakened in ophthalmoplegic forms of acute idiopathic polyneuritis, as well as rostral-dorsal midbrain lesions.

J. If the underlying cause is amenable to treatment, the ocular condition may require little attention. Temporary reading aids can be useful.

References

Hollister LE. Complications of therapeutic drugs. Clin Pharmacol Ther 1964; 5:323.

Mann AM, Heseltine GFD. The desmethyl metabolite of imipramine (G-35020) in treatments of depression, further clinical experience. Can Med Assoc J 1963; 88.

Mazow ML, France TD, Finkelman S, et al. Acute accommodative and convergence insufficiency. Trans Am Ophthalmol Soc 1989; 87:158.

PDR 1992; 46:652.

PDR 1992; 46:1196.

PDR 1992; 46:952.

PDR 1992; 46:1435.

Tasman W, Glaser JS, Bachgusli B, eds. Duane's clinical ophthalmology. Philadelphia: JB Lippincott, 1989:13.

von Graefe, DE. Systems of ophthalmologic motility and strabismus. Henry Kimpton, 1973; 6:706.

ABNORMAL AMPLITUDES OF CONVERGENCE

Malcolm L. Mazow, M.D., F.A.C.S.

A. See paragraph A on p 204.

B. See paragraph B on p 204.

C. True paralysis of convergence demands a work-up to find the cause. Fortunately, total paralysis of convergence is a relatively rare condition. It may be caused by a lesion in the occipital lobe or brain stem, usually in the region of the superior colliculi. It was first described by Parinaud in 1838 as a failure of convergence, typically coming on suddenly with crossed diplopia of a comitant type when the eyes view an object at near.

D. Poor subjective and/or objective near point of convergence suggests convergence insufficiency syndrome. This entity occurs with or without accompaniment of a near exophoric deviation and abnormal convergence/divergence amplitudes. Often an abnormal near point of accommodation accompanies the above findings. Asthenopic symptoms are related to prolonged use of the eyes, necessitating moving detail work further away. The asthenopia is significant enough to create headaches. Divergence amplitude and passive amplitudes may be changed sufficiently to create symptoms along with the abnormalities in the convergence amplitudes. Such individuals must be evaluated monocularly to ascertain whether symptoms are binocular and not from some other cause. If symptoms persist monocularly, other nonfusional evaluation is needed.

E. Appropriate management of convergence insufficiency, including sustained near point of convergence exercises, associated with the build-up of convergence amplitudes and the appreciation of diplopia, often leads to relief of the symptoms. The addition of orthoptic exercises and the use of base-out orthoptic training prism, as well as base-in prism, for the relief of symptoms, have all been used in treatment. On rare occasions, when all of the above fail and a significant exophoric deviation or intermittent exotropia at near exists (which really excludes the convergence insufficiency syndrome), surgery may be considered. This should be undertaken with great reluctance. Most convergence insufficiency patients can be cured or relieved of their symptoms with appropriate exercises and/or prism therapy.

F. Habitual excess of convergence or even spasm of convergence due to tonic innervational influences is usually associated with an orthophoria for distance and normal lateral movements of eyes. The causes may be divided into three types: (1) an increase of convergence associated with increase of accommodation and miosis; (2) a primary type of convergence in association with spasm of accommodation and constriction of the pupils; (3) convergence excess following insufficiency or divergence (see paragraphs G, H, and I).

G. An increase of convergence associated with increase of accommodation and miosis is the most common of the clinical pictures and is called spasm of the near reflex. It is often found in uncorrected hypermetropes, whose excessive accommodation becomes a life-long habit. Rarely, early presbyopes, while making their attempts to see close without the aid of plus lenses, develop this particular condition.

H. A primary type of convergence excess in association with spasm of accommodation and constriction of the pupils may arise from irritative lesions in the superior colliculi, described by Parinaud as retractory nystagmus, convergence excess, and inability to elevate the eyes. An hysterical convergence spasm with miosis accommodation occurs in young adolescent females and to a lesser extent in males. This is similar and does not have pathologic causation.

I. The symptoms of convergence excess may be bothersome as a result of the loss of divergence. These patients must be evaluated for bilateral sixth cranial nerve palsy.

J. Treatment of convergence excess is directed toward elimination of the cause. Refractive error should be corrected, as well as any significant heterophoria. During the period of convergence excess, near work should be limited to a minimum. Near material should be held at such a distance as to decrease the amount of convergence and accommodation needed. This curtailment of near work obviously limits some of the activities of the patient but should relieve symptoms.

K. The synkinesis of the interrelationship between divergence and convergence can be seen to work together very closely, and weakness of one or the other usually is accompanied by a concomitant problem with the fellow. It is very common, therefore, to see a spasm of the near reflex. The management, after elimination of the causative factors, is the use of strong cycloplegics such as atropine. This parasympatholytic agent may allow the return to normalcy of accommodation.

Individuals with a weakness of accommodation associated with a weakness of convergence are treated appropriately with clearing of the near image to allow the management of the convergence weakness. Weakness of convergence is often related only to poor accommodation, and once the accommodation has been corrected the convergence ability returns and the symptoms are relieved. The close relationship of the mechanisms of near may result in asthenopic complaints related to one or both, directing the evaluation and leading to proper diagnosis, therapy, and relief of symptoms.

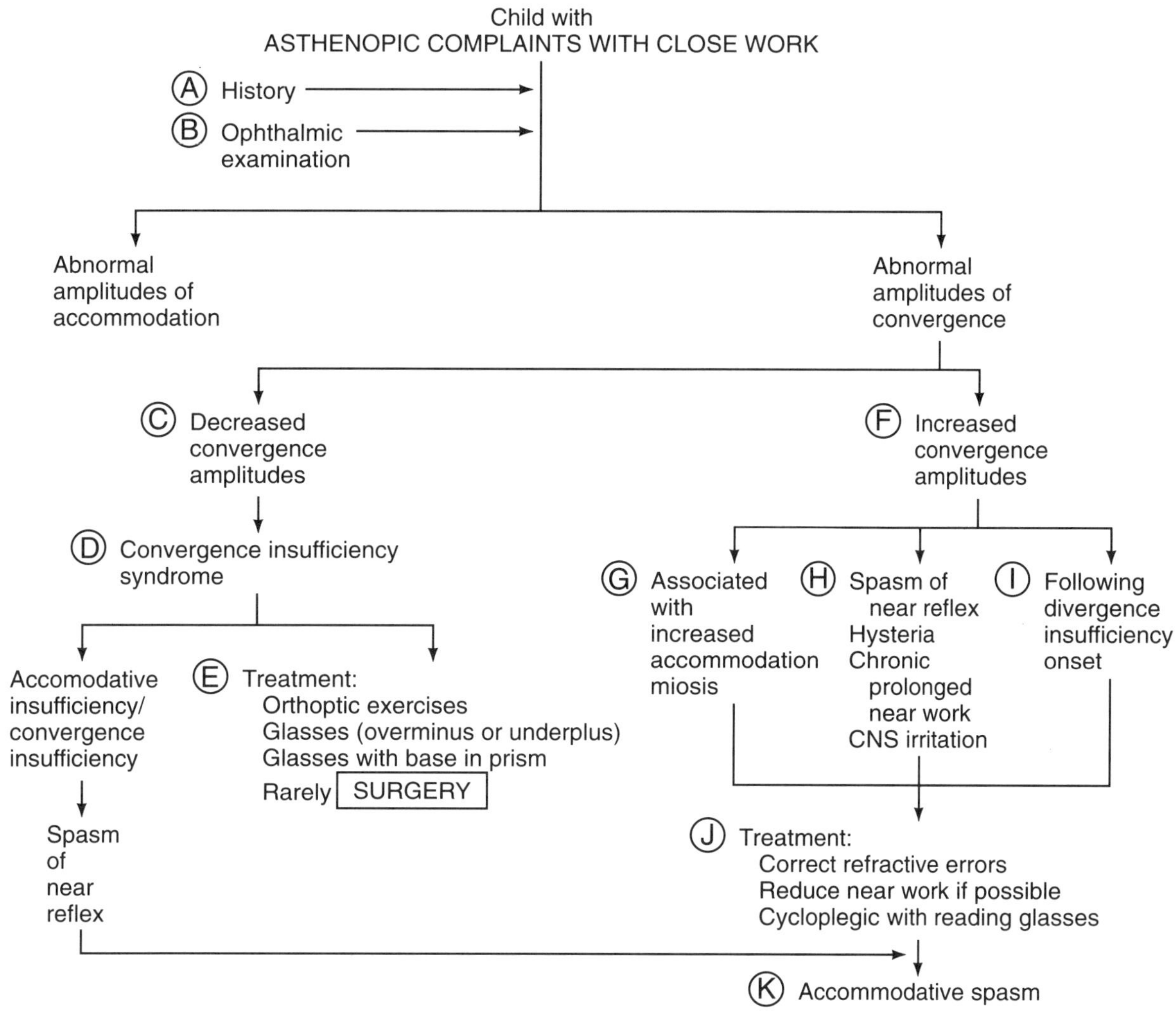

References

Cherington M. Botulism: Ten year experience. Arch Neurol 1974; 30:432.

Irvine G. A survey of esophoria and ciliary spasm. Br J Ophthalmol 1947; 31:289.

Mazow ML. Convergence insufficiency syndrome. Curr Ocular Ther 1990; 3:471.

Mazow ML. The convergence insufficiency syndrome. J Pediatr Ophthalmol 1971; 4:243.

EVALUATION OF ASTHENOPIA IN CHILDHOOD

Andrea Cibis Tongue, M.D.

The preceding two chapters deal with the theoretical background and diagnosis of accommodative and convergence abnormalities that may give rise to difficulty with close work. This chapter presents a clinical approach to the evaluation of pediatric asthenopic complaints. Asthenopia (eye discomfort, eye strain, headaches, brow aches, and so forth with near visual tasks) is a subjective complaint that is not measurable. Diagnosis of visual abnormalities depends on the history, ophthalmologic examination, objective measurements of convergence and accommodation, and evaluation of subjective symptoms. Children with complaints of blurry vision, headaches when reading, not being able to see the words, eye pain, and similar problems are often referred for evaluation of possible vision problems.

A. History should elicit whether complaints occur only during school or during certain classes. Does the child voluntarily read for pleasure without complaints? Are there reading difficulties, dyslexia, or other learning disorders (p 192)? If a child performs other near vision tasks, developing asthenopic symptoms with reading only, a functional cause may be suspected.

B. A complete eye examination is indicated, with particular attention paid to motility, refraction, and accommodative/convergence ability.

C. A prolonged alternate cover test at near with and without accommodative targets is performed. Exophoria may not be uncovered without the use of a nonaccommodative target and prolonged cover test. Esophoria or intermittent esotropia may not be detected if only a nonaccommodative target such as a penlight is used.

D. Convergence and divergence ability at near is tested with a prism bar or rotary prism. Greater than 20 diopters of convergence and 6 to 15 diopters of divergence at near is the norm. Note the amount of prism at which recovery of single vision occurs. A patient with divergence of 10 diopters who does not recover fusion until 2 diopters of base-in prism are reached may have difficulty with divergence amplitudes. Usually recovery is reached within 5 prism diopters of divergence. Observe the patient's eyes, looking for the break point and refusion point. Do not depend solely on subjective answers. Divergence amplitude, both distance and near, should be checked before convergence amplitudes are tested. Amplitudes may be tested by using a prism bar or rotary prism, allowing for a smooth transition from one prism power to the next.

E. Convergence insufficiency may be seen in patients with intermittent exotropia or exophoria at near, rare in children. Usually accommodative convergence is sufficient to keep the eyes straight for near. More commonly, convergence insufficiency is seen as an isolated entity. Fortunately, it responds quite rapidly to orthoptics. Because of its rapid response to push-up or prism exercises, a functional cause may be responsible. Unless accommodative amplitudes are decreased as well, plus lenses are not of any help because they decrease the accommodative convergence stimulation. Isolated accommodative and convergence abnormalities with ominous underlying cause are fortunately rare.

F. Near point of convergence is best tested by having the patient read aloud to the examiner 20/40 or 20/30 size letters (near equivalents). This enables the examiner to be certain that the child is indeed fixing on the target and is accommodating and stimulating convergence. The target is moved slowly toward the patient's nose until it is no longer decipherable. Because of the relative sparsity of letters that fit on a fixation target for near (especially if presented in the desirable vertical row), the target can initially be presented at a fairly close range. It is also best to use targets that have different letters on each side so that with repeated tests new letters are used. This tests both convergence and accommodation. Normal values are between 2 and 8 cm from the eye. (An inexpensive target can be made by pasting a row of small letters on a tongue blade.) Convergence can also be tested with a nonaccommodative target such as a penlight. To test fusional convergence, a red filter is placed over one eye using a penlight for the target. With the latter two methods, convergence is usually within 10 cm from the eye. Accommodation and convergence should be measured together because this most closely resembles everyday conditions the patient encounters.

G. Accommodation can be measured monocularly. Asymmetric accommodative amplitudes usually indicate anisometropia. Cycloplegic refraction usually reveals this. Unilateral third nerve paralysis or pupillary abnormalities also give asymmetric accommodative amplitudes, with the lesser amplitude on the side of the more dilated pupil or the third nerve paralysis.

H. Accommodative facility—the ability to change accommodation easily—should be tested, particularly if functional complaints are suspected. Having the patient read while putting −2.00 lenses in front of the eye and then removing them, repeating this cycle three times within 30 seconds, gives useful information regarding the patient's accommodative abilities. If the patient easily performs this task, subnormal accommodation is probably not the culprit. If accommodative spasm is suspected, the test is repeated using +2.00 and plano lenses; again a

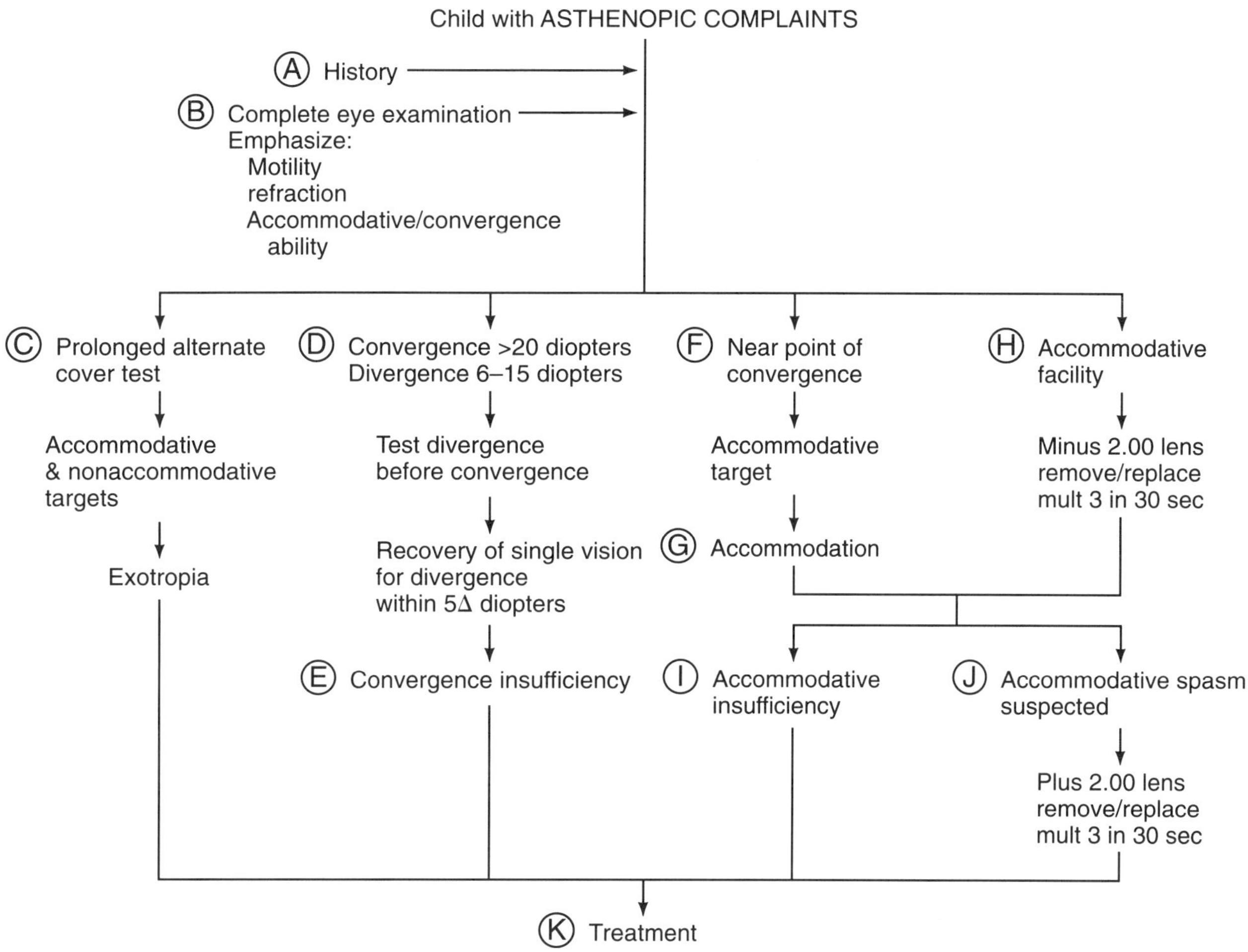

normal response is completion of the cycle three times within 30 seconds.

I. Subnormal accommodation is rare in children. There is, however, a subgroup of accommodative esotropes with a high AC/A ratio who actually have subnormal accommodation and who require bifocals not only to control the esotropia but to provide clear vision at near. Attempts to wean these patients out of bifocals often fail, with continued complaints of near vision difficulty, even if the esophoria/esotropia has resolved. Subnormal accommodation (and convergence) may also follow a closed head injury. Children complaining of difficulty seeing after traumatic injuries involving the CNS or trauma to the head should be screened to see if convergence and accommodation are normal.

J. Accommodative spasm occurs rarely in childhood and is more likely to be encountered in older children. Pupillary miosis, convergence excess (with occasional frank esotropia), and pseudomyopia may complete the clinical picture. Cycloplegia is essential to make the diagnosis. Cycloplegia and bifocal wear may be required to treat the condition.

K. Treatment is directed toward correction of anisometropic or ametropic refractive errors that are likely to cause asthenopia. A cycloplegic refraction should be performed before prescribing lenses. Significant hyperopia and pseudomyopia may be uncovered only after cycloplegia. Patients with true myopia rarely complain of near vision difficulties unless they have astigmatism, anisometropia, or a very high myopia.

Patients with accommodative insufficiency may benefit from orthoptics and/or the wearing of plus lenses for near. Orthoptic exercises include work with plus/minus flipper lenses while reading. Convergence insufficiency usually responds to orthoptic treatment as well. Reading with increasing amounts of base-out prism and convergence push-up exercises are often helpful. Accommodative spasm may be treated with bifocals and cycloplegics if necessary.

Reference

Rosner J, Rosner J. Pediatric ophthalmology. 2nd ed. Stoneham, MA: Butterworth, 1990.

ACUTE OPTIC NEURITIS IN CHILDHOOD

Lois J. Martyn, M.D.

A. Optic neuritis classically presents with sudden or rapidly progressive loss of vision occurring within a period of hours or days. One or both eyes may be affected. Vision loss is usually severe but sometimes mild. There may be associated (concurrent or antecedent) symptoms such as headache, retrobulbar pain, or discomfort on eye movement or palpation. In children the history may vary and may be misleading. Parents of nonverbal children may notice only a change in the child's affect, behavior, or performance. Fearful children may try to conceal their problem. Unilateral or mild vision changes may pass unnoticed. The insidiously progressive vision loss of a tumor or degenerative disease may suddenly become apparent and be misinterpreted as the acute vision loss of optic neuritis.

B. Clinical examination must provide evidence of impaired optic nerve function. Signs consistent with the diagnosis of optic neuritis include reduced visual acuity in one or both eyes, visual field changes (usually central or centrocecal scotoma or generalized depression), altered color vision, impaired contrast sensitivity, and attendant afferent pupillary dysfunction. Documentation of vision and pupillary changes can be difficult in children, but every attempt must be made to differentiate the signs of optic neuritis from those of intracranial tumor or other disorders affecting the visual pathways. Also, proof of organic impairment of optic nerve function is crucial in distinguishing children with optic neuritis from those with feigned or psychogenic visual symptoms (p 180).

C. Classifying optic neuritis on the basis of the ophthalmoscopic findings provides information about the predominant site of involvement and, to some extent, the pathogenesis and significance of the process. Retrobulbar neuritis is rare in children. Its occurrence in any age group raises concern about the possibility of multiple sclerosis (MS) although other causes must be considered. Papillitis is the form of optic neuritis most often seen in children. It is more often bilateral than unilateral; the two eyes may be affected simultaneously or sequentially. Primary considerations are parainfectious processes, Devic's neuromyelitis optica, MS, and occasionally toxic insults. Neuroretinitis, characterized by swelling of the disc(s) and retina, often with a prominent macular star, is usually associated with infection and parainfectious syndromes, although other causes have been reported. In many cases, no cause can be identified.

D. All forms of optic neuritis in children warrant thorough investigation. Neuroimaging, preferably gadolinium-enhanced MRI, is indicated to exclude a mass lesion or signs of increased intracranial pressure and to look for evidence of demyelinating disease, particularly MS. Examination by a pediatric neurologist to detect signs of multifocal or generalized neurologic disease is essential. Electrophysiologic tests, specifically electroencephalography, visual evoked potentials, brain stem auditory evoked potentials, and somatosensory evoked potentials, may be helpful. Examination of CSF for increased cells, protein, immunoglobulins, oligoclonal banding, and myelin basic protein may provide clues to parainfectious and demyelinating degenerative processes. Not to be overlooked is the importance of the general physical examination. A variety of systemic diseases including leukemia, diabetes, collagen vascular disorders, sarcoidosis, and local and disseminated infections must be excluded, and a number of tests including complete blood count, erythrocyte sedimentation rate, antinuclear antibodies, human leukocyte antigen, FTA-ABS, cultures and viral titers, and sinus and chest radiographs may be needed.

E. Of major concern is the possibility of MS. Incidence figures vary, but overall the risk for MS in a child with acute optic neuritis is relatively low. Possible indicators for MS include unilateral optic nerve involvement, female sex, presence of oligoclonal immunoglobulin and increased myelin basic protein in the CSF, and T-cell responsiveness to myelin antigens in the serum. Also to be considered is Devic's neuromyelitis optica (DNMO), a demyelinating disorder characterized by the association of optic neuritis, usually bilateral papillitis, and transverse myelitis. Some investigators have suggested that DNMO may be a form of MS. Rarely, other demyelinating disorders, such as Schilder's disease, may present with optic neuritis.

F. Of special importance is parainfectious optic neuritis. It may occur as a complication of rubeola, rubella, mumps, varicella, pertussis, mononucleosis, and other infectious diseases or as a complication of vaccination against measles, mumps, and rubella. It is usually characterized by bilateral papillitis with profound vision loss occurring 1 to 3 weeks following an illness or vaccination; rarely visual symptoms may precede other signs of infection. Accompanying neurologic signs are infrequent; in some cases there may be signs of coexistent encephalitis. CSF examination may show pleocytosis and increased protein. Spontaneous recovery within a matter of weeks is usual; in some cases there is residual optic atrophy and some degree of permanent visual loss. Parainfectious optic neuritis is thought to be an immunologically mediated demyelination process. Treatment with high-dose systemic corticosteroids may be of benefit in some cases.

Acute optic neuritis may also occur with direct infection of the optic nerve or retina, with infection of the paranasal sinuses, and with a host of systemic infections. Whenever possible, treatment with specific antimicrobial therapy should be instituted.

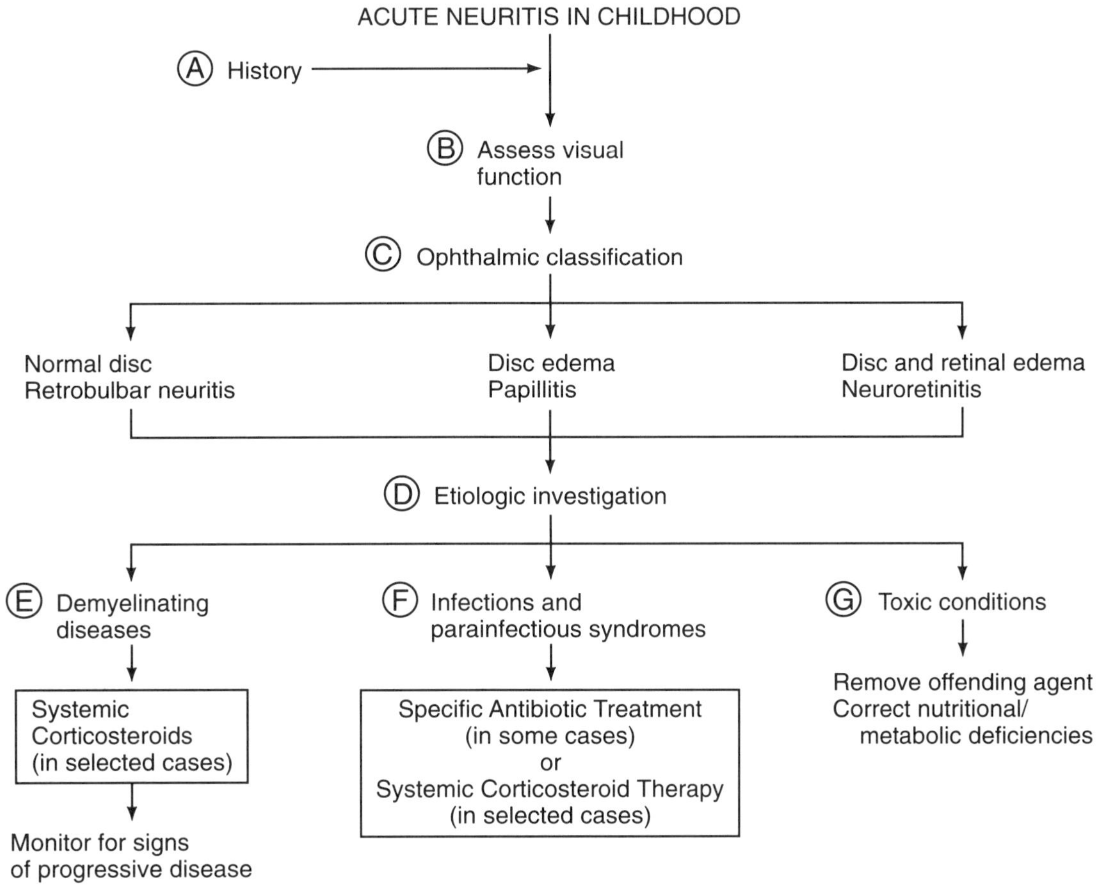

G. A number of drugs and toxins, physical agents, and certain nutritional deficiencies may cause indolent optic neuropathy characterized by progressive optic atrophy and loss of vision, but few produce the typical clinical picture of acute optic neuritis. Well documented is the acute optic neuritis, usually bilateral papillitis, that may occur in some patients on long-term, high-dose chloromycetin therapy. In most cases recovery occurs with prompt withdrawal of the drug; some patients are left with optic atrophy and permanent impairment of vision.

References

Farris BK, Pickard DJ. Bilateral postinfectious optic neuritis and intravenous steroid therapy in children. Ophthalmology 1990; 92:339.

Kriss A, Francis DA, Cuendet F. Recovery after optic neuritis in childhood. J Neurol Neurosurg Psychiatry 1988; 51:1253.

Taylor D. Optic neuropathies. In: Taylor D, ed. Pediatric ophthalmology. Boston: Blackwell Scientific, 1990:473.

Taylor D, Cuendet F. Optic neuritis in childhood. In: Hess RF, Plant GT, eds. Optic neuritis. Cambridge: Cambridge University Press, 1986:73.

Weiss AH, Beck RW. Neuroretinitis in childhood. J Pediatr Ophthalmol Strabismus 1989; 26:198.

PSEUDOTUMOR CEREBRI IN CHILDREN

Rosa Ana Tang, M.D.
Donna S. Burrows, M.D.

A. In a child who presents with headache, dizziness, blurred vision, diplopia, and particularly irritable behavior, the possibility of increased intracranial pressure must be immediately entertained. A history is obtained of the time, course of onset of symptoms, and prior medical conditions.

B. On examination the finding of bulging fontanels in the neonate (or younger child), visual loss, and/or associated cranial nerve palsies should prompt a detailed neurologic examination.

C. The confirmation of positive findings in the neurologic examination (i.e., papilledema (see p 50), cranial nerve palsies (see pp 100, 102, 104)) should direct further evaluation and treatment.

D. The finding of papilledema should prompt an urgent search for a structural lesion with increased intracranial pressure and/or compression of the brain stem. Neuroimaging (CT or MR scan of brain) is requested on an emergency basis to determine the presence of a mass lesion (see p 284).

E. If a mass lesion is present, immediate neurosurgical consultation is obtained.

F. If neuroimaging studies are negative, a lumbar puncture is in order to establish the diagnosis of increased intracranial pressure and exclude the possibility of meningitis or encephalitis.

G. If the only finding is increased intracranial pressure, with CSF chemistries, cultures, and cell cytology negative, a diagnosis of idiopathic intracranial hypertension may be entertained. Associated conditions such as cystic fibrosis, sinus thrombosis, and otitis media need to be searched for. A history of head trauma or ingestion of steroids or tetracycline needs to be specifically sought. If no associated condition is found, the term *idiopathic intracranial hypertension* or *pseudotumor cerebri* is applied as a diagnosis of exclusion. Measures to decrease the intracranial pressure and its effects on vision are instituted and can be medical (diuretics, steroids) or surgical (lumboperitoneal shunt, optic nerve sheath [ONS] fenestration) depending on the severity of the symptoms (headaches, visual loss).

H. Further evaluation of infectious or infiltrative causes includes the following laboratory studies to establish a specific diagnosis: complete blood count with a differential, sedimentation rate, rapid plasma reagin test, and specific infectious agent titers (ELISA, Lyme disease, TORCH). Additional studies are indicated by further specific findings.

I. Further evaluation of toxic or metabolic causes of papilledema includes laboratory studies such as blood and urine toxicology screens, SMA 20, and a CBC with differential. Results of these tests may indicate the need for additional studies.

References

Baker RS, Carter D, Hendrick EB, Buncic JR. Visual loss in pseudotumor cerebri of childhood, a follow-up study. Arch Ophthalmol 1985; 103:1881.

Couch R, Camfield PR, Tibbles JAR. The changing picture of pseudotumor cerebri in childrèn. Can J Neurol Sci 1985; 12:48.

Szenasy J, Paraicz E. Benign intracranial hypertension of uncertain origin. Acta Pediatr Hung 1979; 20:285.

Wall M. Idiopathic intracranial hypertension. Neurol Clin 1991; 90:73.

Welsberg LA, Chutorian AM. Pseudotumor cerebri of childhood. Am J Dis Child 1977; 31:1243.

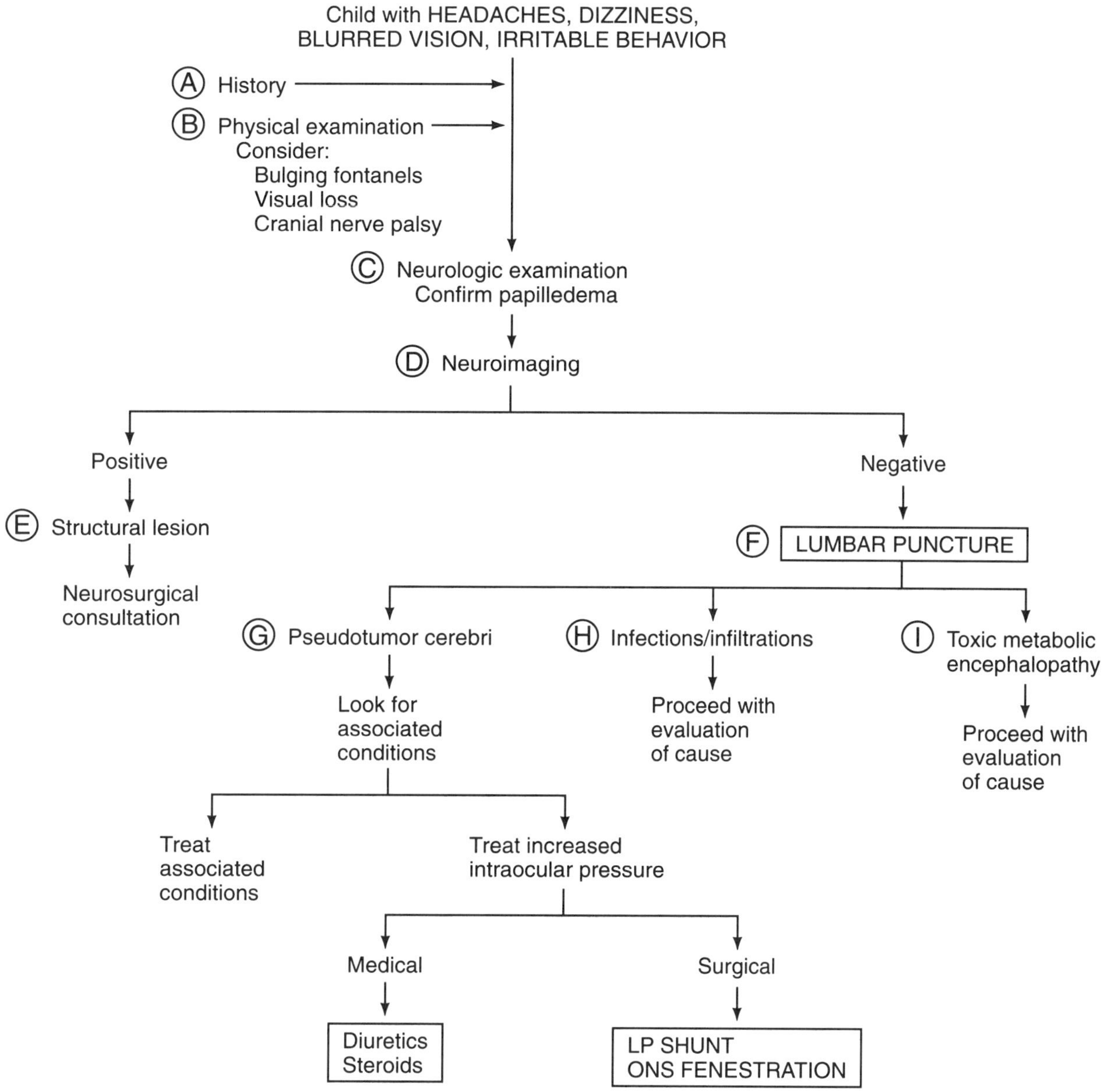
Child with HEADACHES, DIZZINESS,
BLURRED VISION, IRRITABLE BEHAVIOR
(A) History
(B) Physical examination
Consider:
Bulging fontanels
Visual loss
Cranial nerve palsy
(C) Neurologic examination
Confirm papilledema
(D) Neuroimaging
Positive
(E) Structural lesion
Neurosurgical consultation
Negative
(F) LUMBAR PUNCTURE
(G) Pseudotumor cerebri
Look for associated conditions
Treat associated conditions
Treat increased intraocular pressure
Medical
Diuretics
Steroids
Surgical
LP SHUNT
ONS FENESTRATION
(H) Infections/infiltrations
Proceed with evaluation of cause
(I) Toxic metabolic encephalopathy
Proceed with evaluation of cause

IRIDOCYCLITIS IN JUVENILE RHEUMATOID ARTHRITIS

Hamid Sajjadi, M.D.
William A. Godfrey, M.D.

A. Juvenile rheumatoid arthritis (JRA) is a relatively common chronic childhood inflammatory disease. It may represent a group of diseases with similar clinical characteristics and multiple causes. JRA has been divided into three clinical subsets: (1) polyarticular: most common (50%); in this subset, uveitis is uncommon (5% develop iridocyclitis); (2) pauciarticular: next in frequency (40%); in this subset iridocyclitis is very common (75 to 95% of all iridocyclitis that is associated with JRA); and (3) systemic onset (Still's disease): least common (10%); in this subset uveitis is rare (1%).

The pauciarticular type has two subgroups that are associated with a high incidence of iridocyclitis: (a) the classic antinuclear antibody (ANA)–positive group with chronic iridocyclitis and (b) the HLA-B27–positive group; the latter tends to follow a clinical course of acute recurrent episodes of iridocyclitis, as seen in the spondyloarthropathies. This includes juvenile-onset ankylosing spondylitis, Reiter's (reactive) arthritis, and other HLA-B27–associated disease that may present as JRA. In the more classic JRA with iridocyclitis and positive ANA, patients frequently do not recall history of joint involvement. When such involvement is present, the knee is most commonly affected. The iridocyclitis may be insidious with few symptoms, and patients may be found to have asymptomatic posterior synechiae and cataracts. Disease is usually bilateral and has characteristics of a chronic nongranulomatous inflammation. Vitreous cells are usually present. Underlying mechanisms remain obscure.

B. Initial laboratory evaluation may include antinuclear antibodies, erythrocyte sedimentation rate, HLA-B27, rheumatoid factor, and radiography of appropriate joints. An evaluation can best be carried out by a pediatric rheumatologist. ANA is positive in 88% of JRA with uveitis. Rheumatoid factor–positive juvenile-onset rheumatoid arthritis with iridocyclitis is very rare. Radiographs of the joints may reveal minor changes not clinically evident. Patients with pauciarticular disease, positive ANA, and no iridocyclitis should have a slit-lamp examination every 3 to 4 months. When iridocyclitis has been present but is quiet, examinations are suggested every 1 to 3 months. Children with polyarticular disease and negative ANA who have no ocular inflammation should be examined yearly. Specialty laboratory work-up in cases of difficult diagnosis could include evaluation for HLA-DR5, HLA-DR8, and HLA-DPW2, but their clinical significance and diagnostic interpretations are complex.

C. Differential diagnosis is outlined in Table 1. When pauciarticular joint disease, positive ANA, posterior synechiae, cataract, and band keratopathy are present, diagnosis is easily established. In less clear situations, an additional diagnosis to consider may be sarcoidosis. Skin lesions, chest radiographic findings, high angiotensive converting enzyme levels, and positive serum lysozymes may help confirm a diagnosis of sarcoidosis. Pars planitis usually has a pars plana membrane but may be confused with the iridocyclitis seen with JRA. A pediatric rheumatologist is helpful in clarifying systemic involvements.

D. Treatment of the iridocyclitis includes the following:
   1. Cycloplegia/mydriasis is useful in acute phases to prevent posterior synechiae. Frequency of use may be decreased as inflammation subsides, but maintenance with a dose at bedtime on a chronic basis may be needed. Obviously patients require near vision spectacles or bifocals owing to prolonged cycloplegia, but this is often neglected.
   2. Nonsteroidal anti-inflammatory drugs (NSAIDs) may be used on a chronic basis to decrease the need for oral corticosteroids. Naproxen has been used in childhood arthritis. It is available in suspension form for use in twice-daily dosage. Alternatively, tolmetin may be used if no contraindication exists. Switching NSAIDs may show a change in response. Reye's syndrome with aspirin and fatal hepatotoxicity with indomethacin in children have been reported. Long-term NSAID treatment may lessen chances of cystoid macular edema (CME) in postoperative lensectomy/vitrectomy cases.
   3. Corticosteroids: (a) Topical: Prednisone acetate 1% is used as needed up to every hour in acute cases and rapidly tapered according to response. (b) Systemic: Oral prednisone may be necessary in dosages as clinically indicated. This is best done under the observation of a pediatric rheumatologist. (c) Periodic retroseptal or subtenons corticosteroids should be considered before the use of systemic steroids in the older child who can tolerate these without systemic anesthesia.
   4. If significant inflammation persists despite maximally tolerated topical and systemic steroid use, antimetabolite drugs should be considered in consultation with a pediatric rheumatologist.

E. Chronic inflammation and peripheral anterior synechiae (PAS) formation may lead to secondary glaucoma. If medical management is unsuccessful, a filtering procedure may be necessary. Glaucoma specialist consultation may be indicated because the glaucoma in these patients is sometimes very difficult to manage.

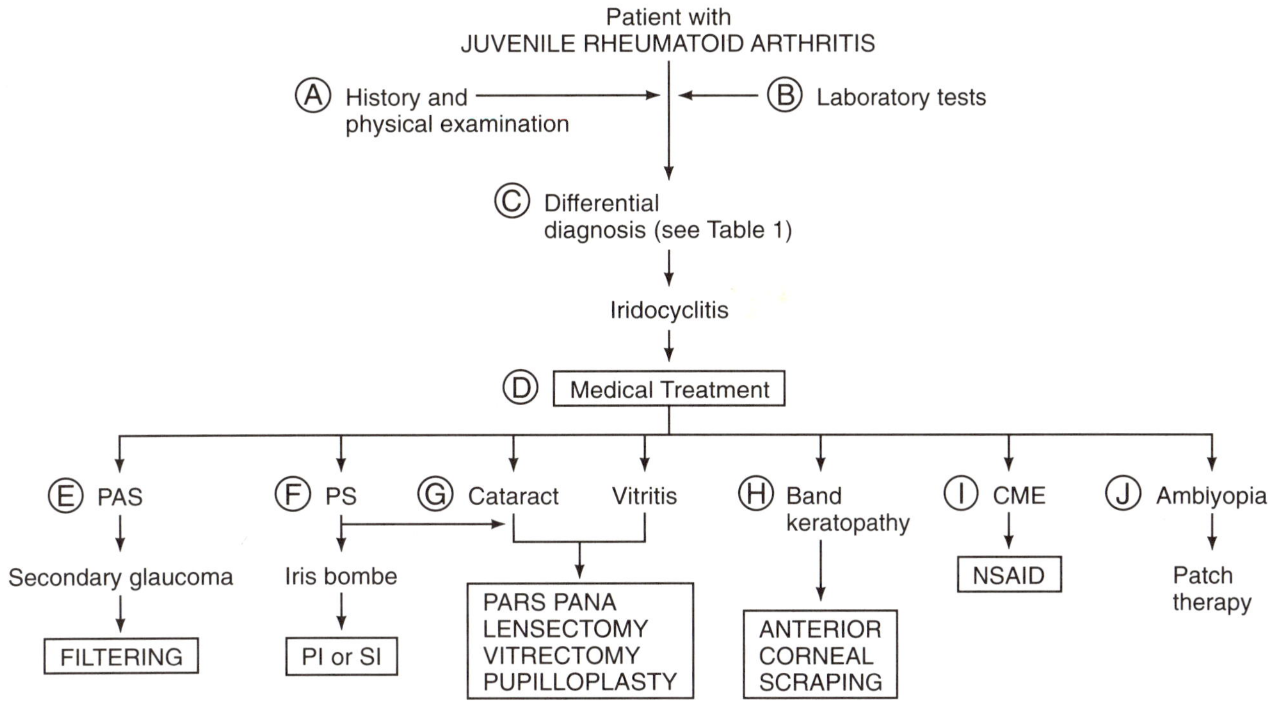

F. A certain number of JRA patients form extensive posterior synechiae (PS), despite adequate mydriatic and cycloplegic therapy. If the patient presents with iris bombe, an iridectomy may be indicated. Despite ease of YAG iridotomy, some surgeons still prefer a surgical sector or peripheral iridectomy. YAG laser iridotomy usually induces more inflammation, and closure of iridotomy is common.

G. When cataract surgery becomes necessary, pars plana pupilloplasty, lensectomy, membranectomy, and near-total vitrectomy, if carried out uneventfully, seem to produce the least long-term problems. Many complications were associated with the classic needle aspiration of cataracts or extracapsular cataract extractions. The pars plana approach offers advantages over an anterior approach in that hemorrhage is more easily controlled in a closed system and a better removal of vitreous debris, including cyclitic membrane, results in less postoperative residual inflammation. The chances of secondary membrane formation are reduced compared with an anterior approach to lensectomy/vitrectomy. Better drug penetration after a near-total vitrectomy may allow lowering of drug dosage.

H. Band keratopathy can be both a cosmetic and symptomatic problem. Although treatment with either EDTA-assisted or simple superficial scraping with a No. 15 BP blade is effective, recurrences are frequent in severe cases.

I. Cystoid macular edema may occur in the chronic severe cases, especially postoperatively. NSAIDs may have some beneficial prophylactic and therapeutic role. More severe inflammation may benefit from NSAIDs for longer periods.

J. The resultant amblyopia from the preoperative optical axis opacity or inappropriate refractive correction is often overlooked after surgery with a clear media. Even in the presence of partial optical axis opacities (e.g., band keratopathy, vitreous debris) or CME, amblyopia is often present and patients benefit from treatment.

TABLE 1 Differential Diagnosis of Nontraumatic Chronic Anterior Uveitis in Children

More common
Juvenile rheumatoid arthritis (JRA)
Ankylosing spondylitis (presents as a type of JRA)
Less common
Sarcoidosis
Herpes simplex keratouveitis
Pars planitis (usually does not form posterior synechiae)
Rare
Psoriatic arthritis
Behçet disease
Vogt-Koyanagi-Harada syndrome
Tuberculosis
Fuchs heterochromic iridocyclitis (usually does not form posterior synechiae)

References

Brostoff J, Scadding GK, Male D, Roitt I. Clinical immunology. London: Gower Medical Publishing, 1991.

Godfrey WA. Chronic iridocyclitis. In: Duane TD. Clinical ophthalmology. Philadelphia: Harper & Row; 1991.

Kanski JJ. Juvenile arthritis and uveitis. Surv Ophthalmol 1990; 34:253.

Olson NY, Lindsely LB, Godfrey WA. Nonsteroidal antiinflammatory drug therapy in chronic childhood iridocyclitis. Am J Dis Child 1988; 142:1259.

Rosenbery AM. Uveitis associated with juvenile rheumatoid arthritis. Semin Arthritis Rheum 1987; 16:158.

RETINOPATHIES AND NYCTALOPIA

Thomas B. Connor, Jr., M.D.
Elias I. Traboulsi, M.D.

A. Difficulty or inability to see at night (nyctalopia) may be a presenting symptom in a number of ocular and systemic conditions. In a child, clues to the presence of nyctalopia are difficulty navigating in unfamiliar, dark places such as movie theaters, inability to see the stars in the sky, or a need to leave lights on at home during the night. Because many of the disorders featuring nyctalopia are genetic, questions about similarly afflicted family members may prove helpful. The two most useful pieces of data in the assessment of the child with nyctalopia are (1) the child's general health and developmental profile and (2) the ophthalmoscopic appearance of the ocular fundus. This last piece of information may narrow the investigation considerably, sometimes clinching the diagnosis. For example, although very uncommon, the Mizuo phenomenon, a fundus color change of yellow-green sheen in a light-adapted patient, is diagnostic of the Oguchi disease in a nyctalopic patient. In evaluating the patient with night blindness, it is the ophthalmologist's responsibility to identify treatable conditions, monitor for potential associated problems, and counsel the patient and family on genetic issues and prognosis.

B. Congenital stationary night blindness (CSNB) is the most common hereditary, nonprogressive retinal dystrophy associated with nyctalopia. Visual acuity varies from normal to less than 20/200. There are several varieties of CSNB. Two types are associated with normal fundi and are differentiated into type I and type II depending on electroretino-graphic (ERG) and electro-oculographic (EOG) findings; type III is associated with high myopia, nystagmus, and low vision.

C. ERG and EOG are frequently abnormal in patients with nyctalopia. Patterns of abnormalities help support or exclude various diagnoses in the evaluation.

D. It is unusual to find a normal ERG and EOG in a healthy child with good vision, a normal-appearing fundus, and nyctalopia. Dark adaptometry may be needed to confirm or refute the presence of nyctalopia. Dark adaptometry is a psychophysical test of the ability of photoreceptors to increase their sensitivity in the dark.

E. Vitamin A deficiency may be the most important cause of nyctalopia to detect because it can be associated with other systemic problems, and it is a treatable disorder. Conjunctival and corneal changes such as Bitot spots and xerosis as well as flecked retinal appearance may be present but are not necessary to make the diagnosis of vitamin A deficiency–associated retinal dystrophy. Dietary deficiency as well as disorders of fat metabolism and intestinal absorption may be the cause. Such situations may be present in inflammatory bowel disease, celiac disease, cystic fibrosis, intestinal bypass surgery, malnutrition, and eating disorders. Nyctalopia may even be the presenting symptom in these disorders. Serum vitamin A levels confirm the diagnosis. Vitamin A supplementation and co-ordinated care with the child's pediatrician and other physicians often leads to reversal of the nyctalopia and the ophthalmic findings.

F. Neurologic, developmental, or physical abnormalities often accompany fundus abnormalities in patients with systemic disease. Nyctalopia may coexist with the peripheral pigmentary fundus changes or may precede them. Early in the disease process, the fundus may appear normal.

G. The nyctalopic child may have an isolated, progressive retinal degeneration. Symptoms may predate typical fundus changes, in which case color vision and electrophysiologic testing are helpful in verifying the presence of an abnormality.

H. Ptosis, ophthalmoplegia, and Christmas-tree cataracts are the typical ocular findings in myotonic dystrophy, but a pigmentary retinopathy and a stellate pattern maculopathy may also be present and can rarely be associated with nyctalopia. The ERG is almost always abnormal, with reduced B-wave amplitude and reduced scotopic responses.

I. Characteristic peripheral chorioretinal islands of gyrate atrophy are striking. They are typically bordered by pigment clumps and display sharp, scalloped borders adjacent to normal retina. Hyperornithinemia results from a deficiency in ornithine aminotransferase. Pyridoxine supplementation and an arginine-free diet reduce serum ornithine levels and may halt the progression of the retinopathy.

J. Extraocular abnormalities that accompany peripheral retinopathies associated with systemic conditions are typically quite conspicuous. The ophthalmologist may play an important role in unifying the ocular findings with the systemic abnormalities by considering the diagnoses on the decision tree. Some of these disorders such as Kearns-Sayre syndrome may have systemic abnormalities such as cardiac conduction defects which are clinically silent on presentation.

K. Although Bassen-Kornzweig syndrome, or abetalipoproteinemia, may present with ptosis and strabismus, nyctalopia with a peripheral pigmentary retinopathy may bring patients with this disease to the attention of the ophthalmologist. Deficiency of the fat-soluble vitamins A and E results from the abetalipoproteinemia. Supplementation with both vitamins may improve retinal function.

Continued on page 218

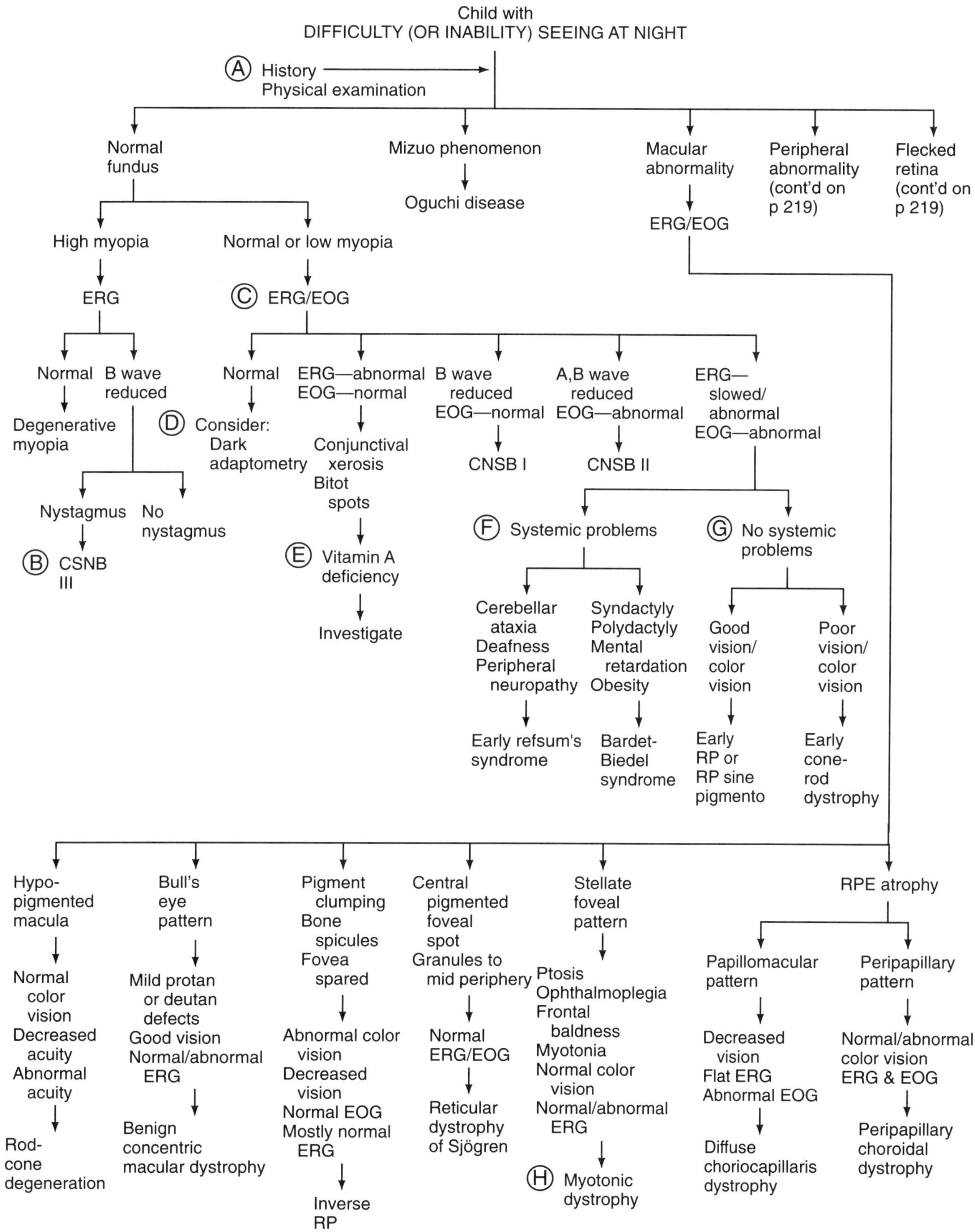
Child with
DIFFICULTY (OR INABILITY) SEEING AT NIGHT
(A) History
Physical examination
Normal fundus
Mizuo phenomenon
Oguchi disease
Macular abnormality
ERG/EOG
Peripheral abnormality (cont'd on p 219)
Flecked retina (cont'd on p 219)
High myopia
ERG
Normal
Degenerative myopia
B wave reduced
Nystagmus
(B) CSNB III
No nystagmus
Normal or low myopia
(C) ERG/EOG
Normal
(D) Consider: Dark adaptometry
ERG—abnormal EOG—normal
Conjunctival xerosis
Bitot spots
(E) Vitamin A deficiency
Investigate
B wave reduced EOG—normal
CNSB I
A,B wave reduced EOG—abnormal
CNSB II
ERG—slowed/abnormal EOG—abnormal
(F) Systemic problems
Cerebellar ataxia
Deafness
Peripheral neuropathy
Early refsum's syndrome
Syndactyly
Polydactyly
Mental retardation
Obesity
Bardet-Biedel syndrome
(G) No systemic problems
Good vision/color vision
Early RP or RP sine pigmento
Poor vision/color vision
Early cone-rod dystrophy
Hypo-pigmented macula
Normal color vision
Decreased acuity
Abnormal acuity
Rod-cone degeneration
Bull's eye pattern
Mild protan or deutan defects
Good vision
Normal/abnormal ERG
Benign concentric macular dystrophy
Pigment clumping
Bone spicules
Fovea spared
Abnormal color vision
Decreased vision
Normal EOG
Mostly normal ERG
Inverse RP
Central pigmented foveal spot
Granules to mid periphery
Normal ERG/EOG
Reticular dystrophy of Sjögren
Stellate foveal pattern
Ptosis
Ophthalmoplegia
Frontal baldness
Myotonia
Normal color vision
Normal/abnormal ERG
(H) Myotonic dystrophy
RPE atrophy
Papillomacular pattern
Decreased vision
Flat ERG
Abnormal EOG
Diffuse choriocapillaris dystrophy
Peripapillary pattern
Normal/abnormal color vision
ERG & EOG
Peripapillary choroidal dystrophy

L. The accumulation of phenothiazine derivatives in the retinal pigment epithelium (RPE) is responsible for the granular and pigmentary fundus changes as well as the nyctalopia of phenothiazine retinopathy. The chief offending agent has been Mellaril (thioridazine), and this toxic retinopathy has been reported after as little as 1 to 3 months of therapy. Prognosis is excellent if the medication is discontinued early in the course of the disorder.

M. Panophthalmic findings may be present in metallosis bulbi, primarily pigment changes from metal deposition and secondary inflammation. Chalcosis secondary to a retained intraocular copper foreign body may yield corneal pigmentation, hypopyon, and a sunflower cataract; siderosis secondary to intraocular iron may yield rust spots on the iris, cornea, or lens as well as a pigmentary retinopathy. A history of penetrating ocular injury as well as signs of occult trauma should be explored in evaluating the child with nyctalopia.

N. Goldmann-Favre vitreoretinal dystrophy displays a pigmentary peripheral retinopathy or opaque, dendritic vessels and retinoschisis. It is an autosomal recessive disorder associated with preretinal membranes, posterior vitreous separation, and posterior subcapsular cataracts. The incidence of retinal detachments may be increased.

O. Retinitis pigmentosa (RP) is the most common cause of progressive nyctalopia. It comprises a group of progressive pigmentary retinopathies initially subclassified according to mode of inheritance and pattern of pigmentary changes. Autosomal dominant RP is now classified according to the type of mutation in the rhodopsin or other affected genes. Symptoms may predate fundus changes, and associated cystoid macular edema and cataract may contribute to visual loss. Useful vision is usually preserved until late in the course of the disease.

References

Berson EL. Retinitis pigmentosa and allied diseases: Applications of electroretinographic testing. Int Ophthalmol 1981; 4:7.

Carr RE. The night blinding disorders. Int Ophthalmol Clin 1969; 9:971.

Drack AV, Traboulsi EI. Systemic associations of pigmentary retinopathy. Int Ophthalmol Clin 1991; 35.

Gans M, Taylor C. Reversal of progressive nyctalopia in a patient with Crohn's disease. Can J Ophthalmol 1990; 25:156.

Jiminez-Sierra JM, Ogden TE, Van Boemel GB. Inherited retinal diseases. St Louis: CV Mosby, 1989.

Neugebauer MA, Vernon SA, Brimlow G, et al. Nyctalopia and conjunctival xerosis indicating vitamin A deficiency in cystic fibrosis. Eye 1989; 3:360.

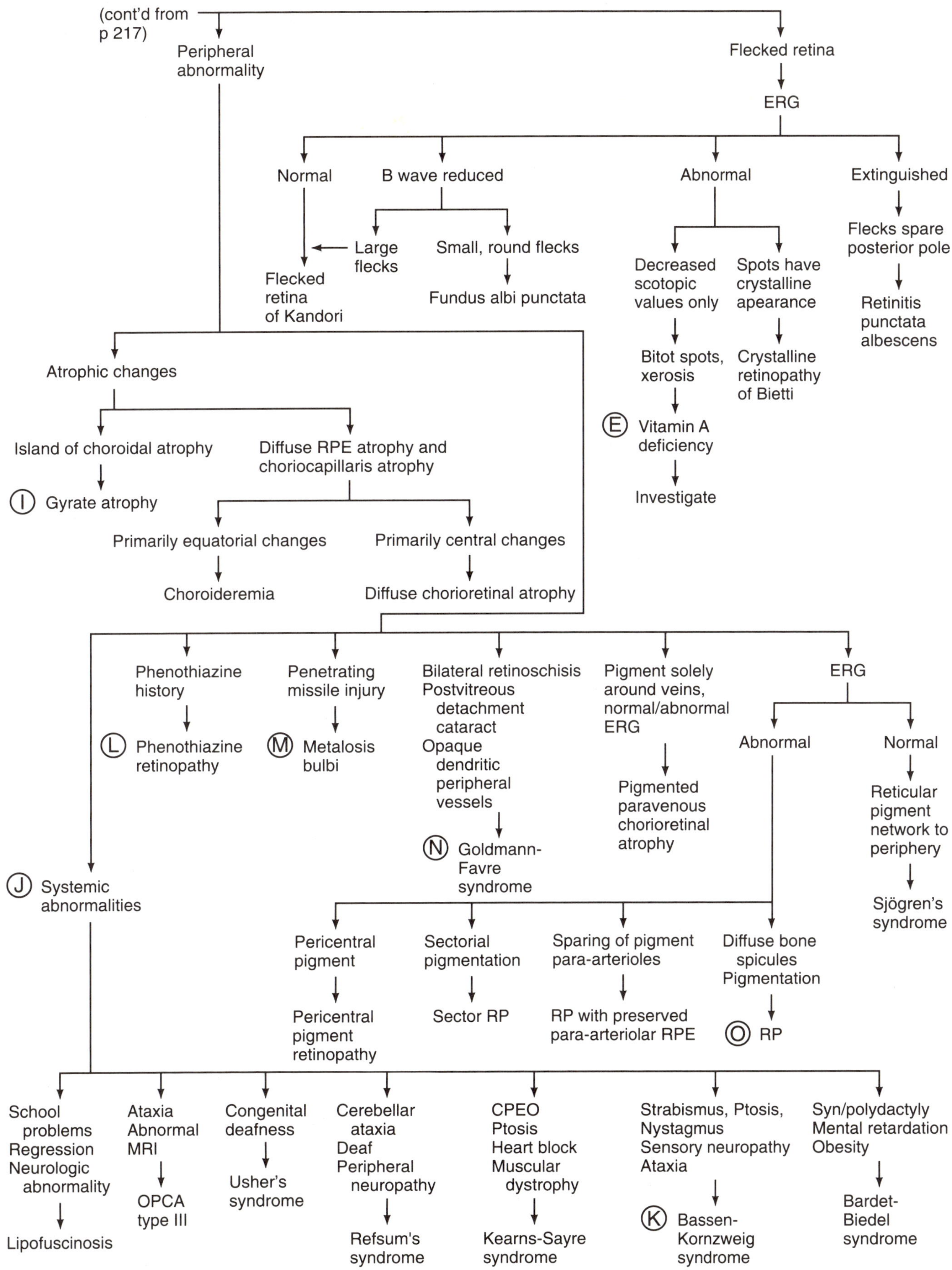
(cont'd from p 217)
Peripheral abnormality
Flecked retina
ERG
Normal
B wave reduced
Abnormal
Extinguished
Large flecks
Small, round flecks
Flecked retina of Kandori
Fundus albi punctata
Decreased scotopic values only
Spots have crystalline apearance
Flecks spare posterior pole
Bitot spots, xerosis
Crystalline retinopathy of Bietti
Retinitis punctata albescens
E Vitamin A deficiency
Investigate
Atrophic changes
Island of choroidal atrophy
Diffuse RPE atrophy and choriocapillaris atrophy
I Gyrate atrophy
Primarily equatorial changes
Primarily central changes
Choroideremia
Diffuse chorioretinal atrophy
Phenothiazine history
Penetrating missile injury
Bilateral retinoschisis
Postvitreous detachment cataract
Opaque dendritic peripheral vessels
Pigment solely around veins, normal/abnormal ERG
ERG
L Phenothiazine retinopathy
M Metalosis bulbi
N Goldmann-Favre syndrome
Pigmented paravenous chorioretinal atrophy
Abnormal
Normal
Reticular pigment network to periphery
Sjögren's syndrome
J Systemic abnormalities
Pericentral pigment
Sectorial pigmentation
Sparing of pigment para-arterioles
Diffuse bone spicules Pigmentation
Pericentral pigment retinopathy
Sector RP
RP with preserved para-arteriolar RPE
O RP
School problems
Regression
Neurologic abnormality
Lipofuscinosis
Ataxia
Abnormal MRI
OPCA type III
Congenital deafness
Usher's syndrome
Cerebellar ataxia
Deaf
Peripheral neuropathy
Refsum's syndrome
CPEO
Ptosis
Heart block
Muscular dystrophy
Kearns-Sayre syndrome
Strabismus, Ptosis,
Nystagmus
Sensory neuropathy
Ataxia
K Bassen-Kornzweig syndrome
Syn/polydactyly
Mental retardation
Obesity
Bardet-Biedel syndrome

ANTERIOR AND INTERMEDIATE UVEITIS

Conrad L. Giles, M.D.

A. Childhood anterior uveitis without history of trauma is relatively rare. Trauma history is usually clear-cut and the necessary treatment of short duration, constituting the usual standard nonspecific anti-inflammatory measures. Absence of such history requires a diagnostic program. Intensity of the program depends on the response of the patient's inflammatory disease. Anterior segment flare and cells in older age groups can be the result of noninflammatory disorders such as vascular insufficiency, but most inflammatory signs in the anterior segment represent a true inflammatory state. Careful daylight examination of iris color makes certain that no difference exists between the two eyes, important in ruling out the presence of Fuchs' heterochromic iridocyclitis. A lighter iris in the inflamed eye associated with characteristic lattice keratitic precipitates eliminates the need for additional diagnostic studies. Careful examination of the cornea for lesions causing keratouveitis is important.

B. Depending on severity of the inflammation, corticosteroid therapy includes local prednisolone acetate 1% drops given as frequently as every 30 minutes. Initial dilatation should be accomplished with 1% atropine, usually required no more frequently than every 6 hours. Attempts to break synechiae early in the course of the illness should be vigorous and may necessitate a general anesthetic and subconjunctival injection of 1:1000 epinephrine in the affected quadrants.

C. Prompt resolution of inflammatory episodes occurs frequently. Although a healthy youngster may have some underlying causative factor, the single most important asymptomatic disease is juvenile rheumatoid arthritis (JRA). Therefore, antinuclear factor (ANF) should be obtained. Pauciarticular (four or fewer joints involved at onset of the disease) ANF-positive disease identifies youngsters most at risk for developing relatively asymptomatic anterior uveal disease. This is especially true in girls under age 10. ANF-positive patients require rheumatology consultation and follow-up every 3 months. If the test is negative, the youngster, once tapered from steroids and mydriatic agents, should be examined in 3 months and then re-examined only as necessary.

D. Often, a specific diagnosis is suggested during the initial history. Systemic disorders already present in the youngster at the time of the episode which fit into this category include juvenile diabetes, Kawasaki disease, childhood exanthems, and regional enteritis. Presence of smoldering disease, unresponsive to therapy, demands further evaluation to elucidate other diagnostic possibilities. Even though associated disorders may little alter the use of the nonspecific anti-inflammatory agents in diseases of unknown origin, a vigorous attempt should be made to identify possible associated disorders. Their diagnosis aids in predicting the course of the illness and more importantly, the possibility of adding therapeutic agents to the nonspecific regimen. The pediatrician should be at the center of this evaluation. With a general physical examination, several serologic and radiographic studies should be considered, including the antinuclear antibody, serum lysozyme, FTA-ABS, HLA, and ELISA studies for Lyme disease. Radiographic studies should include chest and sacroiliac spine and a gastrointestinal series. Skin tests should include a tuberculin and a Kveim test. When abnormal physical findings point to a specific cause, confirmatory laboratory studies only are necessary. When a specific cause is defined (tuberculosis, syphilis, Lyme disease), specific therapy should be started.

E. Intermediate uveitis (IU) in children is a relatively rare, chronic inflammation of unknown cause primarily involving retinal vessels and the peripheral portions of the retina and uveal tract. Usual findings are peripheral retinal vasculitis, anterior vitreous cellular response, and vitreous exudation, with varying amounts of snowbanking. Band keratopathy, posterior subcapsular cataract, optic neuritis (papillitis), significant cystoid macular edema, and vitreous hemorrhage are common. The nature of IU demands that therapy occur simultaneously with evaluation. IU syndrome, while identifying anatomic location for the inflammation, can be broken into three etiologic categories: classic pars planitis syndrome, sarcoidosis, and Lyme disease. Pars planitis, the most common, has no defined cause or associated disorder and is characterized by neovascularization, vitreous hemorrhage, and retinal detachment. The other entities associated with the intermediate segment of the uveal tract—"senile" vitritis, multiple sclerosis, Whipple's disease, and reticulum cell sarcoma—are rarely associated with IU in children. Radiographic studies should be directed toward identification of chest pathology to rule out sarcoidosis. Serologic studies should include the ELISA study for *Borrelia* to rule out Lyme disease and measurement of serum lysozyme in younger children or angiotensin-converting enzyme in older children to rule out sarcoidosis.

F. Local corticosteroids are used only when vision is 20/40 or better and significant anterior chamber (AC) reaction is present. Minimal anterior chamber reaction and vision of 20/40 or better require no treatment. When the vision is less than 20/40 and subretinal exudation, optic nerve papillitis, or disturbing floaters are found, periocular steroids are given weekly (up to six doses) until improvement occurs. If improvement stops and the signs triggering the intervention are not eliminated, reinjection continues until six weekly injections fail to achieve the desired result. Retinal cryopexy should then be applied if steroids fail to produce clinical improvement. Should cryopexy fail

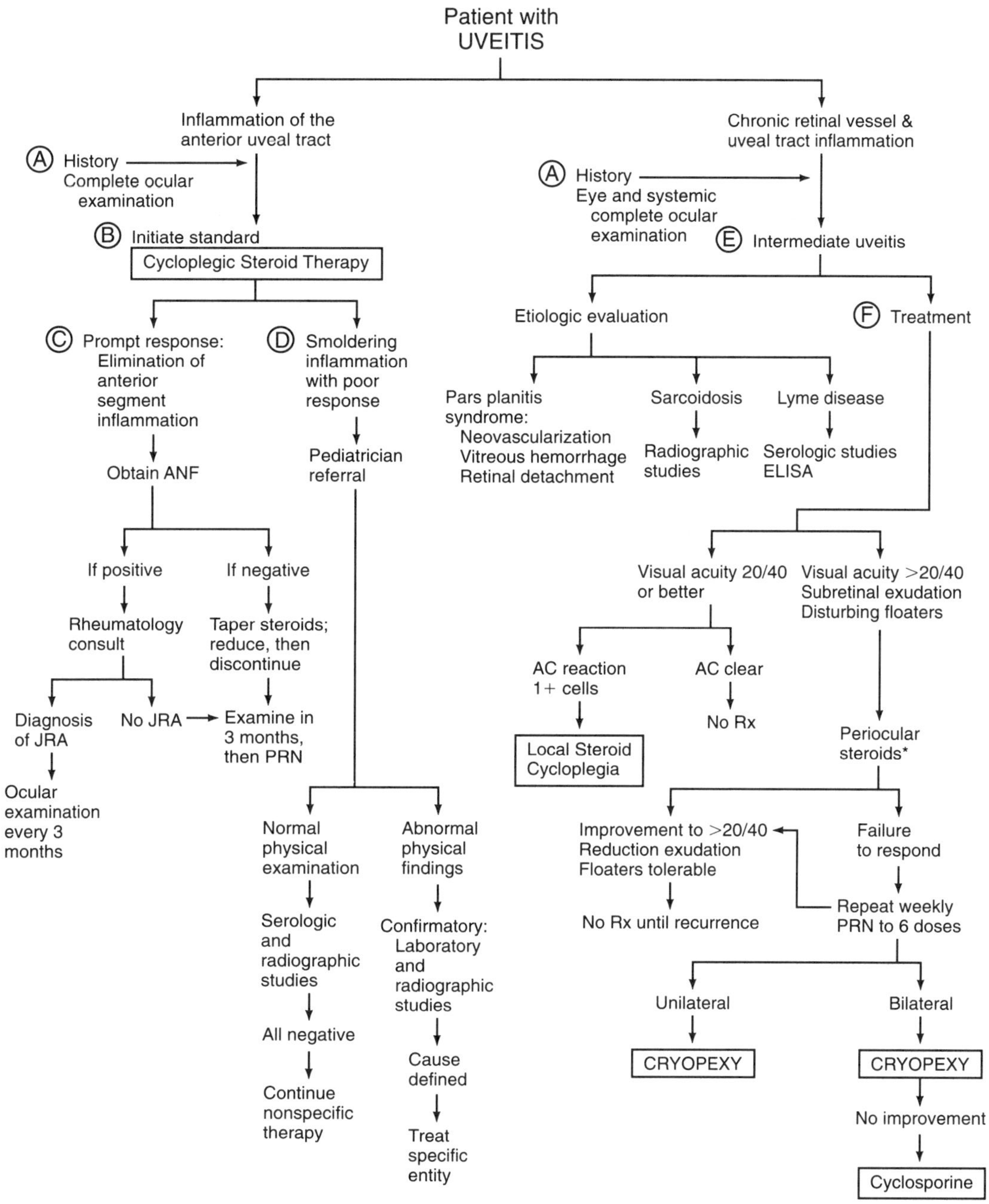

as well and if the disease is bilateral, cyclosporine should then be used. Because of their potential long-term side effects, cyclosporine or other immunosuppressive agents are reserved for bilateral disease.

*Editors' Note: The author of this chapter believes strongly that periocular steroids are the modality of choice. He anesthetizes the patients for each injection. Usually one injection is all that is needed, with repeats months to years apart. He does so because of the severe systemic side effects he has seen from oral steroids. The editors have a different experience based on different patient referrals. Our experience is less with chronic complicated patients and more with newly diagnosed cases. Two to 6 weeks of high-dose (80 mg/day) oral steroids is usually adequate to bring control. Side effects are rare unless frequent re-treatment is needed. Then periocular administration is considered.

References

Aaberg T. The enigma of pars planitis. Am J Ophthalmol 1987; 103:828.

Giles CL. Pediatric intermediate uveitis. J Pediatr Ophthalmol Strabismus 1989; 26:136.

Giles CL. Uveitis in childhood—Part I & Part II intermediate. Ann Ophthalmol 1989; 21:13.

Hoover DL, Khan JA, Giangiacomo J. Pediatric ocular sarcoidosis. Surv Ophthalmol 1986; 30:215.

Kanske JJ. Anterior uveitis in JRA. Arch Ophthalmol 1977; 95:1794.

Knaske JJ, Shun-Shun GA. Systemic uveitis syndromes in childhood—an analysis of 340 cases. Ophthalmology 1984; 91:1247.

O'Connor GR. Doyne lecture: heterochromic iridocyclitis. Trans Ophthalmol Soc UK 1985; 104:219.

POSTERIOR POLE INFLAMMATORY DISEASE

Conrad L. Giles, M.D.

A. The presence of posterior pole inflammatory disease in children poses a significant diagnostic dilemma because of the number of agents that can produce such an inflammation. The anatomic location of the inflammation (choroid versus retinal versus vascular), the extent of the inflammatory focus (focal versus diffuse), and the degree of exudation give the clinician an excellent starting point in attempting to define the cause. The fundus picture enables the ophthalmologist to limit the necessary studies rather than take a "shot-gun" approach to diagnostic evaluation.

Two additional entities that do not lend themselves well to the accompanying chart should be mentioned briefly. Rubella retinitis is the most common ocular feature of the maternal rubella syndrome, being present in 25% to 50% of infants. Unilateral or bilateral pigment deposits, usually limited to the posterior pole, vary from fine, powdery, or granular to more discrete shapes. The retinopathy is benign and nonprogressive and does not interfere with vision unless neovascularization occurs in the macula. Posterior uveitis without vitreous reaction of a mild, degenerative, speckled character is the most striking ocular manifestation of subacute sclerosing panencephalitis (SSP), which is believed to be due to the myxovirus of rubella. SSP occurs most commonly in school-aged children and is marked by changes in behavior and intellectual deterioration.

B. Focal exudative retinitis is most commonly associated with seropositive toxoplasmosis. This lesion is seen usually in association with a healed lesion and sometimes is associated with a vasculitis. The characteristic clinical picture, involving the macular or paramacular areas or the optic nerve and associated with positive serology, calls for anti-*Toxoplasma* therapy with pyrimethamine, sulfadiazine, steroids, and clindamycin. A negative test in patients with this clinical picture dictates the use of steroids alone in treatment.

Peripheral lesions may be observed without treatment. When scarring is not seen in focal exudative retinitis and the lesion has a white moundlike appearance, vitreous biopsy frequently reveals *Candida*. Specific systemic and intravitreal antifungal therapy is then required. Vitrectomy usually accompanies this therapy.

C. Central to the determination of the cause of diffuse exudative retinitis is the immunologic status of the patient. When there is compromise, attempts to isolate a viral agent may yield the viruses of herpes simplex or herpes zoster, HIV, or cytomegalovirus. Specific antiviral therapy can be undertaken. When there is no disturbance in the immunologic status of the patient, diffuse exudative retinitis is usually the result of acute retinal necrosis; vigorous therapy with intravenous acyclovir accompanied by vitrectomy and a 360-degree buckle may be indicated.

D. Diffuse choroiditis (and an associated panuveitis) accompanied by a history of ocular trauma or a prior history of enucleation following ocular trauma is frequently associated with sympathetic ophthalmia. This inflammation responds to the use of corticosteroid and immunosuppressive therapy. The presence of the same clinical picture without panuveitis or a history of trauma accompanied by a salt-and-pepper fundus and associated with diffuse chorioretinitis suggests syphilis. An FTA-ABS study for syphilis should be obtained and, if positive, penicillin therapy should be initiated.

The presence of an exudative retinal detachment, especially when accompanied with vitiligo, suggests the diagnosis of Vogt-Koyanagi-Harada syndrome. Treatment with steroids is indicated.

The classic picture seen in presumed ocular histoplasmosis syndrome (POHS) accompanied with vitreous cellular response suggests the possibility of sarcoidosis, tuberculosis, or syphilis. Appropriate laboratory studies to confirm these entities should be obtained.

E. Vasculitis can be divided into three components. When the vasculitis is primarily arteritic, toxoplasmosis or syphilis is the most likely underlying cause. Involvement of the veins with periphlebitis is most commonly seen in sarcoidosis. Appropriate studies to determine the presence or absence of sarcoid should then be obtained. Occlusive vasculitis accompanied by cotton wool spots with hemorrhages and exudate and associated with aphthous ulcers of the mouth and genitalia suggest Behçet's disease. Treatment with immunosuppressive and corticosteroid agents is indicated.

F. Nonexudative lesions may be primarily choroidal or retinal. POHS syndrome (choroidal in location) may require laser therapy for the hemorrhagic disciform maculopathy. When the nonexudative lesion is primarily retinal and a solitary granuloma is seen, the ELISA test for *Toxocara* should be done. If activity threatens the macula or substantial cellular debris accumulates as a result of this treatment, corticosteriods are indicated.

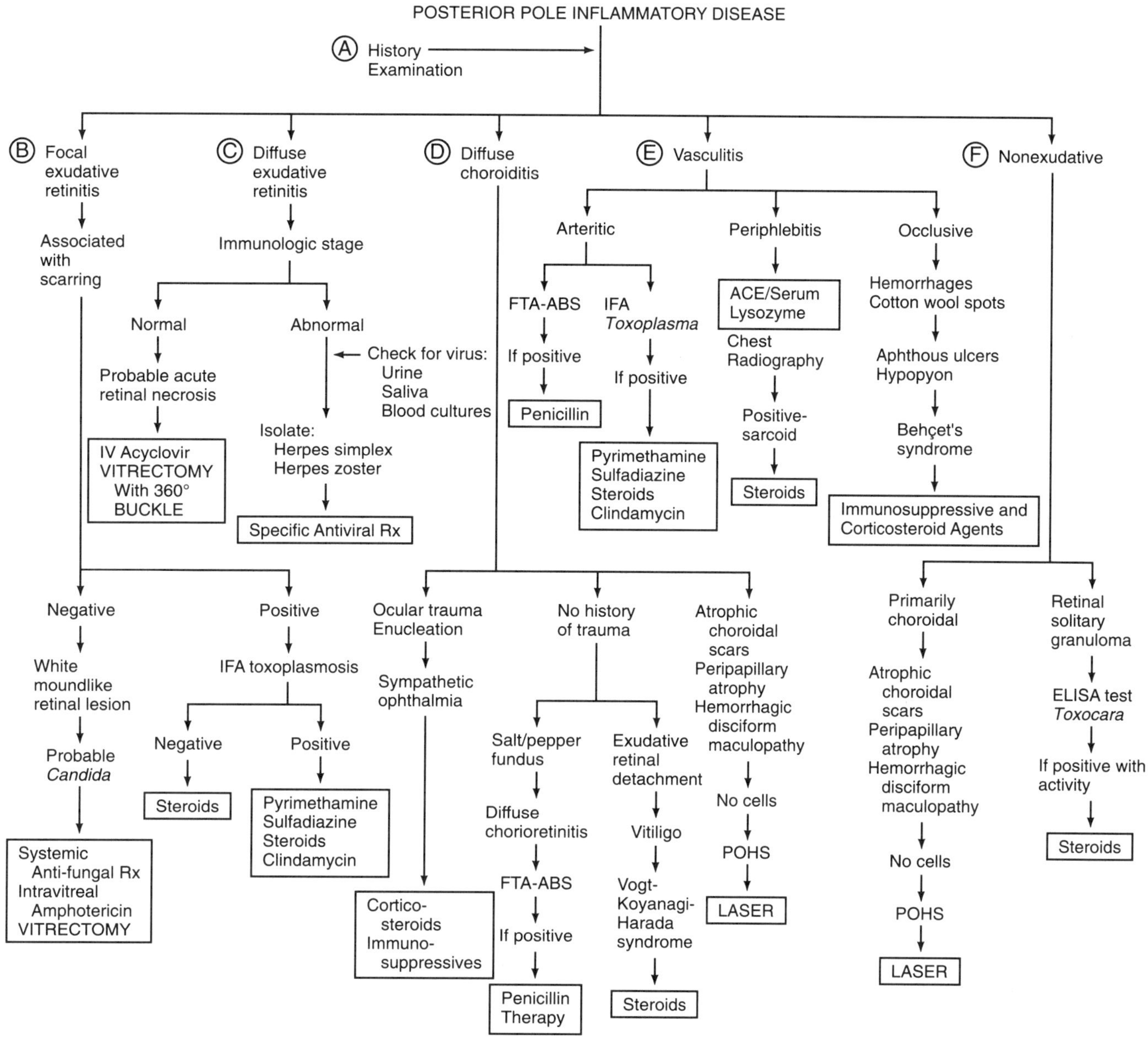

References

Day S. The uveal tract. In: Taylor D, ed. Pediatric ophthalmology. Boston: Blackwell, 1990:276.

Ellis GS, Pakalnes VA, Worley G, et al. *Toxocara canis* infestation: clinical and epidemiological associations with seropositivity in kindergarten children. Ophthalmology 1986; 93:1032.

Giles CL. Uveitis in childhood—Part III. Posterior. Ann Ophthalmol 1989; 21:23.

Lubin JR, Albert DM, Weinstein M. Sixty five years of sympathetic ophthalmia, a clinicopathologic review of 105 cases (1913–1978). Ophthalmology 1980; 87:109.

Noble S, Carr R. Disorders of the fundus; toxoplasma retinochoroiditis. Ophthalmology 1982; 89:1289.

ACQUIRED ESOTROPIA (NONPARETIC)

Andrea Cibis Tongue, M.D.

A. Acquired esotropia (ET) has an onset after 6 months of age. (ET that occurs before 6 months of age is generally referred to as infantile [congenital] [see p 70].) Clinically the most important feature to look for in acquired ET is evidence of abnormal eye movement and therefore incomitance of the deviation. The abnormal eye movement may be due to paresis or mechanical interference. Patients with an acquired ET with evidence of incomitance must have further evaluation to rule out orbital, intracranial, or neurologic disease (see pp 104, 230). Evaluation and treatment therefore depend primarily on clinical findings. Measurement of the deviation in cardinal directions of gaze and at distance and near with accommodative targets, as well as careful evaluation of ductions and versions, is imperative.

B. The most common type of acquired ET is accommodative ET. Usually patients are 2 to 3 years of age. The deviation is often intermittent at first and when measured with an accommodative target is greater at near than at distance. With a nonaccommodative target or if the patient is not making any accommodative effort, the ET may measure the same at distance and at near. Patients may be hyperopic, emmetropic, or myopic, hyperopia being much more common. High hyperopic patients may have a normal accommodative convergence (AC/A) ratio, and their ET can be controlled by distance correction only. With a high AC/A ratio, the refractive error may be normal or even myopic, although most patients are somewhat hyperopic. Correction of the distance refractive error may not eliminate the near ET and may, as in the case of myopia, even aggravate it. Near adds (bifocals) may be necessary for the control of the near ET.

C. Partially accommodative patients achieve only partial control of the ET with hyperopic correction and/or near add. Predisposing factors leading to this nonrefractive ET are unclear. Because most of these patients do not regain full stereopsis or binocularity even after surgery, some may have had pre-existing microtropia or cosmetically inapparent ET that subsequently, because of the uncorrected accommodative component, broke down and led to a larger angle of deviation. It is also not uncommon to observe an increase in the angle of deviation in children who undergo amblyopia treatment. In some this angle again decreases after the visual acuity is equalized and patching is stopped. In others it remains constant, requiring surgical intervention. Interruption of fusion can therefore lead to an increase in or the abrupt manifestation of ET.

Both accommodative and partially accommodative patients show a significant decrease in the magnitude of ET with their basic hyperopic correction or with the addition of bifocals. One need prescribe only the amount of plus near add necessary to control the ET. Empirically in children too young to test with appropriate accommodative targets at near, a +2.50 or +3.00 add is prescribed if the basic refractive correction does not eliminate the near ET. It is imperative, if a residual deviation for distance or near exists, that the child be re-refracted with cycloplegia and that the maximum plus correction be prescribed. Myopic patients should not be overcorrected. Adequate cycloplegic refractions are therefore necessary as part of the work-up of the patient with suspected accommodative or partially accommodative ET.

Myopic patients may show a worsening of the ET when corrected with the basic myopic correction, particularly if corrected with contact lenses, which increase accommodative effort (the opposite occurs with hyperopic contact lenses). Myopes with a high AC/A ratio may not become symptomatically esotropic until switched to a higher spectacle correction or from spectacles to contact lenses. Reading glasses may be required if they wish to continue wearing contact lenses. In some, the ET is controlled after a period of time of contact lens wear. Others benefit from orthoptic intervention, surgical correction, or return to spectacle correction.

D. The first line of treatment for accommodative or partially accommodative ET is optical. If that is not sufficient to achieve control of the deviation, surgery is advisable, particularly if fusion is deemed likely or possible. Patients with partially accommodative ET or with accommodative ET and high AC/A ratio *who have fusion capacity* require a greater amount of surgical correction than their nonfusion counterparts. Patients without fusion but with high AC/A ratios are more likely to become exotropic with time. They frequently manifest a small exotropia (XT) at distance and an acceptably small ET at near. The XT increases with time. The alignment of eyes can be totally manipulated by the amount of plus correction; i.e., less plus straightens the eyes, but eventually the XT increases and requires re-operation. Determining fusion capacity prior to surgery helps establish the amount of surgery needed. This can be done by prism adaptation or sensorimotor evaluation.

Small residual angles of deviation can be treated occasionally by prisms (risk of increasing deviation exists and patients should be monitored) or by orthoptics that can help wean patients from bifocals. An attempt should be made to wean all accommodative ET patients with fusion out of bifocals (those who do not have fusion do not need the bifocal). The plus add can be gradually decreased by +0.50 or +0.75 over a period of 3 to 4 years. A few patients having a high AC/A ratio and an abnormal accommodative amplitude require bifocals to control not only their accom-

Continued on page 226

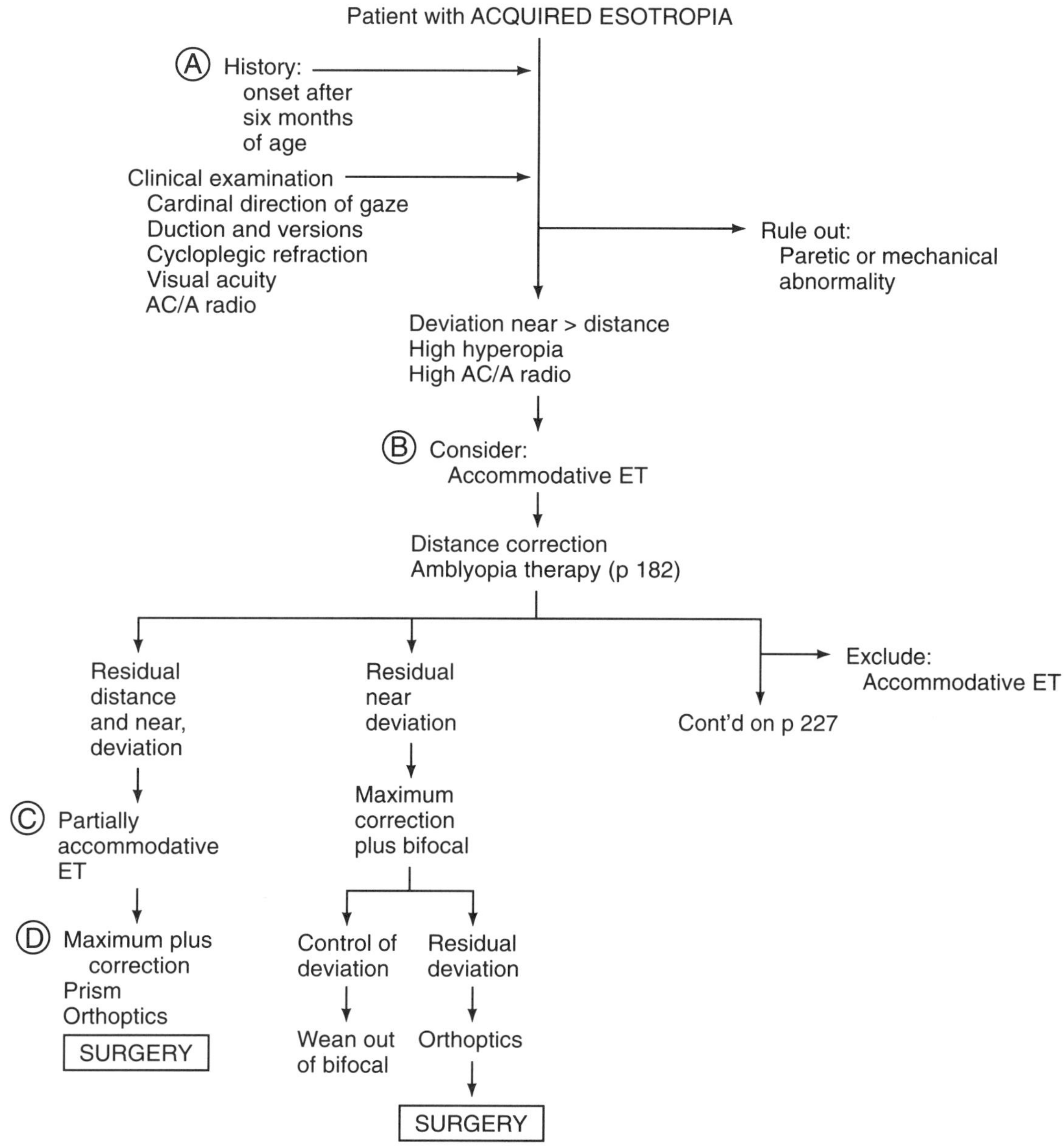
Patient with ACQUIRED ESOTROPIA
(A) History:
onset after six months of age
Clinical examination
Cardinal direction of gaze
Duction and versions
Cycloplegic refraction
Visual acuity
AC/A radio
Rule out:
Paretic or mechanical abnormality
Deviation near > distance
High hyperopia
High AC/A radio
(B) Consider:
Accommodative ET
Distance correction
Amblyopia therapy (p 182)
Residual distance and near, deviation
Residual near deviation
Exclude:
Accommodative ET
Cont'd on p 227
(C) Partially accommodative ET
Maximum correction plus bifocal
(D) Maximum plus correction
Prism
Orthoptics
SURGERY
Control of deviation
Residual deviation
Wean out of bifocal
Orthoptics
SURGERY

modative ET but also premature presbyopia. It is usually not possible to wean them from bifocals or reading glasses. For patients with normal accommodative amplitudes *and good sensory fusion* but an inability to forgo the bifocal add because of persistent ET, surgery is an option. Medial rectus recessions performed for the angle of deviation at near is usually successful. *Surgery is not indicated for a residual near deviation if the patient does not demonstrate good fusion,* because consecutive XT will almost assuredly occur.

E. A few patients have a comitant acquired ET without evidence of an abnormal AC/A or high hyperopia (5% of ET cases). With such patients there is a concern that the deviation may be due to a neurologic lesion, unless there is a history of pre-existing esophoria, microtropia, or amblyopia. In the absence of any symptoms of underlying neurologic problems, surgical correction is advisable. Acute, acquired, nonrefractive comitant ET of adulthood is referred to as Franceschetti ET.

F. Occlusion ET (sudden loss of or disturbance of vision in one eye, particularly patching of one eye) can occur in the myope, the emmetrope, or more commonly the hyperope. One should correct hyperopia of greater than +2.00 to +3.00 if full-time occlusion amblyopia treatment is undertaken.

Cyclic ET is variable, of sudden onset, and manifests on alternate days. With time it may become more constant. There is no evidence of paresis and on the days the patient is straight there may be no evidence of esophoria. Surgery is indicated for the manifest angle of deviation, even when performed at a time when the eyes are straight.

Patients with greater ET at distance than at near should be evaluated for sixth nerve weakness. Bielschowsky-type acute ET is very rare, occurring in myopes (usually women) who have a greater deviation at distance than at near and show abduction weakness. Cause is unknown.

Duane syndrome patients may develop a symptomatic ET. The angle may be incomitant, but features of Duane syndrome such as narrowing of the palpebral fissure on adduction and a history of longstanding abnormal eye movements is helpful in making the diagnosis.

Patients with A or V pattern ET may not be symptomatic early in life. Abnormal head positions may compensate for the deviation. When the child is sufficiently stressed or is unable to maintain the abnormal chin position (up for A patterns, down for V patterns), the ET may become apparent or the child may show signs of diplopia, closing one eye when reading (V pattern) or looking in the distance (A pattern). Measurement of the angle of deviation in all cardinal directions of gaze is therefore imperative.

G. Treatment of nonaccommodative acquired ET consists of correction of refractive errors and any other conditions adversely affecting acuity. Prisms and/or orthoptics are therapeutic possibilities for symptomatic patients with small angle deviations, although prism therapy may gradually increase the deviation. If prism therapy is no longer acceptable and the patient is symptomatic, surgery is advisable. Amblyopia should be treated prior to surgery. After amblyopia treatment, a rare patient may achieve control of the ET without surgery. However, the angle of deviation usually increases with amblyopia therapy. Surgery is indicated if the patient is symptomatic or if fusion is likely.

H. Acute, acquired, nonrefractive comitant ET in childhood is called acute-onset normosensorial ET. Young children may learn to suppress diplopia rapidly and therefore may not be symptomatic. Deferring surgery may lead to permanent loss of fusion capacity. Every attempt should be made to restore normal motor alignment quickly.

References

Lang J. Strabismus. Trans by GW Cibis. Thorofare, NJ: Slack, 1984.

Raab EL, Spierer A. Persisting accommodative esotropia. Arch Ophthalmol 1986; 104:1777.

Cont'd from p 225

(E) Nonaccommodative ET

- (F) Consider:
  - Franceschetti type
  - Occlusion ET
  - Cyclic ET
  - Bielschowski type
  - Breakdown of prior micro- or small-angle ET
  - Esophoria
  - A or V pattern
  - Duane syndrome
  - Adverse response to prism therapy
  - → (G) Eliminate obstacles to clear vision and fusion
    - Correct hyperopia
    - Prism for small angle
    - SURGERY (Includes Option of Oculinum Injection)
- Exclude:
  - Sixth nerve paresis esp. in Bielschowsky-type and Duane syndrome
- (H) Acute-onset normosensorial ET
  - Normal refractive error
  - Normal AC/A
  - Distance and near deviation equal
  - → Glasses
  - → RAPID SURGERY

EXODEVIATION

Michael E. Somers, M.D.

The management and treatment of exodeviations can often be frustrating for both clinician and patient. Whether the deviation is acquired or congenital, any sensory cause must first be corrected. This includes a refractive error (especially myopia and astigmatism), corneal opacity, cataract, or retinal problem. If this has been done and an exodeviation still exists, one must determine if there is a phoria, an intermittent exotropia, or a tropia. This is done through the cover/uncover test and the cross cover test. In addition, motility must be checked for the presence of A or V patterns. Deviations should be measured in both distance and near and the diagnostic positions of gaze.

A. In the acquired form, if a phoria manifests, the patient can be followed. A symptomatic intermittent exotropia can be treated with base-in prism. If symptoms remain despite the prism or if there is a tropia, surgery must be considered.

B. If the patient exhibits a lateral incomitance, surgery should be tailored and the lateral rectus recession should be reduced. If the patient has an A-pattern with overacting superior obliques but demonstrates fusion, some surgeons do superior oblique weakening procedures; others infraplace the lateral rectus muscles. In all these cases, an adjustable suture is best suited for realignment. A slight overcorrection is the goal. The patient should be warned of immediate postoperative diplopia that will gradually lessen over time.

C. With congenital deviations, any sensory causes, as previously listed, need to be ruled out. In addition, any superimposed amblyopia must be treated and corrected. The deviation is divided into either a phoria, intermittent exotropia, or tropia. A phoria can be followed.

D. If an intermittent exotropia develops, it is often helpful to have the parents make a report card of both the amount and the frequency of the turning.

E. If turning occurs more than a third of the day or if a tropia exists that is less than 20 prism diopters (PD), an alternate-patching regimen can be tried. The right eye is patched one day and the left eye the next, and so forth.

F. Alternatively, if this is unsuccessful, one can attempt to stimulate convergence by the prescription of overminus lenses.

TABLE 1 Amount of Surgery Per Unit Deviation

Prism Diopter Deviation	*Amount of Recession*	*Amount of Resection/Recession*
20	5.0	4.0/5.0
25	6.0	5.0/5.0
30	7.0	5.0/6.0
35	7.5	6.0/6.0
40	8.0	6.0/7.0
45		7.0/8.0
50		8.0/10.0

G. If both of these fail or if the deviation is greater than 20 PD, surgery must once again be considered (see B) with the omission of adjustable sutures. The possibility of consecutive esotropia and subsequent amblyopia must be discussed with the parents prior to surgery. See Table 1.

References

Caltrider N, Jampolsky A. Overcorrecting minus lens therapy for treatment of intermittent exotropia. Ophthalmology 1983; 90:1160.

Carlson M, Jampolsky A. Lateral incomitancy in intermittent exotropia: cause and surgical therapy. Arch Ophthalmol 1979; 97:1922.

Freeman R, Isenberg S. The use of part-time occlusion for early onset unilateral exotropia. J Pediatr Ophthalmol Strabismus 1989; 26:94.

Hardesty H, Boynton J, Keenan J. Treatment of intermittent exotropia. Arch Ophthalmol 1978; 96:268.

Helveston E, Ellis F. Pediatric ophthalmology practice. St. Louis: CV Mosby, 1984:50.

Hiles D, Davies G, Costenbader F. Long-term observations on unoperated intermittent exotropia. Arch Ophthalmol 1968; 80:436.

Richard J, Parks M. Intermittent exotropia: surgical results in different age groups. Ophthalmology 1983; 90:1172.

Schlossman A, Muchnick R, Stern K. The surgical management of intermittent exotropia in adults. Ophthalmology 1983; 90:1166.

Scott W, Keech R, Mash J. The postoperative results and stability of exodeviations. Arch Ophthalmol 1981; 99:1814.

von Noorden G. Binocular vision and ocular motility. St. Louis: CV Mosby, 1985:304.

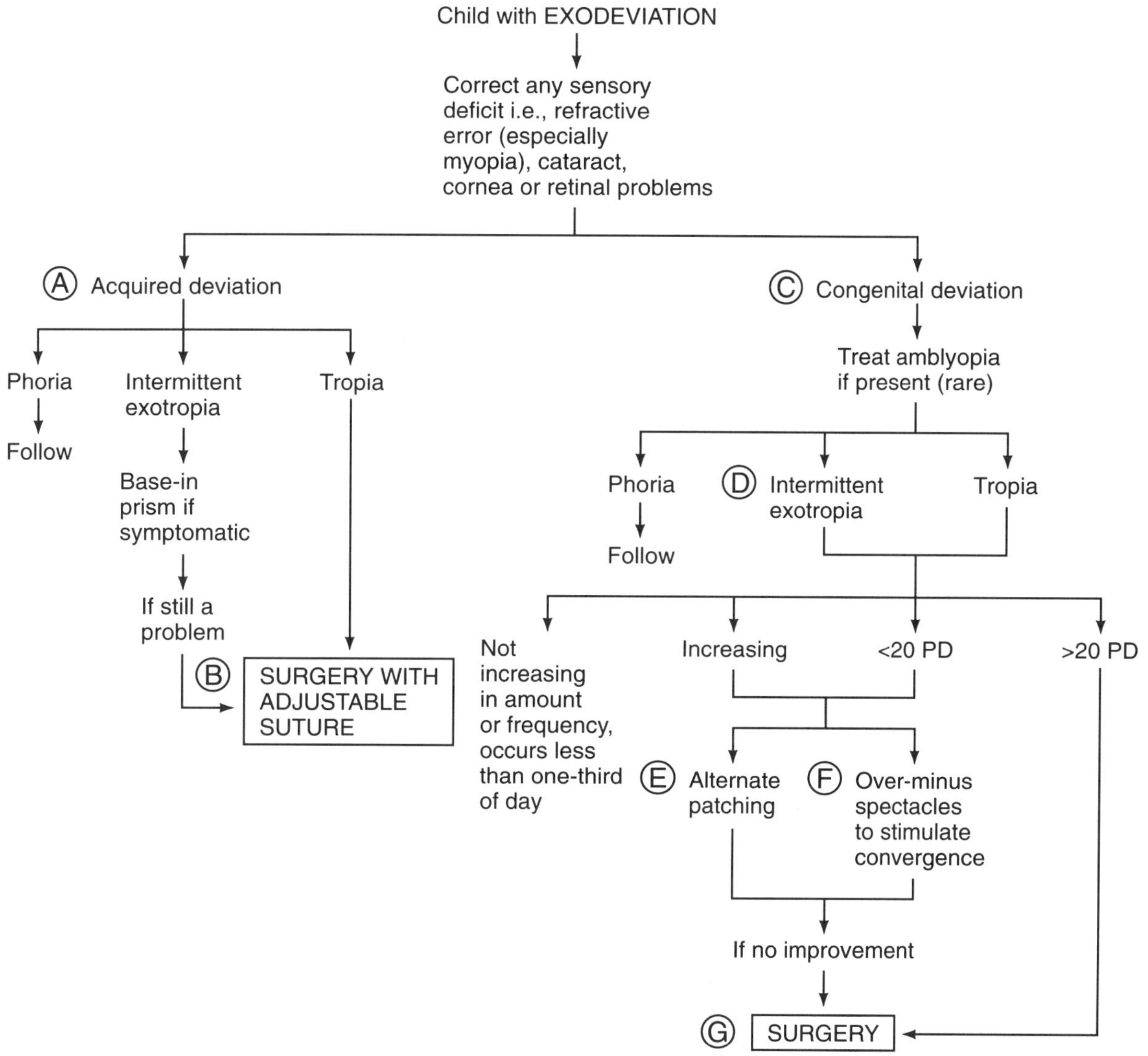
Child with EXODEVIATION
Correct any sensory deficit i.e., refractive error (especially myopia), cataract, cornea or retinal problems
(A) Acquired deviation
Phoria
Follow
Intermittent exotropia
Base-in prism if symptomatic
If still a problem
Tropia
(B) SURGERY WITH ADJUSTABLE SUTURE
(C) Congenital deviation
Treat amblyopia if present (rare)
Phoria
Follow
(D) Intermittent exotropia
Tropia
Not increasing in amount or frequency, occurs less than one-third of day
Increasing
<20 PD
>20 PD
(E) Alternate patching
(F) Over-minus spectacles to stimulate convergence
If no improvement
(G) SURGERY

PARETIC STRABISMUS

Mark J. Greenwald, M.D.

Paretic strabismus characteristically involves limitation of ocular rotation and incomitance of the strabismus deviation. In some cases, however, one or the other of these features is absent. For example, vertical ductions are usually full in fourth nerve palsy, and esotropia comitant with respect to lateral gaze is often seen in bilateral sixth nerve palsy.

A. An excellent method for detecting and documenting deficiency of ocular rotation is the Urist version reflex test. The examiner observes reflections from the surface of each eye created by a light source held in the midline (close to the examiner's nose) as the patient looks as far as possible into each of the secondary gaze positions (left, right, upward, and downward). The location of a reflex from the cornea is quantified (in degrees from its center) as for the Hirschberg estimate of strabismic deviation; a reflex from the conjunctiva is localized by the number of millimeters posterior to the limbus it falls; and a double reflex that straddles the limbus is described as being in the limbal region. Urist measurements can be recorded in a simple diagramatic format (Fig. 1).

B. A divergence insufficiency pattern—esodeviation significantly greater with distance (DT) than near (NR) viewing—is exceptional in association with accommodative or essential (congenital) esotropia (ET) and should be regarded as an indication of a paretic or restrictive problem until proven otherwise. On the other hand, neither lateral rectus (LR) paresis nor medial rectus (MR) restriction can be the primary cause of esotropia with a convergence excess pattern (deviation greater at near than at distance). In such cases, limitation of abduction (ABD) (which may be quite impressive) is attributable to increased MR tone accompanying accommodative or essential esotropia. (Distance/near relations are not helpful in establishing a paretic etiology for exotropia [XT]).

C. Orbital disease may cause either paresis or restrictive change in multiple muscles; combinations inconsistent with palsy of a single cranial nerve (e.g., MR and LR) suggest this possibility. A primary restrictive process in a muscle (Brown's superior oblique [SO] syndrome; orbital fracture with inferior rectus [IR] or other muscle entrapment; Graves' disease, particularly involving the IR or MR) can be difficult to differentiate from paresis of its antagonist; because of secondary contracture, passive rotation (forced duction) may be abnormal in the latter situation as well as the former. With vertical muscle involvement, looking at horizontal alignment in the limited gaze field is often helpful. Brown's syndrome causes exotropia on upward gaze; inferior oblique (IO) paresis, esotropia. Inferior rectus restriction causes esotropia on upward gaze; superior rectus (SR) paresis, exotropia. Demonstration of normal saccadic velocity with movement in the limited direction also suggests a restrictive cause.

D. Mild limitation of adduction (ADD) (often subtle, but detectable with the Urist test) is present in most cases of type 1 (esotropic) Duane's syndrome because of MR-LR co-contraction; abduction (ABA) is similarly reduced in most cases of type II (exotropic) Duane's syndrome because of subnormal innervation of the LR. With simple paresis of either LR or MR, rotation in the direction *opposite* the paretic muscle's field of action is normal, and with primary MR overaction in essential esotropia adduction tends to be greater than normal.

E. Myasthenia gravis should receive particular consideration in the differential diagnosis of exotropia (constant or intermittent, comitant or not) associated with ptosis (unilateral or bilateral, typically quite variable in degree), and also in any case of apparently isolated paresis of the MR, IR, or SR muscle. Cogan's lid-twitch sign (momentary overelevation of the lids with a shift in gaze from downward to upward) is a very helpful diagnostic feature. In addition to a Tensilon test (often equivocal or negative with ocular myasthenia), anti-acetylcholine receptor antibody titers should be included in the evaluation of suspicious cases.

F. Three binary decisions (higher eye right [R] or left [L], greater deviation right gaze or left, greater deviation right head tilt or left) must be made in choosing one from among the eight (2 to the 3 power) cyclovertical muscles whose isolated paresis may cause hypertropia (HT). The Parks three-step test and numerous variations formalize this process. It must be kept in mind that a meaningless result is obtained in any case involving paresis of multiple muscles or primary restriction or overaction. (For clarity, the sequence for right hypertropia only is given in the decision tree; substituting left for right and vice versa yields the left hypertropia scheme.)

G. Primary overaction of the SO may closely mimic (including head tilt variation) ipsilateral IO or contralateral IR paresis and is, in fact, considerably more common than either. Typically (although not always) there is significant esotropia or exotropia in straight-ahead gaze, with A-pattern variation. Primary IO

```
     30°                 15°
      |                   |
10 mm — RE — LR    −15° — LE — 10 mm
      |                   |
    8 mm                 30°
```

Figure 1 Urist measurements of a patient with left N III palsy. Rotation of the right eye is normal, including adduction that results in a light reflex from the temporal limbal region (LR). For the left eye, adduction falls short of the midline by 15 degrees (reflex 2 mm *nasal* to center of cornea). Elevation and depression are also limited. Abduction is normal (reflex from conjunctiva 10 mm posterior to the limbus).

overaction generally does not produce similar confusion.

H. "Double elevator palsy" is diagnosed when hypotropia increases from downward to upward gaze but does not differ significantly between right and left gaze. SR paresis is probably the cause in most cases; simultaneous IO paresis is hard to account for anatomically.

I. The occurrence of secondary IO overaction with SO paresis often results in hypertropia that is greater in upward gaze than in the field of action of the paretic SO. Observation in the oblique gaze positions may then yield the incorrect impression of contralateral SR weakness ("inhibitional palsy of the contralateral antagonist"). For this reason, upward and downward gaze measurements cannot be relied upon to identify a paretic cyclovertical muscle. (Tilt measurements, as pointed out by Bielschowsky, are very consistent and reliable.)

J. In congenital third cranial nerve (N III) palsy the pupil may be spared or may be nonreactive at any diameter from smaller than normal to large. Ipsilateral ptosis frequently accompanies hypotropia, particularly in association with double elevator palsy and palsy of the superior division of N III. Especially when the paretic eye fixates, lid level in relation to cornea may appear normal, but this should not be considered pseudoptosis because the lid as well as the eye is abnormally positioned in relation to the other eye. Ptosis with N III palsy may involve paradoxic elevation of the lid due to aberrant regeneration, particularly with adduction and depression.

K. All four paretic muscles (MR, SR, IR, IO) are on the same side with infranuclear N III palsy; with nuclear lesions, SR involvement is contralateral rather than ipsilateral. The dominant deviation associated with most N III palsies is exotropia. In straight-ahead gaze, vertical deviation may be either hypotropia or hypertropia of the paretic eye, depending on the relative weakness of the IR and SR muscles. The paretic eye is nearly always both hypotropic in upward gaze and hypertropic in downward gaze.

L. Ophthalmoplegic migraine must be considered in the differential diagnosis of acute N III palsy in childhood. Prior to onset there is usually a history of headache, but this may be difficult to obtain from a small child. The family history is typically positive for migraine.

M. Hydrocephalus and posterior fossa brain tumors must always be considered in the differential diagnosis of acute LR paresis in childhood, but its most common cause when the patient appears otherwise healthy is benign transient cranial nerve VI palsy, typically but not always developing after an acute viral illness (and frequently recurrent). Provided that no associated finding indicates increased intracranial pressure (headache, nausea/vomiting, tense fontanelle or increased head circumference in an infant, papilledema), or other focal neurologic deficit (ataxia, facial weakness, dysphagia), close clinical observation alone is justifiable over the period of several weeks, during which recovery usually occurs. An equally valid approach is to obtain neuroimaging at the outset in every case of acute cranial nerve VI palsy.

Binocular function and visual acuity are protected in paretic childhood strabismus when alignment is maintained most of the time with the aid of compensatory head posture that keeps the eyes in a gaze position of minimum deviation; treatment then can be delayed for months or even years without significant harm. If this is not the case, permanent negative sensory consequences may develop within a few weeks of acute onset, and early use of Fresnel prisms to restore fusion until the deviation has stabilized or resolved should be considered. Injection of botulinum toxin into the MR antagonist of a paretic LR is also worth considering. Monocular occlusion should be used sparingly if at all in childhood.

N. Very large amounts of resection (12 mm or more) can safely be done on paralyzed horizontal rectus muscles and may be nearly as effective as transposition procedures when combined with supermaximal recession of the antagonist. Following such surgery it is common to see some rotation into the field of action of even a totally noncontracting muscle, due to the elastic pull of the tightened rectus in synergy with relaxation of the loosened antagonist.

Transposition operations may displace half of each involved muscle, as in the procedures of Jensen (joining adjacent halves of LR and SR/IR with nonabsorbable ligatures) and Hummelsheim (transfer of temporal halves of SR/IR close to the LR insertion) for N VI palsy, or the entire muscle, as in the Knapp procedure (transfer of MR/LR close to the SR insertion) for elevator palsy. The possibility of postoperative anterior segment ischemia should be kept in mind when operating on more than two rectus muscles, and consideration given to preserving the ciliary vessels if such a procedure is necessary.

O. An excellent surgical result can often be obtained by operating on the *normal* eye when a weakened muscle retains enough strength to rotate its eye reasonably well (>20 degrees) into its field of action. Recession of the paretic muscle's yoke and resection of the yoke's antagonist both have their greatest effect in the gaze direction where maximum effect is needed. In contrast, ipsilateral recession/resection is maximally powerful in the gaze direction of minimum deviation and therefore gives a more incomitant result. The amount of surgery done on the normal eye is based on measurement of the *secondary* deviation (paretic eye fixating in the straight-ahead position, prism in front of the nonparetic eye).

P. Selection of a surgical procedure for N IV palsy is based primarily on the specific effect required, particularly in relation to different gaze and head positions. Tightening the paretic SO (tuck, plication) and weakening its antagonist (ipsilateral IO recession, myectomy) both have greater effect on hypertropia in upward (U) than downward (D) gaze and a relatively large increase in effect between straight-ahead and

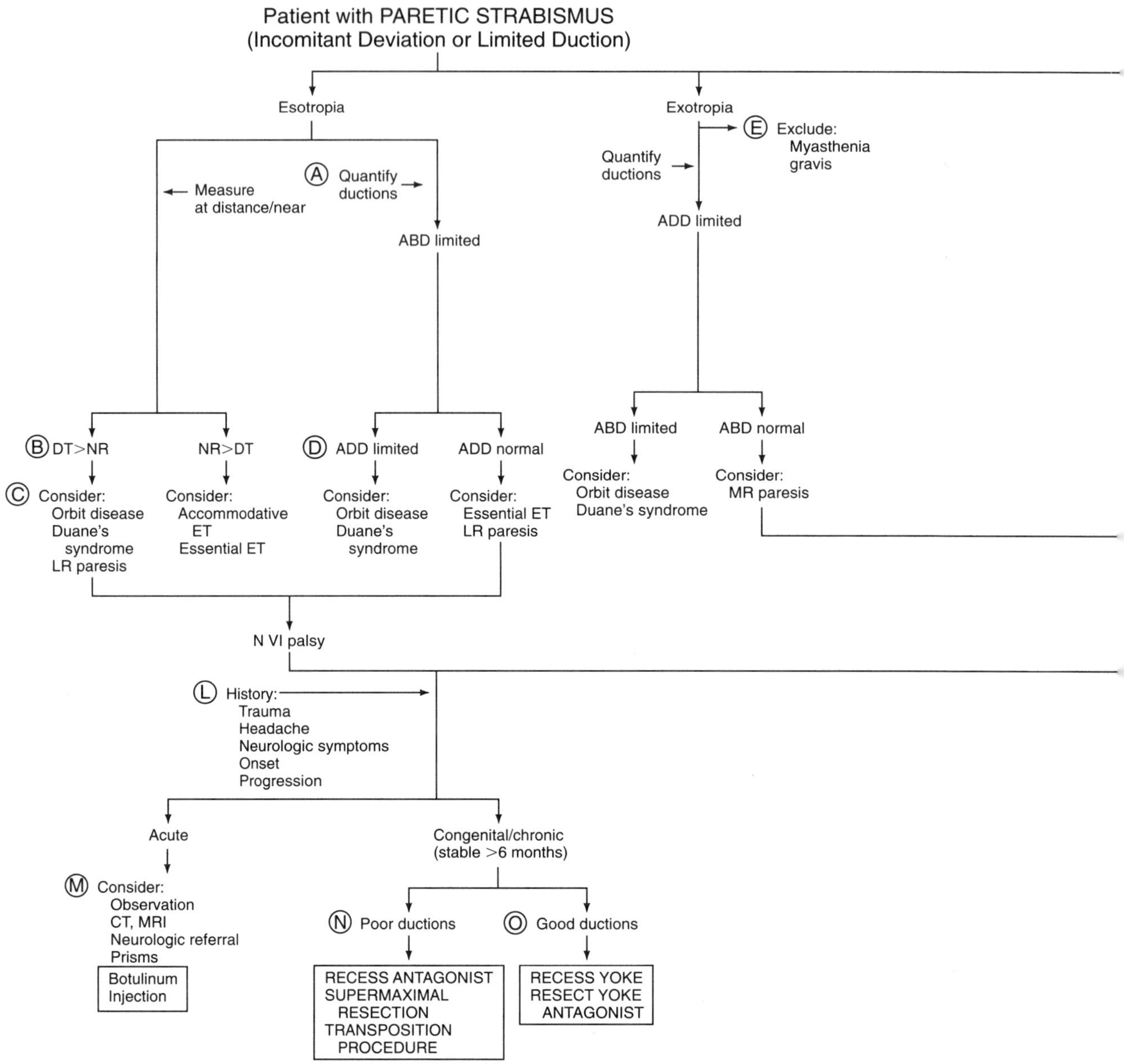

contralateral gaze. Weakening the yoke of the paretic muscle (contralateral IR recession) has greater effect in downward than in upward gaze, with only modest increase in effect between straight-ahead and lateral gaze to the side opposite the paretic muscle. SO tightening is more effective than any other procedure for correcting cyclodeviation, which may contribute to the tendency of some children with congenital SO paresis and little hyperdeviation to maintain a large head tilt. Recession of the ipsilateral SR provides a desirably greater effect with head tilt to the side of the paretic muscle, but has an undesirable increase in effect with gaze to the same side.

Q. IO weakening generally needs no quantification. SO tightening is quantified intraoperatively based on passive rotation of the globe. IR recession requires quantification based on preoperative measurements (from 3 mm for 7 to 10Δ, to 5 mm for 15 to 20Δ) or use of an adjustable suture, making it less suitable for unco-operative children. (Care must be taken to avoid creating noticeable retraction of the lower lid when this operation is performed.) For deviations exceeding 20Δ in straight-ahead gaze, surgery on two muscles is usually necessary.

R. In patients with bilateral N IV palsy (a relatively common complication of closed head trauma), vertical alignment may be virtually normal with straight-ahead gaze (where the right and left depression deficits balance each other); right hypertropia becomes evident with left gaze or with right head tilt, left hypertropia with right gaze or left tilt (as one eye moves out of and the other into the field of action of its SO). Horizontal (abduction) and cyclorotational deficits are additive, tending to cause symptomatic excyclodeviation and V-pattern esotropia, both especially

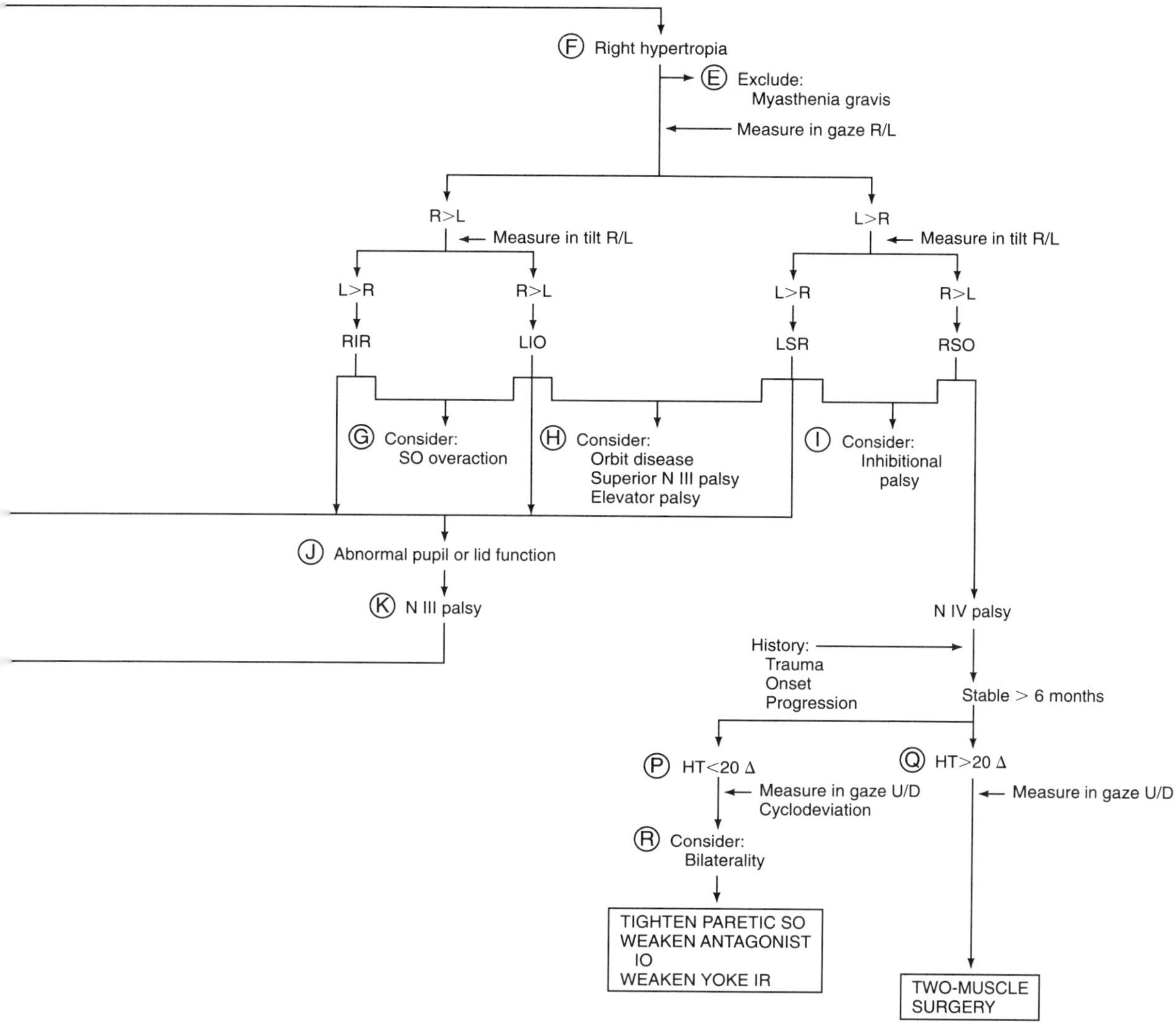

bothersome with downward gaze. Bilateral SO tightening (particularly the Harada-Ito modification, in which only the anterior half of each tendon is displaced) is the corrective procedure of choice. Asymmetric bilateral N IV palsy may be difficult to distinguish from unilateral palsy; cyclodeviation (measured using bilateral Maddox rods) exceeding 10 degrees suggests bilateral involvement.

References

Afifi AK, Bell WE, Bale JF, Thompson HS. Recurrent lateral rectus palsy in childhood. Pediatr Neurol 1990; 6:315.

Ellenhorn N, Lucchese N, Greenwald M. Juvenile myasthenia gravis and amblyopia. Am J Ophthalmol 1986; 101:214.

Folk ER. Strabismus. In: Peyman GA, Sanders DR, Goldberg MF, eds. Principles and practice of ophthalmology. Philadelphia: WB Saunders, 1980; 1777.

Parks MM, Mitchell PR. Cranial nerve palsies. In: Tasman W, Jaeger EA, eds. Duane's clinical ophthalmology. Vol 1. Philadelphia: JB Lippincott, 1986; 19.

Woody RC, Blaw ME. Ophthalmoplegic migraine in infancy. Clin Pediatr 1986; 25:82.

Supported by an unrestricted grant from Research to Prevent Blindness, Inc., New York, New York.

DISSOCIATED VERTICAL DEVIATION

Gerhard W. Cibis, M.D.

A. Dissociated vertical deviation (DVD) refers to a one-eye phenomenon. Double dissociated vertical deviation (DDVD) exists when both eyes show the phenomenon. DVD is a vertical upward displacement of an eye when fusion is suspended. Clinically it is a cosmetic problem. Diplopia is rare. Because of the suspension of fusion, DVD may disrupt efforts at horizontal alignment.

B. Unlike a true hypertropia, no associated hypotropia exists with DVD. This is one way of differentiating inferior oblique overaction from DVD. With the DVD eye in adduction there should be no hypotropia of the other eye. When DDVD is present, a red filter in front of either eye leads to the red image being below the fixation light. This is because the red filter dissociates the eyes, and the eye with the filter makes an upward movement. A prism can be used to measure the amount of deviation in this way. Alternate cover testing with a prism does not measure a DVD because there is no corresponding hypotropia of the other eye. One method of measuring the DVD uses a base-down prism in front of the deviating eye under an occluder. The occluder is then switched to the fixing eye. Base-down prism is added until no downward movement of the deviating eye is observed on switching occlusion. Another method is to simply grade on a scale of 1 to 4, where 1 = slight and 4 = large deviation.

C. Differentiation from inferior oblique overaction is also aided by the DVD remaining elevated when the eye is moved from an adducted position to abduction. With inferior oblique overaction, the elevated eye comes down as it leaves adduction (inferior oblique field of action).

D. There is commonly an associated occlusion nystagmus.

E. DVD is the most common cause of torticollis in the pediatric age group. Usually the tilt is to the side of the more deviated eye.

F. The covered eye manifesting DVD moves down more and more as increasingly stronger neutral-density filters are placed in front of the fixing eye.

G. DVD is ultimately associated with 90% of infantile (congenital) esotropia (ET). The incidence increases with time and is not necessarily present at the time of presentation of the ET. When present, DVD virtually rules out a late acquired ET or partially accommodative ET that has broken down. It is a hallmark of the deviation having been present early in life. It is a cause of further surgery even if the horizontal deviation has been corrected. DVD is less often associated with exotropia. Fusion is usually peripheral and not central, which is why DVD is more common in infantile ET cases than in later accommodative cases. The same is true for exotropia with good fusion; DVD is more common than when fusion is poor. DVD can develop when there is unilateral vision loss, as with cataracts or corneal scarring in early childhood.

H. Therapy is usually surgical. However, when unilateral, forcing the DVD eye to be the fixing eye by blurring or patching the dominant eye can work. Improvement in fusion can also help lessen or eliminate DVD. This can be accomplished with maximum optical methods or surgically for the repair of horizontal deviations. When DVD is present, with horizontal deviations needing surgery, I always also manage the DVD surgically.

Surgical resection of inferior recti and recession of the obliques, although once used, have fallen out of favor except as a second procedure. I prefer a large recession of the superior recti. If only one eye is actually involved, the risk of postoperative hypotropia is great. Frequently the other eye develops DVD. Therefore, with unilateral or highly asymmetric cases, I recess the superior rectus of worse eye 10 mm and that of the other eye 5 mm with a posterior fixation suture (PFS). For bilateral cases, a 10-mm superior rectus recession is preferred. With modest asymmetric cases, one can recess 3 to 5 mm with PFS and place a PFS in the other eye without removing the muscle. Esswein et al recently reported best long-term results with large (7 to 10 mm) recessions. The problems to consider are DVD developing on the other side and hypotropia if large unilateral surgery is done.

With 10-mm recessions the tip of the insertion of the superior oblique is at 9 mm. I once did hang-loose 10-mm recessions but found a case in which the muscle came to rest on the oblique and not on the sclera. Since then we have sewn the muscle directly onto the sclera 10 mm from the original insertion.

References

Burian GM, von Noorden GK. Binocular vision and ocular motility: Theory and management of strabismus. 3rd ed. St Louis: CV Mosby, 1985.

Esswein MB, von Noorden GK, Coburn A. Comparison of surgical methods in the treatment of dissociated vertical deviation. Am J Ophthalmol 1992; 113:287.

Lang J. Strabismus. Trans. by GW Cibis. Thorofare, NJ: Slack, 1983.

Magoon E, Cruciger M, Jampolsky A. Dissociated vertical deviation: An asymmetric condition treated with large bilateral superior rectus recession. J Pediatr Ophthalmol Strabismus 1982; 19:152.

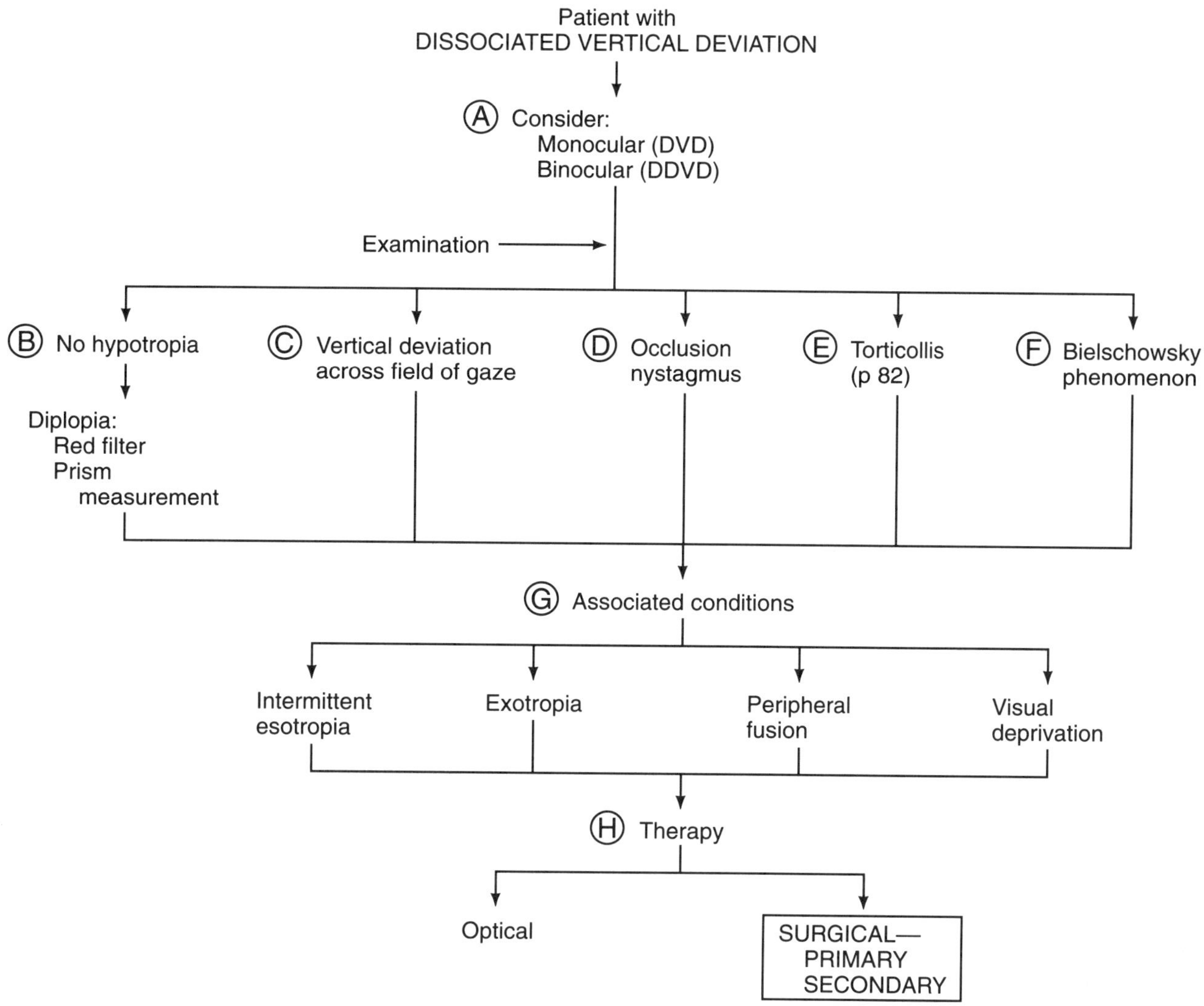
Patient with
DISSOCIATED VERTICAL DEVIATION
(A) Consider:
Monocular (DVD)
Binocular (DDVD)
Examination
(B) No hypotropia
Diplopia:
Red filter
Prism
measurement
(C) Vertical deviation
across field of gaze
(D) Occlusion
nystagmus
(E) Torticollis
(p 82)
(F) Bielschowsky
phenomenon
(G) Associated conditions
Intermittent
esotropia
Exotropia
Peripheral
fusion
Visual
deprivation
(H) Therapy
Optical
SURGICAL—
PRIMARY
SECONDARY

DIPLOPIA

Gerhard W. Cibis, M.D.

A. Whether binocular or monocular diplopia is claimed, the first step is to rule out a pseudodiplopia. Blurred vision is often misinterpreted as double vision. Blurring from refractive or organic reasons needs to be ruled out or properly treated. Physiologic diplopia is the child voicing normal observation that adults have learned to take for granted. The best way to demonstrate physiologic diplopia is to ask the subject to hold their two index fingers in front of them, one a foot or so in front of the other. When looking at the more distant finger the closer one appears double and vice versa. In daily life we learn to ignore this normal, physiologic diplopia.

B. Monocular diplopia is rare. When it occurs and is not pseudodiplopia, look for an explanation in anatomic order from the front to the back: tear film, distorted cornea (lid tumor), polycoria, dislocated lens, vitreous cyst, retinal detachment or elevation.

C. Double vision in children is a very different symptom from that in adults. Children are often not observant and fail to notice diplopia. A child's ability to suppress compared with an adult's alters the amount of time a child manifests diplopia. A 3-year old with acute traumatic palsy may suppress and lose double vision within days to weeks of the trauma. Rather than voice diplopia (i.e., "I see two Mommies"), children close one eye or develop a head turn to get the second image as far away as possible from the first.

D. Binocular diplopia is due to misalignment of the eyes in relationship to each other. This can occur acutely or represent an old, long-standing condition. Because of the ability to suppress in children, diplopia may be transient.

E. Day-to-day variability is common with myasthenia gravis. Proper work-up includes edrophonium (Tensilon) testing and acetylcholine receptor antibody determination. Myasthenia can mimic any cranial nerve palsy and cause ptosis and nystagmus. There is no pain and pupils are normal.

F. Incomitant strabismus means that the deviation is different in different positions of gaze. This implies a neurogenic cause, although inflammation and orbital scarring from trauma or disease can be at fault. Acquired Brown's syndrome has been described with juvenile rheumatoid arthritis (pp 220, 222). Thyroid ophthalmopathy can occur in childhood. Pseudotumor is more common. Myositis can be diagnosed by CT appearance of the muscles. In children, sixth nerve palsies can be caused by tumors but also by viral illness. With postviral sixth nerve palsy, recovery usually occurs in a few weeks. Multiple recurrences have been documented.

G. Comitant strabismus is the same in all directions of gaze. A non-neurogenic etiology is implied.

H. Acute-onset normosensorial esotropia is just that. No significant hyperopia is present. If it fails to resolve within 3 months, surgery is indicated to preserve fusion, which is normal at the onset. Microtropes degenerating to a larger angle because of decreased fusion and exotropes becoming less intermittent may have diplopia during the process of drifting to a larger angle of deviation than their retinal adaptation.

I. Properly corrected accommodative esotropia (ET) with fusion causes double vision when no longer properly corrected. Similarly, those with convergence insufficiency may complain of diplopia at near. We give the full cycloplegic refraction. Bifocals are used when the AC/A ration is high. When, despite maximum glasses, a residual deviation of greater than microtropia persists either at distance, near, or both, surgery is indicated. These cases are then partially accommodative. Posterior fixation sutures are used for high AC/A ratio cases. Orthoptic exercises can help with accommodative and convergence insufficiency and divergence excess (see pp 108, 110).

J. Old deviations that suddenly manifest diplopia do so through a breakdown of their existing situation. When comitant, an increasing angle should be measured with prism adaptation test, and prism glasses or surgery should be prescribed (see p 188). A breakdown of control in accommodative esotropia leads to a nonaccommodative component. When this exceeds microtropia values, surgery is indicated. Posterior fixation sutures on the medial recti are useful if the patient is aligned at distance but not at near despite +3.00 diopter bifocals. Broken-down microtropia is common in adults but less so in children. Prism adaptation testing is done, and prism glasses are prescribed or surgery is done (see chapters on prisms).

K. Incomitant strabismus of long standing can change, leading to diplopia. It is common for Duane's syndrome patients to develop more and more medial rectus constriction, leading to a need for increasing head turn. When the head turn can no longer be comfortably or practically maintained, a complaint of diplopia is elicited. The same mechanism leads to increased deviations with complaints of diplopia in all other forms of long-standing incomitant strabismus.

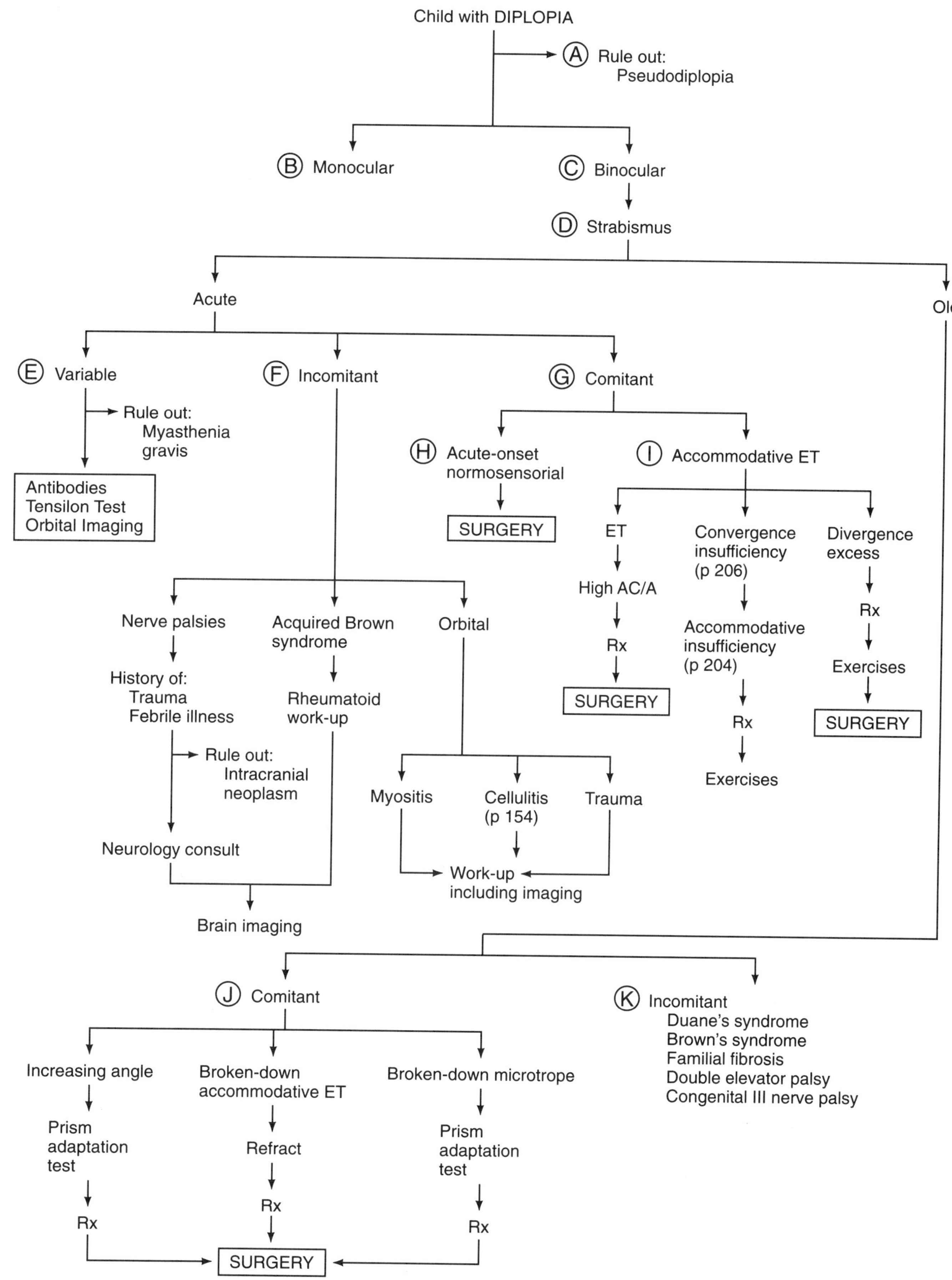

References

Burian GM, von Noorden GK. Binocular vision and ocular motility: Theory and management of strabismus. 3rd ed. St. Louis: CV Mosby, 1985.

Lang J. Strabismus. Trans. by GW Cibis. Thorofare, NJ: Slack, 1983.

Parks MM. Atlas of strabismus surgery. Philadelphia: Harper & Row, 1983.

POST-SURGICAL STRABISMUS MANAGEMENT

Gerhard W. Cibis, M.D.

A. Prior to surgery the accommodative status and its influence on the deviation must be known. If exotropic with high hyperopia, the deviation may need more surgery because with correction an increase in exotropia (XT) from loss of accommodation convergence is to be expected. Esotropic deviations can be expected to improve with hyperopic glasses. Postsurgery glasses can be used to manipulate accommodation and provide alignment. In case of XT overcorrection, less plus and more minus are used. Up to 3.00 diopters of minus overcorrection or plus undercorrection can be tolerated. With esotropia plus is pushed as needed.

B. The sensory status should be tested, or based on the type of deviation, understood before surgery and used to help in post-surgery management. Suppression, abnormal retinal correspondence, and fixation scotoma determine the surgical outcome. Infantile esotropes at best end up microtropic. Eyes with abnormal retinal correspondence (ARC) at modest angles of less than 20 diopters have a strong sensory push to return to that deviation.

C. Esotropic overcorrection following XT surgery is desirable up to 15 diopters. Even if worse on the first postoperative visit, wait up to 3 weeks. If it fails to improve push plus lenses, even bifocals, and part-time alternate patching. Phospholine iodide is used if there is no improvement. Oculinum to an overacting medial rectus muscle can be used if the deviation persists up to 1 month after surgery without improvement. Prisms are useful in maintaining fusion but have the detriment of retaining the patient in the esotropic position. Measures to avoid suppression and even amblyopia should be taken early by part-time patching, allowing stimuli for binocularity the remainder of the time. The amount of patching varies but should not be more than half time unless one is battling a deep amblyopia. Incomitant deviations need to be evaluated for the possibility of slipped muscle. This may include imaging techniques and forced duction tests and may require visual inspection of the operated muscle in another procedure.

D. Check patient 1 week after starting drops. If the deviation goes to microtropia or orthotropia, the drops are used for a total of 6 months. During that time the brain adapts to the new position and when drops are stopped, it is hoped that retinal adaptation is strong enough to maintain alignment. If, despite the drops, a greater than microtropic angle persists, the drops are stopped and further surgery is indicated. We wait 6 weeks after the last drops used before doing surgery because of the potential anesthesia effect. I use phospholine iodide 0.125% and do not increase the amount if the patient fails to respond. Neo-Synephrine can be used to avoid pupillary cyst formation. Phospholine iodide drops are usually used in conjunction with glasses. Use of phospholine iodide as a test for the accommodative component to esotropia rather than giving glasses is not valid.

E. The choice of repeat surgery depends on what was done and the current status. It is not adequate to treat reoperation in the same way as virgin cases. One has to choose between redoing or undoing the original surgery versus working on previously unoperated muscles.

Most over- or undercorrections are not due to crippling of the muscle. Major contractures can occur with time, and these need to be appreciated by saccadic analysis, range of motion, and forced duction tests on the table or in the office. If a clear incomitance or restriction is found, it needs to be addressed. If comitance exists without evidence of constriction, operating on previously unoperated muscles is more predictive than re-operating on the same muscle. My first choice for undercorrected ET is to resect the lateral recti 5 mm each for deviations of up to 35 diopters, more if beyond that. The previous medial recession enhances the effect of the lateral resection. Similarly, I prefer to recess the medials on overcorrected lateral rectus recessions for exotropia. The amount depends on the dioptric deviation and amount of previous surgery.

F. With exotropic overcorrection following ET surgery there is less time to wait than with ET after XT surgery. However, the principles are the same. Push minus lenses (up to 3 diopters). Maximize sharpness of vision with refraction. Patch alternately up to half time. If all that fails, perform surgery. Minus lens overcorrection for consecutive or residual XT is not a permanent solution but can buy time for fusion to develop and then further surgery. Oculinum is usually not needed. Minus lenses are feasible only in young patients with good accommodation.

G. Undercorrections do not benefit from waiting, as do overcorrections. Immediate maximum plus glasses in the case of ET or overminused glasses in the case of XT are needed to achieve alignment. If the residual deviation is less than 15 diopters ET, phospholine iodide drops alone or glasses alone can be used. If there is significant hyperopia (more than 1 diopter), glasses should be strongly considered and bifocals given if the accommodative convergence-accommodation ratio is high. If maximum measures fail to reverse the undercorrection in 2 months, further surgery is indicated. In the case of XT undercorrection that normalizes with overminus glasses, use these for 6 months to achieve fusion and then re-operate. It is critical to recognize that if fusion is not present or not obtainable (too old), a small angle residual that is cosmetically fine need not be further addressed.

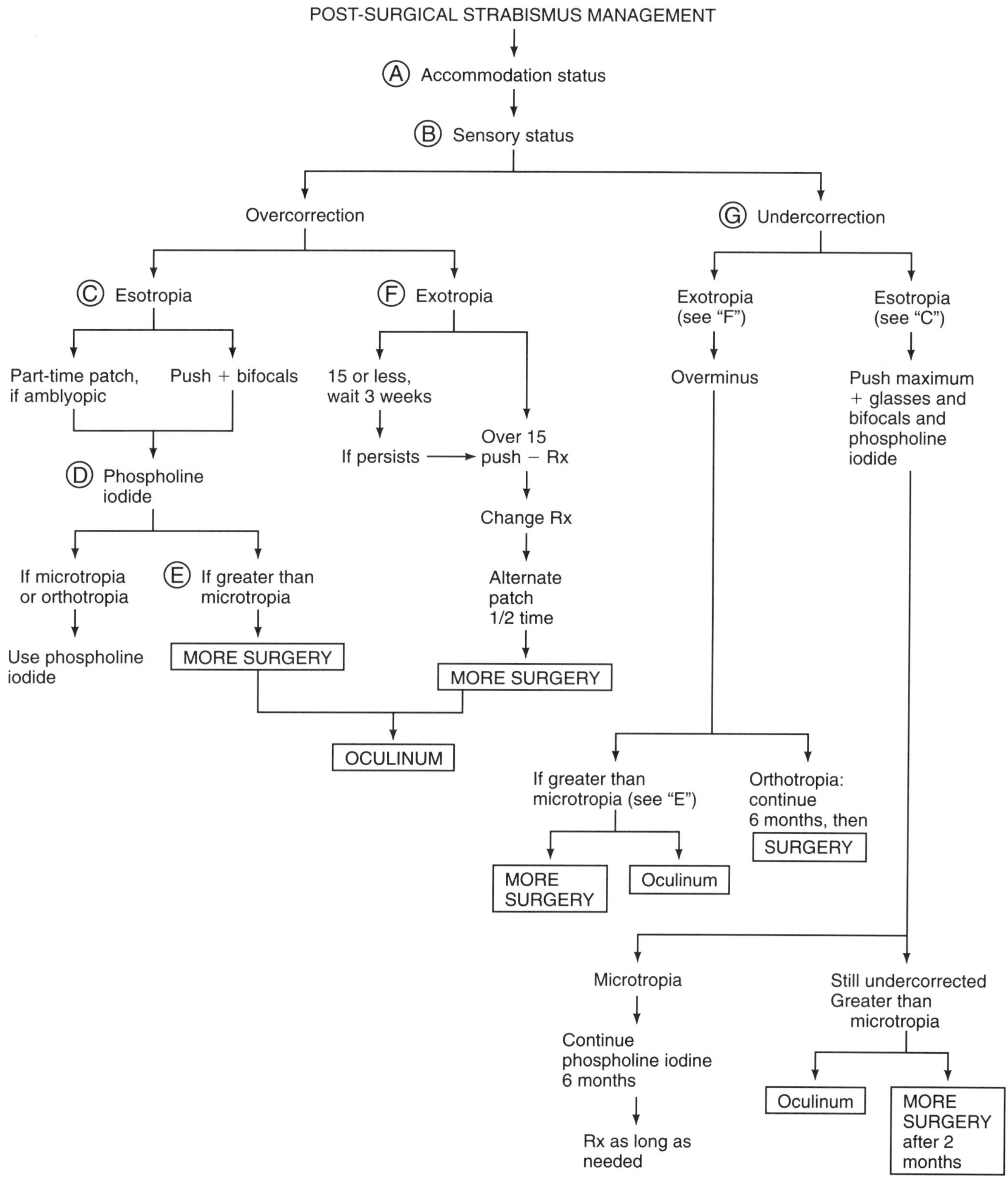

References

Cibis GW. Postsurgical management of strabismus. In: Spaeth GL, Katz LJ, Parker KW, eds. Current therapy in ophthalmic surgery, Philadelphia: BC Decker, 1989:291.

Lang J. Strabismus. Trans. by GW Cibis. Thorofare, NJ: Slack, 1983.

Parks MM. Atlas of strabismus surgery. Philadelphia: Harper & Row, 1983.

Von Noorden GK. Binocular vision and ocular motility: Theory and management of strabismus. 3rd ed. St. Louis: CV Mosby, 1985.

HEADACHES

Andrea Cibis Tongue, M.D.

This chapter is limited to headaches that are chronic or recurrent and are attributed by the patient, patient's family, or primary care physician to eye or eye muscle problems.

A. Because headache is a subjective complaint, history is the key investigative tool in determining its cause. It is important to elucidate the onset, frequency (daily, weekly, monthly, rarely), duration, severity of pain, pattern of occurrence (e.g., Do the headaches occur randomly during the day? Always at the same time? During school? Never on weekends?), association with any specific activity, prodromal or concurrent signs or symptoms, treatment, and treatment results. Localization of the headache is helpful primarily in observing the type of response the child gives to the question. Children with functional complaints often have a difficult time and hesitate before showing or telling where their head hurts. Medical history of recurrent sinus infections, hay fever, a previous shunt for hydrocephalus, neurologic abnormalities such as ataxia, newly developed clumsiness, generalized malaise, weight loss, and kidney disease is important. Has the patient experienced any abnormalities of vision? It is important to know what clinical and laboratory studies have been performed specifically because of the headache complaint.

The information obtained aids in making a clinical judgment about the severity of the headaches and possible medical implications. Headaches that recur in a predictable pattern (e.g., at the same time each day, never on weekends, or only on weekends) and respond relatively readily to no treatment or to mild analgesics are not likely to be medically significant headaches. They may be functional complaints or tension headaches. Questioning the child directly as to what he or she thinks is causing the headaches may be illuminating. There may be problems at school or an aversion to certain activities at school. Alternatively, the child may get headaches on weekends when obliged to visit the "other" parent and family. A child may be overprogrammed or concerned about parental expectations. Some children get headaches when hungry. Occasionally sensitivities to certain food products such as nitrites, monosodium glutamate, and insecticides trigger headaches. There is no reason to assume that children cannot develop true tension headaches. Usually these headaches have been present for months, sometimes years, before the patient presents for an examination.

B. If an ophthalmologist determines that the headaches are not visually related and are not due to any underlying medical problem, an ophthalmologic examination appropriate for the child's age and previous eye care is in order. A comprehensive examination may be performed if the child has never had one before. A more abbreviated examination may be done if all initial parameters such as visual acuity (both distance and near), pupils, external examination, motility, and undilated fundus examination are normal. Reassurance that there are no significant vision system abnormalities and discussion with the patient and parent about possible other causes, including tension headaches and functional headaches, are usually helpful. The pediatrician should be informed that the patient was seen for headaches and what has been discussed with the family.

C. If the headaches are severe and medically significant or if they appear to be visually induced or aggravated, a comprehensive ophthalmologic evaluation is indicated. If increased intracranial pressure is suspected, particular attention needs to be directed toward a neuro-ophthalmologic examination with emphasis on visual acuity, visual fields, optic nerves, and sixth nerve function. All eye examinations include visual acuity, pupil function, external examination, a screening motility examination, and funduscopy. Refraction is carried out if the acuity (distance or near) is subnormal to determine if refractive errors are responsible for subnormal vision.

D. If all parameters are normal and the medical history is unremarkable but the headaches are severe, recurrent, or associated with nausea, vomiting, or prodromal symptoms, migraines are the most likely cause. The patient should be referred to the primary care physician or neurologist for further management and evaluation. The diagnosis of migraine is one of exclusion and is based predominantly on the presenting symptoms. Other conditions that may present with severe headaches and no signs of CNS problems are sinus infections, headaches secondary to intermittent increased intracranial pressure, and hypertension. Cluster headaches or histamine headaches are rare in childhood but can occur. These children should also be referred to the primary care physician.

E. If ophthalmologic findings are abnormal (e.g., papilledema, optic atrophy, uncorrected subnormal visual acuity, acquired nystagmus, sixth nerve paresis), immediate referral for comprehensive medical and neurologic evaluation with appropriate imaging studies is advisable. Elevated intracranial pressure, intermittent or chronic, and hypertension need to be considered. Intracranial space-occupying lesions and pseudotumor cerebri enter the differential diagnosis.

F. Occasionally headaches are secondary to eye disease such as chronic uveitis, bullous keratopathy, phthisis, or acute angle closure glaucoma. Treatment is directed toward the alleviation or amelioration of the underlying ocular disease.

G. Evaluation of headaches related to visual tasks (e.g., reading, doing homework) needs to include a complete sensorimotor evaluation and visual acuity eval-

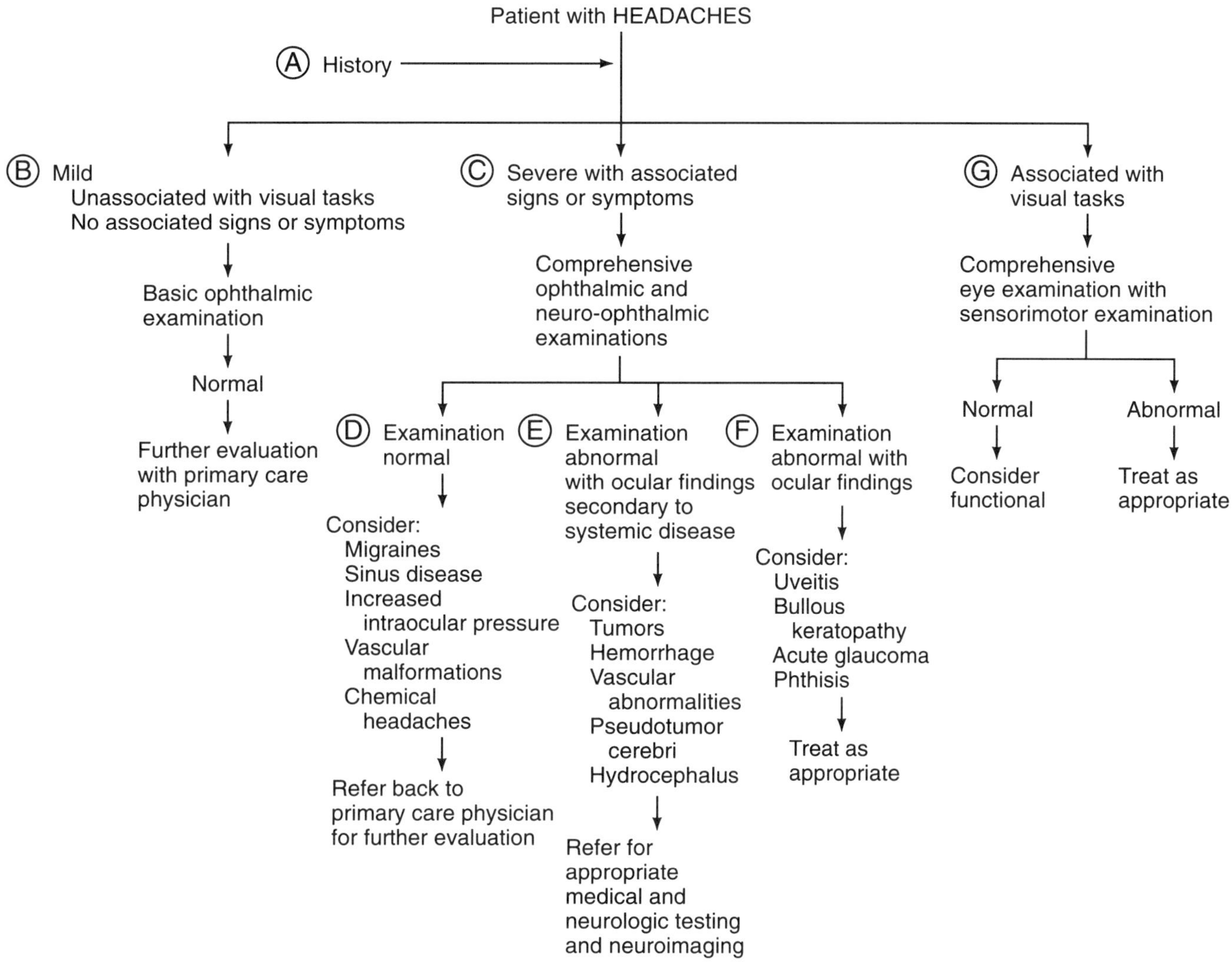

uation at near. Alternate cover tests to detect phorias, prism convergence, and accommodative amplitudes should be done. Cycloplegic refraction to uncover significant ametropia, especially hyperopia and anisometropia, should be performed. Correction of refractive errors is indicated if visual acuity is subnormal without correction at distance or at near or if the accommodative amplitude is subnormal. Clinical judgment is used when the refractive errors are borderline. If the physician believes that the headaches are not due to refractive errors or ametropia and the refractive findings are a borderline hyperopia or decreased accommodative amplitude, a trial with nonprescription reading glasses may be indicated. Patients with subnormal convergence amplitudes usually respond rapidly to orthoptics directed toward the improvement of the convergence amplitudes. Accommodative amplitudes can sometimes be helped by a short course of orthoptics as well (see p 204). If no ocular or sensorimotor abnormalities are found, functional headaches or tension headaches should be considered. The child who complains of headaches with visual tasks often has reading or learning difficulties. Headaches also appear to be more common among young adolescent girls, usually ages 10 to 12 years. They seem to disappear spontaneously without treatment intervention. If comprehensive ophthalmologic and sensorimotor examinations are normal, the patient should be reassured that all findings are normal.

References

Raskin NH. Headache. 2nd ed. New York: Churchill Livingstone, 1988.

Taylor D. Headaches. In: Taylor D, ed. *Pediatric ophthalmology*. London: Blackwell Scientific Publications, 1990: 702.

EYE PAIN

Andrea Cibis Tongue, M.D.

A. Eye pain, like headache, is a subjective symptom. When accompanied by objective signs such as tearing, obvious light sensitivity, conjunctival injection or chemosis, lid swelling, proptosis, or a history of acute ocular trauma or recent eye surgery, diagnosis is facilitated. Eye pain unaccompanied by any external signs of abnormality is more difficult to evaluate. History of onset of pain, duration, frequency, pattern of occurrence, and apparent severity is most helpful in trying to elucidate the cause. As with headaches in the absence of clinical findings, clinical judgment must be exercised as to need for further investigative studies. The examiner needs to determine whether the pain is an acute episode, recurrent, or chronic. If possible, one should ask the child what the pain feels like: Is it scratchy? Sharp? Felt when closing or opening the lids or looking around? Does it feel like something is in the eye, or is the pain a dull headache-like pain? Does light exposure exacerbate or aggravate the pain?

B. External examination of the eye and ocular adnexa may be most rewarding, and abnormalities are most likely to be found on slit-lamp examination. Particular attention should be paid to the lids, the type of bulbar injection, pupil size (miotic in cases of ciliary spasm, i.e., uveitis, iritis) and whether proptosis is present or not. Slit-lamp examination is necessary to detect signs of uveitis, subtle corneal changes, and keratoconjunctivitis. If corneal epithelial lesions are suspected, instillation of fluorescein or rose bengal dye makes detection easier. Funduscopy is performed if posterior lesions or abnormalities are suspected. Pain from intraocular problems without any concomitant external signs of injury or disease are rare, however. If increased intraocular pressure is suspected, perform tonometry.

C. Acute persistent eye pain of sudden onset is usually secondary to a corneal injury such as abrasion, keratitis, or foreign body. Accompanying signs are tearing, light sensitivity, and injection of the globe. Fluorescein may facilitate the detection of corneal epithelial defects. Foreign bodies may lodge in the conjunctiva of the upper tarsus and usually cause vertical linear abrasions. Lid eversion is necessary to reveal these hidden foreign bodies.

Keratitis accompanied by acute severe eye pain is usually the result of contact lens overwear, burn, or chemical injury of the cornea. Infectious keratitis such as herpes simplex and herpes zoster may present initially as pain without any signs of keratitis. Corneal ulcers may give rise to an acutely painful eye.

Bullous keratopathy with rupture of the bullae may lead to acute pain. Usually the underlying ophthalmic disease is known and readily recognized. Some corneal dystrophies and degenerations are also accompanied by recurrent epithelial erosions and pain.

Ocular contusions may cause acute pain secondary to traumatic iritis. Hyphema may or may not be present. Acute elevation of intraocular pressure secondary to a hyphema can cause severe pain and vomiting. Other ocular conditions can give rise to acute glaucoma and acute eye pain. Usually the underlying conditions such as dislocated lenses, retrolental fibroplasia, and prior intraocular surgery (i.e., cataract extraction) are known and readily recognized.

Painful acute iritis is rare in childhood and usually seen in older children. Iritis secondary to juvenile rheumatoid arthritis is rarely painful in the early stages.

Pseudotumor of the orbit may present with acute pain, particularly with movement of the eye. Other space-occupying lesions of the orbit may cause pain if there is rapid expansion. Referred pain from the CNS is rare in children. Optic neuritis may be associated with pain on eye movement as well. Periorbital and orbital cellulitis may be associated with acute pain. Dacryoadenitis and dacryocystitis may present with acute pain and swelling in the affected gland or lacrimal sac area, respectively. Hordeolum presents with localized erythema and swelling of the lid and is often accompanied by complaints of acute pain exacerbated by touch.

D. Some conditions give rise to pain that may be present for days or weeks before ophthalmologic help is sought. This type of pain, often seen in patients with keratoconjunctivitis, is usually less severe than the acute pain of a corneal abrasion and tends to have a slightly more insidious onset. Keratoconjunctivitis may be viral or bacterial in origin. Exposure keratitis and keratitis secondary to trichiasis may also result in chronic discomfort.

E. Recurrent pain episodes may be due to recurrent erosions, keratitis, keratoconjunctivitis, hordeolum, uveitis, or uncontrolled glaucoma. However, in the absence of any external signs of ocular pathology, the most likely diagnosis is functional. Usually parents give a history of the child complaining about pain, but the pain does not appear severe, does not last long, and is unaccompanied by tearing or redness. Reassurance that no abnormalities are noted and tincture of time usually ameliorate the pain complaints. If the pain episodes appear to be severe and debilitating, migraines, histamine headaches, or retrobulbar lesions need to be considered and appropriate referral for further studies is indicated.

F. Chronic debilitating ocular pain is unusual in childhood without underlying ocular disease such as phthisis or chronic uveitis in a prephthisical eye. Treatment with topical steroids may be helpful, but enucleation is sometimes the only definitive treat-

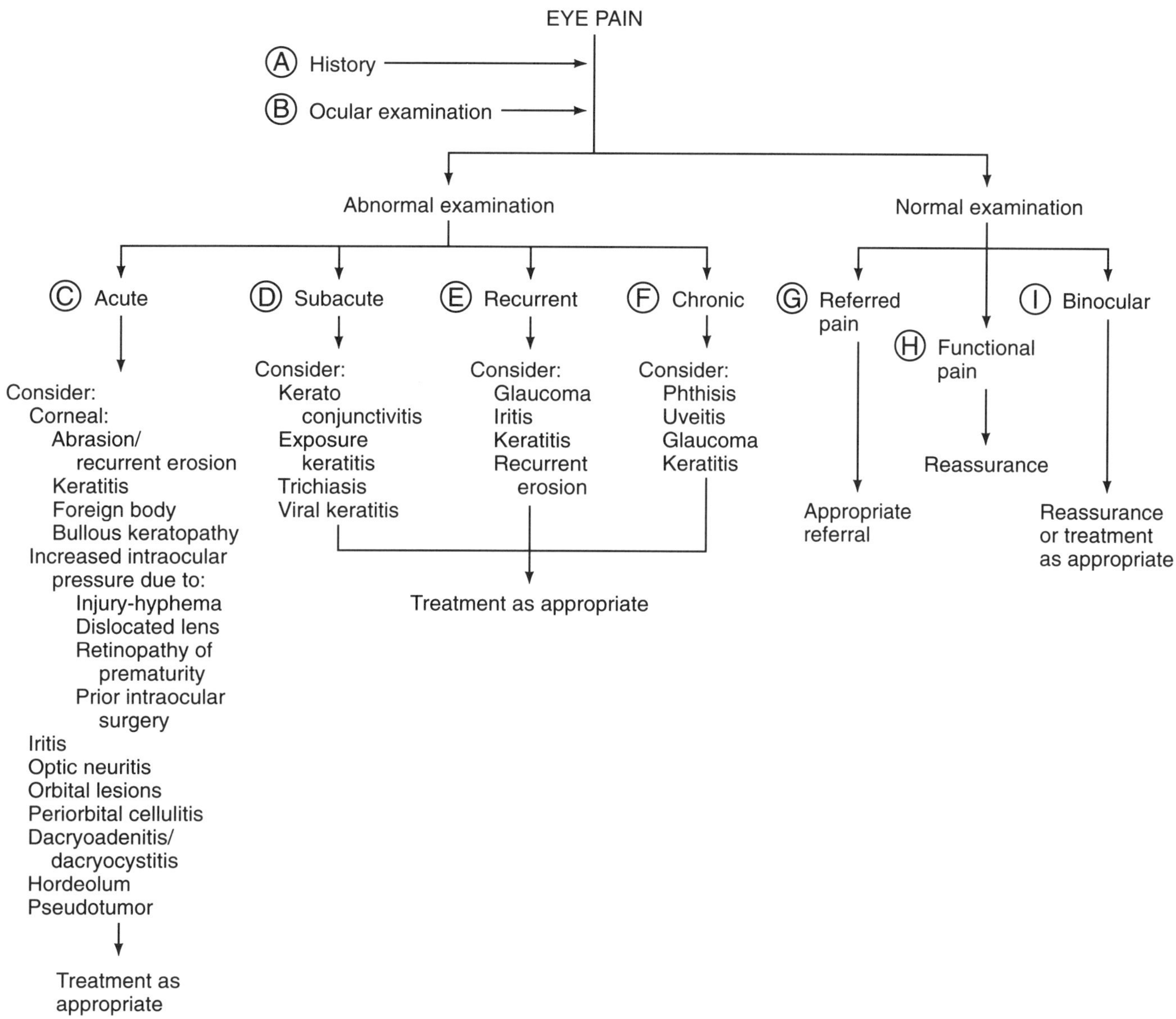

ment. Some patients with glaucoma may be sensitive to pressure elevations, and if the pressures are high and uncontrolled, they suffer from eye pain.

G. Severe acute ocular or periocular pain unaccompanied by any detectable signs on ophthalmologic examination may be secondary to intraorbital or retro-orbital pathology. Tumors or space-occupying lesions may press on the fifth cranial nerve, causing recurrent trigeminal neuralgia of short duration. If a child appears to have severe pain of this type, careful neuroradiologic imaging of the fifth cranial nerve is indicated. Cluster or histamine headaches are also recurrent and may last for minutes only but are usually accompanied by tearing and injection of the eye and are rare in childhood.

H. The most common complaint of eye pain without accompanying signs is self-limited and probably functional. Parents usually report that a young preschool child complains of an eye hurting. However, the child does not appear to be in severe distress and there is no redness, tearing, or light sensitivity. Usually the child states that the eye hurts and resumes normal activities within minutes. The ophthalmologic examination is normal. When functional pain is suspected, conservative observation is indicated. Parents should be instructed not to question the child about whether the eye hurts, but simply to note the frequency of occurrence. They should also not show any undue concern or excessive sympathy when the complaint is voiced. If the episodes become more frequent or appear to be of increasing severity, re-evaluation is indicated.

I. Binocular eye pain or discomfort with reading or school work may be a complaint voiced by the school-aged child. In the absence of refractive errors, anisometropia, phorias, convergence insufficiency, and subnormal accommodative amplitudes, functional eye pain or aesthenopia is to be suspected. Significant refractive errors should be corrected; plus lenses may be prescribed if the child has subnormal accommodative amplitudes; orthoptics may be helpful in cases of convergence insufficiency. These, however, are unusual causes of eye pain or discomfort in childhood. The most frequent cause is functional or tension.

Reference

Taylor D. Pediatric ophthalmology. Cambridge, MA: Scientific, 1990:686.

MIGRAINES IN CHILDREN

Phillip L. Pearl, M.D.
Benjamin M. Frishberg, M.D.

Migraine is a recurring headache lasting 4 to 72 hours with at least two of the following features: unilateral location, pulsating quality, moderate or severe intensity, aggravated by activity, and associated with either photophobia and phonophobia or nausea and/or vomiting. It may be associated with an aura, typically visual, that builds up over minutes and lasts less than 1 hour. The incidence of migraine in children approached 6% in one large study, whereas the incidence of other headache types was 38% in 7 year olds and 70% in 15 year olds.

A. Although the acute onset of a new headache may represent a child's first migraine, other important considerations include subarachnoid hemorrhage, meningitis, concussion, sinusitis, systemic infection, toxic reaction, glaucoma, and hypertension. Chronic unremitting headaches do not represent migraine and require thorough evaluation to rule out tumors, arteriovenous malformation, hydrocephalus, pseudotumor cerebri, infection, vasculitis, and psychiatric causes. An imaging study, either MRI or CT with contrast, would likely be included in the evaluation of most unremitting chronic headaches. The examination should include funduscopy, cranial nerves, sinus palpation, blood pressure, a check for meningismus, and a brief general physical examination. Any ill-appearing patient deserves a more thorough examination.

B. The definition of migraine is outlined in the introduction. Other common historic features include a positive family history, motion sickness, specific triggers, ice pick pain, and ice cream headaches. The most common type of headache in children is the episodic tension headache. These headaches last from 30 minutes to 7 days, are not associated with nausea and vomiting, may have either photophobia or phonophobia but not both, are typically bilateral, nonthrobbing, and mild to moderate in severity, and worsen with physical activity. Any headache pattern falling outside the definition of migraine or tension headaches should be strongly considered for cranial reimaging (MRI or CT with contrast).

C. Worrisome features of childhood headaches include awakening with headache, personality change, headaches always on the same side, prolonged aura, aura occurring during or after the headaches, or any significant change in headache pattern. Any atypical or worrisome features should lead to a cranial imaging study (MRI or CT with contrast).

D. Abortive therapy may be instituted with the use of combination analgesics such as acetaminophen with codeine or acetaminophen with butalbital and caffeine (Fioricet), or with vasoconstrictor agents such as Midrin and Cafergot. Nonsteroidal anti-inflammatories such as naproxen sodium (Anaprox) are also often effective. If nausea and vomiting are a problem, metoclopramide (Reglan) or promethiazine (Phenergan) may be very helpful. The key to abortive therapy is immediate treatment at the onset of symptoms.

E. Prophylactic agents are used daily to prevent migraine. Calcium-channel blockers such as verapamil and nifedipine and beta-blocking agents such as propranolol and metoprolol are often very effective in substantially reducing the frequency and intensity of headaches. Other agents that may be useful in children include cyproheptadine (Periactin), phenytoin, valproic acid, and amitriptyline.

F. Nonpharmacologic therapies include life-style adjustments, regular meal and sleep habits, and avoidance of activity overload. Biofeedback therapy may be useful. Psychotherapy is indicated in the setting of a disturbed home life or other psychopathology. Reassurance that children with migraine frequently enjoy remission within 6 months is a mainstay of treatment.

G. Ophthalmologic abnormalities that may be seen as part of migraine include visual field defects indicating migraine-related stroke, unilateral pupillary mydriasis that may be benign or related to subtle oculomotor nerve palsy, and complete or partial oculomotor nerve palsy. Ophthalmoplegic migraine is a distinctly rare syndrome and is a diagnosis of exclusion. Any patient with a focal neurologic or neuro-ophthalmologic deficit requires an appropriate imaging study, either MRI or CT with contrast, as well as referral to an appropriate specialist (neurologist, neuro-ophthalmologist, neurosurgeon).

References

Barlow CF. Headaches and migraine in childhood. Philadelphia: JB Lippincott, 1984.

Bille B. Migraine in school children. Acta Pediatrica 1962; 51(Suppl 136).

Forsythe I, Hockaday JM. Management of childhood migraine. In: Hockaday JM, ed. Migraine in childhood. London: Butterworths, 1988:63.

Oleson J. The classification and diagnosis of headache disorders. Neurol Clin 1990; 793.

Rothner AD. Diagnosis and management of headache in children and adolescents. Neurol Clin 1983; 1:511.

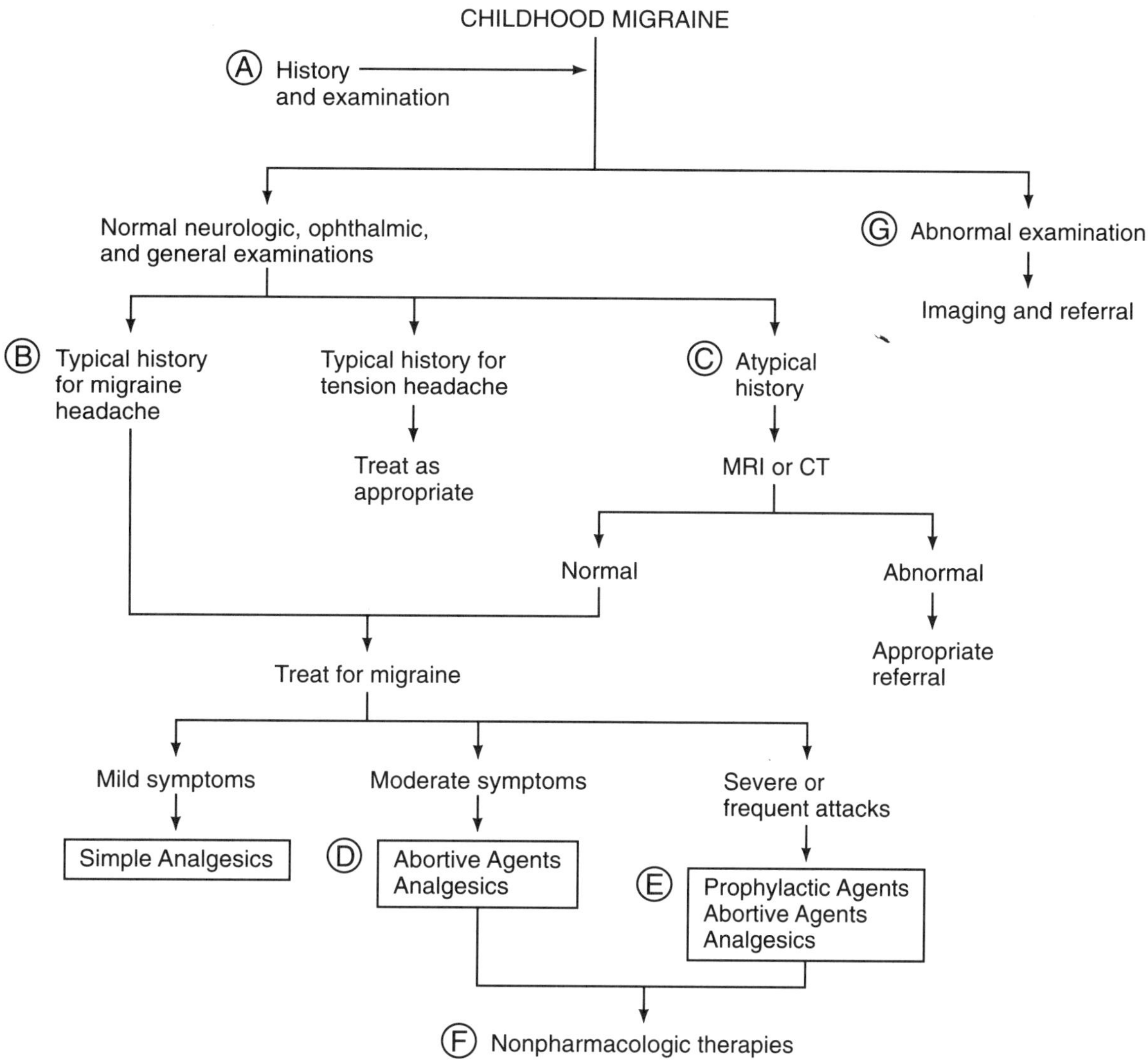
CHILDHOOD MIGRAINE
(A) History and examination
Normal neurologic, ophthalmic, and general examinations
(G) Abnormal examination
Imaging and referral
(B) Typical history for migraine headache
Typical history for tension headache
Treat as appropriate
(C) Atypical history
MRI or CT
Normal
Abnormal
Appropriate referral
Treat for migraine
Mild symptoms
Moderate symptoms
Severe or frequent attacks
Simple Analgesics
(D) Abortive Agents Analgesics
(E) Prophylactic Agents Abortive Agents Analgesics
(F) Nonpharmacologic therapies

THE RED EYE

Merrill L. Stass-Isern, M.D.

A. The red eye may have many possible causes, with minor to major vision-threatening capabilities. A careful history including information on trauma, possible foreign bodies, allergies, a history of systemic diseases (e.g., juvenile rheumatoid arthritis [JRA]), contact lens use, family eye health, and prior surgery should be reviewed. Slit-lamp examination provides the most diagnostic clues.

B. A history of a foreign body may not always be present, especially in the younger child. Slit-lamp examination along with eversion of the eyelid is mandatory. Corneal burring should be performed for residual rust rings. Cycloplegia, topical antibiotics, and pressure patching are recommended for any residual deficits following removal or burring.

C. When other causes have been eliminated and conjunctivitis is the diagnosis, a good history as well as physical examination helps pinpoint the cause. For example, other family members with "pink eye" incriminates adenovirus (epidemic keratoconjunctivitis); systemic allergies with watery, burning eyes point to an allergic cause. Bacterial conjunctivitis is usually associated with a mucopurulent discharge (p 164). Parinaud's oculoglandular syndrome causes a unilateral granulomatous follicular conjunctivitis associated with preauricular and submandibular lymphadenopathy. The cause is usually unknown but may be associated with cat-scratch fever. The patient usually has fever, malaise, and a mucopurulent discharge. The diagnosis usually requires conjunctival biopsy. Treatment is then tailored to the specific causative agent.

D. Blepharitis may cause a secondary conjunctivitis (p 162). A bacterial cause as well as demodex and phthiriasis of the lid should be considered. A vesicular lesion may herald a primary herpetic eruption. Treatment with trifluorothymidine (Viroptic) is reasonable (p 170).

E. A keratitis may be seen in association with a retained foreign body, secondary to exposure as occurs with seventh cranial nerve palsies, following radiation therapy, or in association with conjunctivitis such as that which occurs with adenovirus, chlamydial, or staphylococcal marginal ulcerative disease. Typical dendritic eruption occurs with herpes simplex and herpes zoster. Involvement of the tip of the nose (Hutchinson's sign) often precedes ophthalmic involvement in herpes zoster. Treatment for herpes simplex is topical Viroptic. Steroids are avoided and cycloplegia may relieve photophobia and ciliary spasm. Treatment for herpes zoster is systemic Zovirax as well as topical cycloplegia and a topical antibiotic-steroid combination.

Occasionally a corneal ulcer is the cause of a red eye. This is associated with pain and commonly results from misuse of contact lenses. It requires immediate culturing and Gram's stain. Frequent topical antibiotics should be tailored to Gram's stain and ultimately to culture results.

F. Ninety percent of endophthalmitis cases occur after trauma or an elective surgery. Occasionally endogenous endophthalmitis occurs, such as from subacute bacterial endocarditis (SBE). Intense pain, photophobia, and diminished vision are present. Preorbital edema, an intense conjunctival reaction, uveitis, and corneal edema are associated with endophthalmitis. Prompt diagnostic taps of the anterior chamber and/or vitreous are necessary to salvage the eye. Topical subconjunctival and/or intravitreal antibiotics are then used according to bacterial type (pp 248, 250, 252).

G. A subconjunctival hemorrhage is painless. A history of an upper respiratory infection with sneezing and coughing or a Valsalva-type mechanism should be elicited. Most frequently, no specific cause is found. A bleeding diasthesis should be checked. No treatment is necessary because spontaneous resolution occurs. Occasionally, subconjunctival hemorrhages may be associated with a conjunctivitis, the most frequent offender being adenovirus.

H. A history of JRA or other arthropathies, ulcerative colitis, sarcoidosis, or trauma may help pinpoint a cause. Both anterior and posterior cells should be checked for (pp 214, 220).

I. Clinically, children with glaucoma present with epiphora, photophobia, and blepharospasm. Examination may reveal increased corneal diameter, corneal edema, and conjunctival injection. An evaluation under anesthesia (EUA) is usually required for the diagnosis. The glaucoma can be primary congenital, associated with congenital anomalies, or secondary to trauma (pp 312, 314, 316).

References

Cobo LM. Oral acyclovir in the therapy of acute herpes zoster ophthalmaicus: An interim report. Ophthalmology 1985; 92:1574.

Jones DB. Initial therapy of suspected microbal corneal ulcers. II: Specific antibiotic therapy based on corneal smears. Surv Ophthalmol 1979; 24:105.

Macke IA. Neuroparalytic (neurotrophic keratitis). In: Black CJ. Symposium on C.L. St Louis: Mosby–Year Book 1973; 125.

Wear DJ. Cat scratch disease bacilli in the conjunctiva of patients with Parinaud's oculoglandular syndrome. Ophthalmology 1985; 92:1282.

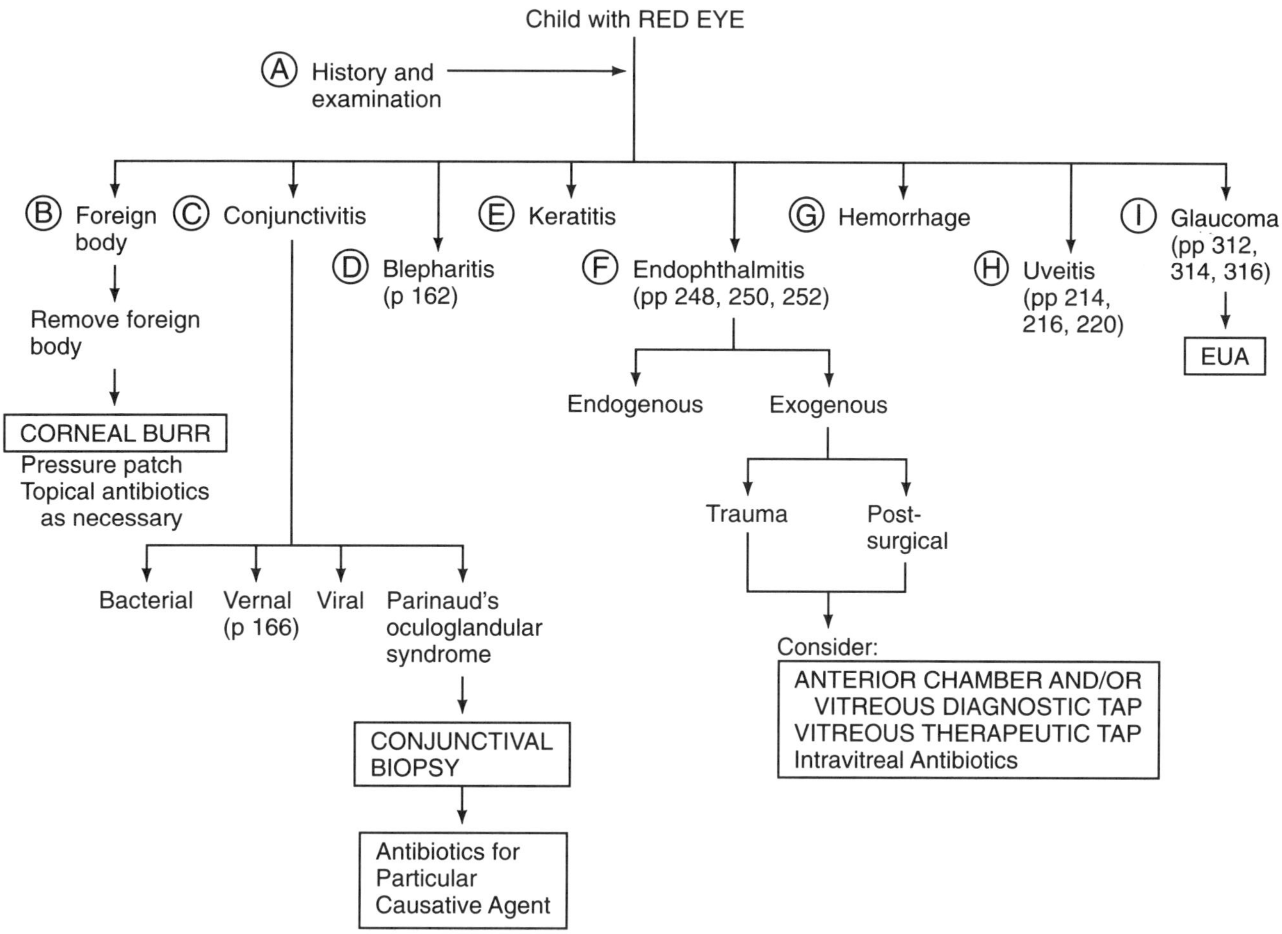
Child with RED EYE
(A) History and examination
(B) Foreign body
Remove foreign body
CORNEAL BURR
Pressure patch
Topical antibiotics as necessary
(C) Conjunctivitis
Bacterial
Vernal (p 166)
Viral
Parinaud's oculoglandular syndrome
CONJUNCTIVAL BIOPSY
Antibiotics for Particular Causative Agent
(D) Blepharitis (p 162)
(E) Keratitis
(F) Endophthalmitis (pp 248, 250, 252)
Endogenous
Exogenous
Trauma
Post-surgical
Consider:
ANTERIOR CHAMBER AND/OR VITREOUS DIAGNOSTIC TAP
VITREOUS THERAPEUTIC TAP
Intravitreal Antibiotics
(G) Hemorrhage
(H) Uveitis (pp 214, 216, 220)
(I) Glaucoma (pp 312, 314, 316)
EUA

CLINICALLY SUSPECTED ENDOPHTHALMITIS

Roy D. Brod, M.D.
Harry W. Flynn, Jr., M.D.

A. A detailed history and ophthalmologic examination are important in all cases of clinically suspected endophthalmitis. The history of a preceding, predisposing event and the time course of symptom onset are important in categorizing the type of endophthalmitis into known subgroups. The subgroups (acute postoperative, delayed-onset postoperative, post-traumatic, and endogenous) are important in determining the initial management approach. The classic symptoms of endophthalmitis include ocular pain, loss of vision, and floaters, and the presenting signs often include lid edema, conjunctival injection, and anterior chamber and vitreous inflammation with hypopyon and fibrin formation. Other, more specific, ophthalmologic findings may be helpful in predicting a specific causative agent.

B. Acute postoperative and post-traumatic endophthalmitis typically occur within days after intraocular surgery or trauma. The time course and degree of inflammation depend primarily on the causative organism. *Staphylococcus epidermidis,* the most common organism isolated from cases following cataract surgery, produces a less fulminant inflammatory response than other gram-positive or gram-negative organisms. *Bacillus cereus* is the most common cause of post-traumatic endophthalmitis. This ubiquitous gram-positive rod produces a rapidly progressive destructive form of endophthalmitis. Rapid diagnosis and treatment are crucial in preventing severe visual loss in these two forms of endophthalmitis.

C. Once a diagnosis of acute exogenous endophthalmitis is suspected, the degree of ocular involvement should be assessed. Slit-lamp biomicroscopy and indirect ophthalmoscopy are used to determine the degree of anterior and posterior segment inflammation. When a severe anterior segment inflammatory reaction obscures visualization of the posterior segment, ultrasonography can be useful in assessing the degree of vitreous involvement and the status of the retina (attached or detached).

D. If the inflammatory response involves only the anterior chamber, a conservative initial approach to treatment is prudent. Because a noninfectious cause is likely in such cases, topical corticosteroids and cycloplegics should be used as the initial management approach. Frequent observation is crucial to detect a worsening course, which is indicative of an infection. If the anterior chamber inflammatory reaction worsens without evidence of vitreous involvement, a diagnostic anterior chamber tap is performed. If vitritis is seen during the course of topical corticosteroid therapy, a diagnostic pars plana vitrectomy in addition to an anterior chamber tap is recommended. Depending on the degree of suspicion for an infectious cause, topical, periocular, and intraocular antibiotics and steroids can be administered.

E. The degree of vitreous inflammatory response is important in determining the appropriate therapeutic option at this point. When moderate (no fundus detail but red reflex present) or severe (no red reflex) vitritis is observed, an immediate pars plana vitrectomy combined with intraocular and periocular antibiotics and steroids is indicated for both diagnosis and therapy. The vitreous specimen should be sent to the laboratory for bacterial stains and culture. In most cases of acute postoperative endophthalmitis, the organism is unknown at the time of surgery and broad-spectrum antibiotic coverage is required. A recommended intraocular antibiotic regimen includes vancomycin 1.0 mg/0.1 cc and ceftazidime 2.25mg/0.1cc. In addition, 400 μg of dexamethasone sodium phosphate per 0.1 cc is also injected into the vitreous cavity. Periocular injections of vancomycin 25 mg, ceftazidime 100 mg, and dexamethasone sodium phosphate 4 to 12 mg are also administered. Postoperative treatment with topical antibiotics and corticosteroids is begun approximately 24 hours after therapy (the next morning). Dosages used are for adults. Pediatric dosages may be modified according to weight.

If only mild vitritis is present at initial examination (detailed fundus view possible), topical corticosteroids, antibiotics, and close observation and a diagnostic vitreous tap are appropriate management options depending on the index of suspicion for infectious endophthalmitis. If the inflammatory response worsens during the course of observation, one can proceed with a diagnostic and therapeutic pars plana vitrectomy combined with appropriate corticosteroid and antibiotic therapy, as mentioned above.

References

Flynn HW Jr, Pflugfelder SC, Culbertson WW, et al. Recognition, treatment and prevention of endophthalmitis. Semin Ophthalmol 1989; 4:69.

Greenwald MJ, Wohl LG, Sell CH. Metastatic bacterial endophthalmitis: A contemporary reappraisal. Surv Ophthalmol 1986; 31:81.

Mieler WF, Ellis MK, Williams DF, Han DP. Retained intraocular foreign bodies and endophthalmitis. Ophthalmology 1990; 97:1532.

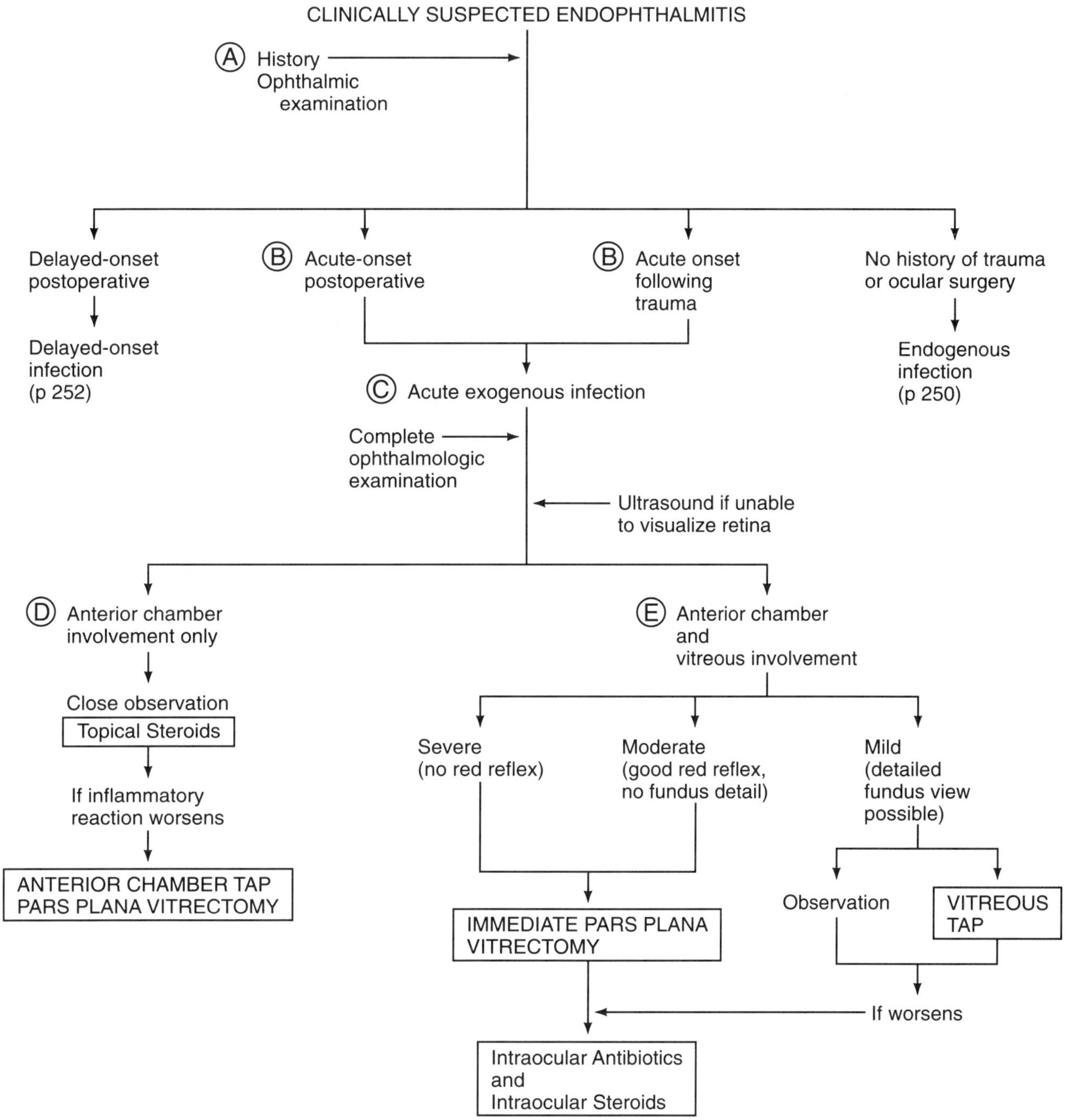
CLINICALLY SUSPECTED ENDOPHTHALMITIS
Ⓐ History
Ophthalmic examination
Delayed-onset postoperative
Delayed-onset infection (p 252)
Ⓑ Acute-onset postoperative
Ⓑ Acute onset following trauma
No history of trauma or ocular surgery
Endogenous infection (p 250)
Ⓒ Acute exogenous infection
Complete ophthalmologic examination
Ultrasound if unable to visualize retina
Ⓓ Anterior chamber involvement only
Close observation
Topical Steroids
If inflammatory reaction worsens
ANTERIOR CHAMBER TAP
PARS PLANA VITRECTOMY
Ⓔ Anterior chamber and vitreous involvement
Severe (no red reflex)
Moderate (good red reflex, no fundus detail)
Mild (detailed fundus view possible)
Observation
VITREOUS TAP
IMMEDIATE PARS PLANA VITRECTOMY
If worsens
Intraocular Antibiotics and Intraocular Steroids

SUSPECTED ENDOGENOUS ENDOPHTHALMITIS

Roy D. Brod, M.D.
Harry W. Flynn, Jr., M.D.

A. A detailed history, physical examination, and appropriate laboratory studies, particularly blood cultures, are crucial in confirming the diagnosis of suspected endogenous endophthalmitis. A high index of suspicion must be maintained, especially when one or more predisposing conditions are identified (see Table 1).

B. Fungi are a more common cause of endogenous endophthalmitis than bacteria, and *Candida* is the most common fungus isolated in endogenous endophthalmitis. Clinical features that help distinguish fungal from bacterial infection include slow onset, fluffy yellow or white vitreous opacities, and, particularly in the case of *Candida* infection, creamy white chorioretinal infiltrates.

C. The treatment of fungal endophthalmitis depends on two factors: the presence or absence of fungemia or other organ involvement and the location and degree of the ocular inflammatory response. When systemic infection is identified, intravenous amphotericin B is often the drug of choice and should be administered by an infectious disease specialist. When chorioretinal infiltrates are present with only minimal vitreous involvement, local ocular therapy (other than topical corticosteroids) may not be needed. On the other hand, when moderate to severe vitritis is observed, a pars plana vitrectomy combined with intraocular instillation of amphotericin B (5 μg) is recommended.

D. In the absence of systemic fungal infection, when only chorioretinal infiltrates with no or mild vitritis is present, an oral antifungal agent (azole compounds) may be curative. We prefer either ketoconazole or fluconazole. In very mild cases, observation without any treatment may suffice because spontaneous resolution may occur. If a more severe vitritis is present, pars plana vitrectomy and intraocular amphotericin B (5 μg) are recommended. Patients are also treated with either fluconazole or ketoconazole postoperatively.

TABLE 1 Predisposing Factors for Endogenous Endophthalmitis

Intravenous hyperalimentation	Malignancy
Prolonged antibiotic therapy	Diabetes mellitus
Systemic corticosteroids	Massive trauma
Immunosuppressive therapy	Hepatic insufficiency
Abdominal surgery	Cardiac abnormality
Hemodialysis	Prematurity
Acquired immunodeficiency syndrome	Genitourinary manipulation

E. Endogenous bacterial endophthalmitis is a rare cause of ocular inflammation but must be considered in debilitated persons, especially those with known systemic infection or immunosuppression. This form of endophthalmitis also occurs in intravenous drug abusers, and attention to this during the history and physical examination is important. The clinical features are similar to those of acute postoperative bacterial endophthalmitis and include rapid onset of both anterior chamber and vitreous inflammation and, in some cases, a chorioretinal abscess.

F. As with the other subgroups of endophthalmitis, the treatment varies with the degree of infection. In all cases of endogenous bacterial endophthalmitis, systemic antibiotic therapy is indicated and should be tailored to the specific bacteria when possible. Again, an infectious disease specialist should be consulted to help determine the appropriate systemic antibiotic. In cases with chorioretinitis and minimal vitritis, intravenous antibiotic therapy may be the only treatment necessary. These patients must be followed closely, however, and a worsening course may require a diagnostic and therapeutic pars plana vitrectomy, as well as intraocular and periocular antibiotics and steroids.

G. When moderate to severe vitritis occurs in suspected endogenous bacterial endophthalmitis, systemic therapy should be supplemented with local ocular therapy, including pars plana vitrectomy and intraocular and periocular antibiotics and steroids. Cultures of a vitreous specimen should be obtained to confirm the causative organism.

H. One must also consider other causes of vitreous cellular infiltration, including toxocariasis, toxoplasmosis, uveitis secondary to juvenile rheumatoid arthritis, par planitis retinoblastoma, and old vitreous hemorrhage, in the differential diagnosis.

References

Brod RD, Clarkson JG, Flynn HW Jr, Green EW. Endogenous fungal endophthalmitis. In: Tasman W, Jaeger EA, eds. Clinical ophthalmology. Vol. 3. Philadelphia: JB Lippincott, 1991.

Flynn HW Jr, Pflugfelder SC, Culbertson WW, et al. Recognition, treatment and prevention of endophthalmitis. Semin Ophthalmol 1989; 4:69.

Greenwald MJ, Wohl LG, Sell CH. Metastatic bacterial endophthalmitis: A contemporary reappraisal. Surv Ophthalmol 1986, 31:81.

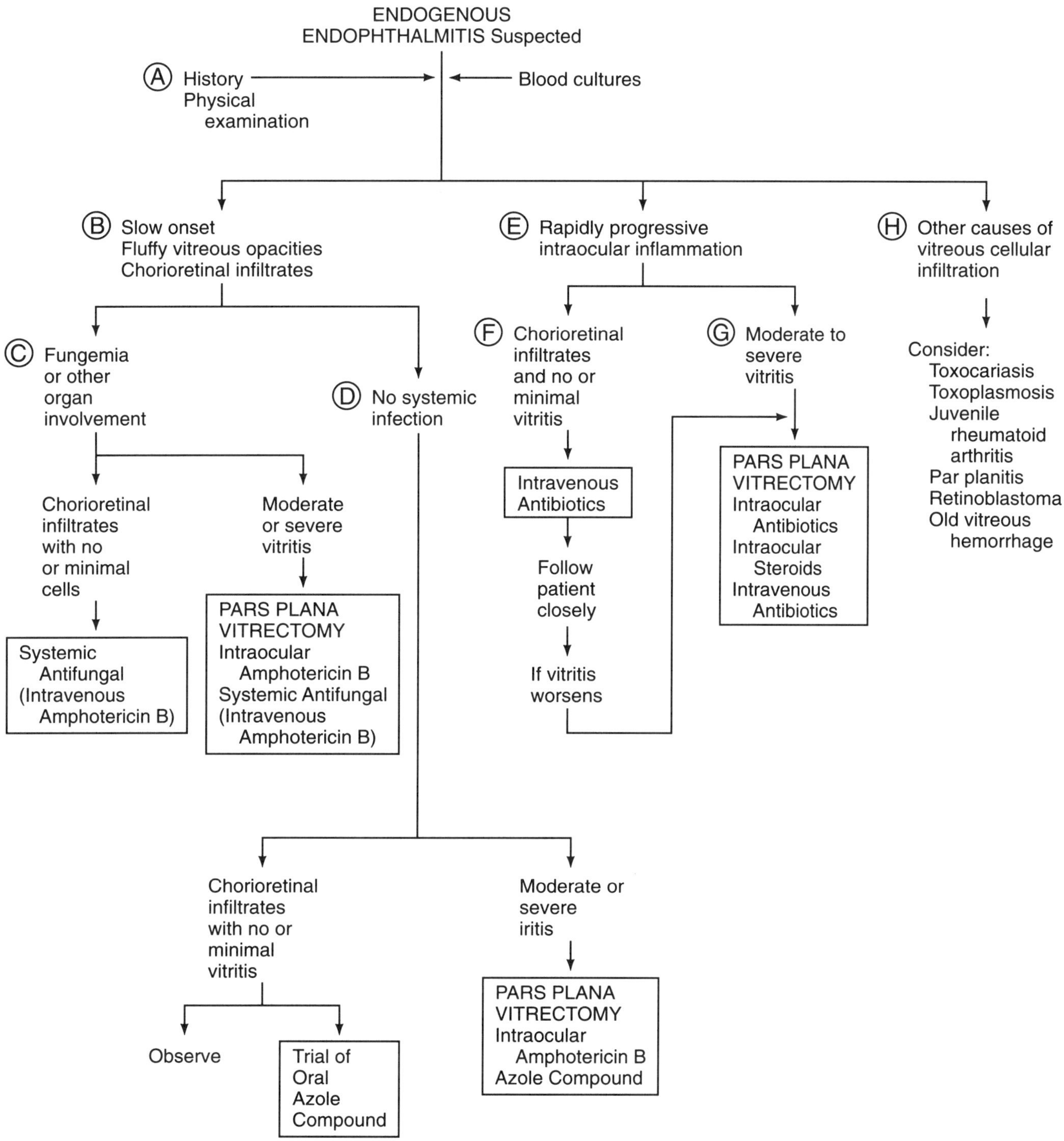
ENDOGENOUS ENDOPHTHALMITIS Suspected
(A) History
Physical examination
Blood cultures
(B) Slow onset
Fluffy vitreous opacities
Chorioretinal infiltrates
(C) Fungemia or other organ involvement
Chorioretinal infiltrates with no or minimal cells
Systemic Antifungal (Intravenous Amphotericin B)
Moderate or severe vitritis
PARS PLANA VITRECTOMY
Intraocular Amphotericin B
Systemic Antifungal (Intravenous Amphotericin B)
(D) No systemic infection
Chorioretinal infiltrates with no or minimal vitritis
Observe
Trial of Oral Azole Compound
Moderate or severe iritis
PARS PLANA VITRECTOMY
Intraocular Amphotericin B
Azole Compound
(E) Rapidly progressive intraocular inflammation
(F) Chorioretinal infiltrates and no or minimal vitritis
Intravenous Antibiotics
Follow patient closely
If vitritis worsens
(G) Moderate to severe vitritis
PARS PLANA VITRECTOMY
Intraocular Antibiotics
Intraocular Steroids
Intravenous Antibiotics
(H) Other causes of vitreous cellular infiltration
Consider:
Toxocariasis
Toxoplasmosis
Juvenile rheumatoid arthritis
Par planitis
Retinoblastoma
Old vitreous hemorrhage

DELAYED-ONSET POSTOPERATIVE ENDOPHTHALMITIS

Roy D. Brod, M.D.
Harry W. Flynn, Jr., M.D.

A. Delayed-onset endophthalmitis is a postoperative inflammatory response occurring more than 3 weeks after surgery. This broad category of postoperative endophthalmitis is broken down into two subgroups based on observed clinical findings. These two categories include cases with or without an observed external entry site.

B. Careful inspection of the surgical ocular wound is important in identifying features that may predispose to entrance of bacteria into the eye. These wound changes include filtering blebs, suture abscesses, vitreous-wick syndrome, and wound fistula. In this category of delayed-onset postoperative endophthalmitis, the degree of vitritis is important in guiding therapy. If the vitreous inflammation is mild or moderate, management includes culturing the wound abnormality and broad-spectrum periocular and topical antibiotic administration. Close observation is required to identify and appropriately manage a worsening course. If severe vitritis is present, one should proceed with a diagnostic and therapeutic pars plana vitrectomy, intraocular and periocular antibiotics, and steroids. The surgical wound abnormality is cultured and surgically repaired.

C. When there is no visible observed external entry site, several possible causes for the postoperative intraocular inflammation exist. A detailed ophthalmologic examination may in some cases give clues to the cause.

D. Fluffy white vitreous opacities and chorioretinal infiltrates are typical clinical findings in fungal endophthalmitis. In the presence of these clinical features, fungal infection must be considered. If the vitritis is mild, either the eye can be closely observed or empirical treatment with an oral antifungal agent can be begun. We prefer either ketoconazole or fluconazole in these cases. If the inflammatory response worsens or if the patient presents with a moderate or severe initial inflammatory response, a diagnostic and therapeutic pars plana vitrectomy is indicated. The fluffy white vitreous opacities should be specifically removed and sent for fungal stains and culture. The results of the fungal smear are helpful intraoperatively, especially if fungal elements are seen. In such cases, intravitreal amphotericin B (5 μg) is injected. If the stains are negative for fungal elements but a high index of suspicion for fungal endophthalmitis remains, amphotericin B can be injected into the vitreous cavity. If there is uncertainty as to whether infection is bacterial or fungal, both amphotericin B and broad-spectrum antibiotics are injected. The use of intraocular steroids in fungal infection is controversial, although no clear evidence exists that it has a deleterious effect.

E. A smoldering, chronic, mild to moderate inflammatory response in the presence of large keratitic precipitates and a white capsular plaque is typical of *Propionibacterium acnes* infection. Infection with this anaerobic gram-positive, pleomorphic bacillus is increasingly recognized as a cause of delayed-onset chronic endophthalmitis. In suspected cases the initial management approach should include a pars plana vitrectomy with selective removal of the white capsular material combined with intraocular and periocular vancomycin and dexamethasone sodium phosphate. In cases refractory to this initial management approach a total capsulectomy combined with intraocular lens removal or exchange may be curative.

F. Retained lens material following cataract surgery may lead to phacoanaphylactic uveitis. This diagnosis should be suspected when retained lens fragments are observed in either the anterior or posterior segment. When mild to moderate inflammation is present, topical corticosteroids are recommended. If the inflammatory response is more severe, a pars plana vitrectomy combined with the removal of the retained lens material should be performed.

G. When a nonspecific cellular inflammatory response occurs weeks after intraocular surgery, infection with bacteria of relatively low virulence is likely. It is difficult, if not impossible, to distinguish this from other causes of uveitis. The recommended treatment approach in these cases includes a trial of topical corticosteroids initially. If the inflammatory response worsens during treatment, a diagnostic pars plana vitrectomy with or without intraocular antibiotic injection should be considered.

References

Flynn HW Jr, Pflugfelder SC, Culbertson WW, et al. Recognition, treatment and prevention of endophthalmitis. Semin Ophthalmol 1989; 4:69.

Fox GM, Joondeph BC, Flynn HW Jr, et al. Delayed-onset pseudophakic endophthalmitis. Am J Ophthalmol 1991; 111:163.

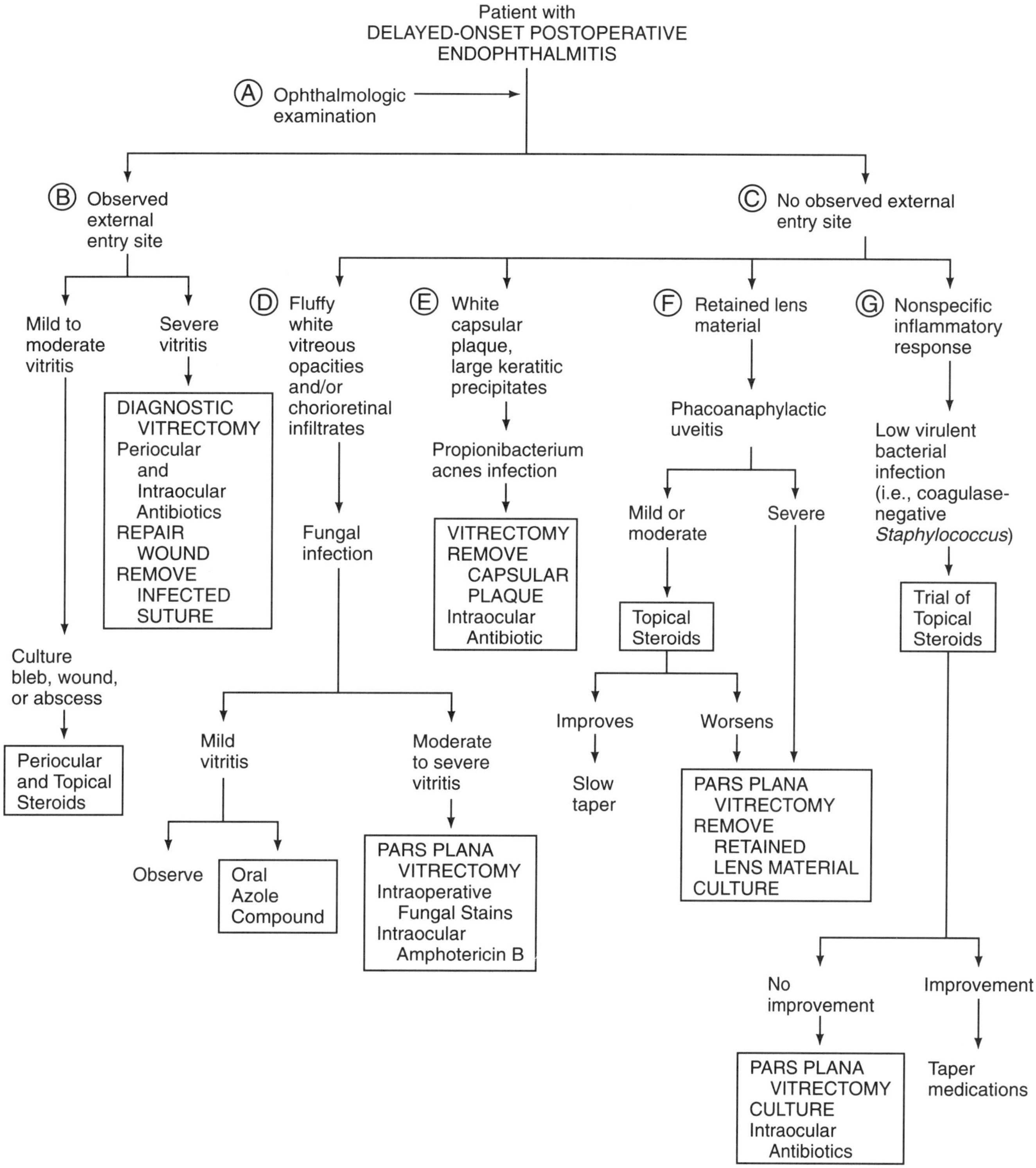
Patient with
DELAYED-ONSET POSTOPERATIVE ENDOPHTHALMITIS
(A) Ophthalmologic examination
(B) Observed external entry site
Mild to moderate vitritis
Severe vitritis
DIAGNOSTIC VITRECTOMY
Periocular and Intraocular Antibiotics
REPAIR WOUND
REMOVE INFECTED SUTURE
Culture bleb, wound, or abscess
Periocular and Topical Steroids
(C) No observed external entry site
(D) Fluffy white vitreous opacities and/or chorioretinal infiltrates
Fungal infection
Mild vitritis
Observe
Oral Azole Compound
Moderate to severe vitritis
PARS PLANA VITRECTOMY
Intraoperative Fungal Stains
Intraocular Amphotericin B
(E) White capsular plaque, large keratitic precipitates
Propionibacterium acnes infection
VITRECTOMY
REMOVE CAPSULAR PLAQUE
Intraocular Antibiotic
(F) Retained lens material
Phacoanaphylactic uveitis
Mild or moderate
Severe
Topical Steroids
Improves
Slow taper
Worsens
PARS PLANA VITRECTOMY
REMOVE RETAINED LENS MATERIAL
CULTURE
(G) Nonspecific inflammatory response
Low virulent bacterial infection (i.e., coagulase-negative Staphylococcus)
Trial of Topical Steroids
No improvement
PARS PLANA VITRECTOMY
CULTURE
Intraocular Antibiotics
Improvement
Taper medications

CONTACT LENSES

Andrea Cibis Tongue, M.D.

A. Indications for contact lens wear in children are no different from those in adults. Many preteens and teens choose to switch from spectacles to contact lenses for cosmetic reasons. Some very young children are put in contacts because of sports activities, special self-esteem concerns, or unilateral aphakia. Unilateral aphakia should be corrected with a contact lens whenever possible because spectacle correction causes a significant aniseikonia. The same is true for the correction of high nonaxial anisometropia. Some patients with unilateral or bilateral high refractive errors achieve better visual acuity with contact lenses than with spectacles.

Lenses should not be prescribed solely to retard myopia. There are no definitive data that contact lenses slow the progression of myopia. Patients generally tolerate small refractive changes better with contact lenses than with glasses and therefore may not need to have their contact lens power changed as frequently as they would with glasses. However, patients who experience substantial increases of their myopic refractive error do so with or without contact lenses.

B. The fitting of contact lenses in children is the same as that in adults. Contacts are fit by trial, with the initial lens choice based on the patient's keratometry readings and refractive error. Multiple lens choices are now available, and astigmatic patients can be fitted with soft or rigid gas-permeable lenses. Contact lens filters should have lenses of different parameters and materials available in order to achieve the best possible fit in their patients.

A few patients do not achieve an acceptable visual acuity level or develop problems secondary to contact lens wear. Problems such as giant papillary conjunctivitis (GPC) and keratitis in soft contact lens wearers may be minimized by using disposable lenses and having the patient wear them for only 2 weeks. Frequent enzyme cleaning and more frequent replacement of the lens may be necessary if a disposable lens is not used. Switching to a gas-permeable lens from a soft contact lens may also be helpful.

C. Young children should not be expected to clean and take care of their contact lenses; that should be a parental responsibility. The choice of a soft or gas-permeable lens for fitting initially may depend partly on the practitioner's preferences and experiences. Cleaning methods are relatively comparable but still slightly more involved with soft lenses than with gas-permeable lenses. The life expectancy of the lenses is comparable, although soft lenses sustain deposits more readily and there is a higher incidence of GPC. Gas-permeable lenses are easier to insert and correct small to moderate astigmatic refractive errors, whereas spherical soft lenses usually do not. Extended wear of lenses is not recommended in children, except for cases of unilateral aphakia in infancy if insertion and removal is difficult for the parent and traumatic for the infant. Most parents, however, master the technique of insertion and removal if the benefits of daily removal and the potential complications of extended wear are explained to them.

D. All patients who wear contact lenses should be warned that contact lenses are foreign bodies on the eye and that complications can occur which could result in loss of vision and potentially even loss of the eye. Proper hygiene and prompt attention to any symptoms decrease the risk of serious complications. Teenagers particularly need to warned not to wear their lenses if they develop pain, redness, tearing, irritation of the eyes, or decreased vision. If symptoms persist after the lenses are removed or recur when the lenses are worn, the patient needs to be seen by an ophthalmologist. Proper hygiene and care of the lenses need to be re-emphasized as well.

E. Evaluation of complications requires a thorough external examination and a history of the contact lens care products and procedure the patient uses. The history needs to establish the onset, duration, and frequency of symptoms, thereby allowing the ophthalmologist to make an educated guess as to the cause of the problem.

Visual acuity assessment, external examination, slit-lamp examination with fluorescein, keratometry, evaluation of tear film, and Schirmer test are the most informative parts of the ophthalmologic examination. The lenses need to be examined as well to look for deposits, tears, or defects. The tarsal conjunctiva of the upper lid particularly should be examined when GPC is suspected or symptoms such as injection, discomfort, and tearing are present. The cornea needs to be evaluated with and without fluorescein. Soft contact lenses may cause a keratitis of the superior cornea, hidden by the lid and not easily appreciated without fluorescein. Punctate keratitis at 3 and 9 o'clock in rigid gas-permeable lens wearers is also often not appreciated unless fluorescein is used.

Keratometry readings are helpful not only to follow the corneal curvature changes but to evaluate the clarity of the mires. Distorted mires indicate a problem with fit. In case of decreased visual acuity, refraction with and without contacts should be performed. If visual acuity is correctable to 20/20 over the contact lens, the visual change is due to a refractive change. If the acuity cannot be corrected to 20/20 over the contact, one needs to consider a problem with the contacts themselves, such as coating, or changes in the cornea, such as irregular astigmatism or corneal edema secondary to hypoxia.

Conjunctival injection may be due to an allergic reaction to the solutions used to clean or soak the contact lenses. The preservative thimerosol has been

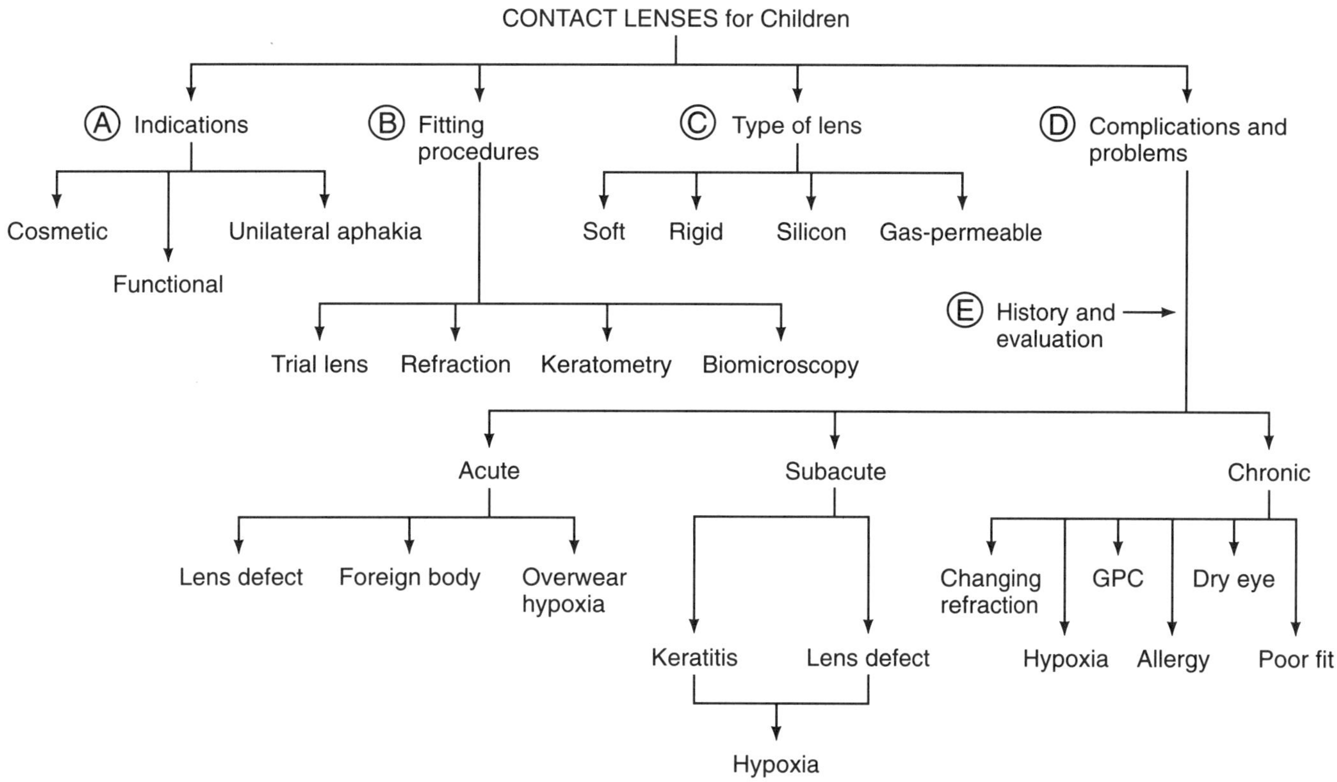

associated with allergic symptoms such as red, itchy eyes and has been implicated in the development of GPC in some patients. Injection of the conjunctiva may also be secondary to corneal hypoxia and keratitis and keratoconjunctivitis. Discomfort that occurs immediately upon insertion of the lens is usually secondary to a foreign particle or material on the lens or a torn or chipped lens. Corneal abrasions from the insertion process may also occur. Removal and rinsing of the lens usually removes the foreign material and the lens is comfortable upon reinsertion. If pain persists, abrasion or a lens defect should be suspected. Pain that develops after some hours of wear is usually secondary to hypoxia or keratitis sicca. Pain from superficial keratitis may not be appreciated until after the contact lens is removed, and pain from contact lens overwear may not occur until hours after removal. Patients with corneal ulcers usually complain of pain that has been present for a day or several days and worsens with time.

References

Eyeglasses for Infants and Children. Special Considerations. American Academy of Ophthalmology Public Education Brochure 6/90.

Halberg GP. Contact lenses for infants and children. In: Robison H. Pediatric ophthalmology. 2nd ed. Philadelphia: WB Saunders, 1983:1280.

Tongue A. Refractive errors in children. Pediatr Clin North Am 1987; 34:1425.

REHABILITATIVE CARE OF THE PEDIATRIC LOW VISION PATIENT

Donald C. Fletcher, M.D.
Mary Warren, M.S., OTR

After optimal medical and surgical options are exhausted, many children are left with a permanent reduction in vision. Their medical care is not complete until appropriate rehabilitation issues have been addressed and the best possible functional results obtained.

A. The functional history is different from a diagnostic interview. Here the focus is on consequences of vision loss rather than causes and cures. What is the impact of the visual deficit on the life of the individual? Ask questions about real-life tasks that the child is likely to encounter such as ability to ride a bicycle, play Nintendo, read the blackboard, participate in sports, or read a comic book. It is imperative to have parents in attendance and to listen to their input on the problems being encountered. It is also often helpful to have the child's school or special education teacher attend or offer input on the problems he or she has noted.

B. As the child ages, new and different visual tasks are encountered with differing visual demands. Periodic review allows for appropriate rehabilitation to be encouraged as it becomes indicated. It is also important to stress that even though the level of visual loss is permanent, other eye conditions may be encountered that further threaten remaining vision.

C. Small print access and other detailed close work are frequently encountered problems for the visually impaired. A valuable asset of children is their high accommodative amplitude. By holding the print or other task close to the face, sufficient magnification is often afforded to allow resolution. Parents should be reassured that this does not hurt the eyes. When this is not sufficient, additional magnification can be provided with low vision devices. High plus spectacles may be helpful and are often necessary for teenagers who could manage without them until they started to lose accommodative amplitude. Highest levels of magnification are accomplished by using video magnification systems (CCTV). Where print is not reasonably accessible using vision enhancement, vision substitution is necessary. For those requiring vision substitution, Braille is a useful skill, but these children should also be introduced to computers early in life. An excellent array of computer access technology is available for those with visual impairments.

D. Distance detail features of the environment are frequently difficult for the visually impaired youngster to appreciate. Children may not complain of difficulties in early youth because they may not be aware of what they are missing. An inexpensive pocket monocular telescope is often a useful device for the low-vision child to explore the world of distant objects. It also provides an inconspicuous, socially acceptable way for the teenager to spot signs.

E. Orientation and mobility difficulties are frequently a problem for children with decreased vision. Visual field deficits are traditionally recognized as the major culprit in travel difficulties. Decreased contrast sensitivity may also be a significant cause of problems for individuals with full peripheral fields. The instruction of a skilled orientation and mobility specialist is invaluable for these children; safe and effective travel is possible for the visually impaired child. Occupational therapists may also provide valuable input for the multiply handicapped child.

F. Although acquisition of daily living skills often receives less emphasis than the achievement of academic proficiency, mastering these skills is critical to achieving an independent life style and successfully entering competitive employment. Training should begin early with emphasis on acquiring age-appropriate skills. The preschool-aged child should receive instruction in basic self-care skills such as dressing, toileting, and eating. In adolescence, the emphasis should be placed on homemaking skills such as making a bed, preparing simple meals, clothing care, and laundry and on the skills needed to function independently in the community such as money management, use of public transportation, and shopping. Proper grooming and manners should be strongly emphasized at all ages because these skills are critical for peer acceptance. Acquisition of daily living skills provides the child with a sense of self-esteem and the confidence to pursue academic and career goals.

References

Faye EE. The low vision child. In: Clinical low vision. 2nd ed. Boston: Little, Brown & Company, 1984:437.

Hritcko T. Assessment of children with low vision. In: Jose RT, ed. Understanding low vision. New York: American Foundation for the Blind, 1983:105.

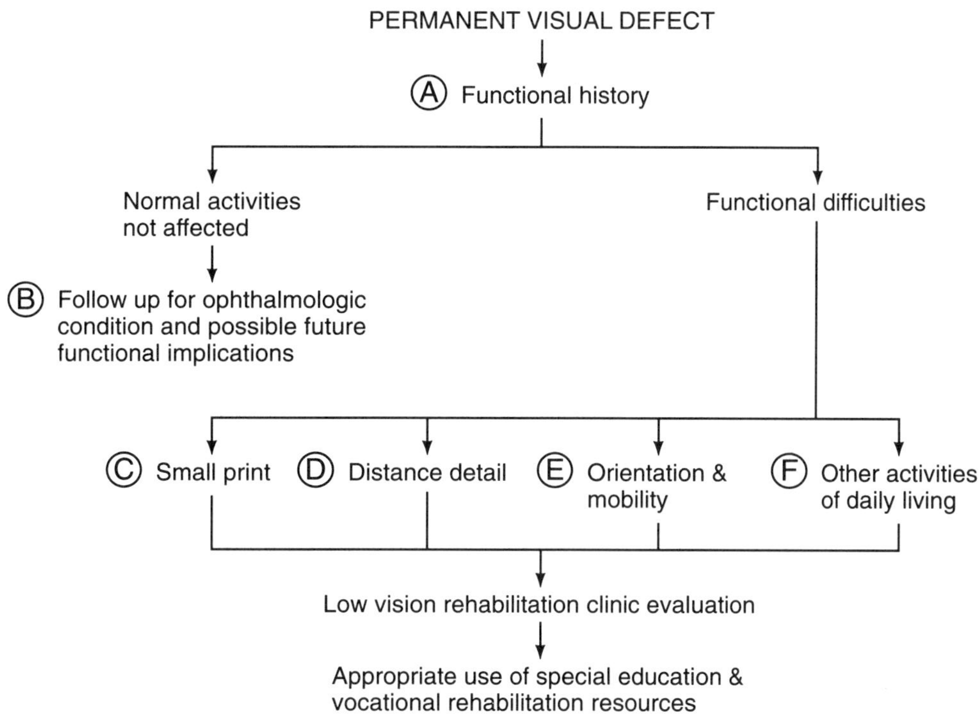
PERMANENT VISUAL DEFECT
(A) Functional history
Normal activities not affected
(B) Follow up for ophthalmologic condition and possible future functional implications
Functional difficulties
(C) Small print
(D) Distance detail
(E) Orientation & mobility
(F) Other activities of daily living
Low vision rehabilitation clinic evaluation
Appropriate use of special education & vocational rehabilitation resources

EYE TRAUMA

Susan H. Day, M.D.
John B. Jeffers, M.D.

A. Acute trauma involving the eye or affecting vision usually requires that an ophthalmologist be consulted. The severity of the injury often does not parallel the severity of the eye's appearance to an untrained observer. Often, a history indicates the nature of the trauma, which helps ascertain the most probable injury. Symptoms of visual involvement may provide a quick assessment of the area of injury.

B. Blunt trauma may be difficult to assess owing to the presence of lid swelling. Nevertheless, the globe itself must be very carefully examined because significant pathology may be present as well. When examination of more posterior structures is prevented by anterior pathology, other diagnostic tests such as ultrasonography, radiography, or neuroradiologic imaging may be indicated.

C. Sharp trauma often occurs as a consequence of common objects such as sharpened pencils, elastic book straps with metal fasteners, coat hangers, and compasses. It is critical to measure acuity of each eye because the path of the sharp object may affect the "uninvolved" side. In general, injuries related to sharp trauma require surgical exploration more often than those with blunt trauma.

D. A chemical splash in the eye is one of the most potentially devastating injuries one can suffer. Time is of the essence and therefore only a brief history of the fact that a chemical was involved need be obtained. This is one situation in which a visual acuity measurement is not obtained before any ocular examination.

E. In a hospital setting immediate treatment consists of irrigating the eye with either physiologic saline or lactated Ringer's solution. This may be accomplished with IV bottles and tubing such that a forceful stream can be maintained. Irrigation washes out the chemical

Continued on page 260

TRAUMA TO THE EYE

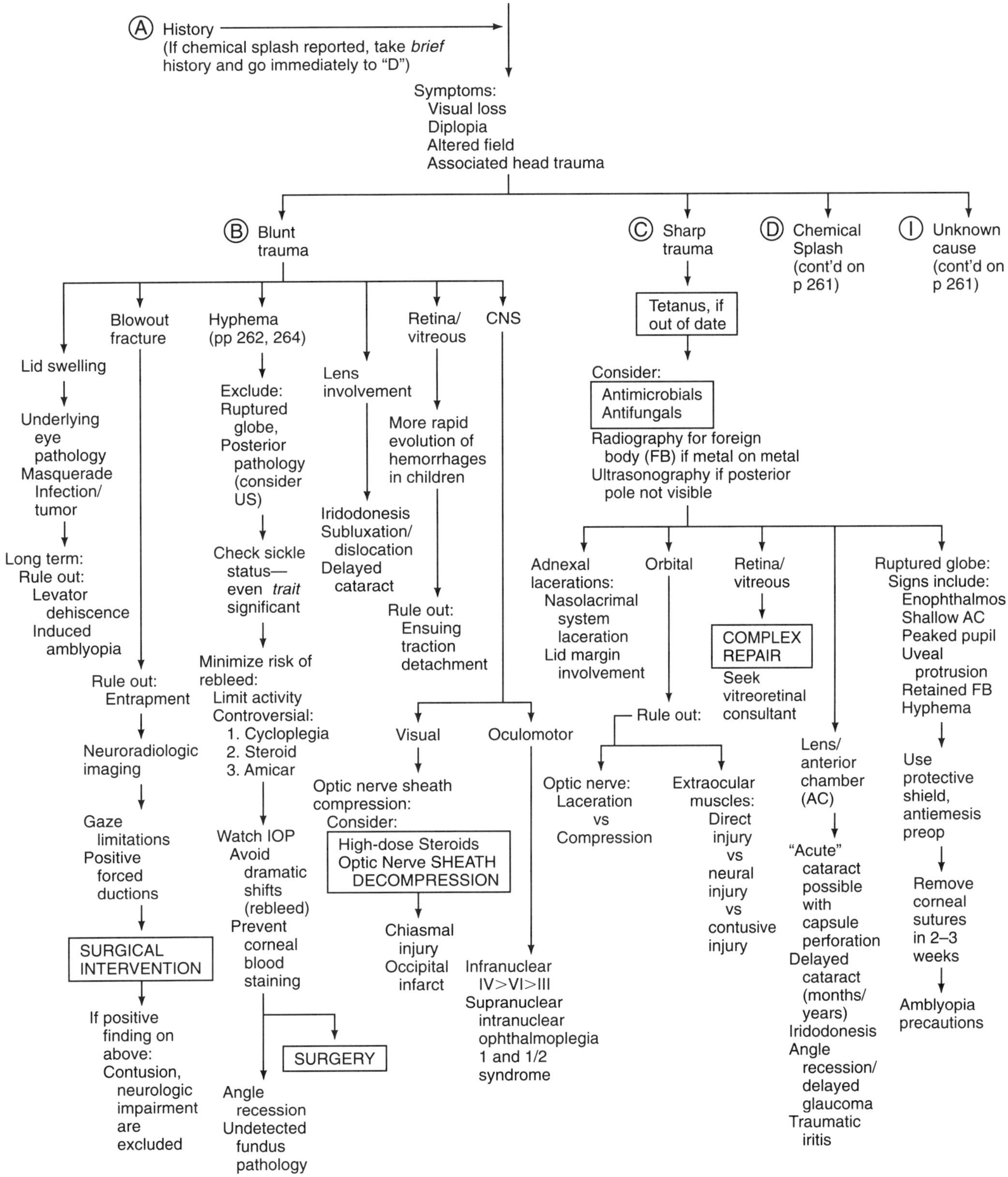

and the flushing mechanism of the stream removes particulate matter. It is essential that the upper lid be everted and cul-de-sac swept with a moist cotton-tip applicator to remove solid matter. The irrigant also dilutes the chemical. If IV fluids are not available, any liquid may be used, such as water from a specialized irrigating mechanism like a shower, fountain, or faucet, milk, iced tea, and so forth. Irrigation should be carried out for at least 30 minutes and a pH of 7.0 obtained. If the pH measures over 7.0, continued irrigation is necessary. Treatment may require 10 to 20 liters of fluid.

F. A more elaborate history of the events of the injury are then obtained, along with visual acuity (VA) measurement. If the patient is not ambulatory and cannot be measured by the Snellen chart, a near vision card or some form of measurable print (e.g., medication box) may be used while the patient is on a stretcher. An external and slit-lamp examination is then performed to evaluate the severity of the injury.

G. If the damage is considered mild to moderate with no conjunctival blanching, suggesting vascular integrity, the individual may be treated on an outpatient basis. The treatment involves topical cycloplegia, an antibiotic ointment, and application of a pressure patch for 24 hours. An analgesic of choice may be used as needed for pain. If the intraocular pressure (IOP) is elevated, consider utilizing a beta blocker.

H. If the ocular damage is considered severe, with conjunctival blanching suggesting vascular impairment, the individual should be treated on an inpatient basis. There may be need to debride necrotic tissue, followed by the instillation of cycloplegic, use of antibiotic ointment, and pressure patching. Some experts believe that topical steroids this early are not indicated. If the intraocular pressure is elevated, one would consider using a beta blocker. In the severe case, mechanical lysis of conjunctival adhesions with a glass rod may be necessary. A collagenase inhibitor may be helpful in severe cases.

I. When adults have not directly observed the occurrence of the injury or when the physical findings are not consistent with the history, other causes must be considered. Nonaccidental injury, bleeding dyscrasias, and rare tumors may present as an initial concern about possible trauma.

Reference

Grin TR, Nelson LB, Jeffers JB. Eye injuries in childhood. Pediatrics 1987; 80:13.

(cont'd from p 259)

- (B) Blunt trauma (see p 259)
- (C) Sharp trauma (see p 259)
- (D) Chemical splash
  - Symptoms:
    - Pain
    - Blurred vision
  - (E) Immediate treatment:
    - Irrigate with saline
    - Flush
    - Remove particulates
    - Evert upper lid
    - Sweep cul-de-sac
  - Test pH
    - pH>7.0
      - Continue irrigation → pH=7.0
    - pH=7.0
      - (F) Elaborate history
        - VA measurement
        - External examination
        - Slit-lamp examination
        - (G) Mild/moderate involvement, No conjunctival blanching
          - Outpatient therapy
          - Topical cycloplegia
          - Antibiotic ointment
          - Pressure patch for 24 hrs.
          - [Analgesic prn]
          - If elevated IOP, consider: [Beta Blockers]
        - (H) Severe involvement, conjunctival blanching
          - Inpatient therapy
          - Debride necrotic tissue
          - Cycloplegia
          - Topical antibiotic ointment/steroids
          - Pressure patch
            - If elevated IOP, consider: [Beta Blockers]
            - If severe
              - Mechanical lysis of adhesions
              - Collagenase inhibitors
- (I) Unknown cause
  - Rule out: Nonaccidental injury (p 108)
  - "Spontaneous hyphema"
    - Rule out:
      - Unsuspected trauma
      - Juvenile xanthogranuloma
      - Leukemia
  - "Raccoon eyes"
    - Rule out:
      - Neuroblastoma
      - Child abuse
  - Blindness/head injury
    - Rule out injury as red herring
    - Consider: Bilateral papillitis
      - Post-infectious
      - Post-immunization

TRAUMATIC HYPHEMA

Paul E. Romano, M.D., M.S.O.

A. Traumatic hyphema (TH) is a hemorrhage into the anterior chamber (AC) of the eye resulting from blunt trauma (simple, i.e., without corneal or scleral laceration). The size of the TH may vary from microscopic, visible by slit microscope as only a small crescent of dark blood in the inferior angle, to 100%, an "eight-ball" hyphema with complete filling of the AC with dark blood (resembling the black No. 8 billiard ball). Larger TH may extend into the posterior chamber (PC) and vitreous body. Because the incidence of rebleeding, visual loss, and other complications is not directly related to hyphema size, age, or race, all THs are treated the same.

The TH comes from torn vessels at the iris root. The greatest danger is from rebleeding episodes. These occur most frequently between the second and fourth day following trauma when the clot retracts.

Do not acutely dilate the pupil at the initial examination! This can and does precipitate rebleeding. If absolutely necessary, use atropine (see H below). *Acute dilatation is absolutely contraindicated.** Use ultrasonic echography, CT, or MRI as an alternate method of posterior pole examination.

B. Rule out (posterior) rupture of the globe. Signs include enophthalmos, pseudoblepharoptosis, marked softness of the globe, very low intraocular pressure (IOP), and subconjunctival bleeding. Use CT or MRI to confirm. A ruptured globe is a surgical emergency and must be repaired directly without regard to any coincidental TH.

C. Because the history of trauma is not always reliable, especially in very young children, consider the possibility of a *spontaneous hyphema* misidentified as traumatic. Retinoblastoma can present as a spontaneous hyphema. Juvenile xanthogranuloma can also present with a spontaneous hyphema.

D. Rule out sickle cell anemia or trait. In sickle disease or trait, the increased IOP results in a decreased perfusion pressure within vessels of the optic nerve and retina, with subsequent sludging and sickling of red blood cells in these vessels. The result of this is obstruction of flow and infarction of neuronal tissue. Therefore increases of IOP must be treated much more aggressively in children with sickle cell disease or trait. IOP must be measured frequently from presentation; if IOP exceeds 24 mm Hg for 24 hours, surgical intervention and "washout" are indicated.

E. The purpose of the initial treatment is to prevent rebleeding. Rebleeding and its complications are primarily responsible for poor outcomes in most reported series. Complications include glaucoma, optic atrophy, corneal blood staining, secondary amblyopia, and strabismus. All treatment items reduce the probability of a rebleed, without incurring significant medical risk. This treatment regimen prevents rebleeding in the critical 2- to 4-day postbleed period. It is *not* suspended or altered if the hyphema disappears before day 5.

F. *Hospitalization* for all patients *under the age of 18 years is mandatory*. In the hospital, recurrent accidental trauma from peers and siblings can be prevented, as well as accidental self-trauma. Hospitalization greatly improves adherence and compliance with medication and supportive treatment. It facilitates observation and follow-up examinations. It endorses the seriousness of a TH to the patient and family members. The expense of 6 days of hospitalization is justified on cost-benefit analysis.

G. Oral systemic prednisone or antifibrinolytics (aminocaproic acid [ACA]) greatly reduce or eliminate rebleeding (many studies). We recommend Yasuna's prednisone regimen; it is as effective in preventing rebleeds as ACA is but is much less expensive and has fewer contraindications and side effects. Note that the first dose should be a full day's medication of 0.6 mg/kg (a loading dose). It should be given as soon as possible—at the time of the initial examination and diagnosis in the emergency room or eye clinic (see Editorial note).

H. We recommend against pupil dilatation for 6 days or more. Examination of the posterior pole for retinal or choroidal trauma can be delayed. The best treatment for retinal/choroidal trauma is systemic steroids, which are already being given as treatment for TH (another reason to use steroids instead of ACA).

I. The antiplatelet effect of acetysalicylic acid (ASA) causes rebleeding. *ASA is absolutely contraindicated.*

J. Tonometry is unnecessary: One need treat IOP only when it is so high that one does not need a tonometer to recognize it. (An initial and transient [24 to 48 hours] mild IOP rise is common owing to angle blockage by red blood cells.) A healthy optic nerve can stand, without irreversible damage, an IOP of 50 mm Hg for 5 days, 45 for 7 days, or 35 for 14 days. A lesser IOP increase should therefore only be

---

*Editiorial note: The editors believe that several aspects of Dr. Romano's treatment regimen are controversial and would like to comment on the following points:

1. We routinely dilate all hyphemas with atropine 1%. We have yet to see this cause a bleed at the time of examination. Dr. Romano is warning against the use of rapidly acting dilating drugs such as Cyclogyl, Mydriacyl, and Neosynephrine.
2. Although there are many reported studies that agree with Dr. Romano's use of oral prednisone for the treatment of hyphema, it has not proven efficacious with our patients.
3. We routinely use Amikar (aminocaproic acid) and find that it does reduce the incidence of rebleed. Dosage: 50 mg/kg orally every 4 hours up to maximum daily dosage of 30 g/day. Continue for 5 days. Discontinue evening of 5th day. Observe, day 6.

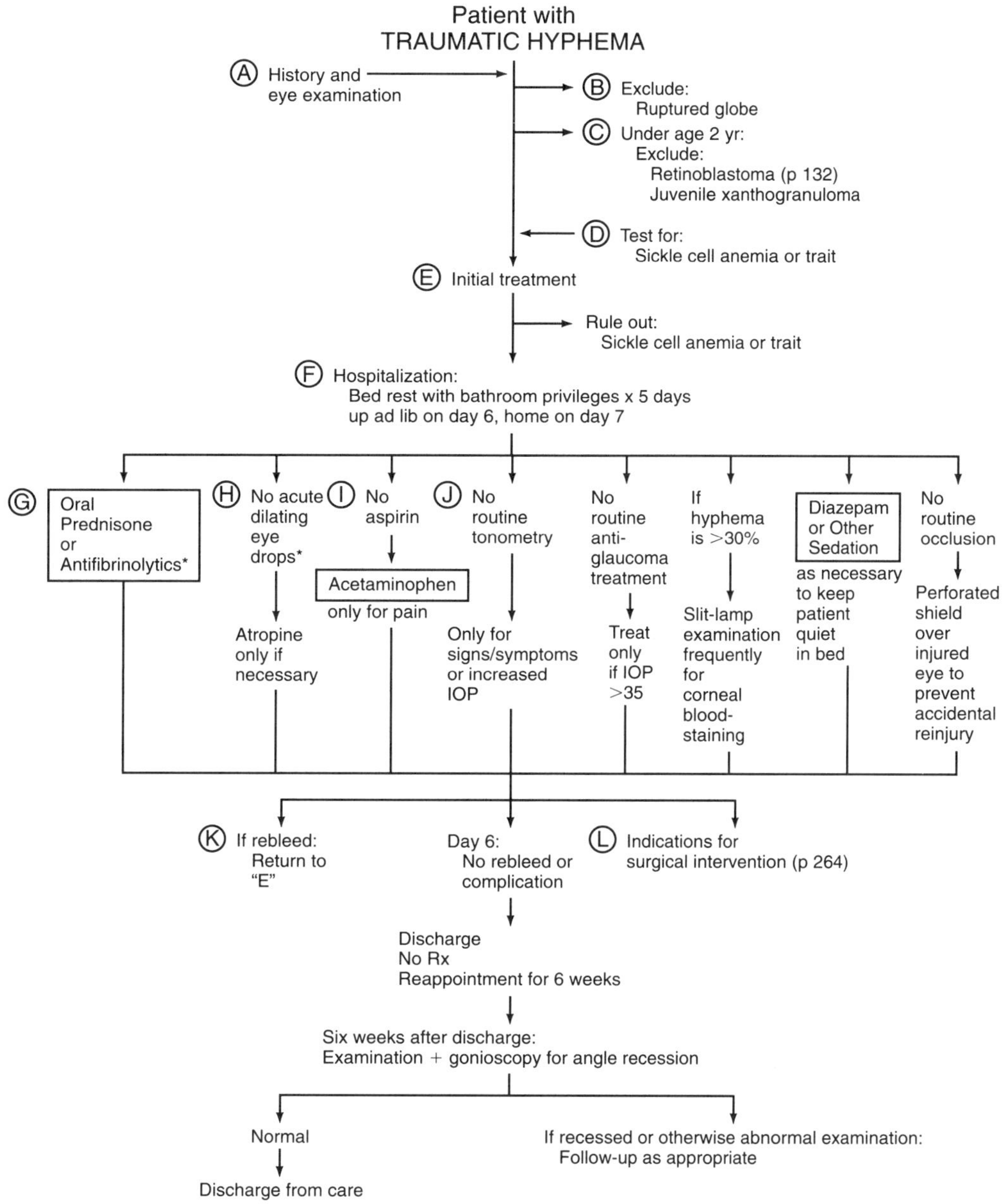

observed (not treated). If it exceeds those limits, use acetazolamide first. Acetazolamide must be used very cautiously in children with sickle cell disease or trait because it lowers the pH in the anterior chamber, increasing the propensity of hemoglobin (as red blood cells) to sickle. Methazolamide may be a better choice than acetazolamide because it raises the intracameral pH. Many topical IOP drugs cause iris movement, root stretching, and vascular congestion, any of which can lead to a rebleed. Considering the trauma of tonometry and the struggle one may encounter in performing tonometry in a child, we consider tonometry to be contraindicated, at least for the normally uncooperative younger child. However, if signs or symptoms suggest increased IOP, pressure must be measured.

K. If a rebleed occurs, start the protocol over again at the first day.

L. Indications for surgical intervention are discussed in the following chapter.

References

Farber MD, Fiscella R, Goldberg MF. Aminocaproic acid versus prednisone for the treatment of traumatic hyphema: A randomized clinical trial. Ophthalmology 1991; 98:279.

Goldberg MF. The diagnosis and treatment of sickled erythrocytes in human hyphemas. Trans Am Ophthalmol Soc 1978; 76:481.

Romano PE, Shuster JN. Traumatic hyphema. In: Fraunfelder FT, Roy FH, eds. Current ocular therapy 3. Philadelphia: WB Saunders, 1990:384.

Sears ML. Surgical management of black ball hyphema. Trans Am Acad Ophthalmol Otolaryngol 1970; 74:820.

Yasuna E. Management of traumatic hyphema. Arch Ophthalmol 1974; 91:190.

TRAUMATIC HYPHEMA NOT RESPONSIVE TO MEDICAL THERAPY

Paul E. Romano, M.D., M.S.O.

A. *Surgery is rarely needed for traumatic hyphema (TH). Medical therapy must be attempted first!* Surgery is difficult and replete with complications and poor visual results. Look for the indications described here.

B. Greater than 50% hyphema (up to "8-ball") for 4 days, without evidence of clearing, is associated with serious anterior chamber (AC) problems: extensive peripheral anterior synechiae, fibrin membranes, occluded/secluded pupil, and their sequelae.

C. Recurrent and/or uncontrollable rebleeding in spite of full medical treatment regimen. Rebleeding rarely occurs after any AC washout operation. Surgery tends to be curative.

D. Vision deprivation (any amblyogenic situation especially in children <6 years of age; consider to age 10 years); sequelae are loss of binocular vision and secondary strabismus at any age caused by (a) Corneal blood staining: once initiated, it is difficult to stop and impossible to remove by anything less than corneal transplant. Otherwise, it takes 2 years to clear spontaneously. (b) Vitreous blood staining: This creates retinal hazards and is a possible indication for vitrectomy.

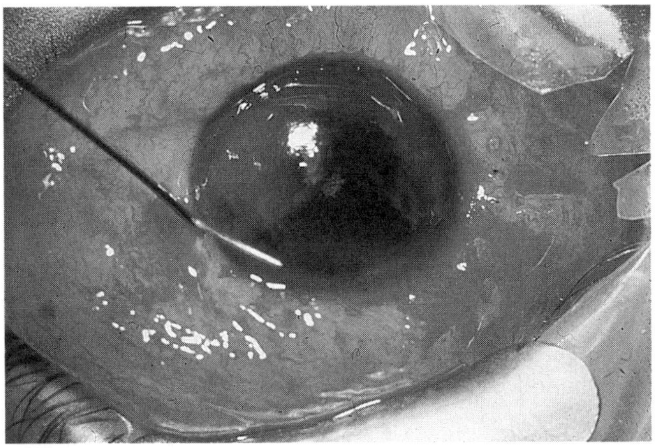

Figure 1 Attempt to wash out traumatic hyphema with chronic pressure elevation.

E. Increased IOP per se: >50 mm Hg for 5 days; >45 mm Hg for 7 days; >35 mm Hg for 14 days.

F. The surgery of choice is trabeculectomy ab externo and "washout." This gives an adequate AC access and avoids problems seen in children from wider limbal cataract extraction–type incisions. Trabeculectomy cures and prevents further IOP elevation. It provides safe, excellent, maneuverable access to AC without instruments entering the AC. (Very poor AC visibility typical of complicated unresolved TH creates a very high chance of surgical disaster, including accidental iridectomy, lens trauma, and cataract.) The "washout" can be partial and incomplete. It is *not* necessary to remove all the blood from the AC for surgery to be effective. Simply direct a forceful stream of fluid into the AC from the outside. It is unnecessary and hazardous to invade the AC with the irrigator tip or with Ocutomes or vitrectomy instruments to extract all clots. This can instead cause rebleeding.

G. All patients and parents need to be warned about the possibilities of further problems with glaucoma, cataracts, and retinal detachments.

References

Farber MD, Fiscella R, Goldberg MF. Aminocaproic acid versus prednisone for the treatment of traumatic hyphema: A randomized clinical trial. Ophthalmology 1991; 98:279.

Goldberg MF. The diagnosis and treatment of sickled erythrocytes in human hyphemas. Trans Am Ophthalmol Soc 1978; 76:481.

Romano PE, Shuster JN. Traumatic hyphema. In: Fraunfelder FT, Roy FH, eds. Current ocular therapy 3. Philadelphia: WB Saunders, 1990:384.

Sears ML. Surgical management of black ball hyphema. Trans Am Acad Ophthalmol Otolaryngol 1970; 74:820.

Yasuna E. Management of traumatic hyphema. Arch Ophthalmol 1974; 91:190.

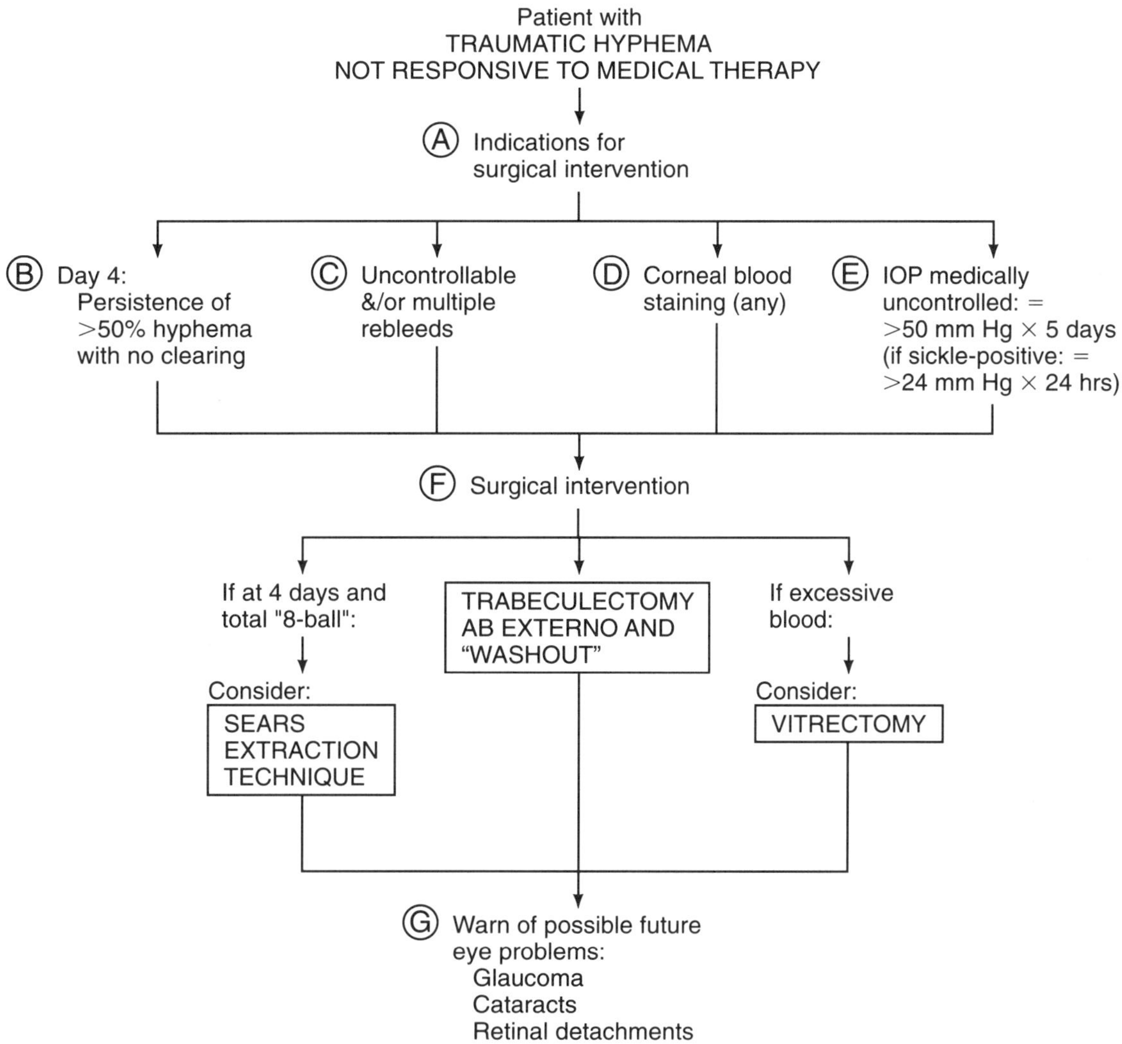
Patient with
TRAUMATIC HYPHEMA
NOT RESPONSIVE TO MEDICAL THERAPY
(A) Indications for surgical intervention
(B) Day 4: Persistence of >50% hyphema with no clearing
(C) Uncontrollable &/or multiple rebleeds
(D) Corneal blood staining (any)
(E) IOP medically uncontrolled: = >50 mm Hg × 5 days (if sickle-positive: = >24 mm Hg × 24 hrs)
(F) Surgical intervention
If at 4 days and total "8-ball":
Consider:
SEARS EXTRACTION TECHNIQUE
TRABECULECTOMY AB EXTERNO AND "WASHOUT"
If excessive blood:
Consider:
VITRECTOMY
(G) Warn of possible future eye problems:
Glaucoma
Cataracts
Retinal detachments

PEDIATRIC EYE SAFETY

John B. Jeffers, M.D.

A. Adequate protective eyewear for children in school (e.g., shop, laboratory) must meet or exceed ANSI Z87.1 (American National Standards Institute). Polycarbonate eye or face protection for sports activities must meet or exceed ASTM (American Society for Testing and Materials) standards.

B. **Contact lenses offer no eye protection.** Plano (no prescription) polycarbonate sports goggles should be worn for sports and plano safety spectacles for shop and laboratory activities. Under dusty/misty working conditions, contact lens wear may be contraindicated.

C. Polycarbonate is at least eight times stronger than any other material. If a complex prescription cannot be made of polycarbonate, then it should be made from CR-39 (plastic) with 3-mm center thickness. An added advantage of polycarbonate lenses is that they filter ultraviolet rays.

D. Goggles are safer than streetware glasses.

E. For laboratory, shop, and home, goggles (cover or cup) or industrial safety spectacles should be worn. Sideshields should always be attached to safety spectacles.

F. For protective eyewear to be effective, it must be appropriate and properly fitted. An experienced optician should be consulted. Some children have very narrow facial features that are difficult to fit. An excellent merchandising ploy has been the introduction of "neon colored" nose and temple cushions on some sports goggles, which has lessened the resistance of children to wearing sports goggles.

G. The functionally one-eyed child or one with eye disease that may result in weakened ocular tissue should always protect the eyes with appropriate eyewear. The functionally one-eyed child is one whose better eye corrects to 20/20 and whose worse eye corrects to less than 20/50. Full-time daily eye protection is essential. Use polycarbonate lenses, prescription or nonprescription, of 2-mm center thickness in a sturdy frame with a posterior lip to prevent dislodgement of lenses into the eye. If the strength of a prescription does not lend itself to be ground into polycarbonate, then CR-39 plastic should be used.

For sports or recreational activities (gym/recess) polycarbonate sports goggles with 3-mm center thickness should be worn. In sports that require a helmet and faceguard or shield, the sports goggles should be worn underneath.

TABLE 1 Organizations Standards for Protective Eyewear

Streetwear and industrial safety glasses/goggles/shields	American National Standards Institute (ANSI Z87-1) 1430 Broadway New York, NY 10018 (212) 354-3300
Baseball polycarbonate faceguard	American Society for Testing and Materials (ASTM F910-86) 1916 Race Street Philadelphia, PA 19103 (215) 299-5400
Racquet sports goggles	ASTM (F 803-88) Address as above
Hockey helmets and faceguards	ASTM (F513-86) Amateur Hockey Association of the United States (AHAUS) Hockey Equipment Certification Council (HECC) Canadian Standards Association (CSA)
Literature available from: American Academy of Ophthalmology P.O. Box 7424 San Francisco, CA 94120-7424 "Eye Safety for Children" National Society to Prevent Blindness 500 East Remington Road Schaumburg, IL 60173 1-800-221-3004 Request educational materials	

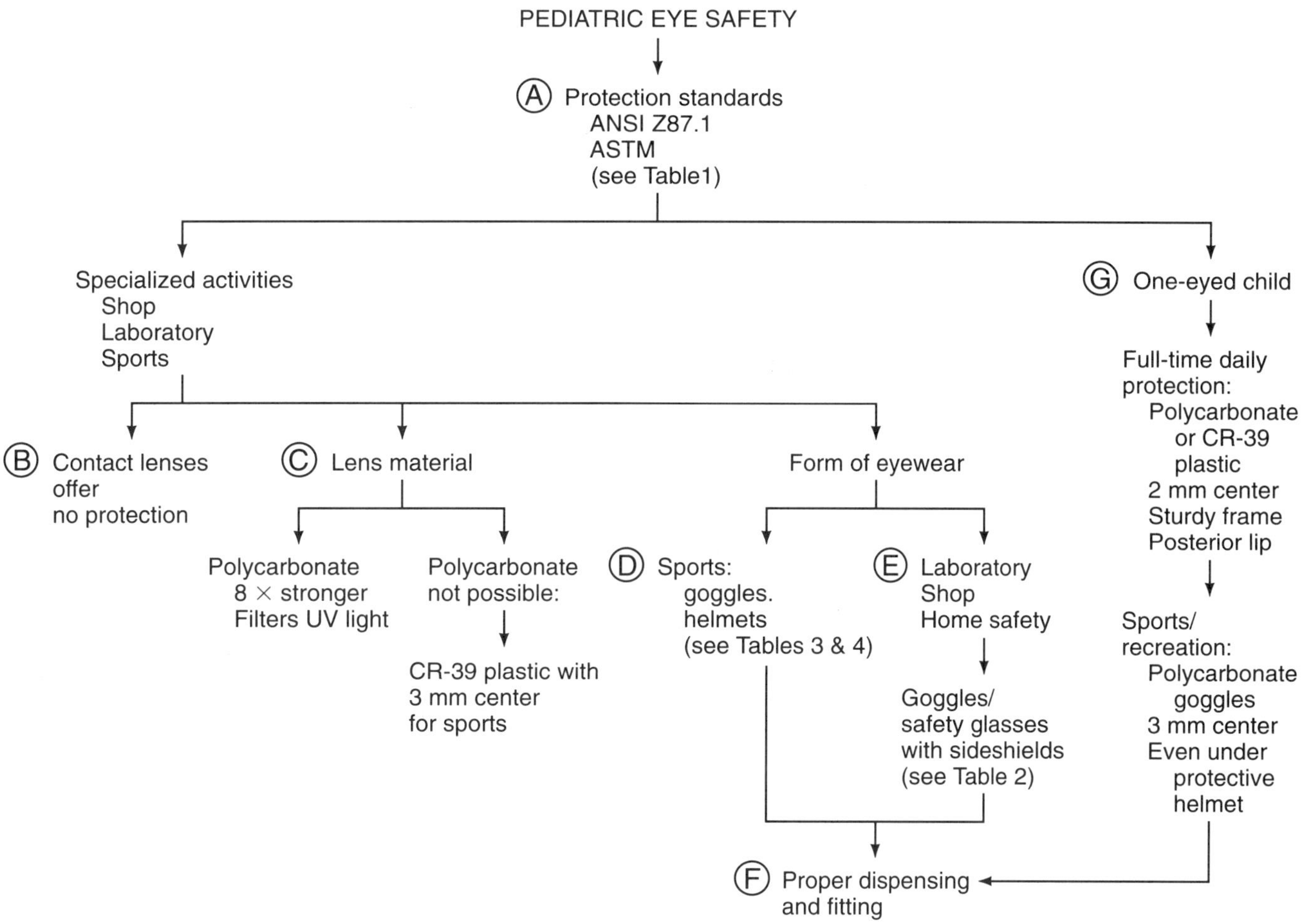

TABLE 2 Eye Injury Prevention

Activity	*Available Protection*
School	
A. Laboratory	
1. Splash (chemical, hot)	Goggles (cover or cup)
2. Explosion (glass)	Goggles (cover)
3. Laser	ANSI Z136.1 eye protectors
B. Shop (machinery)	
1. Woodworking	Industrial-strength spectacles (sideshields/cover goggles
a. Sawing	ANSI Z87.1)
b. Hammering	Industrial-strength spectacles (sideshields)
c. Chemical (solvents)	Goggles (cover or cup)
2. Metal	Industrial-strength spectacles (sideshields) and cover
a. Cutting	goggles
b. Hammering	Industrial-strength spectacles (sideshields)
3. Auto repair	Industrial-strength spectacles (sideshields) and cover goggles
4. Welding	Welding helmet with filter shield over industrial-strength spectacles
Home	
A. Chemicals	
1. Oven cleaner	Goggles (cover or cup)
2. Drain cleaner (alkali)	Goggles (cover or cup)
B. Hot splashes (grease)	Goggles (cover or cup)
C. Lawn/hedge work	Cover goggles
D. Hammering	Industrial-strength spectacles (sideshields)

Continued on page 268

TABLE 3 Sports Eye Injury Prevention

Activity	*Best Available Protection*	*Eye Injury Risk*	*Company (from Table 4)*
Baseball/softball	Batting helmet with polycarbonate face guard* (also for base running)	High	A
	Polycarbonate sports goggles for fielding		B, D, E, F, G, H
Basketball	Polycarbonate sports goggles	High	B, D, E, F, G, H
Racquetball, squash, badminton, tennis, handball	Polycarbonate sports goggles†	High	B, D, E, F, G, H
Football	Helmet with polycarbonate shield*	High	C
Hockey			
1. Organized ice	Helmet with full face protection*	High	
2. Unorganized ice or street hockey	Polycarbonate sports goggles		
	Goalie: helmet with full face (wire) protection. *Note:* Molded goalie mask can be penetrated by ball.		
Soccer	Polycarbonate sports goggles	High	B, D, E, F, G, H
Volleyball	Polycarbonate sports goggles	High	B, D, E, F, G, H
Lacrosse (boys'/men's)	Helmet with full face protection*	High	B, D, E, F, G, H
Lacrosse/field hockey (girls'/women's)	Should wear polycarbonate sports goggles (are discouraged from wearing)	High	B, D, E, F, G, H
Track and field	Streetwear (polycarbonate preferable)‡	Low	J, K
Skiing	Polycarbonate ski goggles	High	B
Cycling	Streetwear (polycarbonate preferable)‡	Low	J, K
Swimming/water sports	Polycarbonate swim goggles	High	B, D, F
Boxing/wrestling/full-contact martial arts	None available	Very high eye risk without available protection	

*One-eyed child should *also* wear polycarbonate sports goggles (also child who has history of intraocular surgery/eye disease that may weaken ocular tissue).
†Lenseless goggles ineffective.
‡ANSI 287 acceptable but polycarbonate is stronger material.

TABLE 4 Pediatric Sports Safety Eyewear

Model	*Prescription Capable*	*Company Name, Address, and Phone Number*
A. Polycarbonate Face Guard* (baseball)	No	Face Guard Incorporated P.O. Box 8425 Roanoke, VA 24014 800-336-9683
B. Essex	No	LSP Leader Sports Products, Inc. 675 N. Margaret St. Suite 14 Plattsburg, NY 12901 800-847-2001
Troy	Yes	
Albany	No	
Westport Jr. Champ (Swim)	No	
C. Vision Plus (Football)	No	LSP Leader Sports Products, Inc.
D. Jr. Rec-Specs (neon colors)‡	Yes	Liberty Optical 380 Verona Avenue Newark, NJ 07104 800-444-5010
Pro-Guard	Yes	
All-Pro	Yes	
Sport Goggle	Yes	
Swim goggles	Yes	
E. Action Eyes	Yes	Black Knight (Viking Sports) 5355 Sierra Road San Jose, CA 95132 800-283-2635
F. Regent	No	Ektelon 8929 Aero Drive San Diego, CA 92123 800-854-2958
Swim goggles	No	
Interceptor	No	
G. Sports Specs	No	Herslof Optical 12000 W. Carmen Avenue Milwaukee, WI 53225 800-558-7073
H. R.E.P.* (small and large)	Yes	Eagle Eyewear P.O. Box 486 Whitehouse, NJ 08888 908-236-9300
J. American Optical Safety Division of Cabot Safety	Yes	14 Mechanic Street Southbridge, MA 01550 800-982-2828
K. Titmus Company	Yes	P.O. Box 191 Petersburg, VA 23804 800-446-1802

*Tints available: plain, smoke
†Kids "love" neon colored nose and temple cushions—are more apt to wear

IMAGING APPROACH TO THE CHILD WITH PROPTOSIS WITHOUT INFECTION

Thomas L. Slovis, M.D.
John D. Baker, M.D.
Cristie Becker, M.D.

A. When a child presents with unilateral proptosis, a contrast-enhanced CT scan (CECT) should be the first imaging study. The major considerations are those of a mass.

B. When no mass is seen, there are many reasons for the presence or appearance of proptosis. A larger eye may result from unilateral megophthalmos with no pathology, congenital glaucoma, or a high degree of unilateral myopia. Pseudoproptosis may occur from the contralateral eye being smaller or microphthalmic, ptosis, or retraction of the contralateral eye as in Duane syndrome. Exophthalmos caused by thyroid disease, although common in adults, is seen infrequently in children.

C. MRI is the ideal tool to evaluate the extent of tumor, as the orbital apex, optic canal, and chiasm are easily seen. The technical factors important in MRI are:
   1. Planes of scan—sagittal, axial with appropriate angle for the nerve and chiasm, and coronal
   2. Pre- and postcontrast—gadolinium scans
   3. Head coil and 5-mm section
   4. Types of images
      a. T1—Short relaxation time (TR) and excitation time (TE), an anatomic image. The CSF appears black.
      b. T2—Long TR and TE, pathologic image. The CSF appears white.
      c. Fat suppression techniques after gadolinium

   In general, our MRI approach to the child with an orbital mass (almost any location) would be the following sequence: Sagittal T1 and axial T2 runs are done first. The best plane or planes to demonstrate the pathology are selected for pregadolinium T1 imaging. Then the postgadolinium T1 scans and fat suppression images are done in the best plane(s). In most instances the best plane is angled axial.

D. Masses within the orbit are arbitrarily divided by their anatomic location. Many masses are found in more than one location. The intraconal region is that between the four rectus muscles and the anterior extent is the globe. The most common intraconal lesion is an optic nerve glioma. Twenty-five to 50% of children with optic nerve glioma have neurofibromatosis, but only 15% of neurofibromatosis patients develop optic nerve glioma(s) (Fig. 1). However, if only type 1 neurofibromatosis is considered, the incidence of optic nerve glioma is much higher; bilateral optic nerve glioma is pathognomonic of neurofibromatosis type 1.

   Once the diagnosis of an enlarged optic nerve is made on CT, MRI is the best test to fully define the

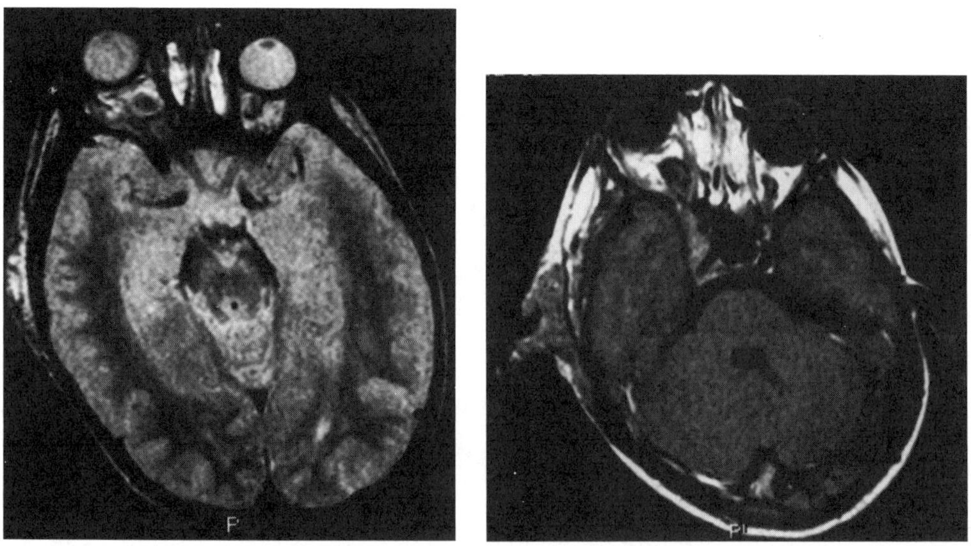

A B

Figure 1 Neurofibromatosis type I with optic nerve glioma. *A,* Axial T2 MR image reveals proptosis of the right globe and a large tortuous right optic nerve within the orbit and in the optic canal. *B,* Postgadolinium T1 axial scan reveals not only the enlarged nerve (nonenhancing) but also the enlarged abnormal right cavernous sinus.

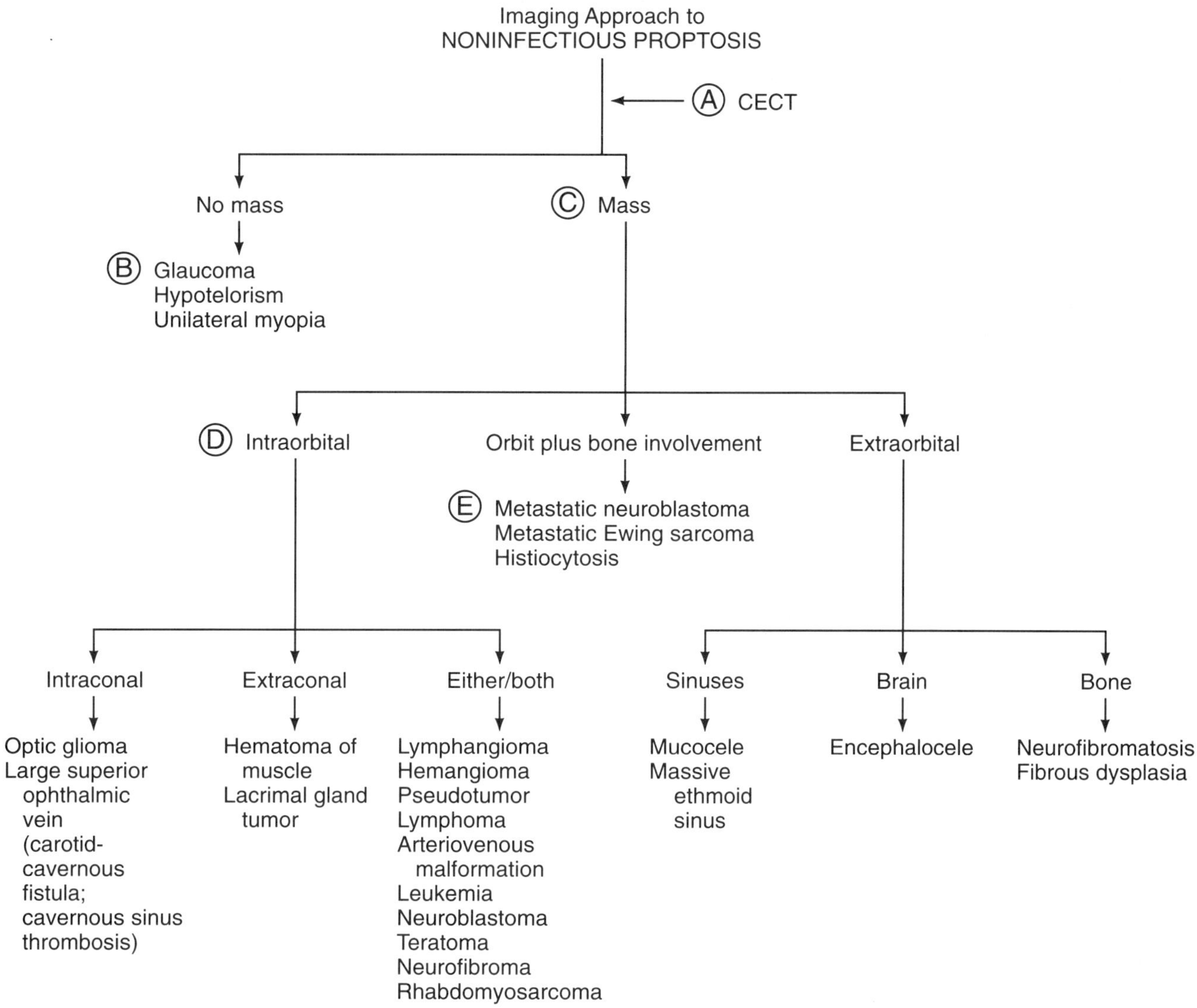

extent of disease. The signal intensity of the glioma is similar to that of gray matter on T1 images and variable on T2 images. Up to 50% of tumors (or part of them) enhance with gadolinium (see Newton et al.). The extraconal space is that portion of the orbit lateral to the lateral rectus and medial to the medial rectus. Frequently, lesions in this location involve the preseptal space (as in hemangioma, Fig. 2).

Rhabdomyosarcoma is the most common primary malignant tumor of the orbit in childhood (Fig. 3). It may arise from the undifferentiated mesenchymal cells that form muscles of the orbit or, as often is the case, may involve both the orbit and sinuses, making the primary site of origin difficult to determine. Embryonal rhabdomyosarcoma is the most common cell type in children. Although this tumor is most often seen in the extraconal space, when it becomes large it may involve both spaces. Because this tumor may extend in any direction, including intracranial, MRI is the best imaging tool for full evaluation.

The majority of lesions involve either or both the intraconal and extraconal spaces. One such lesion is lymphoma (Fig. 4).

E. The most common lesion to involve the bone and extraconal orbit is metastatic neuroblastoma (Fig. 5).

Continued on page 272

A

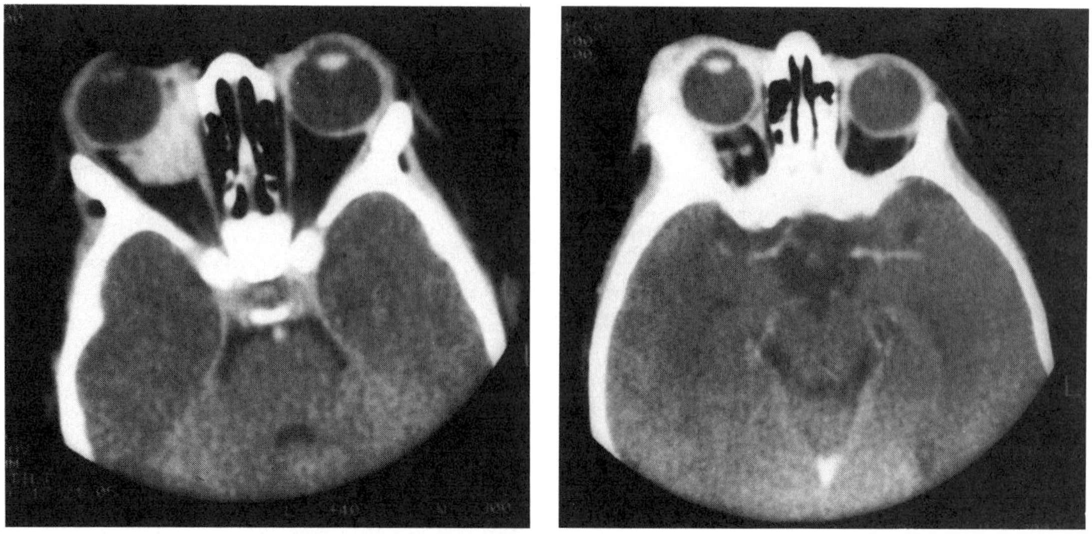

B

C

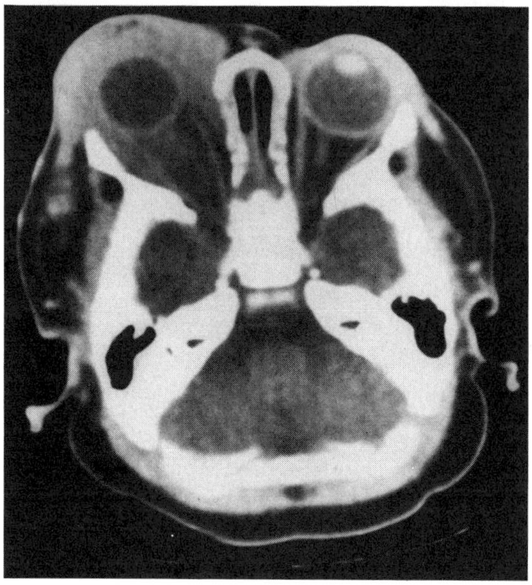

Figure 2 Hemangioma in three separate patients demonstrating the multiple sites of involvement. *A,* Axial CT scan shows a right intraconal hemangioma enhancing brightly. *B,* Diffuse right extraconal preseptal hemangioma with enhancement on an axial CT. *C,* A nonenhanced axial CT scan showing right preseptal, extraconal, and intraconal hemangioma.

A

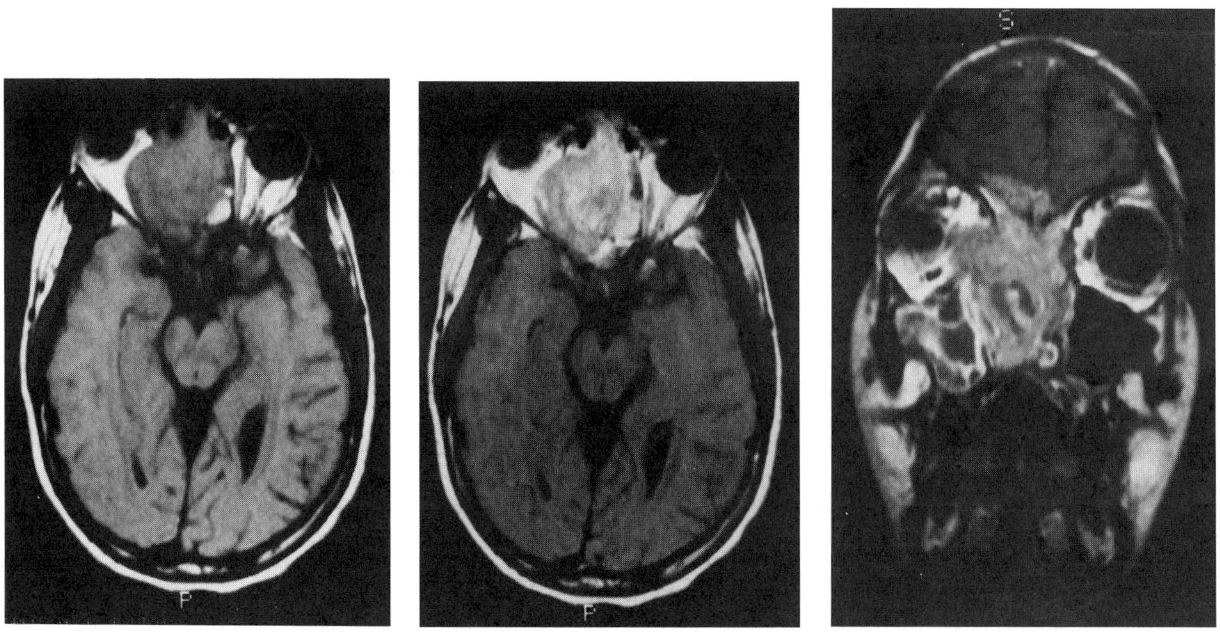

B, C

Figure 3 Rhabdomyosarcoma. *A,* Axial MR scan with T1 imaging. The large orbital-ethmoidal right sinus rhabdomyosarcoma is seen with intracranial invasion. *B* and *C,* Axial and coronal gadolinium-enhanced T1 images show the lesion greatly enhancing.

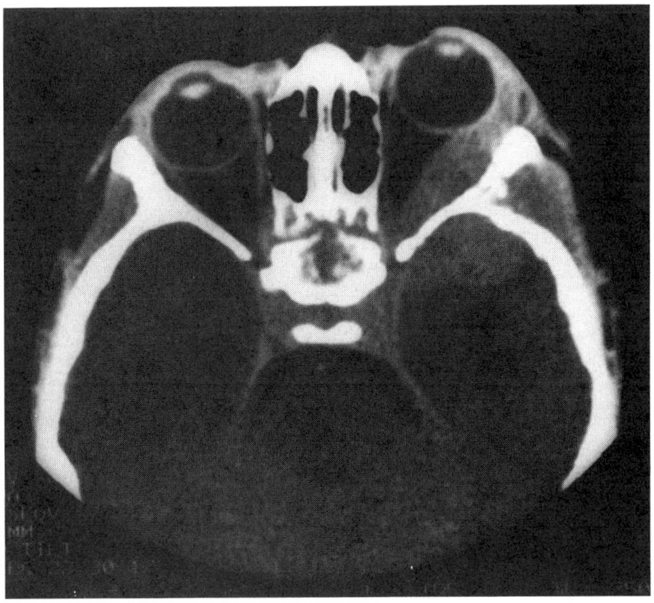

Figure 4 Lymphoma. Axial CECT scan shows homogeneous extraconal mass on the left with preseptal involvement and extra-axial involvement of the left middle cranial fossa.

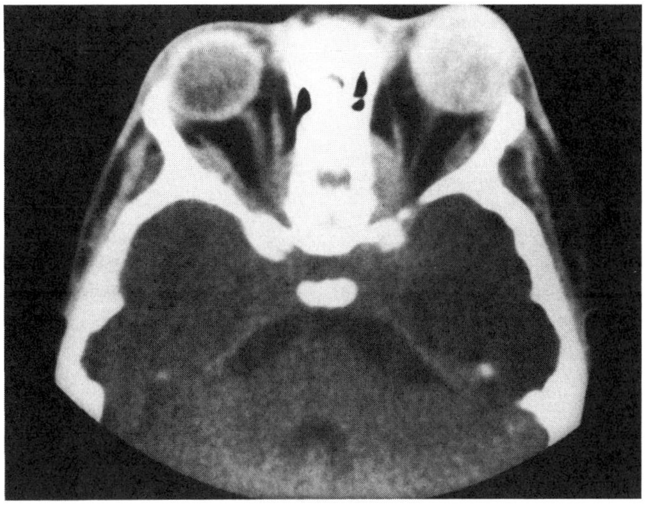

Figure 5 Metastatic neuroblastoma. There are bilateral extraconal masses. Proptosis is noted on the left side with glaucomatous changes of the globe.

References

Flanders AE, Espinosa GA, Markiewicz DA, Howell DD. Orbital lymphoma: role of CT and MRI. Radiol Clin North Am 1987; 25:601.

Lallemand DP, Brasch RC, Char DH, Normal D. Orbital tumors in children. Radiology 1984; 151:85.

Nelson LB, Calhoun JH, Harley RD. Pediatric ophthalmology. 3rd ed. Philadelphia: WB Saunders, 1991.

Newton TH, Bilaniuk LT. Radiology of the eye and orbit. In: Modern neuroradiology. New York: Raven Press, 1990.

Shields JA. Diagnosis and management of orbital tumors. Philadelphia, WB Saunders, 1989.

Vade A, Armstrong D. Orbital rhabdomyosarcoma in childhood. Radiol Clin North Am 1987; 24:701.

AN IMAGING APPROACH TO INFECTION OF THE PEDIATRIC ORBIT

Thomas L. Slovis, M.D.
John D. Baker, M.D.
Cristie Becker, M.D.

A. The cause of an acutely swollen eye in a child is frequently related to a traumatic event (see algorithm for trauma). Periorbital (preseptal) and orbital (postseptal) cellulitis may arise from trauma with secondary infections of the skin surrounding the orbit. Staphylococci and streptococci are the usual organisms. Other important historical information is the presence of an upper respiratory infection. Cellulitis of the pediatric orbit frequently (60%) follows paranasal sinus infection. In this instance the history of nasal or orbital discharge is quite helpful. The most common organisms causing paranasal sinus–orbital infection are staphylococci, streptococci, and *H aemophilus influenzae*. Dacryocystitis is a rare cause of preseptal or postseptal cellulitis.

B. The physical examination focuses on determining the site of involvement: Is the process limited to the lid or are the globe and orbit involved? Because the lid is swollen and lid motion is restricted, the first step is to open the lid (with fingers, lid retractors, or cotton-tip applicators) and visualize the globe. The presence of a quiet conjunctiva, full range of extraocular movement, and normal pupil reaction means that the process is preseptal. However, an injected swollen conjunctiva, proptosis of the globe, and limitation of extraocular movements are all signs of globe and orbital involvement. Abnormal pupil response and decreased visual acuity also signify orbital involvement and increase the urgency of the problem.

C. The treatment of preseptal, periorbital cellulitis is the administration of intravenous antibiotics. Imaging studies are restricted to paranasal sinus plain films (to detect the source of the infection). If the lid swelling does not improve in 48 to 96 hours, further studies, including a CT scan, are indicated.

D. The CT examination needs to be performed meticulously to delineate fully orbital pathology.

Continued on page 276

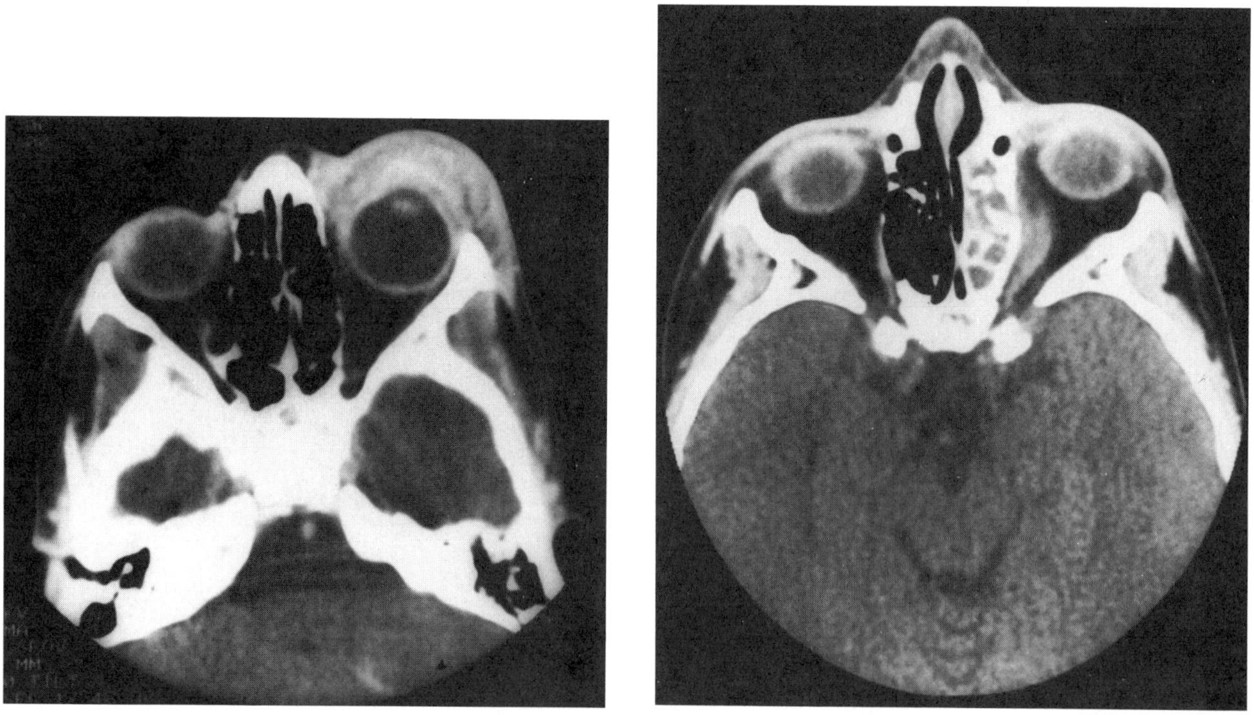

A B

Figure 1 Preseptal and postseptal cellulitis. *A,* Preseptal (periorbital) cellulitis. This child had enough swelling of the left eye that proper clinical examination could not be done. The axial CT scan reveals swelling of the left lid, but the tarsal plate is not violated and the position of the globe is not proptotic. The sinuses are clear. Note that all the swelling is superficial and preseptal. *B,* Postseptal (orbital) cellulitis. There is opacification of the right ethmoid air cells on this nonenhanced axial CT scan. The medial rectus muscle is deviated laterally with ill-defined density between it and the lamina papyracea

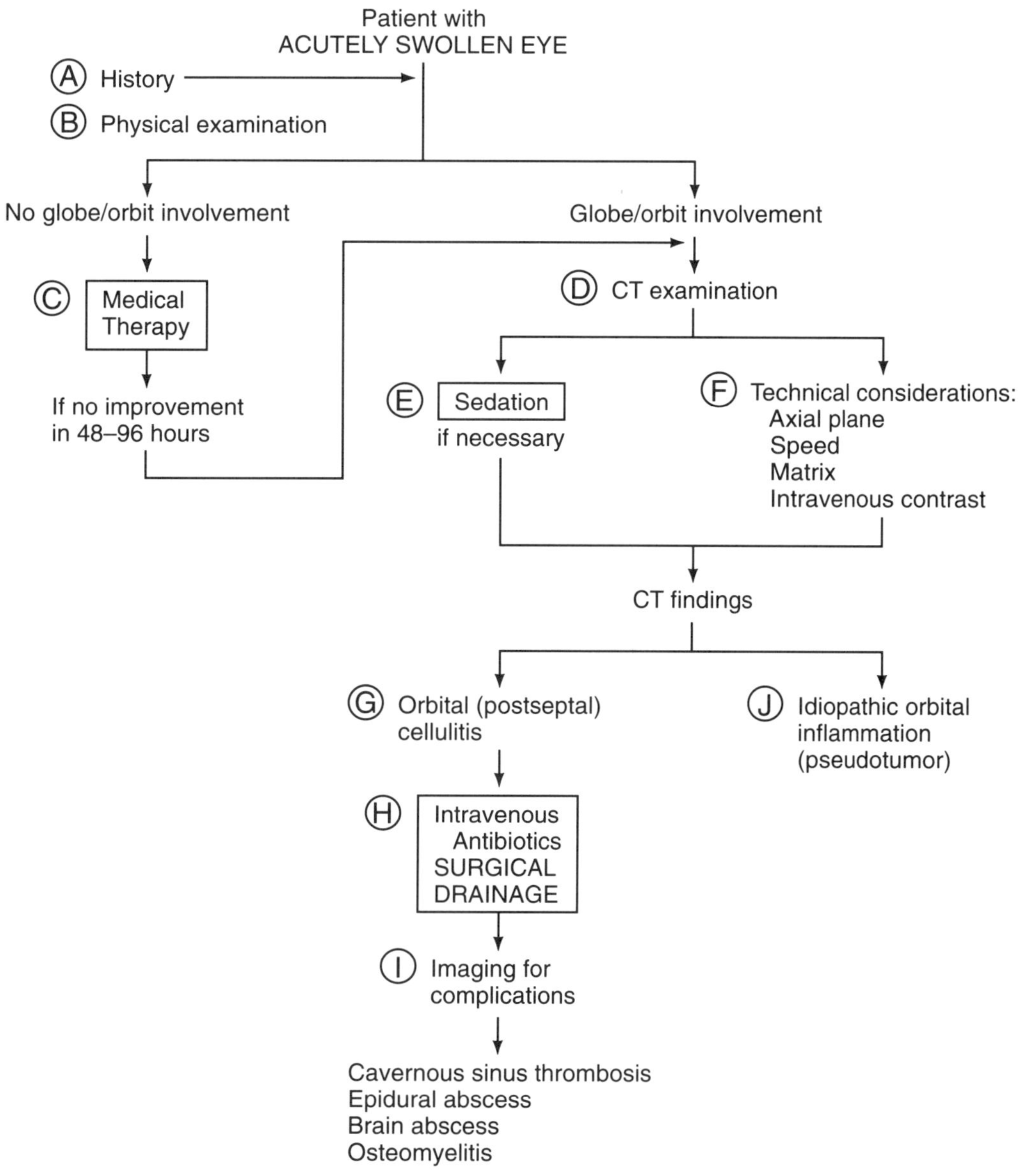
Patient with
ACUTELY SWOLLEN EYE
(A) History
(B) Physical examination
No globe/orbit involvement
(C) Medical Therapy
If no improvement in 48–96 hours
Globe/orbit involvement
(D) CT examination
(E) Sedation if necessary
(F) Technical considerations:
Axial plane
Speed
Matrix
Intravenous contrast
CT findings
(G) Orbital (postseptal) cellulitis
(H) Intravenous Antibiotics
SURGICAL DRAINAGE
(I) Imaging for complications
Cavernous sinus thrombosis
Epidural abscess
Brain abscess
Osteomyelitis
(J) Idiopathic orbital inflammation (pseudotumor)

E. If the child cannot lie completely still for the examination (up to 15 minutes) or if he or she is frightened by noise or the scanner, he or she must be sedated. Proper sedation demands monitoring with a minimum of nurse and/or physician and pulse oximetry. Various drug regimens have been successful, including oral chloral hydrate in the younger (<18 months) child, intravenous Nembutal, and intravenous Versed.

F. The examination for infection of the orbit is performed in the axial plane with 3-mm-thick, 3-mm-contiguous slices. The axial plane is best for showing deviation of the medial rectus muscle and for evaluation of the spread of infection to the brain. When necessary, coronal images may be obtained for small lesions at the inferior and superior areas of the orbit. Sections are obtained at the fastest possible speed (2 seconds or less) and with the highest resolution matrix (512 × 512). The study field extends from the floor of the maxillary sinuses to the top of the frontal calvarium so that both sinus disease and intracranial involvement may be detected (see below). The images are "targeted," that is, enlarged to fill the frame. Intravenous contrast is necessary for detecting intracranial extension of the inflammatory process. Therefore we use contrast once the diagnosis of orbital (postseptal) cellulitis is made and we are searching for the complications (see below). Hard-copy images are obtained with both soft tissue windows and bone windows. The examination is obtained with standard algorithm.

G. The CT findings of orbital cellulitis begin with the evaluation of the paranasal sinuses, particularly the ethmoids. These sinuses are separated from the medial orbit only by the extremely thin lamina papyracea. Because the bone offers little protection, infection easily spreads to the orbit. "The lack of lymphatic drainage of the orbit and the lack of valves in the ophthalmic venous system also allow easy bacterial invasion of the orbit" (Gonzalez et al). The first findings then may be sinus opacification. The orbit becomes edematous with swelling of the muscle and sclera. A soft tissue density is seen between the periosteum and the medial rectus muscle (although the density may be anywhere in the orbit, depending on the origin of the infection). With time the phlegmon may become an abscess with low-density center and contrast-enhancing walls. There is proptosis and of course lid swelling (Fig. 1). It is uncommon in children to see intraconal involvement in orbital (postseptal) cellulitis. When this happens, the fat becomes mottled in appearance and normal soft tissue planes between the optic nerve, fat, and muscles are obliterated.

H. The treatment of orbital cellulitis involves intravenous antibiotics and surgical drainage of abscesses. Intravenous antibiotics at meningitis dosage should be started as soon as possible. A subperiosteal abscess should be drained when clearly demonstrated on CT. Orbital abscesses are more difficult to drain and usually respond to intravenous antibiotics and so may be watched. Decreased visual acuity and abnormal pupil reaction usually signify compression of the optic nerve by orbital pressure and are clinical signs of potential complications.

I. The major complications of orbital (postseptal) cellulitis are intracranial extension and osteomyelitis. The latter is always present with extension from a frontal sinusitis. Once again the major imaging tool is contrast-enhanced CT. This time a brain study is done, with particular attention to the routes of spread—through the orbital apex and into the cavernous sinus, from hematogenous spread into the meninges or brain, or by direct extension from a sinus to the epidural space. In most instances, 3- to 5-mm axial sections before and after contrast are done through the frontal brain and cavernous sinuses. The rest of the brain can be studied with 10-mm slices (Fig. 2). When deemed clinically important, a bone scan may be used to diagnose osteomyelitis of the face or calvarium.

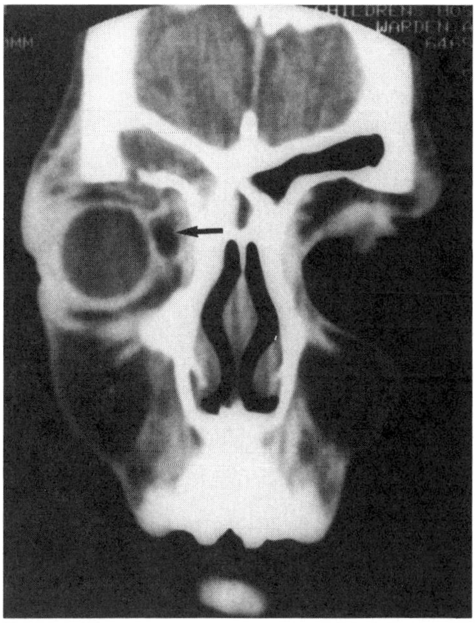

A

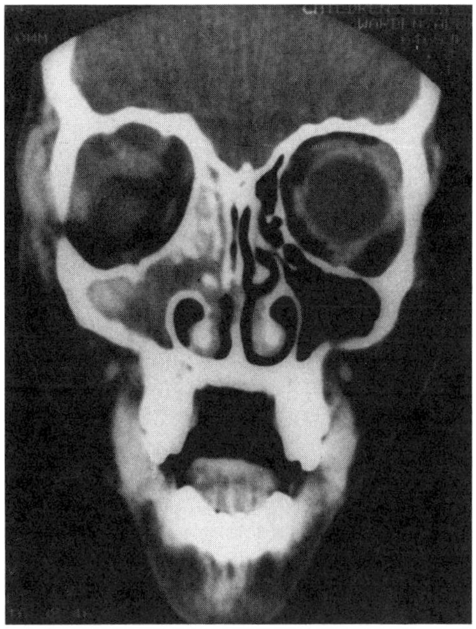

B

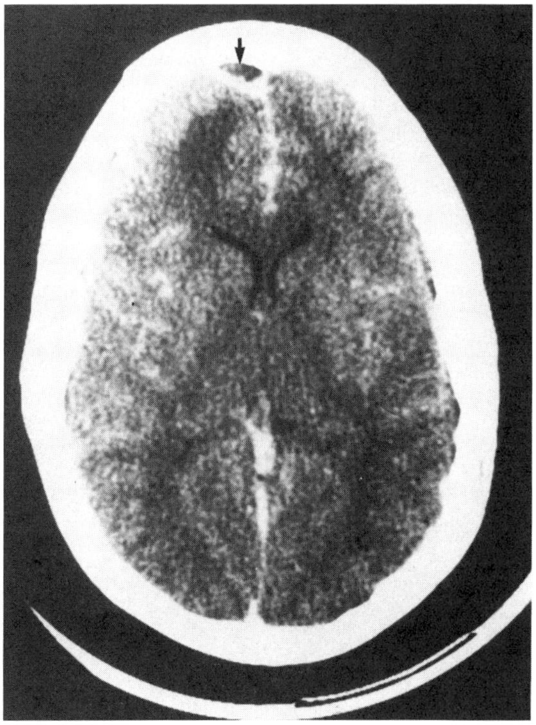

C

Figure 2 Complications of postseptal (orbital) cellulitis. *A,* Coronal CT scan showing opacification of the right frontal sinus. There is density superiorly and medially in the right orbit, and the globe is deviated laterally. The low-density area medial to the orbit represents a large abscess *(arrow). B,* Another coronal view of the same child shows right ethmoid and maxillary sinus involvement. The large mass superior to the right globe is seen again. A lower attenuation region superiorly also represents abscess. *C,* Contrast-enhanced CT of the brain. A small epidural abscess *(arrow)* is visible immediately behind the right frontal sinus.

J. Idiopathic orbital inflammation—orbital pseudotumor—is distinctly uncommon in children. The CT findings include uveal-scleral thickening (the halo appearance), enlargement of the optic nerve and/or extraocular muscles, and frequently intra- or extraconal poorly defined density. The involvement of muscle groups may be spotty. There is proptosis but no sinus involvement. The lacrimal gland may be involved.

References

Bilaniuk LT, Zimmerman RA, Newton TH. Magnetic resonance imaging: Orbital pathology. Radiology of the eye and orbit. New York: Raven Press, 1990.

Curtin HD. Pseudotumor. Radiol Clin North Am 1987; 25:583.

Flanders AE, Mafee MF, Rao VM, Choi KH. CT characteristics of orbital pseudotumors and other orbital inflammatory processes. J Comput Assist Tomogr 1989; 13:40.

Gonzalez CF, Becker MH, Flanagan JC. Diagnostic imaging in ophthalmology. New York: Springer-Verlag, 1986.

Hopper KD, Sherman JL, Boal DKB. Abnormalities of the orbit and its contents in children: CT and MR imaging findings. AJR 1991; 156:1219.

Slovis TL, Towbin RB, Kuhns LR. Pediatric application of CT and MR. Curr Opinion Radiol 1990; 2:534.

Weber AL, Mikulis DK. Inflammatory disorders of the paraorbital sinuses and their complications. Radiol Clin North Am 1987; 25:615.

Wells RG, Sty JR, Gonnering RS. Imaging of the pediatric eye and orbit. RadioGraphics 1989; 9:1023.

IMAGING APPROACH TO THE CHILD WITH ORBITAL TRAUMA

Thomas L. Slovis, M.D.
John D. Baker, M.D.
Cristie Becker, M.D.

A. The history provides the first clue as to whether imaging is necessary. When there is the possibility of penetrating injury (sharp object) or of retained foreign body (FB) (e.g., BB pellet), some imaging is almost mandatory. However, when there is blunt trauma to the eye, the need for imaging depends greatly on the physical examination and visual acuity. The most important aspects are whether the posterior as well as the anterior segment of the eye can be visualized and whether there is any evidence of penetration through the cornea or conjunctiva. The presence of a full range of motion indicates that the extraocular muscles are intact.

B. No history of penetrating injury or retained foreign body is present. The anterior and posterior segments of the eye can be visualized, the extraocular movements are full, and there is no evidence of corneal or conjunctival laceration.

C. CT is indicated when there is a history of penetrating injury or retained foreign body or the examiner cannot see within the eye and examine the retina because of hyphema or traumatic cataract formation. Additionally, CT should be done when the examiner is able to see within the eye but there is corneal or scleral perforation. When a conjunctival laceration is present, imaging is not required if the retina can be examined underneath the laceration. If a conjunctival laceration is accompanied by limited extraocular movements or an inability to examine the retina in the area of the laceration, imaging is required.

D. The CT findings of ruptured globe are smaller globe and irregular shape (flat tire sign). Orbital hemorrhage CT findings are hematoma of muscle—hyperdense muscle (see Figure 1) and intra- or extraconal density. There will be discontinuity at the nerve in CT findings of avulsion of the nerve. MR is better for the intracanalicular portion of the nerve if no contraindication exists such as a metallic FB. For retinal detachment, do ultrasonography (US) and see leukocoria discussion.

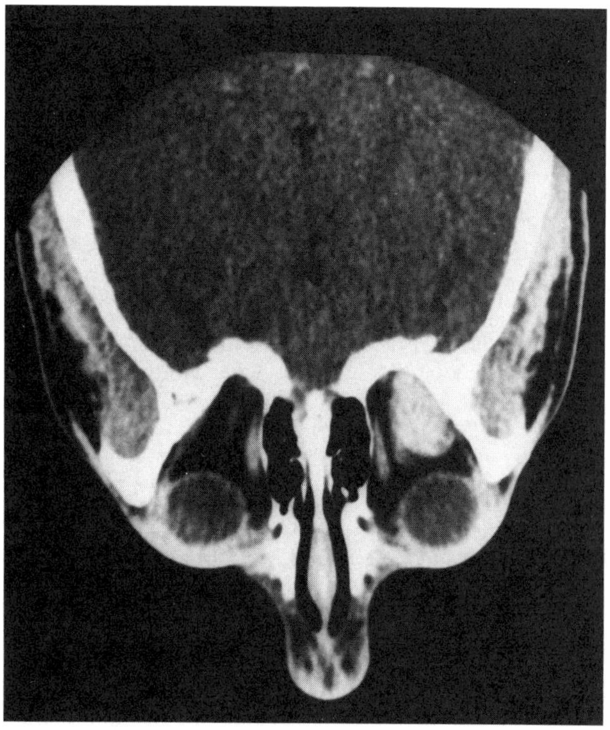

A

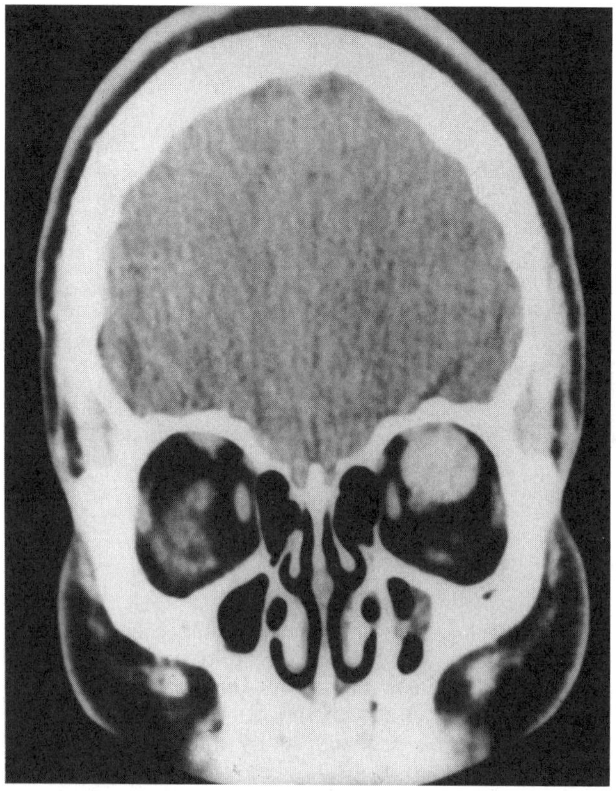

B

Figure 1 Hematoma of the superior rectus: *A,* Axial CT section shows dense mass in the superior aspect of the left orbit. *B,* Coronal section confirms the mass and shows it to be the superior rectus muscle. This healed without treatment.

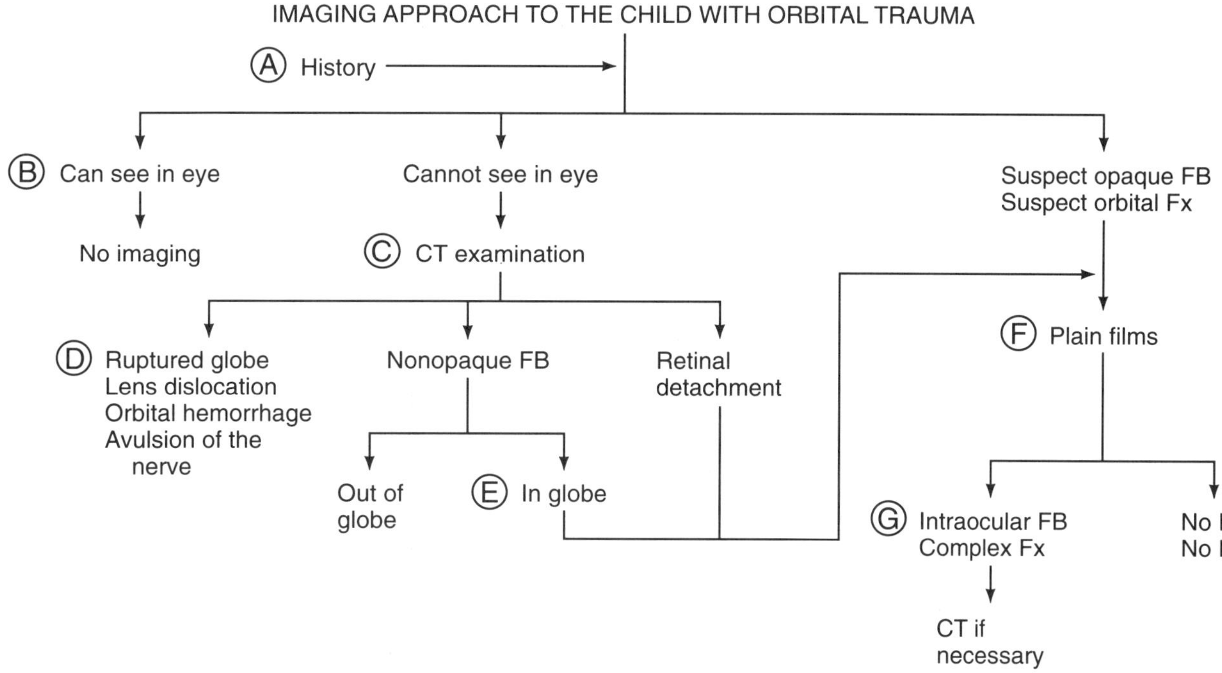

E. FB may cause retinal detachment. US is the best and easiest modality for detecting this abnormality (see Leukocoria algorithm).

F. The first imaging procedure for the suspicion of an opaque retained foreign body is the plain film series. At least two views 90 degrees apart are necessary (a frontal and a lateral film). If no foreign body is found, no further imaging may be necessary. However, if an intraocular foreign body is detected or if one is seeking a nonopaque foreign body, CT is the appropriate test. CT is also the best and most appropriate test to screen for intracranial injuries and facial and sinus fractures.

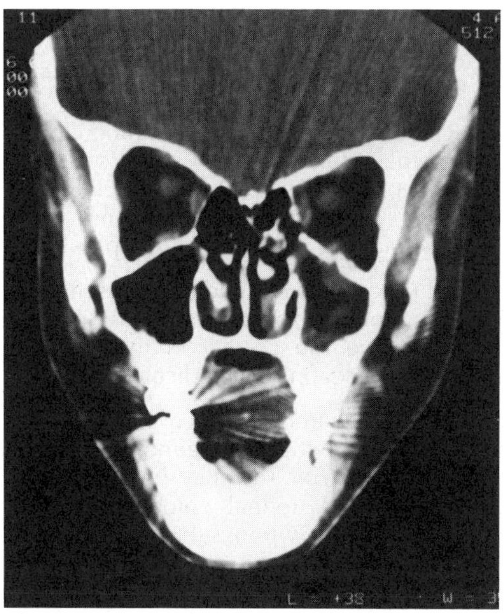

Figure 2 Fracture of the floor of the orbit—blow-out fracture. Coronal view of a child with a fracture of the floor of the left orbit. Note the different shape of the inferior rectus muscle, clearly a sign of entrapment. This is best seen on coronal views.

1. Sedation as in previous algorithm
2. Axial sections are obtained with 3 to 5 mm interval and thickness. Soft tissue algorithm with both soft tissue and bone windows obtained on hard copy.
3. No contrast is necessary and in fact is contraindicated because we are looking for bleeding and/or FB.

Severe facial trauma with possible fracture (Fx) of the bony orbit is another indication for imaging. Although plain films are much less sensitive than CT, plain radiography is usually a good initial imaging procedure. If the films are negative and the clinical suspicion is low, the examination can end. If CT is necessary for orbital fractures, the examination should be done in both axial and coronal plains. A bone algorithm should be used and then computerized images derived for a standard algorithm. Three-dimensional imaging is now readily obtainable with CT and is of tremendous help in complex facial injuries. These images are obtained by getting contiguous 3-mm cuts through the entire area of concern (use low MA to decrease radiation) and then having the information reconstructed by the computer.

G. Blowout fractures are best viewed with coronal CT (see Fig. 2). The indications for the CT examination are based on clinical findings. The asymptomatic patient with a floor fracture does not necessarily need CT.

References

Gonzalez, CF, Becker MH, Flanagan JC. Diagnostic imaging in ophthalmology. New York: Springer-Verlag, 1986.

Koornneef L, Zonneveld FW. The role of direct multiplanar high resolution CT in the assessment and management of orbital trauma. Radiol Clin North Am 1987; 25:753.

Spoor TC, Nesi FA. Management of ocular, orbital, and adnexal trauma. New York: Raven Press, 1988.

IMAGING APPROACH TO THE CHILD WITH LEUKOCORIA

Thomas L. Slovis, M.D.
John D. Baker, M.D.
Cristie Becker, M.D.

A. In evaluating a child who presents with a "white pupil"—leukocoria—the diagnosis of retinoblastoma must be confirmed or excluded. When retinoblastoma is excluded from the differential diagnosis, the cause must be sought. If the ophthalmologist cannot rule out the diagnosis of retinoblastoma by history and/or physical examination, CT scanning is the first imaging study.

B. The CT examination needs to be performed with the same general guidelines of sedation and technical factors described in the algorithm for infection of the pediatric orbit. However, the following modifications are noted:
   1. Because we are looking for calcium, a nonenhanced scan is vital prior to intravenous enhancement.
   2. Both axial and coronal sections are important to detect intraorbital spread.
   3. The contrast-enhanced CT study should include enough of the brain to evaluate pathways of intracranial extension. When the tumor is bilateral, complete CT and MRI of the brain are mandatory to rule out trilateral retinoblastoma (see below); because it is so easy to do a complete study, we recommend complete CT on all patients with retinoblastoma (see Pesin and Shields).
   4. Hard copy of both soft tissue and bone windows for osseous involvement should be obtained.

C. Retinoblastoma is the most common intraocular malignancy in childhood. In a large series by Howard et al, it accounted for 265 of the 500 patients who presented with leukocoria (53%). Retinoblastoma arises from the neural layer of the retina, is most often unilateral (66 to 75%), and most often represents a spontaneous mutation. When bilateral, the genetic form of the disease is frequently present. Ninety-eight percent of children with retinoblastoma present before the age of 3 years. CT is the best test to confirm the ophthalmologic findings and to initiate the search for the extent of disease. The findings on CT (Fig. 1) include the following: (1) Intraocular mass (isodense or hyperdense). (2) Calcification of the mass (90%). The calcification may be single or multiple. (3) When the mass is large enough, retinal detachment can occur. (4) The tumor enhances mildly to moderately.

D. The differential diagnosis of intraocular calcification includes retinopathy of prematurity (ROP), toxocariasis, and optic head drusen. A more serious and difficult consideration is retinal astrocytoma (astrocytic hamartoma), which may be present before the manifestations of tuberous sclerosis. These lesions are usually found in children older than 3 years.

E. Once retinoblastoma is diagnosed, the extent of tumor must be defined. Spread of tumor beyond the globe occurs via two mechanisms—directly with involvement of the optic nerve and into the subarachnoid space with further spread to the meninges of the brain and spinal cord and hematogenously into the emissary veins to orbital tissue. Contrast-enhanced CT is excellent for detecting these routes of spread. In the at-risk child with bilateral tumor, a third primary must be considered—midline malignancy or trilateral retinoblastoma. Because of its multiplanar potential, MR becomes the next imaging test. It must be understood that MRI is *not* best for the initial evaluation because it cannot detect calcium and its resolution is much poorer than that of CT (MRI cannot detect 3- to 4-mm lesions).
   1. Sedation as with CT.
   2. Technical
      a. Planes of scan—sagittal, axial, and coronal.
      b. Contrast-enhanced—gadolinium.
      c. Use head coil and 5-mm sections.
      d. Types of images
         1) T1—short relaxation time (TR) and excitation time (TE)—an anatomic image. The CSF appears black.
         2) T2—long TR and TE—a pathologic image. The CSF appears white.
         3) Fat suppression techniques after gadolinium.
   3. MR findings of the primary intraocular tumor:
      a. Moderately increased signal on T1.
      b. Hypointense on T2.
      c. Subretinal fluid is hyperintense on T2, thus separating it from the retinoblastoma.

   In a small percentage of children with retinoblastoma, the lesion metastasizes beyond the globe/orbit and CNS to involve the bones. In this group nuclear medicine bone scanning is indicated.

F. If the anterior chamber is clear, a cataract can be diagnosed. When the ophthalmologist can see the fundus clearly, he or she may be able to make the diagnosis of ROP, retinal coloboma, or persistent hyperplastic primary vitreous (PHPV). Once assured of the diagnosis and having eliminated retinoblastoma from consideration, supplemental imaging with ultrasonography (US) may give additional information (see US technical discussion below—K and Fig. 2).

G. If a cataract is present, US may more fully visualize the

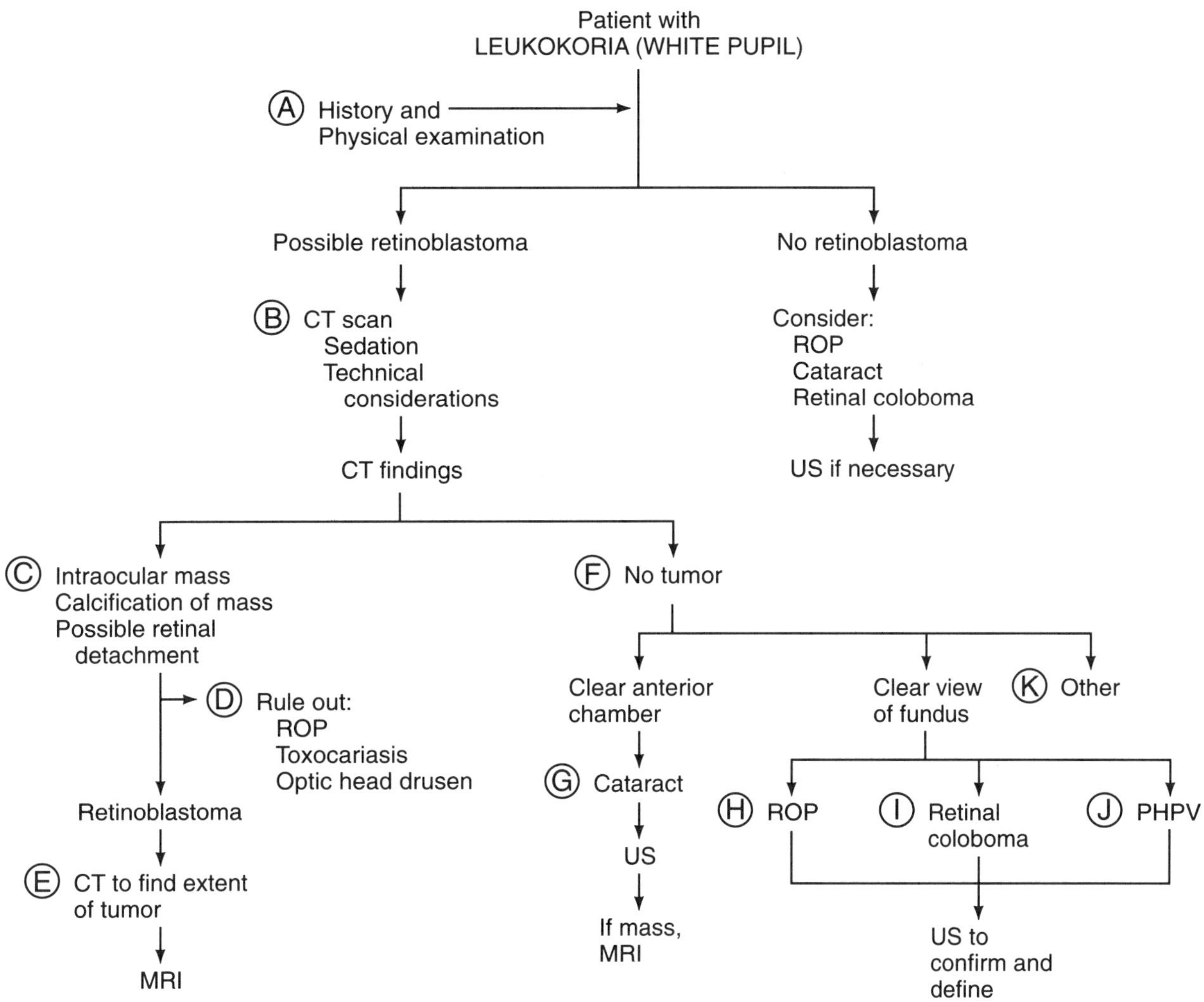

posterior segment. If a mass is then identified, CT is indicated.

H. In ROP, the fundus picture is usually diagnostic. The diagnosis is bolstered by the history of premature birth and a birth weight of less than 1300 g. When total retinal detachment is present, US (real-time and color-flow) is the initial imaging modality of choice.

I. Retinal coloboma is a diagnosis of retinal examination. Large colobomata of the nerve and posterior pole may be confirmed with US; they also have characteristic findings on CT.

J. The diagnosis of PHPV involving the anterior or mid-portion of the eye is usually made by clinical examination. The eye is smaller and there may be cataract formation, retrolental mass or membrane, and prominent ciliary processes. US demonstrates the persistent hyaloid vessel or remnant and, with color-flow Doppler, shows the vascularity.

K. The differentiation of the remaining diseases that can cause leukocoria is based on the results of the CT and US evaluation. Recently MRI has been suggested as a useful modality in separating these entities (Table 1). A common feature of all these entities can be the presence of retinal detachment. Therefore it may be impossible to separate these diseases and anomalies by imaging.

For US to be helpful, several technical aspects need to be considered. The examination must include both real-time and color-flow Doppler investigations. The parameters on color-flow Doppler must be such that there is minimal wall filter and the lowest possible velocity. In most instances the child can be studied without sedation. US is most useful in diagnosing retinal detachment and defining the vascular supply to the lesion. This may aid in following various treatment modalities.

(Continued on p. 283.)

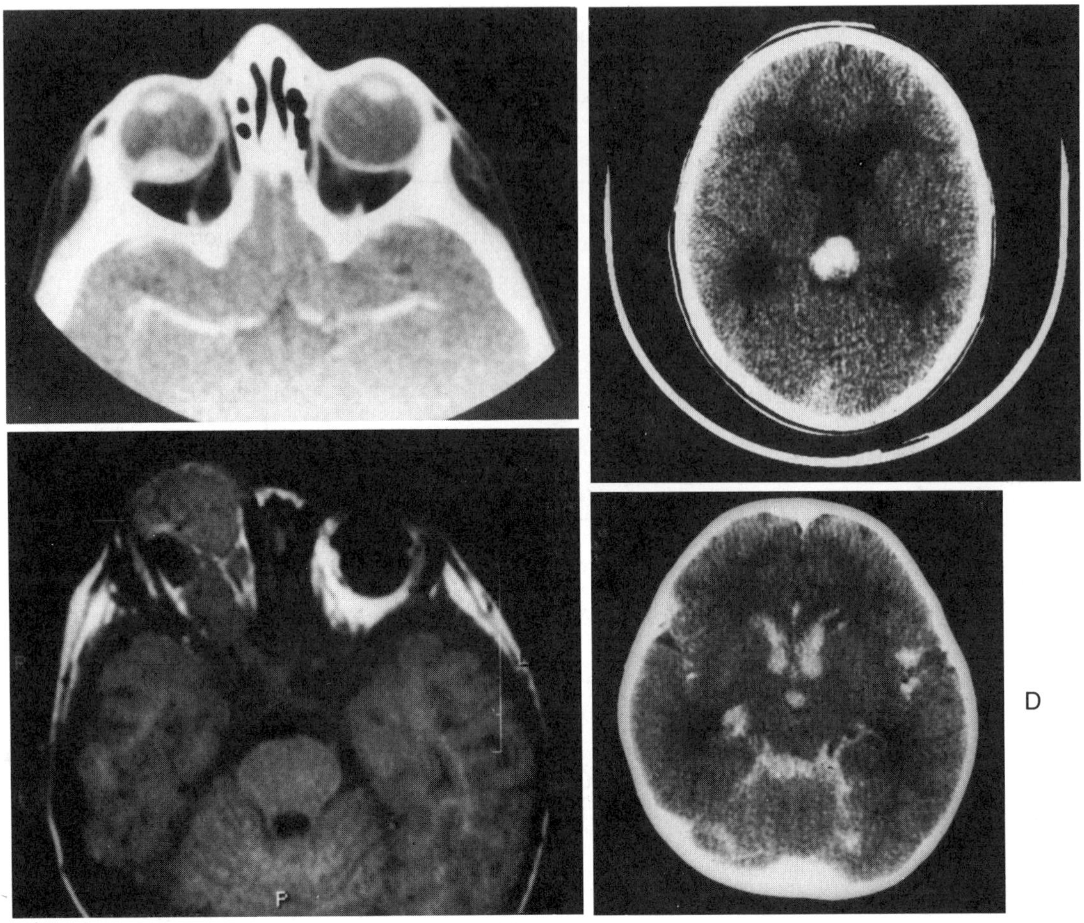

Figure 1 Retinoblastoma. *A,* Contrast-enhanced axial-section CT reveals a mass of the posterior retina with calcification. *B,* Complications of retinoblastoma include both intraorbital and intracranial spread. This T1 MR image shows involvement of the globe after enucleation, with tumor tracking back along the nerve through the optic canal. *C,* Enhancing pineal mass representing trilateral retinoblastoma on axial CT scan. *D,* CT on the same child as *C* reveals ependymal and meningeal spread of tumor, as seen by avid enhancement.

TABLE 1 Comparison of US, CT, and MRI

Entity	*US*	*CT*	*MRI*
Normal			
Vitreous	No echoes	Hypodense	Hypointense T1
Retina*	Cannot see	Cannot see	Cannot see
Retinal detachment			
Subretinal fluid	No echoes	Hyperdense	Hyperintense T1 and T2
Retina	Echogenic	Cannot see except by the contrast difference between retina and subretinal fluid	Cannot see except by the contrast difference between retina and subretinal fluid
Vasculature	Defines it	Cannot see	Cannot see
PHPV			
Small eye	Yes	Yes	Yes
Anterior chamber	Cannot define	Flat and lens is small	Flat and lens is small
Vitreous	Hypoechoic	Hyperdense	Hyperintense T1 and T2
Hyaloid stalk	Defines it	Seen only by the difference in contrast with the dense or intense vitreous	Seen only by the difference in contrast with the dense or intense vitreous
Vascularity	Defines it	Not seen	Not seen
Toxocariasis			
Mass	Nonspecific	Nonspecific	Isointense to hyperintense T2; if this is verified, may be a way to separate from retinoblastoma
Coats' disease			
Retinal detachment	All modalities nonspecific		

*As a distinct and separate structure.

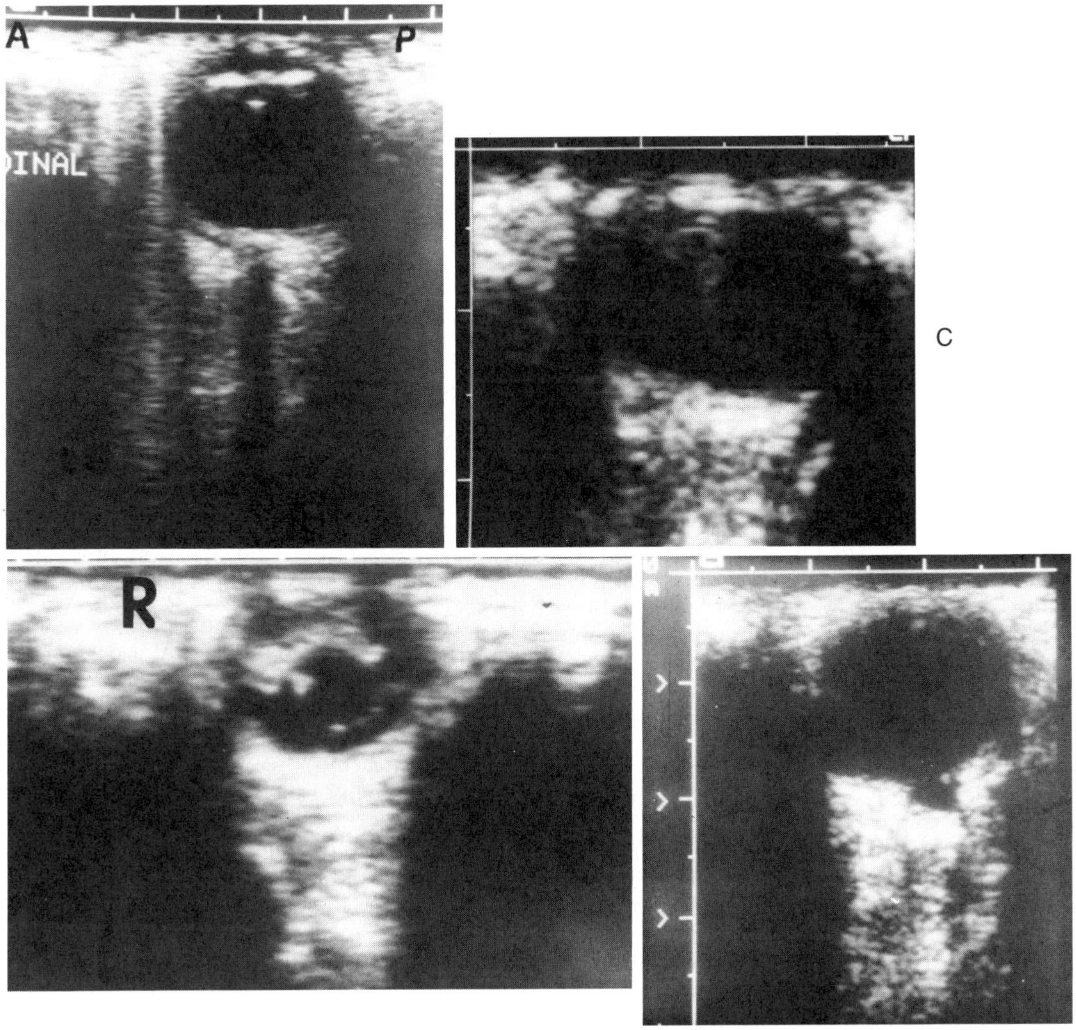

Figure 2 Ultrasound evaluations. *A,* Normal real-time sonogram of an orbit depicting the anterior chamber, lens, and posterior chamber with anechoic vitreous. In this particular scan, the optic nerve is well seen silhouetted by the retrobulbar fat. Normal color-flow Doppler image would delineate the ophthalmic artery extending from posterior lateral to anterior medial (by convention, viewer's left is medial). Some arterial flow to the lacrimal gland comes from the lacrimal artery. A small amount of flow would be seen in the retinal artery. In a normal color-flow Doppler image of the vascularity to the retina. Only spectral Doppler imaging defines whether arteries or veins are involved. *B,* Ultrasonogram of a young infant with retinopathy of prematurity. The retina is elevated although still fixed posteriorly, and subretinal fluid is present. *C,* Real-time ultrasonogram shows the thick stalk in a child with PHPV. A color-flow Doppler image would show normal retinal vascularity and then specific vascularity in the stalk, confirming the persistent hyaloid vessel. *D,* Ultrasonogram of a child with a retinal coloboma showing the large retinal defect.

References

Erickson SJ, Hendrix LE, Massaro BM, et al. Color Doppler flow imaging of the normal and abnormal orbit. Radiology 1989; 173:511.

Gardner TW, Zaparackas ZG, Naidich TP. Congenital optic nerve colobomas: CT demonstration. J Comput Assist Tomogr 1984; 8:95.

Hopper KD, Katz NNK, Dorwart RH, et al. Childhood leukokoria: Computed tomographic appearance and differential diagnosis with histopathologic correlation. RadioGraphics 1985; 5:377.

Mafee MF, Peyman GA. Retinal and choroidal detachments: Role of magnetic resonance imaging and computed tomography. Radiol Clin North Am 1987; 25:487.

Mafee MF, Goldberg MF, Choen SB, et al. Magnetic resonance imaging versus computed tomography of leukocoric eyes and use of in vitro proton magnetic resonance spectroscopy of retinoblastoma. Ophthalmology 1989; 96:965.

Mafee MF. Orbital pathology in magnetic resonance imaging. In: Newton TH, Bilaniuk LT, eds. Radiology of the eye and orbit. New York: Raven Press, 1990.

Wong AD, Cooperberg PL, Ross WH, Araki DN. Differentiation of detached retina and vitreous membrane with color flow Doppler. Radiology 1991; 178:429.

HIGH-RESOLUTION SURFACE-COIL MRI OF THE PEDIATRIC EYE

Hong-Ming Cheng, O.D., Ph.D.
Kameran Lashkari, M.D.

A. Improvement of signal-to-noise ratio is achieved by using small-diameter surface coils. These coils can be either transmitter-receivers or receivers that collect signals from only the eye-orbit region. Transceiver coils of 2 to 5 inches in diameter are commercially available (although coils of <3 inches are prohibited for eye imaging); smaller receiver coils are usually home-made. Receiver coils are preferred because they do not involve potential energy deposition (heat) to the eye as with the transceiver; the radiofrequency is transmitted using the main body coil. Further improvement of the signal-to-noise ratio can be achieved by averaging signals (normally the number of excitation, NEX, is 1; the improvement is by a factor of — N); however, this increases the scan time by a factor of N and may be undesirable in some pediatric cases.

B. Increase in resolution is accomplished using a small field of view (FOV) (e.g., 8 cm) with the thinnest possible slices (for spin-echo 3 mm, and for GRE 0.7 mm). For a 256 × 256 display (with 256 each of frequency-encoding data points and phase-encoding steps), the in-plane resolution is therefore 0.31 × 0.31 mm (i.e., 80 mm/256). FOVs of less than 8 cm are available on some imagers; however, because an increase in resolution reduces signal intensity in each voxel, compensations such as increasing slice thickness and/or the number of averages may have to be implemented concurrently. If a 256 × 128 matrix is selected, the scan time is half that of 256 × 256, but the image quality often is acceptable.

C. Selection of imaging modes, such as T1- or T2-weighted spin-echo imaging, is achieved by selecting interpulse delay (or repetition time, TR) and echo time (TE), and in gradient-recalled-echo (GRE) the tip angle in addition (for example, 30 degrees for T1- and 70 degrees for T2-weighted imaging).

The T1 and T2 of ocular tissues are proportional to proton density (i.e., water content). T1 and T2 decrease in the following order: vitreous, aqueous humor > cornea > lens cortex > choroid + ciliary body–iris > lens nucleus > sclera. Lens nucleus and sclera have extremely short T2s that do not permit echo generation and therefore appear dark. If TE of less than 20 msec is available, it should be used to allow more signal generation.

T1-weighted spin-echo images provide the best contrast; at a TR of 400 to 600 msec and TE of 20 to 30 msec, tissues with short T1 (e.g., lens cortex and choroid) appear bright and those with long T1 (e.g., the vitreous and aqueous) appear dark. In this mode, the ciliary body, posterior aqueous chamber, choroid, and sclera can all be differentiated. The retina itself, on the other hand, is not resolvable unless detached; in this case, the subretinal fluid provides contrast because it has shorter T1 than the vitreous. Noncontrast T1-weighted imaging is particularly useful in delineating anatomy and ocular anomalies, especially with media opacity. These include anterior segment anomalies, angle closure, nanophthalmos, posterior cysts, and anophthalmia. Optic nerve anomalies including hypoplasia, aplasia, and large colobomatous lesions (morning glory syndrome) may be discerned. Further, the insertion sites and thickness of extraocular muscles also may be measured.

D. The T1 contrast agent gadolinium diethylenetriamine penta-acetic acid (Gd DTPA) is useful for the detection of intraocular lesions with increasing vascularity, leaky vessels, and stagnant blood flow, as in melanoma, retinoblastoma, choroidal hemangioma, and osteoma, and also may be useful for the detection of breakdown of the blood-ocular barrier. The administration dose is 0.1 mmol/kg by intravenous push followed by saline flush. Normally the ciliary body and choroid also are enhanced by Gd DTPA and can be used as the basis of comparison. If necessary, signal intensity in the region of interest can be measured using software resident in the imager.

Although T1-weighted imaging usually provides superb anatomy, further improvement is possible by suppressing fat signals. This is done by selectively saturating the fat resonance with radiofrequency. Because of the short T1 of the orbital fat, it is usually the brightest region on the image. Fat suppression is desirable in that the reduction of orbital fat signals increases the dynamic range of ocular images and permits a better view of the orbital anatomy. The superimposition of fat on tissue is usually referred to as the "chemical-shift artifact," and with fat suppression, measurement of ocular/orbital dimensions can be better achieved. Similarly, if the fat region only is examined (e.g., intravitreal silicone oil and orbital fat in Graves' disease), the water resonance can also be suppressed.

With T2-weighted imaging (e.g., TR/TE = 2000/60 msec), both the aqueous and vitreous appear bright because of the long T2, whereas other intraocular tissues appear dark. This mode is useful for detecting intravitreous nonferrous foreign bodies and choroidal lesions and in $H_2{}^{17}O$-enhanced imaging for the quantitation of water diffusion.

Two other imaging modes that are of limited use at preset time are (1) proton-density mapping using long TRs and short TEs that allow determination of tissue hydration; for example, an increase in water content is noted in incipient cataracts; and (2) diffusion imaging, which determines the motion of water (self-diffusion) in tissue; it is not yet clinically applica-

Continued on page 286

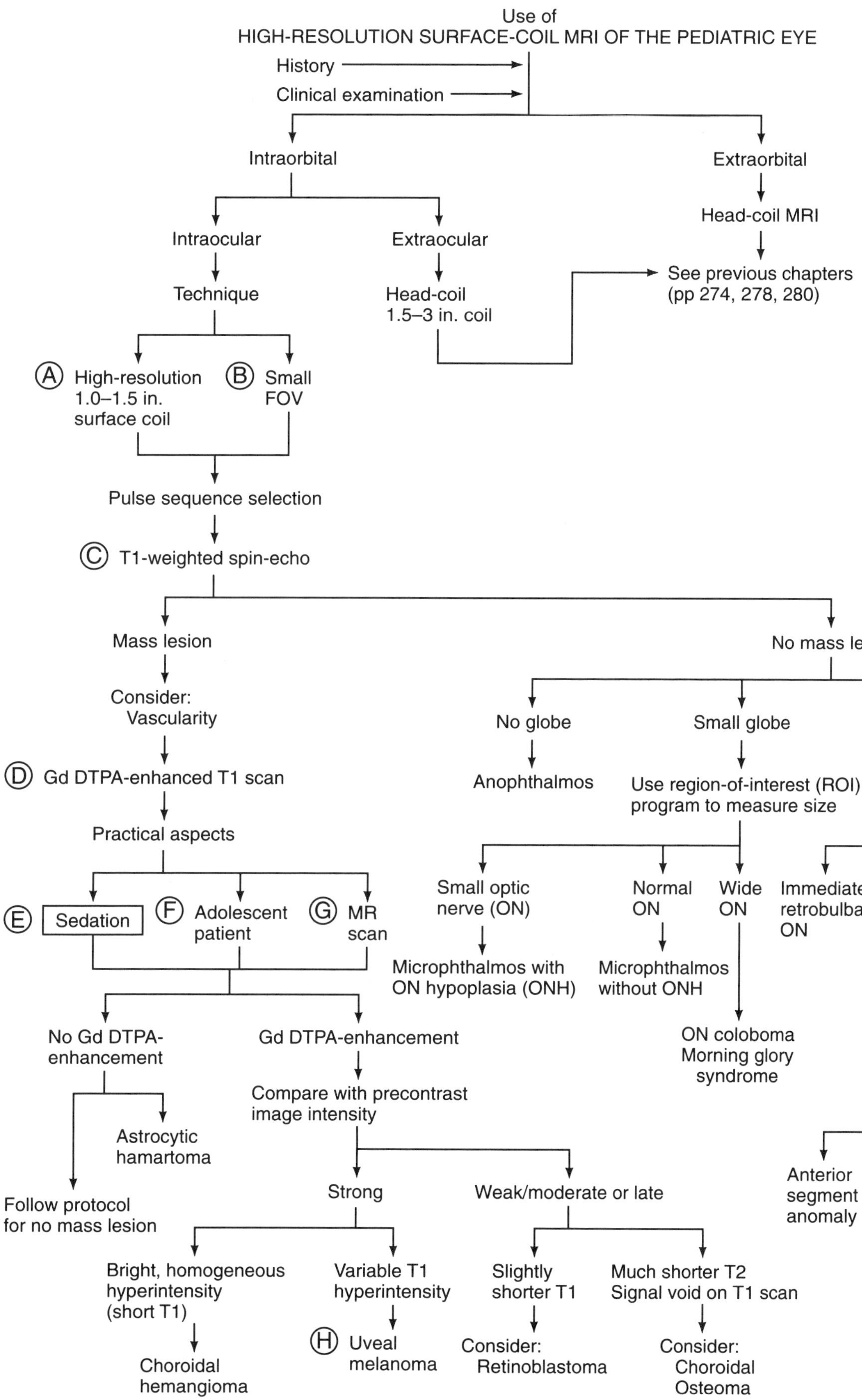
Use of
HIGH-RESOLUTION SURFACE-COIL MRI OF THE PEDIATRIC EYE
History
Clinical examination
Intraorbital
Extraorbital
Head-coil MRI
See previous chapters (pp 274, 278, 280)
Intraocular
Extraocular
Technique
Head-coil 1.5–3 in. coil
A High-resolution 1.0–1.5 in. surface coil
B Small FOV
Pulse sequence selection
C T1-weighted spin-echo
Mass lesion
No mass lesion
Consider: Vascularity
D Gd DTPA-enhanced T1 scan
Practical aspects
E Sedation
F Adolescent patient
G MR scan
No Gd DTPA-enhancement
Gd DTPA-enhancement
Astrocytic hamartoma
Follow protocol for no mass lesion
Compare with precontrast image intensity
Strong
Weak/moderate or late
Bright, homogeneous hyperintensity (short T1)
Choroidal hemangioma
Variable T1 hyperintensity
H Uveal melanoma
Slightly shorter T1
Consider: Retinoblastoma
Much shorter T2 Signal void on T1 scan
Consider: Choroidal Osteoma
No globe
Anophthalmos
Small globe
Use region-of-interest (ROI) program to measure size
Normal/large globe
Small optic nerve (ON)
Microphthalmos with ON hypoplasia (ONH)
Normal ON
Microphthalmos without ONH
Wide ON
ON coloboma Morning glory syndrome
Immediate retrobulbar ON
Small or no ON
ON hypoplasia ON aplasia
Nl ON
Anterior segment anomaly
Posterior segment anomaly

ble because of the difficulty in controlling ocular motion.

Recent development of fast imaging methods is based on GRE and echo-planar techniques; the latter requires retrofitting of gradient hardware. The image acquisition time is much shorter than spin-echo (seconds versus minutes); the ocular images, however, are usually degraded by the susceptibility effect from air-tear fluid interface, and the anterior segment therefore is poorly defined. Despite this shortcoming, GRE still is the method of choice for the detection of vitreous hemorrhages and accentuation of uveal melanomas. Fast imaging techniques are useful primarily for functional imaging for the measurements of water diffusion, blood flow, and blood oxygenation.

E. We prefer to sedate pediatric subjects under 12 years of age. The drug of choice is pentobarbital because of its rapid onset and short duration of action. Usually an intravenous dose of 2 to 6 mg/kg in divided doses is recommended; this produces adequate sedation. We have not observed spontaneous or REM eye movements in these patients under sedation. Therefore, superb image quality may be obtained. Monitoring of vital signs and close observation are strongly recommended. Monitors that are compatible with the magnetic environment are commercially available and should be used.

F. If sedation is not used, as in the case of older children, the patient is asked to fixate at a stationary visual target, usually a black spot, 5 mm in diameter, painted on a piece of paper taped on top of the magnet cavity directly in the line of sight of the patient.

G. Following the general precaution of removing metallic objects, the patient is positioned supine in the magnet. The surface coil is installed on an overhead carriage with the coil directly above the eye to be scanned. Alternatively the coil can be positioned over the nose bridge so that both eyes can be scanned at the same time, although the image quality of the latter may be poor because the eye may lie partially outside the active volume of the coil. To localize the eyes, a prescan sagittal head scan is done using an FOV of around 20 cm in the T1-weighted multislice spin-echo or GRE mode. Once the eye of interest is identified, graphic prescription is applied to select the imaging plane (either axial or coronal) and slice thickness (in the spin-echo mode, we recommend 3 mm). The pulse sequence parameters are then entered. An FOV of 8 cm or smaller (when available) is recommended. T1- or T2-weighted imaging is then performed. Fast imaging sequences can be used when available. Because the sound from gradient movements tends to be startlingly loud, earplugs must be worn.

H. Uveal melanoma is very rare in pediatric patients.

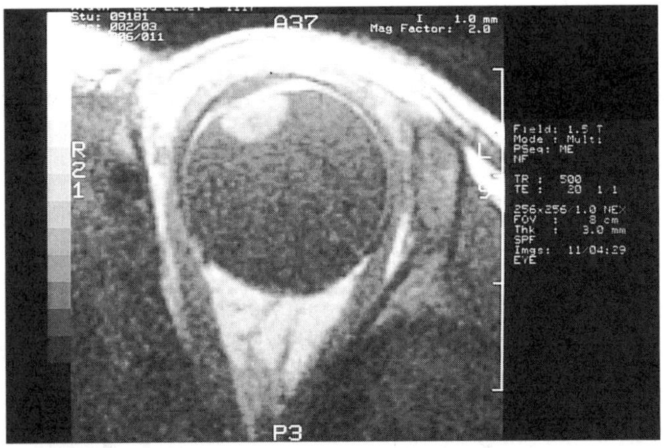

Figure 1 T1-weighted MR image of an infant eye with optic nerve aplasia; only the sheath is seen. Eye is approximately 18 mm in diameter with a very shallow anterior chamber and a small oval-shaped lens. The ciliary body is flat and continuous with the iris. Signal intensity of the choroid is segmented, with lower intensity in the posterior region. Image was acquired with TR/TE = 500/20 msec; image resolution was 0.3 × 0.3 mm in-plane with a 3-mm slice thickness.

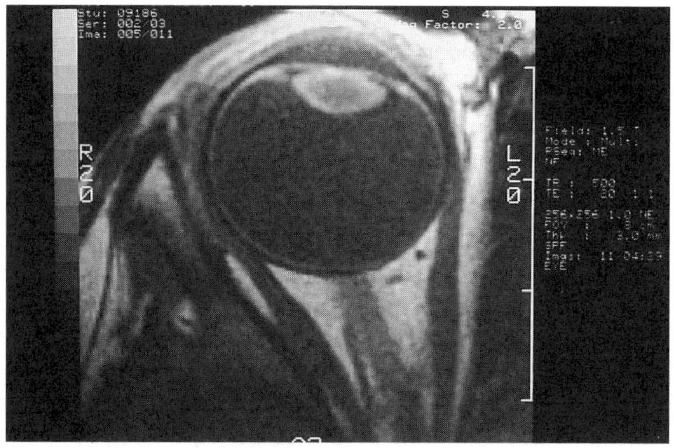

Figure 2 MR image of a normal eye using the same parameters as those in Figure 1.

References

Cheng HM. Magnetic resonance imaging of the human eye in vivo. Optom Vis Sci 1991; 68:976.

Cheng HM. Nuclear magnetic resonance studies of ocular tissues. Med Sci Res 1988; 16:441.

Cheng HM. The fate of water in the soft contact lens immediately after lens placement onto the cornea. Optom Vis Sci 1991; 68:414.

Cheng HM, Kuan WP, Garrido L, et al. High-resolution MR imaging of water diffusion in the rabbit lens. Exp Eye Res 1992; 54:127.

Cheng HM, Kwong KK, Xiong J, Woods BT. Visualization of water movement in the living rabbit eye. Graefe's Arch Clin Exp Ophthalmol 1992; 230:62.

Cheng HM, Yeh LI, Barnett PA, et al. Proton magnetic resonance imaging of the lens. Exp Eye Res 1987; 45:875.

Kwong KK, Kuan WP, Xiong J, Cheng HM. Measurement of water movement in the rabbit eye in vivo using $H_2{}^{17}O$. Magn Reson Med 1991; 22:443.

DIAGNOSTIC TECHNIQUES IN OCULAR INFECTIOUS DISEASE

Merrill L. Stass-Isern, M.D.
David L. Zwick, M.D.

More difficult than choosing a particular culture medium or stain is deciding when an individual's infectious ocular disease needs to be studied. There are no specific guidelines or rules. A sound knowledge of the clinical findings associated with specific viral, bacterial, and fungal infections eliminates the need to study the majority of these diseases. However, once a culture has been obtained, it is important to know the normal flora of the conjunctiva and eyelids so that clinical correlation and treatment are appropriate (see Table 1, p 290). The ensuing two chapters address obtaining specimens, cultures, stains, and rapid diagnostic tests.

A. When obtaining material from the cornea for a culture, topical anesthesia with proparacaine hydrochloride is recommended because it is less bacteriostatic than other agents. Use a Kimura or Lindner spatula sterilized by flaming both before and after use. If neither is available, a No. 15 Bard-Parker blade or a bent 27-gauge needle may be substituted. Direct inoculation onto the medium rather than onto transport medium is important and increases the yield of positive results. The optimal situation is to obtain the specimen prior to antibiotic use. If this is not possible, the laboratory needs to be informed of the type and method of delivery of antibiotic being used. When obtaining a slide for cytology or microbiologic features, immediate fixation with methyl alcohol is recommended to prevent any drying effects. In general, corneal scraping is not valuable for cytology unless a tumor or herpes is suspected.

B. Recognizable organisms many times are not seen from the smear of the exudate; therefore, a conjuctival scraping is recommended. The same principles of anesthesia and use of a platinum spatula are recommended. The scraping should not be so deep as to cause bleeding, which may obscure reading of the slide by peripheral blood elements. One should be able to recognize material on the tip of the spatula. When it is smeared on a slide, as thin a layer as possible is better for identification of individual cells. Immediate fixation is critical. Sterile applicators may be used when obtaining cultures from the conjunctiva. Once again, transport media should not be used.

C. When specimens need to be obtained because of suspected endophthalmitis (p 248), special care and handling of the specimen are imperative. A subconjunctival, retrobulbar, or general anesthetic is appropriate. A small conjunctival peritomy is performed. A 23-gauge, 1-inch needle is passed through the pars plana 3.5 mm posterior to the limbus in the vitreous cavity. (This is for the older child; for the younger child, a proportionately smaller distance from the pars plana is recommended.) Ideally, the needle tip is visualized through the pupil. A small amount of vitreous (0.2 ml) is then withdrawn. Direct inoculation onto culture media should be done. At least three drops of the specimen should be dropped onto each plate. The remaining fluid can be used to prepare slides for staining and direct visualization. If aqueous humor is to be obtained, a 27-gauge needle is passed into the anterior chamber through the limbus, and 0.1 to 0.2 ml is withdrawn. Once again, direct inoculation onto the media is imperative.

D. Blood agar is most useful and is able to support the majority of organisms likely to be isolated in the eye, both bacterial and fungal. Chocolate agar is best for *Haemophilus* and *Neisseria*. General nutrient broths (PABA and trypticase soy) are all-purpose media and are more likely than agar to allow for detection of small numbers of organisms.

E. Thioglycolate broth is an all-purpose medium good for anaerobes and microaerophilic organisms. Cooked meat broth can also be used.

F. Occasionally, one may need to isolate *Mycobacterium tuberculosis* or *Nocardia* species. This is best done with Lowenstein-Jensen medium.

G. Sabouraud dextrose agar with cycloheximide, a saprophytic fungus inhibitor, is best for fungi and yeast while inhibiting bacteria. Brain or beef heart infusion works well for fastidious fungi that fail to grow on Sabouraud's agar. It must contain an antibacterial agent such as gentamicin to inhibit bacterial overgrowth.

H. Viral cultures are expensive and the yield is small. Therefore, case selection is important. These are rarely necessary to diagnosis a herpetic or adenovirus infection. The highest yield occurs with direct inoculation onto a cell line and tissue culture, but, this is rarely possible. Therefore, a transport medium (Hank's medium) is usually used.

I. *Chlamydia* cultures are also expensive and of low yield. *Chlamydia* can be better diagnosed by fluorescein antibody staining (p 292).

J. When acanthamoeba is suspected, it may be cultured on non-nutrient agar overlaid with *Escherichia coli*. The amoeba may be detected by direct wet-mount preparations or a variety of stains. Viable organisms rapidly attach to glass surfaces and hence transport vessels should be shaken gently to dislodge them prior to preparation of cultures or smears.

(Continued on p. 291.)

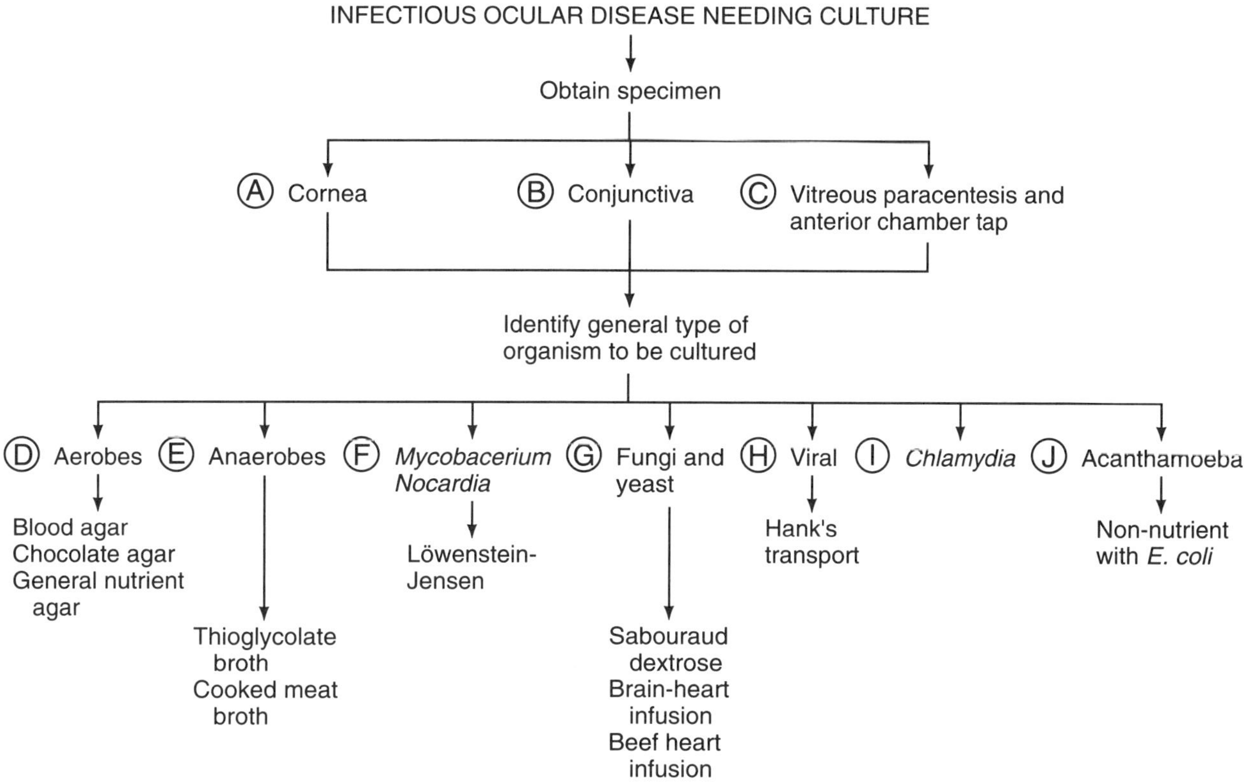
INFECTIOUS OCULAR DISEASE NEEDING CULTURE
Obtain specimen
(A) Cornea
(B) Conjunctiva
(C) Vitreous paracentesis and anterior chamber tap
Identify general type of organism to be cultured
(D) Aerobes
Blood agar
Chocolate agar
General nutrient agar
(E) Anaerobes
Thioglycolate broth
Cooked meat broth
(F) Mycobacterium Nocardia
Löwenstein-Jensen
(G) Fungi and yeast
Sabouraud dextrose
Brain-heart infusion
Beef heart infusion
(H) Viral
Hank's transport
(I) Chlamydia
(J) Acanthamoeba
Non-nutrient with E. coli

TABLE 1 Microorganisms Encountered in Eye Specimens

Organism	*Frequency of Isolation**	*Disease Involvement†*
Absidia spp	C	2
Acanthamoeba spp.	C	3
Achromobacier xylosoxidans	C	1
Acinetobacter spp.	B	2
Acromonium spp.	B	2
Actinobacillus actinomycetemcomitans	C	2
Actinomyces spp.	C	2
Adenoviruses	B	2
Aeromonas hydrophila	B	2
Alternaria spp.	B	2
Arachnia spp.	B	2
Aspergillus spp.	B	2
Aureobasidium spp.	C	1
Azotobacter spp.	C	1
Bacillus spp.	B	2
Bacteroides spp.	C	2
Bifidobacterium spp.	C	2
Blastomyces dermatitidis	B	3
Branhamella (Moraxella) catarrhalis	B	1
Brucella spp.	C	3
Candida spp.	B	2
Chlamydia trachomatis	B	3
Cladosporium spp.	B	1
Clostridium spp.	C	2
Coccidioides immitis	C	3
Corynebacterium diphtheriae	C	3
Corynebacterium spp.	B	2
Cryptococcus neoformans	C	3
Curvularia spp.	B	1
Cytomegalovirus	B	3
Drechlera spp.	B	1
Enterobacteriaceae	B	2
Epstein-Barr virus	C	3
Exophiala jeanselmei	C	1
Francisella tularensis	C	3
Fusarium spp.	B	2
Fusobacterium spp.	C	2
Haemophilus influenzae biotype III *(H. aegyptius)*	B	3
Herpes simplex virus	B	3
Lactobacillus spp.	C	2
Leptospira spp.	C	3
Loa loa	C	3
Measles virus	B	3
Moraxella supp.	B	2
Mucor spp.	B	2
Mumps virus	B	3
Mycobacterium spp.	C	2
Mycobacterium tuberculosis group	C	3
Neisseria gonorrhoeae	B	3
Neisseria meningitidis	B	3
Neisseria spp.	B	1
Nocardia spp.	C	3
Nosemia spp.	C	3
Onchocerca volvulus	C	3
Paecilomyces spp.	B	1
Peptococcus spp.	C	2
Peptostreptococcus spp.	C	2
Poxvirus	C	3
Propionibacterium spp.	B	2
Pseudallescheria boydii	C	3
Pseudomonas spp.	B	2
Rhizomucor spp.	B	2
Rhizopus spp.	B	2
Rubella virus	B	3
Sporothrix schenckii	C	3
Staphyloccus spp.	A	2
Streptococcus spp.	B	2
Taenia solium larvae	C	3
Toxocara spp.	C	3
Toxoplasma gondii	B	3
Treponema pallidum	B	3
Varicella-zoster virus	B	3
Veillonella spp.	C	2

*A-Commonly encountered in clinical specimens; B-occasionally encountered in clinical specimens; C-rarely encountered in clinical specimens.
†1-When present, it is rarely if ever involved in disease production; 2-when present, it is occasionally involved in disease production; 3-when present, it is commonly involved in disease production.

From Balows A, Hausler WJ Jr, Herrimann KL, et al. Manual of clinical microbiology. 5th ed. Washington, DC: American Society for Microbiology Publication, 1991; with permission.

References

Balows A, Hausler WJ Jr, Herrmann KL, et al. A manual of clinical microbiology. 5th ed. Washington, DC: American Society of Microbiology Publication, 1991.

Flynn Jr HW, Pflugselder SC, Culbertson, et al. Recognition, treatment and prevention of endophthalmitis. Semin Ophthalmol 1989; 4:69

Pavan-Langston D. Laboratory techniques in ocular virology. Int Ophthalmol Clin 1975; 15:1.

Petite TH. Management of bacterial corneal ulcers. Symp Ocular Ther 1976; 8:57.

SMEARS, STAINS, AND RAPID DIAGNOSTIC TESTS

Merrill L. Stass-Isern, M.D.
David L. Zwick, M.D.

A. Proceed as in previous chapter under cultures (see p 288).

B. Gram's stain is the most helpful for demonstrating bacteria and yeast.

C. Giemsa stain is useful for demonstrating the presence of chlamydia and fungal elements. It shows hypae and cross walls well.

D. Calcoflur white and acridine orange stains make use of dyes (fluorochromes) and require the availability of a fluorescein microscope and an experienced microbiologist. Calcoflur white binds to the cell walls of fungi and acanthemoeba, enhancing their visibility. Acridine orange binds to nucleic acids of viable and dead bacteria.

E. Periodic acid–Schiff (PAS) and Gomori-methenamine-silver (GMS) can also be used for identification of fungi.

F. Occasionally an acid-fast stain may be needed for identification of mycobacteria and nocardia.

G. Other rapid detection techniques for identifying fastidious or slow-growing microorganisms have been developed. Through the application and recognition of specific monoclonal antibodies on sample smears by immunofluorescent or immunoperoxidase techniques, a growing number of viral, bacterial, and parasitic infections may be diagnosed in a matter of hours. These would otherwise take days to weeks to identify. A wide variety of antibodies is commercially available, but only a few are widely applied. Molecular biologic techniques using in situ and in vivo complementary DNA hybridization probes to various microbes are beginning to find clinical application for specific and rapid diagnosis. It is important to recognize that most of these tests lack the sensitivity of standardized culture techniques and, although quite specific, have not been rigorously evaluated. One should specifically inquire with the local laboratory to determine its capabilities for rapid detection testing. Herpes simplex and *Chlamydia trachomatis* immunostaining tests are most widely available. At our laboratory we have MicroTrak by Syva and Pathfinder by Kallestad for *Chlamydia*.

H. In general, the Giemsa stain delineates cytologic features better than Gram's stain. With herpetic keratitis it may reveal syncitial giant cells with intranuclear inclusions. Gram-negative diplococci of Neisseria can be demonstrated intracellularly in conjunctival epithelium as well as in neutrophils. Intracytoplasmic inclusion bodies found in neonatal inclusion conjunctivitis (chlamydia) stain best with Giemsa stain. They are blue and granular in the cytoplasm near the nucleus. Giemsa stain is also good for demonstrating epithelial tumor cells.

I. The Wright stain is not ideal for ocular cytology, but it may be substituted if a Giemsa stain is not available. It readily stains eosinophils and eosinophilic granules.

J. When looking for intranuclear inclusion bodies seen with herpes, the Papanicolaou stain with methanol fixative should be used. These inclusions appear as either smudged ground-glass nuclei or as eosinophilic nuclear inclusions surrounded by cleared nucleoplasm which imparts the characteristic owl-eye appearance.

References

Balows A, Hausler WJ Jr, Herrmann KL, et al. A manual of clinical microbiology. 5th ed. Washington, DC: American Society of Microbiology Publication, 1991.

Flynn Jr HW, Pflugselder SC, Culbertson, et al. Recognition, treatment and prevention of endophthalmitis. Semin Ophthalmol 1989; 4:69.

Pavan-Langston D. Laboratory techniques in ocular virology. Int Ophthalmol Clin 1975; 15:1.

Petite TH. Management of bacterial corneal ulcers. Symp Ocular Ther 1976; 8:57.

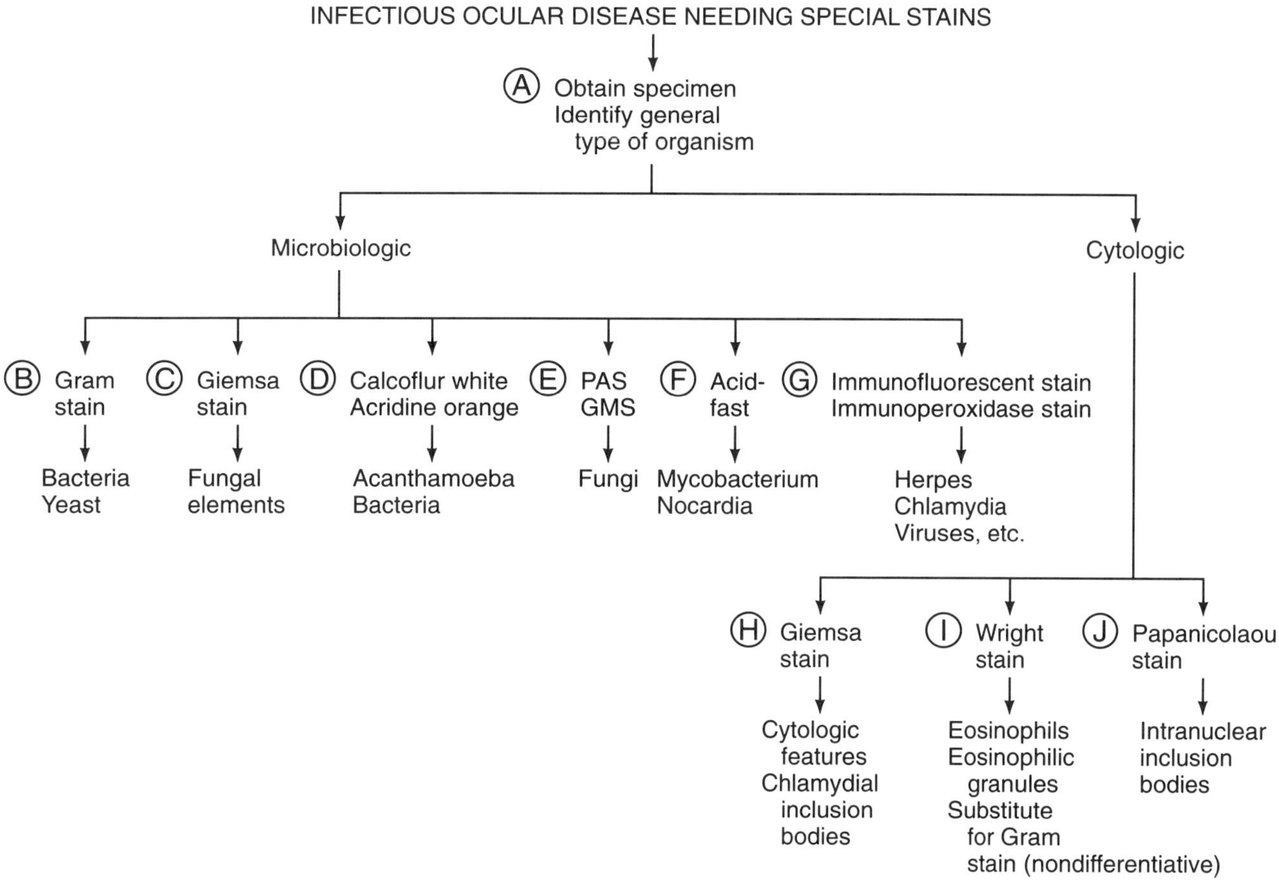
INFECTIOUS OCULAR DISEASE NEEDING SPECIAL STAINS
(A) Obtain specimen
Identify general type of organism
Microbiologic
Cytologic
(B) Gram stain
Bacteria
Yeast
(C) Giemsa stain
Fungal elements
(D) Calcoflur white
Acridine orange
Acanthamoeba
Bacteria
(E) PAS
GMS
Fungi
(F) Acid-fast
Mycobacterium
Nocardia
(G) Immunofluorescent stain
Immunoperoxidase stain
Herpes
Chlamydia
Viruses, etc.
(H) Giemsa stain
Cytologic features
Chlamydial inclusion bodies
(I) Wright stain
Eosinophils
Eosinophilic granules
Substitute for Gram stain (nondifferentiative)
(J) Papanicolaou stain
Intranuclear inclusion bodies

ELECTRORETINOGRAPHY

Donnell J. Creel, Ph.D.

The electroretinogram (ERG) is a mass electrical response of the retina to photic stimulation. A flash of light such as that produced by a strobe lamp elicits a biphasic wave form similar to that shown in Figure 1. The photopic ERG reaches adult form by 3 months of age and the scotopic ERG by 1 year of age. Normal ranges, means, and standard deviations should be compiled by each laboratory. Pattern ERGs are generated using reversing checkerboard patterns or shifting lines. The pattern ERG is generated primarily by ganglion cells. Its clinical use is limited in pediatric ophthalmology.

The flash ERG can be recorded using several methods. The pupil is dilated if low-intensity stimuli are used in the testing procedure. There are a half-dozen commonly used recording electrodes. Speculum electrodes hold the eye open and have a contact lens with a built-in wire that "floats" on the cornea supported by a small spring. Electrodes that limit eye movement and directly contact the cornea record the largest-amplitude, most reliable ERG and are preferred to skin electrodes for that reason. There are also several methods of stimulating the eye. ERGs are most reliable when recorded using a Ganzfeld device to control background illumination and intensity of flash reaching the retina.

A. The ERG can be a valuable adjunct to the evaluation of any retinal problem. Even a normal ERG can be diagnostically significant, such as in cortical blindness and hysteria. In general, a child 5 years or older can be tested using a speculum electrode and a Ganzfeld. Infants older than a few months and children under 5 years of age frequently have to be tested using a sedative or anesthesia.

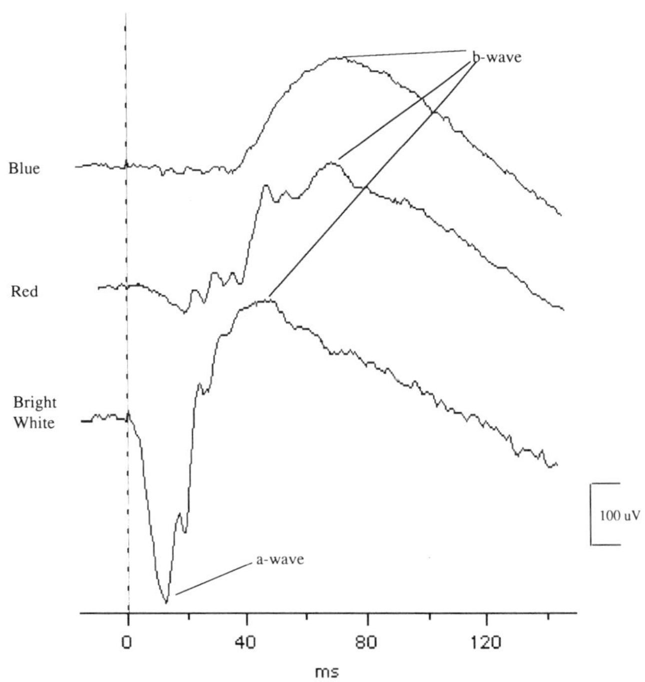

Figure 1 Normal dark-adapted ERG of a 2 year old.

B. The rods in the retina must be dark adapted to test their function adequately. It is more important that the length of dark adaptation be consistent from patient to patient than that the period be a certain length. The recommended time period of dark adaptation is 45 minutes.

C. To isolate rod function, the patient should be dark adapted and the initial stimulus limited to a dim white or preferably blue flash attenuated at least 2 log units compared with the white flash used during photopic testing. The flash intensity should be dim enough that in the normal individual B-wave amplitude is only about 200 μV. Dim stimuli require an analysis time of about 200 msec. Scotopic dim blue flashes presented singularly isolate rod function, providing sensitive evaluation of rod physiology fundamental to detection of many common retinal disorders such as retinitis pigmentosa (RP). In all genetic forms of RP and Leber congenital amaurosis, ERG changes precede visible fundus disease. B-wave amplitude elicited by dim scotopic stimulation is the most sensitive indicator of defective rod physiology and of metabolic dysfunction reflected in the physiology of the retina, such as siderosis, vitamin A deficiency, hypothyroidism, anemia, myotonic dystrophy, the mucopolysaccharidoses, and Batten disease.

D. Some laboratories also use a scotopic red flash that is matched by trial and error addition of neutral-density filters until the ERG produces B waves of the same amplitude as the scotopic dim blue stimulus. The ERG elicited by the scotopic red flash provides a reliability check of the results of the scotopic dim blue ERG and also provides a glimpse of cone physiology. A scotopic intensity series is also used in some laboratories to determine the Naka-Rushton parameters.

E. The ERG produced by scotopic bright white flash stimulation is not definitive if retinal dysfunction is subtle, such as in metabolic disorders or metallosis. The scotopic bright white ERG can be very informative in some disorders such as confirming juvenile retinoschisis by demonstrating the missing B wave and B/A ratio, and to quantitate severe expression of disorders such as RP or cone-rod dystrophy, in which often no recordable ERG response to other stimuli can be elicited. All bright flash stimuli require an analysis time of only 75 to 100 msec.

F. Oscillatory potentials (OPs) that appear on the ascending limb of the B wave following bright white flash stimulation can be isolated by changing the low bandpass on the amplifiers to 100 Hz instead of the usual <1 Hz. The effect of this filter change is to eliminate the slow-rising limb of the B wave, leaving the OPs, which appear as a sinusoidal train beginning

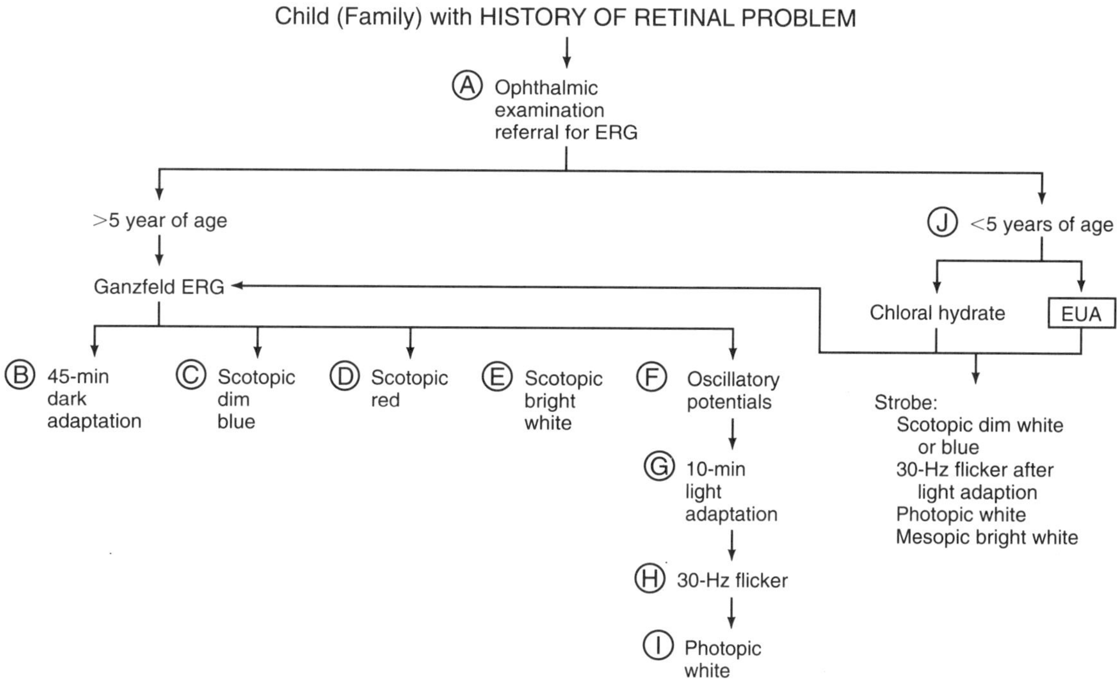

about 15 msec after flash onset. These potentials can be quantitated by power spectral analysis or by measuring the implicit times and peak-to-peak amplitudes of individual components. OPs should be recorded after the scotopic bright white stimulation with about 15 seconds between each flash. OPs are the most sensitive ERG component to vascular changes affecting the diffuse or mid retina. Any disorder that compromises retinal vasculature, such as diabetic retinopathy, central retinal vein or artery occlusion, hypertension, or Takayasu's (pulseless) disease, often demonstrate only reduced OPs in early disease. Reduced OP amplitude is also recorded in retinoschisis, central serous chorioretinopathy, and carriers of congenital stationary night blindness (CSNB). OPs may be prognostic in branch retinal vein occlusion and in early stages of diabetic retinopathy.

G. After the above scotopic tests the patient should be light adapted for about 10 minutes or more with background illumination of about 10 ftL to return the retina to a light-adapted state.

H. Only the cones can recover fast enough to follow a flickering light faster than about 20 Hz. Most laboratories determine whether cones are healthy by recording the ERG following several bursts of 30-Hz flicker. Usually two or three 100-msec time epochs are averaged. The ERG response is a train of B waves. The time to the first peak and interpeak times can be measured along with peak-to-peak amplitude. Reduced amplitude must be interpreted cautiously when ERGs produced by 30-Hz flicker are averaged because photophobia is common in this testing condition. Simply squeezing the eyelids together attenuates the ERG response to flicker.

I. Photopic single white flashes may be presented either before or after 30-Hz stimulation. The ERG produced also reflects cone physiology because the rods have been light adapted and do not contribute to this ERG. The photopic ERG usually has an A-wave implicit time as fast as 10 msec in children and a B-wave implicit time frequently faster than 30 msec. Prolonged B-wave implicit time is sometimes seen early in all forms of RP and may precede detectable rod anomalies. Patients with most cone degenerations have abnormal photopic ERGs and normal or supernormal scotopic ERGs.

J. It is unusual to talk a child less than 5 years of age through an examination using contact lens or speculum electrodes. Skin or scleral electrodes can be used, with their limitations, or the patient can be sedated or anesthetized. Many clinics use chloral hydrate or the three-in-one "cardiac cocktail" to sedate pediatric patients. Chloral hydrate has several limitations including that the patient weighs less than about 15 kg. ERG testing is also sometimes performed as part of a more extensive examination under anesthesia (EUA). In an ERG laboratory the sedated patient can be dark adapted and a more or less normal series of stimuli similar to those in B to I above can be used, although the length of effect of the sedative usually necessitates that the method be abbreviated to just three or four stimuli. Dark adaptation even for a few minutes followed by single flashes of white or blue assesses scotopic ERG function. Photopic single flashes and 30-Hz flicker can be used to evaluate cone function. It is not possible to completely darken the operating room, so abbreviated testing is accomplished under mesopic and photopic light conditions.

References

Fishman GA, Sokol S. Electrophysiologic testing in disorders of the retina, optic nerve, and visual pathway. San Francisco: American Academy of Ophthalmology, 1990.

Heckenlively JR, Arden GB, eds. Handbook of clinical electrophysiology. St. Louis: CV Mosby, 1991.

Weleber RG, Eisner A. Retinal function and physiological studies. In: Newsome DA, ed. Retinal dystrophies and degenerations. New York: Raven Press, 1988.

VISUAL EVOKED RESPONSE

Donnell J. Creel, Ph.D.

The terms *visual evoked response* (VER), *visual evoked potential* (VEP), and *visual evoked cortical potential* (VECP) are synonymous. They refer to electrical potentials recorded from the scalp overlying the visual cortex which have been extracted from the electroencephalogram (EEG) by signal averaging. VERs can provide quantification of visual function and clinically inapparent information.

When recording VERs the diagnostic yield depends upon appropriate selection of visual stimuli. Steady-state VERs are those recorded using stimulation rates of six or more per second. Transient VERs are recorded using rates of less than three per second. Transient pattern VERs have specific components that can be followed during maturation and changes of acuity. Until 25 years ago patients were tested using only a strobe flash, producing a VER that could be recorded over the visual cortices. A flash-evoked VER is reliable in form within the individual but varies considerably between patients. Pattern stimuli produce more reliable VERs, enabling specific components to be evaluated. The most common method is to present a checkerboard pattern on a television monitor. The checkerboard pattern can be made to reverse its black and white checks at various set rates, or a pattern can be made to appear (onset) and disappear (offset). The VER waveform, amplitudes, and peak latencies depend upon the parameters of the stimulus.

Pattern reversal and flash VERs are similar in form in that they both have a major negative component at about 70 msec (N70) and a major positive component at approximately 100 msec (P100), although the flash P100 actually appears around 110 msec. In most individuals the pattern-onset VER is opposite in polarity to flash and pattern reversal VERs. The pattern-onset VER usually includes a positive component at about 80 msec and a large negative component at about 110 msec. An advantage of the pattern-reversal VER is that it has the most consistent form when comparing individuals and has a smaller standard deviation for the P100 component of about 6 msec. The P110 component of the flash VER and the N110 component of the pattern-onset VER have standard deviations of about 10 msec. When infants are tested, the analysis time should be 300 to 600 msec because components of the VERs may have long peak latencies during early maturation. VERs change rapidly in form and complexity during the first 6 months. Children and adults may be tested using an analysis time of 200 to 400 (the editors prefer 300 to 400) msec. It is imperative that each laboratory have their own normative data, particularly when testing pediatric patients, because of variability in this population due to differences in maturation. The VER form resembles that of an adult by early school years, reaching largest amplitude and fastest P100 time of about 95 msec by 7 to 10 years of age. Components of the VER change slowly after this age with a gradual attenuation in amplitude and slowing of the P100 component of about 1 msec per decade.

A. If the history and ophthalmic examination of a pediatric patient raise the possibility of dysfunctional optic nerves, tracts, or cortices, the VER may yield diagnostically useful information. A common clinical referral is the patient in whom the diagnostic question is whether visual problems are due to retinal or more central visual dysfunction. Recording both an electroretinogram (ERG) and VER usually answers this question. Data from VERs and ERGs are particularly helpful in the pediatric population, in which communication and cooperation are often poor.

B. It is important that a patient be tested with refractive error corrected. Select the most powerful stimulus that the visual acuity and cooperation of the patient allow.

C. If the corrected visual acuity of the patient is approximately 20/200 (6/60) or better and he or she does not have nystagmus, the stimulus of first choice is pattern reversal. Check sizes subtending 10 to 20 minutes of arc are the best stimuli for testing foveal vision. Checks of 40 to 50 minutes are superior in evaluating parafoveal function; therefore, using more than one check size increases diagnostic yield. If the resulting VER using the smaller check size is poorly formed, retest using a larger check size of about 60 to 70 minutes. Pattern reversal stimuli are the best choice in cooperative patients with good visual acuity, particularly when testing for possible effects of optic neuritis, hydrocephalus, ventriculitis, cortical hematomas, optic atrophy, or compression of the optic pathways.

D. If the corrected acuity of the patient is approximately 20/200 to 20/400 (6/60 to 6/120) and/or the patient has nystagmus, the preferred stimulus is pattern onset. Pattern-onset or "pattern-flash" stimuli produce a more robust VER than does pattern reversal in these patients. Pattern-reversal stimuli usually exacerbate nystagmus, interfering with the ability of the eye to maintain foveal fixation. Pattern-onset stimuli can also be the most productive stimuli in conditions such as monitoring amblyopia in patients with poor acuity, possible hemispheric asymmetry, or a defect in geniculostriate projections.

E. If the patient's acuity is approximately 20/400 (6/120) or worse, or the patient is uncooperative, unconscious, sedated, or anesthetized, the stimulus of choice is strobe flash or light-emitting diodes (LEDs). Flash stimuli are useful in infants who do not fixate on a pattern. The resulting VER usually detects significant optic atrophy and other abnormalities of the central visual pathways. In most cases of true cortical blindness the flash VER is abnormal, although it is possible to record a normal flash VER. In general, the better the VER, the better the prognosis. The VER is not prognos-

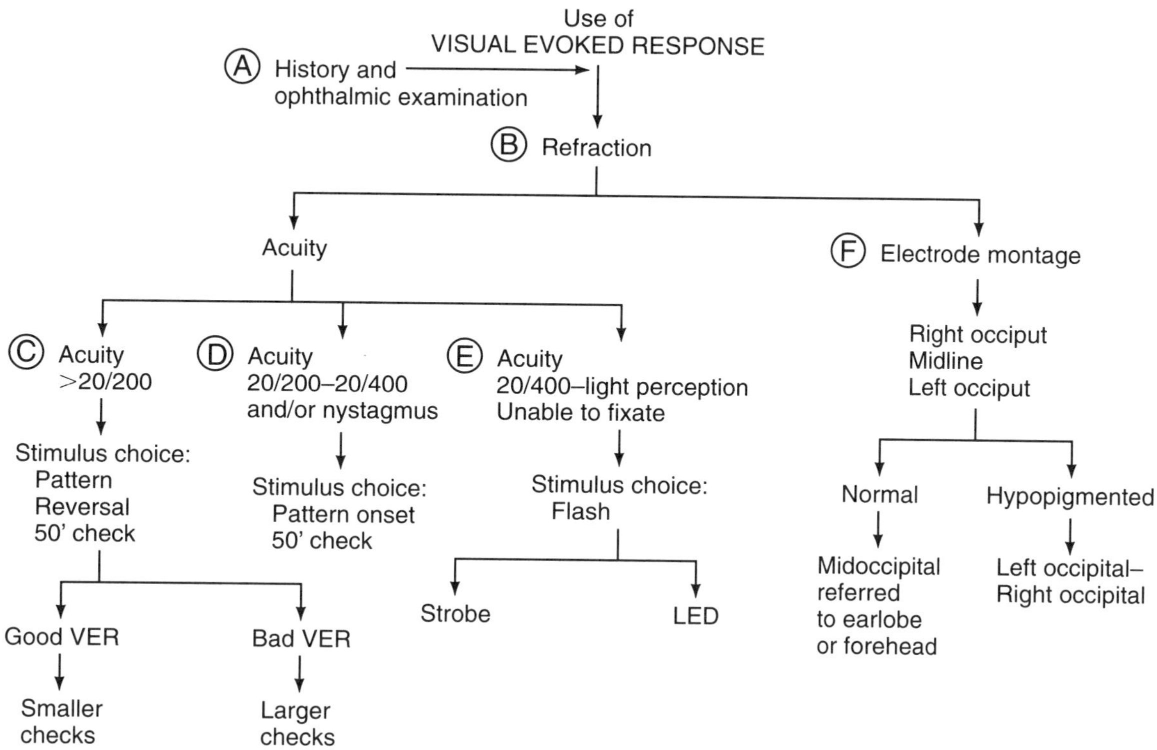

tic in delayed maturation of the visual system except that usually the infant with delayed maturation has a normal flash VER, whereas most cortically blind infants have poor VERs. Flash stimuli produced by LEDs can be useful in some patients. The LEDs are available inside goggles and on discs about 50 mm in diameter. These are more effective than a strobe lamp for monocular stimulation and useful in the operating room when monitoring VERs during surgery because they can be placed over the patient's eyes with the surgical drape over them.

F. Electrode montage should focus on activity at the midline overlying the central pole of the occipital cortex owing to the fact that the macula is projected onto the occipital pole. A recording electrode placed 3 to 4 cm above the inion can be referenced to either central midline, central frontal, or ipsilateral mastoid. The forehead serves as a ground. Other recording sites of interest are 3 to 4 cm left and right of the central occipital electrode. The same reference electrode is used. The left and right occipital electrodes may be referenced to each other on a bipolar montage, which records a "difference" potential. This bipolar montage is especially useful in suspected albinism, in which an excessive proportion of ganglion fibers decussate and erroneously project to the contralateral hemisphere. Normally pigmented individuals have nearly equal innervation of visual cortex from nasal and temporal retinas, so the "difference" potential recorded between hemispheres is similar in form whether stimulating the left or right eye. In contrast, more central retinal ganglion fibers cross to the contralateral hemisphere in albinos, so the "difference" potential recorded between occipital hemispheres changes polarity when results of monocular stimulation are compared.

A VER to hemifield stimulus can be recorded by using a 60-minute check in the left or right side of the television monitor. The pattern projects to either the nasal or temporal retina. Additional recording electrodes are placed 3 to 4 cm temporal to the left and right occipital electrodes. This VER is sensitive to field defects that may not be seen on a full-field VER and is useful in the pediatric patient who cannot perform a visual field examination.

References

Beringer TA, Heider W. Electrophysiology and perimetry in acute retrobulbar neuritis. Documenta Ophthalmol 1989; 71:293.

Creel DJ, Shearer DE, Dustman RE. Visually evoked potential parameters for detecting visual pathology. In: Nodar RH, Barber C, eds. Evoked potentials II. Boston: Butterworth, 1984:237.

Creel DJ, Summers CG, King RA. Visual anomalies associated with albinism. Ophthalmol Paediatr 1990; 11:193.

Fishman GA, Sokol S. Electrophysiologic testing in disorders of the retina, optic nerve, and visual pathway. San Francisco: American Academy of Ophthalmology, 1990.

Regan D. Human brain electrophysiology. New York: Elsevier, 1989.

ELECTROPHYSIOLOGIC ACUITY TESTING

Gerhard W. Cibis, M.D.
Kathleen Fitzgerald, R EP T

Visual acuity information is necessary for diagnostic, classification, therapeutic, educational, genetic, and prognostic purposes. Obtaining visual acuity in nonverbal patients is equally important, so alternatives to the Snellen charts have attracted interest. Numerous methods have been developed which are capable of testing nonverbal infants or an older child unable to communicate (see p 304). Our experience finds electrophysiologic methods, specifically those of sweep visual evoked potential (VEP), to be useful.

A. History combined with examination (B) can diagnose conditions for which acuity can be inferred. An infant with no clinical evidence of vision or pupil reactions, nystagmus of the blind, and no recordable VEP or electroretinography (ERG) does not need acuity assessment. Conversely, a normal infant with central, steady, and maintained fixation (CSM), normal fundi, optokinetic nystagmus, and otherwise normal examination can be inferred to have normal visual acuity for age. The cases between these extreme conditions need differentiation.

B. The examination should be complete, observing fixing and following behavior, nystagmus, and structural defects such as optic nerve hypoplasia (ONH), foveal aplasia, aniridia, cataracts, and ptosis. Clinical evidence for factors that cause poor vision, such as poor fixation in one or both eyes, refractive errors capable of causing unilateral or bilateral amblyopia (p 102), strabismus, and nystagmus should be noted. Documentation of poor visual acuity is especially needed when considering patching, glasses, or surgery. If there are social needs such as school placement, educational approaches, or adoption, the sweep VEP can provide Snellen equivalent acuity in patients unable to communicate.

C. The sweep VEP can provide Snellen values and contrast sensitivity (CS) values. Clinical application of CS has not been fully described in pediatric ophthalmology. Decreased CS in amblyopia when acuity is still normal has been reported. The same is true with glaucoma, cataracts, and other conditions. How to use CS in these situations remains to be elucidated. When practical, CS should be measured whenever sweep VEP is recorded to develop data that is likely to become clinically useful in the future.

TABLE 1 Conditions in Which Sweep VEP is Useful

Ptosis
Hemangioma
Partial cataract
Corneal leukomas
Disc anomalies
Retinal anomalies as with regressed retinopathy of prematurity
Functional vision loss
Unsuccessful patching
Monitoring occlusion therapy

D. The sweep VEP is especially practical in cases of malingering or functional vision loss. The values obtained are evidence of acuity that is indisputably not compatible with the claimed poor level of vision.

E. Patching in amblyopia leads to improvement in fixation patterns not reflected in acuity values. Whereas an amblyopia of two to three lines in the virgin case leads to poor fixation patterns, vision of as little as 20/200 can have good fixation when the patient has had extensive patching. As patching progresses, therefore, fixation pattern assessment is less reliable, and sweep VEP to confirm or refute a good "end point" for patching is indicated. This phenomenon accounts for the common mishap of successful patching in patients <3 years of age with good CSM fixation in each eye suddenly showing two to four lines of amblyopia or worse at age 3 years or older, when acuity values can be verbally derived. Similarly, ptosis patients may show good fixation patterns but may actually have amblyopia as detected by sweep VEP.

F. The sweep VEP has a high intraindividual test reliability of 0.2 octave. This is better than other methods such as forced-choice preferential looking, which was originally reported to be sensitive to 1 octave difference. However, recent reports with abridged Teller acuity cards approach the 0.2-octave level as well. The VEP depends less on subjective decisions than even the abridged Teller method. Subjective bias of the observer is a problem with fixation and behavioral acuity card assessments but is minimal in sweep VEP assessments. If an acuity estimate cannot be obtained using the sweep VEP, behavioral assessments (preferential looking) may yield results.

A transient pattern VEP may be used to estimate acuity by virtue of response amplitude versus check size and gives information about the status of the visual pathway. If this fails, a flash VEP may be used to determine the status of the pathway, but it does not yield acuity estimates other than less than or better than 20/200. The flash VEP provides information on lateralization, which is useful in injuries and congenital brain anomalies as well as albinism.

G. Sweep VEP is labor and equipment intensive and therefore not well suited to screening (p 198).

H. Conditions with risk for amblyopia development can be effectively monitored with sweep VEP (see also Table 1).

I. The sweep VEP is based on discrete Fourier analysis of the steady-state VEP. A contrast-reversed, square wave–generated vertical grating is presented on a television monitor. The gratings reverse at 6 Hz, and during a 10-second period the size of the grating (spatial frequency) decreases to a size well below the acuity threshold. The acuity estimate is obtained by

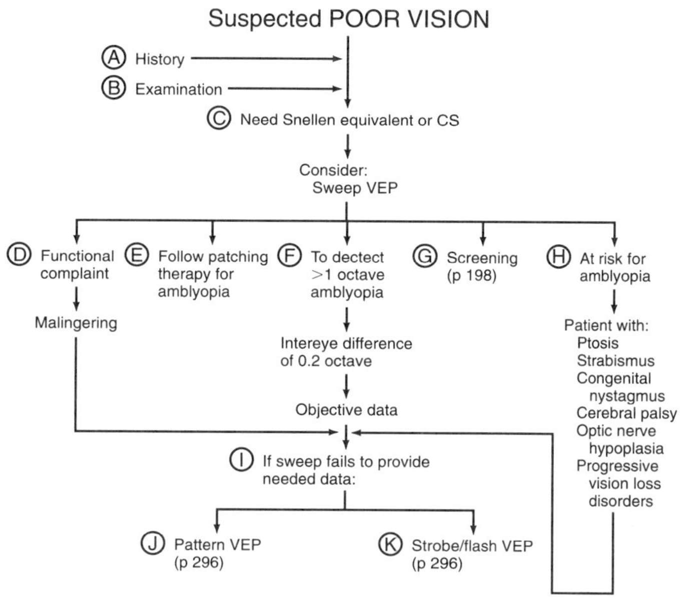

using linear extrapolation to zero amplitude of the VEP versus spatial frequency function (Fig. 1). The response is recorded from electrodes placed over the occipital midline. Three or four trials are obtained for each test condition (binocular or monocular). Fixation on the monitor is required and can be maintained by dangling a small toy or noisemaker in front of the monitor (Fig. 2). When fixation is lost, the recording may be interrupted by pressing a button and resumed when fixation resumes.

J. The pattern VEP is a transient response recorded from electrodes placed over the occipital cortex. The stimulus is usually a high-contrast, slowly reversing (<2 Hz) checkerboard pattern. The check size and contrast remain stationary throughout the 1- to 2-minute trial. Amplitude and latency measurements are obtained from the waveform. Two trials are required for replication of responses. Fixation of the center of the television monitor for the duration of the trial is required.

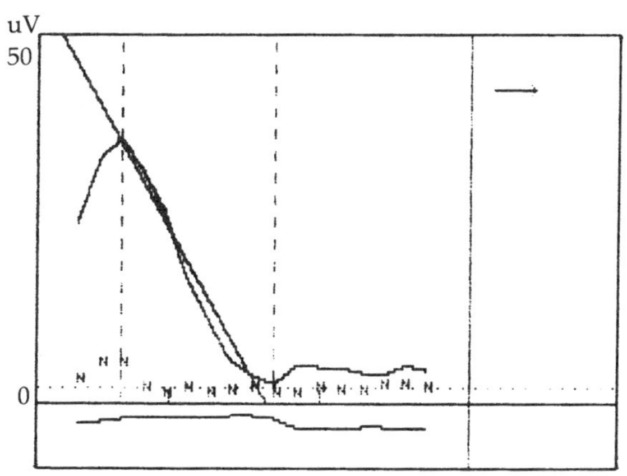

Figure 1 Print-out from sweep VEP. This is from the digital instrumentation for visual assessment (DIVA) system developed at the Smith-Kettlewell Eye Institute. The curved solid line in the upper panel represents the amplitude of the VEP as the spatial frequency is being swept from 1 to 30 cycles per degree. Phase of the response is represented in the small lower panel. The "N" represents the random EEG noise. The slanting regression line indicates the estimated acuity at the intercept of the spatial frequency axis.

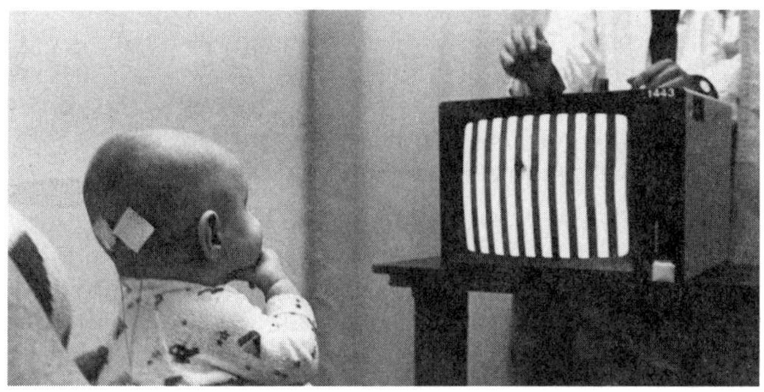

Figure 2 Infant with scalp electrodes in place watching Sweep stimulus. Toy dangled in front of monitor helps fixation.

K. The flash VEP is also a transient response recorded from electrodes placed over the occipital cortex. The stimulus is a strobe light that alternates on-off at a rate of greater than 2 Hz. Amplitude and latency measurements are obtained from the waveform. Two trials are required for replication of responses. Fixation is not required.

References

Birch EE. Visual acuity testing in infants and young children. Ophthalmol Clin North Am 1989; 2:369.

Leguire LE, Rogers GL, Bremer DL. Amblyopia: The normal eye is not normal. J Pediatr Ophthal Strabismus 1990; 27:32.

Norcia AM, Tyler CW. Infant VEP acuity measurements: Analysis of individual differences and measurement error. Electroencephalogr Clin Neurophysiol 1985; 61:359.

Norcia AM, Tyler CW. Spatial frequency sweep VEP: Visual acuity during the first year of life. Vision Res 1985; 25:1399.

Sokol S, Hansen VC, Moskowitz A, et al. Evoked potential and preferential looking estimates of visual acuity in pediatric patients. Ophthalmology 1983; ():552.

Teller DY, McDonald M, Preston K, et al. Assessment of visual acuity in infants and children. Dev Med Child Neurol 1986; 28:779.

CHILDHOOD ONSET OF PROGRESSIVE RETINAL DYSTROPHIES

Gerhard W. Cibis, M.D.

A. Retinal dystrophies diagnosed later in life may have been present from birth, but usually the later diagnosis implies that it is of late onset and therefore progressive. When the electroretinogram (ERG) is fully extinguished at the time of diagnosis, the progressive nature of the disorder and later onset than the first 6 months of life is important in differentiating it from congenital amaurosis of Leber (p 68). The frequent association of retinitis pigmentosa (RP) with systemic disorders requires that these be looked for by history and proper subspecialty examination. Hearing tests, metabolic, genetic, and neurology consultation, and brain imaging, when appropriate, should all be considered. In contrast to findings in the stationary group, ERG waveforms are less helpful in making a specific differential diagnosis. They do, however, divide cases into rod, cone, and rod-cone dystrophies, which have different associated systemic implications.

B. Rod dystrophies are the classic retinitis pigmentosa. They may be associated with other systemic findings, in which case they usually represent a syndrome, or they may occur in isolation. Pure RP is familial. Most cases, however, present sporadically but are recessively inherited. Dominant and sex-linked inheritance exists as well. Specific defects in the rhodopsin gene have been identified as the cause of dominantly inherited RP in 17% of familial cases. Knowledge of the exact rhodopsin defect correlates well with clinical findings as to age of onset and degree and speed of visual field and acuity loss. The most common childhood form of RP is sex-linked recessive; it manifests in the first decade, leading to extensive vision loss by the second decade. It is becoming apparent that many different genetic defects can result in the clinical picture of RP.

C. Rod-cone dystrophies are commonly associated with systemic anomalies. Appropriate medical and genetic work-ups are indicated.

D. Progressive cone dystrophies are not usually symptomatic until later in childhood, unlike achromatopsia. Photophobia and progressive vision loss are the hallmarks. Acquired color vision loss is present. Central scotoma and bull's-eye retinopathy occur. Some cone-rod dystrophies begin as cone disorders and then develop rod involvement.

E. Choroideremia is a sex-linked disorder with abnormal ERG with carrier findings. Gyrate atrophy is associated with hyperornithemia and may respond to vitamin B_6 therapy. Both conditions show lacuna-like areas of pigment epithelial loss.

F. Sex-linked juvenile retinoschisis is not an uncommon condition. There is an abnormal ERG A/B wave ratio with an intact A wave and low-amplitude B wave reminiscent of the Schubert-Bornschein "negative" ERG seen with congenital stationary night blindness (CSNB). The macula shows typical spokelike cystic changes. Schisis is seen in the retinal periphery. The ERG argues a relationship to CSNB in that the retinal split occurs in the plexiform layer. Full-thickness holes are not common. Laser surgery to prevent progression of the schisis is futile. Occasionally retinal buckling can relieve traction. Goldmann-Favre syndrome has an "empty" vitreous space with a decreased to absent ERG (see p 136).

G. Certain drugs can give an acquired retinopathy. Chloroquine, commonly used in rheumatoid disorders, is a major agent. Careful monitoring of visual acuity, visual fields, color vision, retinal sensitivity, ERG, and electro-oculography is advised.

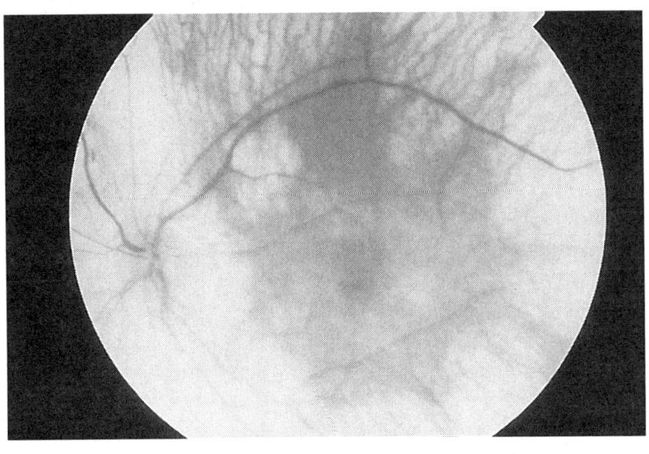

Figure 1 Choroideremia of an affected male. Only an island of macula is spared the degeneration.

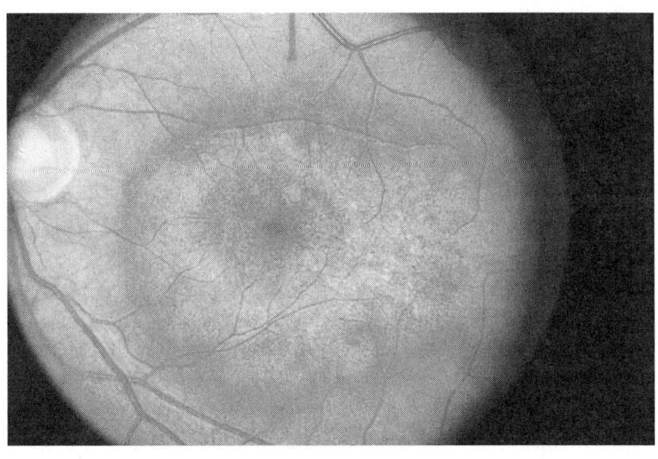

Figure 2 Bull's-eye maculopathy.

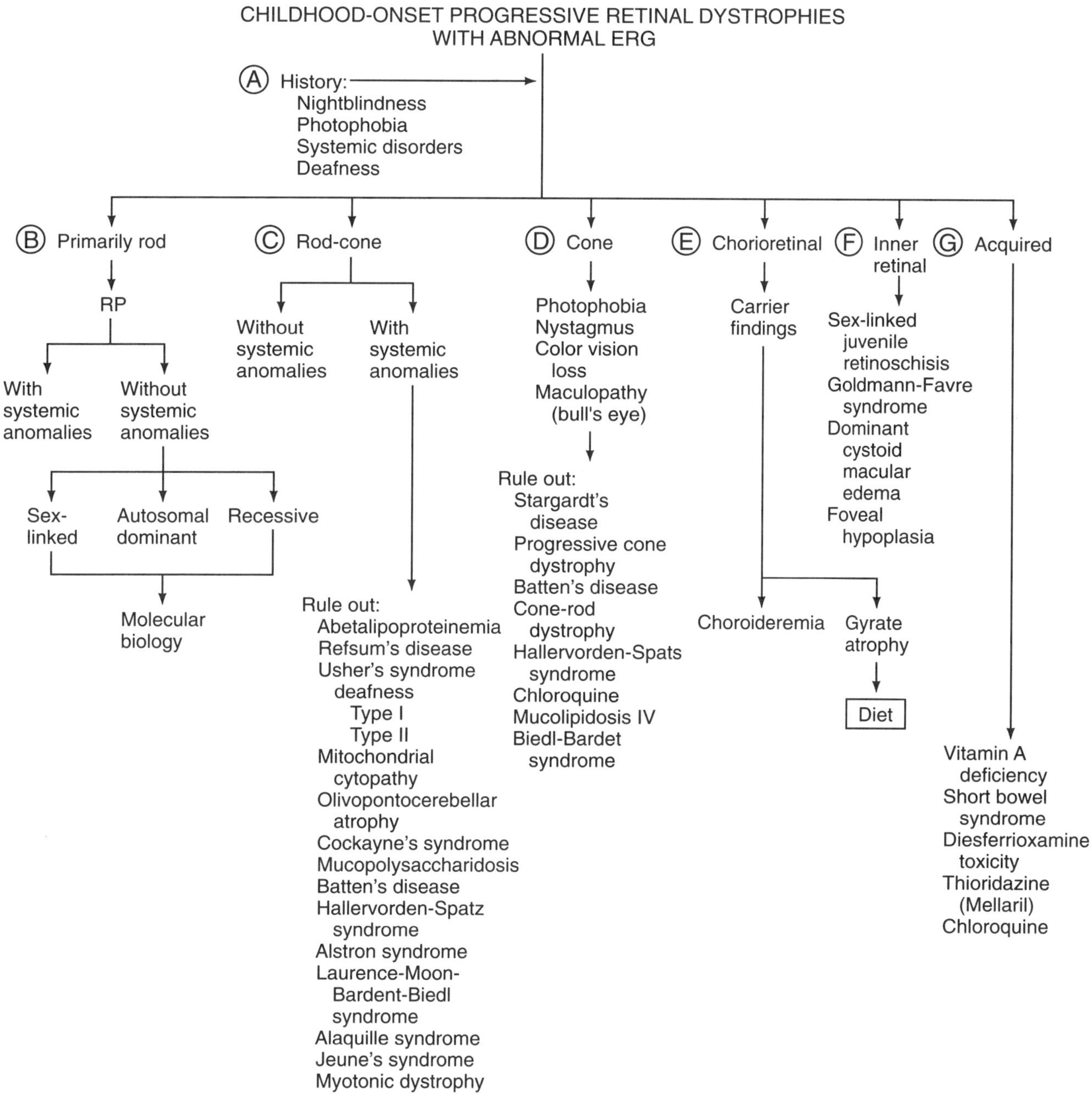

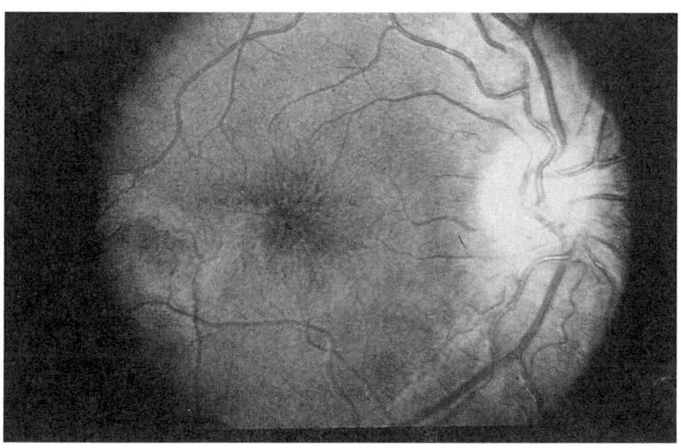

Figure 3 Plicated macula in sex-linked juvenile retinoschisis.

References

Cibis GW, Morey M, Harris DJ. Dominantly inherited macular dystrophy with flecks (Stargardt). Arch Ophthalmol 1980; 98:1785.

Moore A. Inherited retinal dystrophies. In: Taylor D, ed. Pediatric ophthalmology. Boston: Blackwell Scientific, 1990:376.

Newsome DA, ed. Retinal dystrophies and degenerations. New York: Raven Press, 1988.

BIOPSIES AND CYTOPATHOLOGY

Ramesh C. Tripathi, M.D., Ph.D.
Junping Li, M.D.
Brenda J. Tripathi, Ph.D.

A. Conjunctival cytopathology aids in the diagnosis of several types of infection, inflammation, allergy, degeneration, and neoplasia by studying epithelium, inflammatory cells, inclusions, microorganisms, pigment, fibrin, mucus, and crystals present in exfoliative specimens. Culture of responsible microorganisms may be difficult at times, although in some severe destructive processes, the need to identify the causative pathogen is urgent.

B. Inflammatory cells (polymorphonuclear leukocytes) are predominant in bacterial infections. Lymphocytes are present in chronic infections and inflammation. Eosinophils are indicative of allergic reaction. Mononuclear inflammatory cells indicate viral infections (adenoviruses or enteroviruses). Giant cells occur in herpes virus infection. Halberstader-Prowazek inclusion bodies are diagnostic of trachoma. Keratinization of conjunctival epithelium is a feature of keratoconjunctivitis sicca, trachoma, measles, vitamin A deficiency, exposure keratitis, chemical burns, and neoplasia. Exfoliative cytology permits grading of dry eye conditions.

C. Conjunctival biopsy is indicated in many inherited and acquired systemic disorders of carbohydrate, lipid, protein, amino acid, and mineral metabolism, and in local diseases and results of therapeutic approach.

D. Tissue biopsy helps diagnosis of conjunctival diseases such as bacterial, viral, chlamydial, and parasitic infections, ligneous conjunctivitis, juvenile xanthogranulomas, and other granulomatous inflammations; degenerations (xerosis); choristomas (epidermoid and dermoid cyst, dermolipoma); pseudocancerous epithelial lesions (hereditary benign intraepithelial dyskeratosis, pseudoepitheliomatous hyperplasia, squamous papilloma, oncocytoma, myxoma); potentially precancerous epithelial lesions (xeroderma pigmentosum, dysplasia); cancerous lesions (carcinoma in situ, squamous carcinoma, lymphomas); and pigmented lesions (nevus, malignant melanoma).

E. Types of cellular infiltrates in conjunctival cytopathology signify probable causes of inflammation. True membranes that consist of fibrin-fibrovascular tissue with cellular debris attach firmly to underlying epithelium in epidemic keratoconjunctivitis, *Corynebacterium diphtheriae* infection, Stevens-Johnson syndrome, ligneous conjunctivitis, and pneumococcal and staphylococcal infections. Pseudomembranes consisting of loose fibrinous exudate and cellular debris are not adherent to the underlying epithelium and can occur in the same diseases as those that cause true membranes as well as in vernal conjunctivitis, streptococcal infection, and chemical burns.

Fronds or finger-like projections of hyperplastic and acanthotic epithelium with a core of fibrovascular tissue form conjunctival papillae. These are signs of chronic inflammation or irritation. Follicular formation is characterized by focal lymphoid hyperplasia often associated with drug toxicities, allergic conditions, and infections such as trachoma. Epidermoid cysts are composed of an epidermis and a cystic cavity containing keratin and debris. Walls of dermoid cysts are lined by epidermis and contain epidermal appendages, such as hair follicles and sebaceous and sweat glands. The cystic cavity contains keratin, hair shafts, and debris.

Pseudocancerous epithelial lesions exhibit acanthosis, hyperkeratosis, parakeratosis, and dyskeratosis. Cancerous epithelial lesions are evidenced by the loss of cell polarity and maturation, abnormal mitotic figures, and atypia. Malignant lesions invade the basement membrane and deeper stroma. A nevus, the most common lesion, occurs as subepithelial, junctional, compound, or blue nevus or congenital melanocytosis. Cells show normal polarity and are clustered to form nests. In malignant melanoma, normal polarity is lost, and cells are atypical. The overlying epithelium is invaded. Juvenile xanthogranuloma shows diffuse granulomatous inflammatory reactions with histiocytes and Touton giant cells.

F. Systemic diseases such as cystinosis, ochronosis, hypercalcemia, Addison's disease, mucopolysaccharidoses, glycoproteinoses, lipidosis, amyloidosis, dysproteinemias, prophyria, and malignant atrophic papulosis often affect the conjunctiva and cornea. Light microscopy, histochemistry, electron microscopy, and biochemical analyses of the biopsy specimens are of diagnostic value.

G. In cystinosis, cystine crystals are seen in epithelial and fibrocytic cells as membrane-limited, elongated, rectangular, or needle-shaped profiles. Ochronosis exhibits globules, amorphous strands, and curlicues in the superficial corneal stroma and substantia propria of the conjunctiva. Mucopolysaccharidoses often have intracytoplasmic, single membrane-bound vacuoles that contain flocculent or fibrillogranular material. In mucolipidosis, ballooned epithelial cells contain fibrillogranular material and lamellar lipid inclusions. The diagnosis is established by enzyme assay.

H. Corneal biopsy is indicated in local and systemic disorders that often manifest as a cloudy cornea, which could be due to edema, malformations, abnormal deposits, or inflammation.

I. Dystrophy of Meesmann's shows cystic degeneration of individual corneal epithelial cells containing peculiar fibrillogranular material. Map-dot and fingerprint disorders exhibit focal cystic degeneration of epithelial cells with aberrant formation of intraepithelial

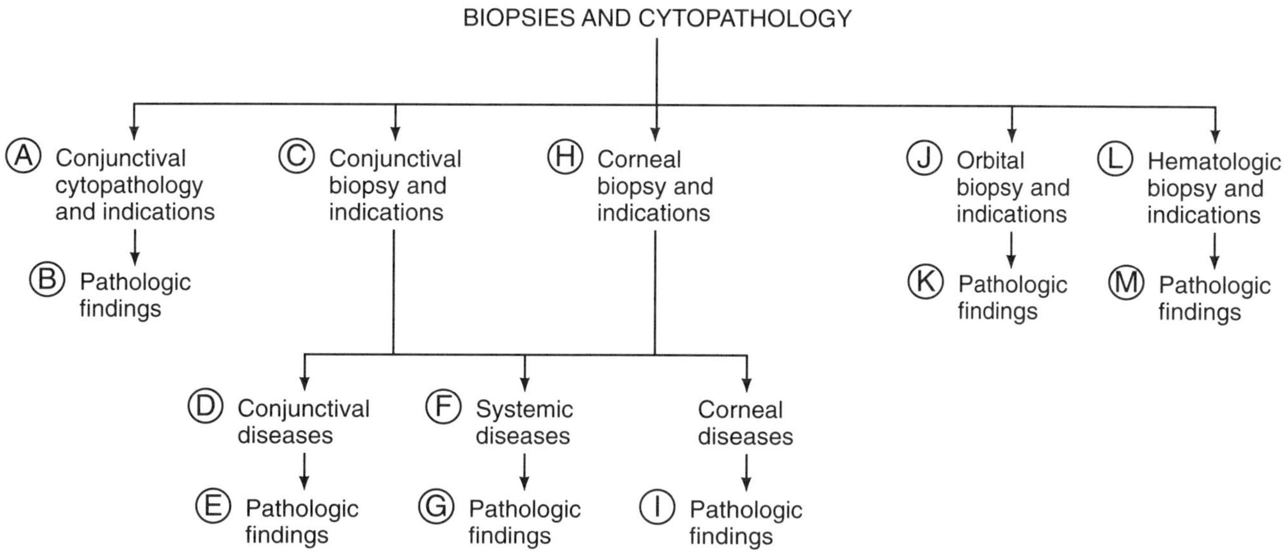

basement membrane and fibrous tissue. In primary gelatinous drop-like dystrophy, confluent nodular amyloid deposits are present in the subepithelial zone. Corneal lesions in Reis-Bückler dystrophy are limited to levels in and around Bowman's layer. The layer is replaced by scar tissue containing masses of noncollagenous fibrillar material. Granular, eosinophilic crystalline stromal deposits are indicative of granular dystrophy. Basophilic deposits, staining positively for mucopolysaccharide, present in and around keratocytes and endothelial cells and are characteristic of macular dystrophy. Focal subepithelial and stromal Congo red-positive, birefringent amyloid deposits are present in lattice dystrophy. Congenital hereditary stromal dystrophy is evidenced by atrophic or absent endothelium, thickened Descemet's membrane, and stroma. In posterior polymorphous dystrophy the "endothelium" is multilayered with ultrastructural characteristics of epithelium. Descemet's membrane is thickened and may show guttate changes.

J. Orbital biopsy is a useful diagnostic tool in inflammatory conditions, pseudotumor, cysts, and neoplasms. In pediatric practice, the frequently encountered orbital disorders for which tissue biopsy is indicated include dermoid, rhabdomyosarcoma, neurogenic tumors, pseudotumor, glioma of the optic nerve, and meningioma.

K. Granulomatous inflammation can be seen in pseudotumor, tuberculosis, and sarcoidosis or as a reaction to fungal and parasitic infections, foreign bodies, and ruptured cysts. Pathologic findings of pseudotumor include collagenization around small blood vessels in the orbital fat, as well as eosinophilic and lymphocytic infiltrates. The fibrous tissue can be either loose with elongated, immature fibroblasts or acellular and hyalinized. Various types of cysts are recognized by the specific epithelium that forms the cyst wall. The embryonal type of rhabdomyosarcoma occurs most commonly in the orbit, and it is composed of long, slender cells with centrally located elongated nuclei. The presence of tadpole cells and cross-striations within the cytoplasm are diagnostic, although these are often difficult to find. Other histologic types of rhabdomyosarcoma are pleomorphic and alveolar.

L. Hematologic biopsy is indicated in sickle cell disease and myeloproliferative and lymphoproliferative diseases, which cause abnormal ocular changes.

M. In sickle cell diseases, blood smear shows decreased erythrocytes, polychromasia, sickle cells, target cells, and Howell-Jolly bodies. In leukemia, depending on the disease process and cell types, blood smear and bone marrow biopsy reveal the specific changes.

References

Bron AJ, Tripathi RC. Corneal disorders. In: Goldberg MF, ed. Genetics and metabolic eye diseases. Boston: Little, Brown & Company, 1974:281.

Garner A. The pathology of tumors at the limbus. Eye 1989; 3:210.

Iliff WJ, Green WR. Orbital tumors in children. In: Jakobiec FA, ed. Ocular and adnexal tumors. Birmingham: Aesculapius Publishing Inc. 1978.

Spencer WH, ed. Ophthalmic pathology. Philadelphia: WB Saunders, 1985.

Stenson S. Cytologic diagnosis. A. The anterior segment cytopathology. In: Karcioglu ZA, ed. Laboratory diagnosis in ophthalmology. New York: Macmillan, 1987:90.

Yanoff M, Fine BS, eds. Ocular pathology. A text and atlas. 3rd ed. Philadelphia: JB Lippincott, 1989.

VISION TESTING IN INFANTS AND CHILDREN

Gerhard W. Cibis, M.D.

A. Vision testing in infants and children can be divided into those that demand verbal co-operation and are therefore age and development limited and those that can be performed without co-operation. The correct reading of a line of letters, identification of picture objects, or direct orientation of the letter E are all cognitive. The question at hand is understood, including the symbolism of the object. This is missing when visual attention or just pointing at or picking up beads or objects without necessarily identifying them is used. With presentation of patterns, as in visual evoked response (VER) or preferential looking (FPL), there clearly is an act of vision that produces a brain wave or a turn of the face to look at the pattern. The brain wave disappears or the face fails to turn to look when the size of the stripe intervals is so small that they are no longer differentiated from a homogeneous background. Snellen equivalents are ascribed to these limits.

B. Numerous efforts to simplify the act of communication between tester and child exist. These include Snellen equivalents using pictures (Allen cards, HOTV test, Parson test). For pictures the child need not know the alphabet. Even simpler is the Parson test, in which only three pictures are presented in all possible positions and the patient is taught to point at the selected of the three. With HOTV the chart contains only those letters in random orientation. The subject has a card with these four letters on it in his lap and is allowed to point to the letter matching the one the tester is pointing to on the main test chart. The crowding phenomenon of amblyopia applies to all tests (see p 102). The illiterate E, when used singly, as with the cube containing E's of different size on each of its six faces, overestimates amblyopic acuities compared with the same test with the letters presented in traditional lines.

C. Nonverbal vision testing covers a wide range of techniques. These range from simple observation of the child's behavior to the presentation of lights or objects to sophisticated electrophysiologic determinations.

D. If the child fixes a pen light centrally (observe the corneal Hirschberg reflex), this implies that he or she is seeing it. Maintained fixation is recorded as central, steady, and maintained (CSM) and is considered normal. It says nothing of actual acuity values. Uncentral, unsteady, and unmaintained fixation (UCUSUM) implies poor vision. Nystagmus and patching therapy for amblyopia make correlation of fixation pattern and actual acuity inaccurate. A small prism held vertically dissociates the eyes and allows for better assessment of fixation of each eye separately. A simpler test is whether the child fixes on and follows lights or toys. This can be accomplished even with less than 20/200 vision. Similarly, the touching or picking up of small beads or objects confirms that they are seen but gives little information as to actual level of vision and is not useful in amblyopia therapy.

We prefer the Brueckner method, in which the Hirschberg corneal reflex and the red fundus reflex are used. This method allows observation of the dynamics of fixation, pupillary movement, and ocular alignment with the background of the fundus reflex, establishing when the patient is truly accommodating the target light as opposed to just looking at it. Even this test is not as accurate as VER (acuity and contrast sensitivity methods) in assessment of vision in the nonverbal infant. The Brueckner red reflex test is a subjective form of amblyopia determination. It gives clinical information based on patient fixation and alignment that allows an estimate of vision but not an exact Snellen acuity number such as 20/30 or 20/100. The test is performed by the clinician looking through an ophthalmoscope, observing both the red reflex coming back from the eye and the pupil behavior. Misalignment of the eye, high refractive errors, media opacities, and other amblyogenic factors can be identified. When the patient fixes the light, the pupil gets smaller and the red reflex darker than when he or she is not fixing. With decreased vision, fixation is not CSM but becomes UCUSUM. The test can be done and documented using a videocamera (see p 202).

E. Grating acuity is used for preferential looking as well as VER testing. Grating acuity consists of alternating white and black stripes or checks. Acuities are reported as relative to spatial frequency, which is reported in cycles per degree. One black stripe and one white stripe equal a cycle. If this cycle subtends 1 degree (60 minutes) of arc, it is reported as 1 cycle/degree. Therefore, if spatial frequency is reported as 30 cycles/degree, each black stripe subtends 1 minute of arc and each white stripe subtends 1 minute of arc, which are the components of the letter **E** at 20/20. Mathematically, 600 divided by spatial frequency gives acuity in Snellen terms.

A major drawback of preferential looking is that acuity does not reach normal adult levels until age 5 years. An adjustment table for age is used. In contrast, acuity distribution is at adult level at 18 months of age with the Parson test and at 6 months of age for VER and digital instrumentation for visual assessment (DIVA) tests. Preferential looking can be time consuming, is variable in older infants who do not co-operate as younger infants do, and difficult to interpret in clinical situations. However, preferential looking can give better results in neurologically damaged patients.

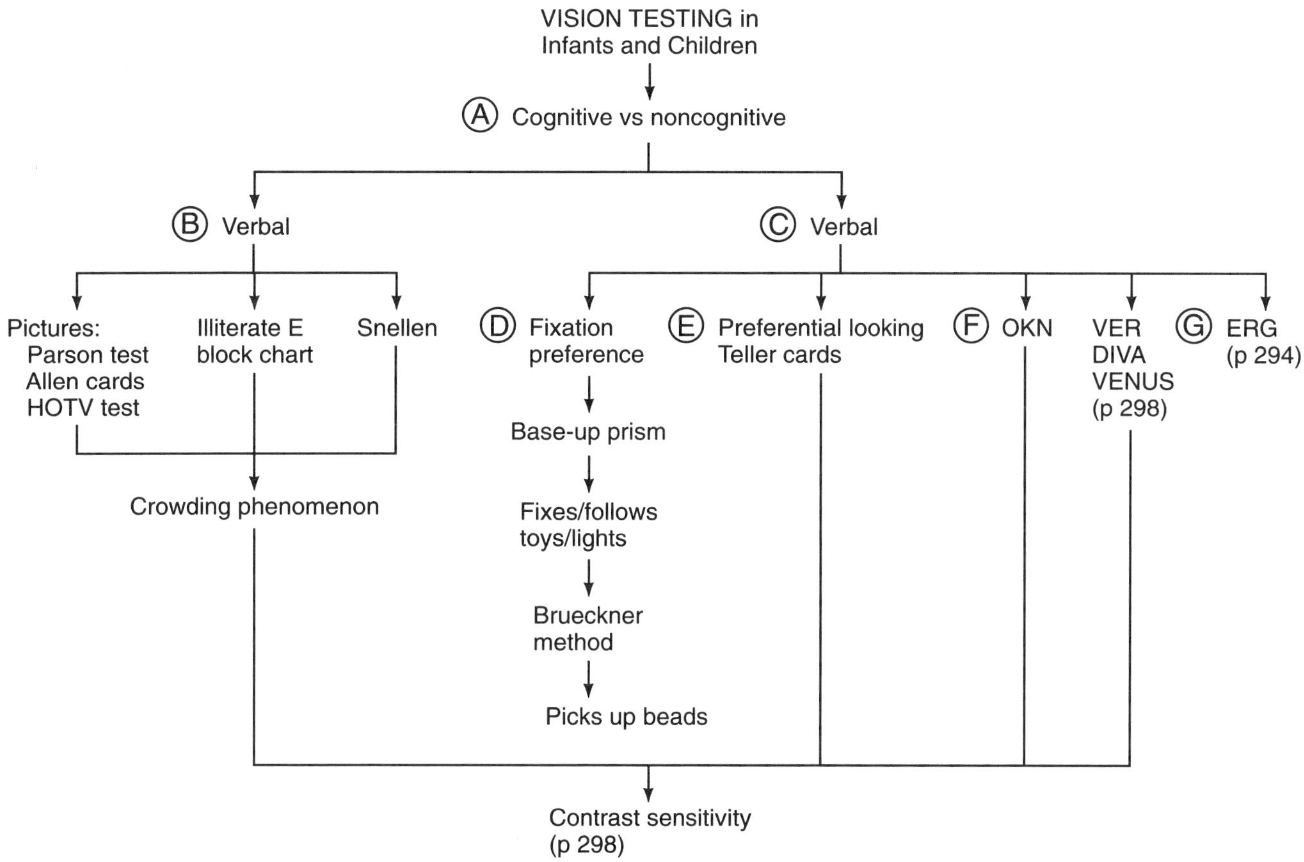

We therefore use both FPL and Sweep VEP (DIVA, VENUS [visual evoked neural universal system]).

F. Optokinetic nystagmus (OKN) can be elicited by presenting targets repetitively moving across the subject's visual field in one direction. The OKN may be positive to large target size with less than 20/200 acuity. Because of the complicated neurologic basis of this test and the difficulty in presenting an environment of varying stripe sizes, OKN is not practical in clinical acuity determination.

G. Electroretinography (ERG) simply tests retinal integrity and says nothing of acuity (see p 294).

References

Cibis GW, Maino JH, Crandall MA, et al. The Parsons visual acuity test for screening children 18 to 48 months old. Ann Ophthalmol 1985; 17:471.

Cibis GW, Mancillas MS. Contrast sensitivity. Curr Opinion Ophthalmol 1991; 2:81.

Cibis-Tongue A, Cibis GW. Brueckner test. Ophthalmology 1981; 88:1041.

Mayer DL, Fulton AB. Preferential looking grating acuitites of infants at risk of amblyopia. Trans Ophthalmol Soc UK 1985; 104:903.

Wright KW, Walonker F, Edelman P. 10-diopter fixation test for amblyopia. Arch Ophthalmol 1981; 99:1242.

SENSORY TESTING IN STRABISMUS

Gerhard W. Cibis M.D.

A. The purpose of sensory testing is to establish the degree and type of binocular co-operation or lack thereof. This is to monitor the result of therapy or to predict the likelihood and type of result that may be anticipated with therapy. Establishment of the sensory status also can help in making a judgment about past status in cases in which that is not clearly known. For example, is an exotropia secondary or primary? If there is suppression without diplopia on overcorrection (by prisms), it is not a primary exotropia, but secondary based on the evidence of esotropia suppression.

B. Ocular alignment or deviation from alignment is determined. Examination of sensory status may be complex in co-operative and verbal patients or highly abbreviated in infants. We find that the Lang random-dot stereogram card can be used with very young children. You can observe children's eyes flick from object to object and confirm fusion that way. At 2 to 3 years of age, they can be asked to name the objects they see. Infants can be tested with monocular optokinetic nystagmus (OKN). A normal OKN when rotating the objects from nasal to temporal is a good indicator of probable fusion after 6 months of age. It is expected to be abnormal in infantile esotropes.

Tests for establishing sensory status are most accurate when they are obtained under conditions of normal vision. Disruption of the two eyes in any way leads to suppression and retinal rivalry that alters the true binocular sensory status. The Bagolini striate lens test is the least dissociating and therefore the best test in this regard. Everything looked at, including the peripheral field, is the same to both eyes except for the two streaks of light. Red-green lenses, as with the Worth four-dot test, are highly dissociating, as are afterimages. These tests can show suppression when there is fusion with the Bagolini lenses. Table 1 lists tests in order of least to more dissociating. The deeper a filter in front of one eye, the more dissociating the effect. Advantage is taken of this to combine use of the Bagolini striate lenses with Bagolini red filter bar to increase dissociation until suppression occurs. The depth of fusion, anomalous retinal correspondence, or suppression can be measured in this way.

C. Monocular OKN, nasal to temporal direction, fails to develop normally if fusion is not present. However, it is normal in the temporal to nasal direction monocularly and both directions binocularly. The polarized glasses "fly" test has monocular clues to fusion that may mask suppression. Random-dot stereograms truly can be seen only if fusion is present. Even microtropes fail the random-dot test rather than get three or four stereo circles, as they do with the "fly" test. Proper refusion movement with a base-out 4-diopter prism implies fusion and lack of suppression. Microtropes fail that test.

D. Anomalous retinal correspondence (ARC) is common with long-standing deviations that occur early in childhood. All microtropes have ARC with a central scotoma. With synoptophores an adaptation between the measured angle and orthotropia can be obtained. This is called unharmonious ARC but is an artifact of testing. True ARC is always harmonious and, in pattern deviations or other variable-angle strabismus such as Brown's syndrome, may adapt to each position. ARC in small angles and microtropes drives the eye back to that position if surgery is done or prisms are given. This is why small angle deviations of 12 to 18 diopters are so difficult to correct. ARC can lead to paradoxic diplopia when a deviation is corrected. Determining the depth of such adaptations prior to surgery can predict the risk of diplopia and the likelihood of suppression developing.

TABLE 1 Dissociation of Test in Decreasing Order

Test		
Bagolini lenses (striate)		
Polarizing glasses/haploscope		
Synoptophore	→	Dissociation
Red filter	→	increases with
Worth four-dot	→	filter density
Negative afterimage		
Positive afterimage		

References

Atkinson J, Braddick O. Development of optokinetic nystagmus in infants: An indicator of cortical binocularity? In: Fisher DF, Monty RA, Senders JW, eds. Eye movements: Cognition and visual perception. Hillsdale, NJ: Lawrence Erlbaum Associates, 1981:53.

Bagolini B, Campos EC. Clinical usefulness of sensory testing in strabismus. Perspect Ophthalmol 1981; 5:61.

Boeden P. Anomalies retinal correspondence refuted. Am J Ophthal 1964; 53:366.

Lang J. Strabismus. Trans. by GW Cibis. Thorofare, NJ:Slack, 1983.

SENSORY TESTING IN STRABISMUS

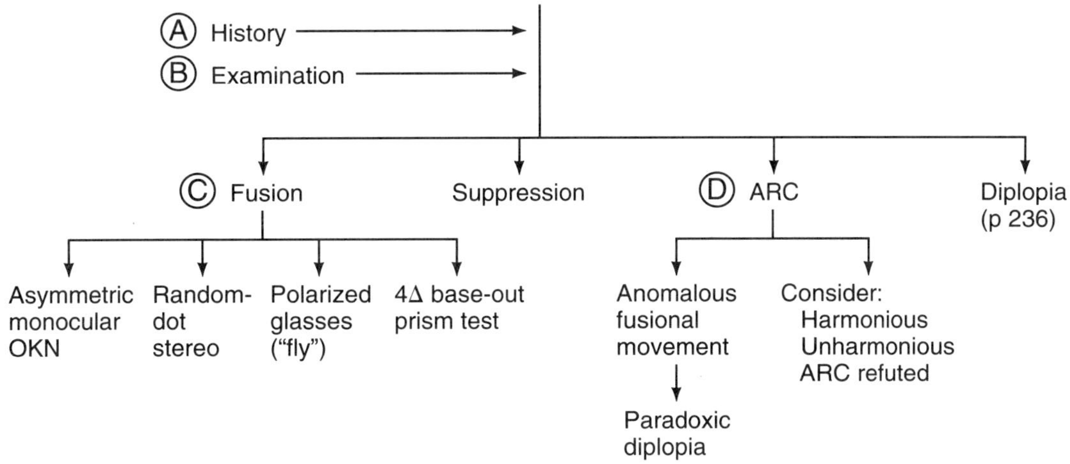

ANESTHESIA

Peter H. Mestad, M.D.

A. The majority of ophthalmologic procedures can be performed on an outpatient basis. A brief history and physical examination are necessary to determine the patient's present medical status, as well as to look for associated congenital anomalies. Laboratory tests, such as a hematology screen and urinalysis, are not routinely necessary and should be ordered only as indicated for each specific patient.

B. Anesthetics used at the present time do not have many of the side effects of earlier agents, negating the need for preoperative medications in most cases. Ophthalmologic phenylephrine solutions should be no stronger than 2.5% concentration.

C. Thiopental and volatile agents, in clinical dose range, may suppress electrophysiologic studies. Induction and maintenance with ketamine and, if needed, a muscle relaxant provides satisfactory conditions for the evaluation. Midazolam, 0.05 to 0.1 mg/kg, decreases the incidence of hallucinogenic reactions attributed to the use of ketamine.

D. Most children undergoing strabismus surgery are healthy, allowing a wide choice in anesthetics. The most popular anesthetic combines a volatile agent, such as halothane or isoflurane, with nitrous oxide and oxygen. Muscle relaxants may be used to facilitate tracheal intubation. Intravenous drugs may also be used for induction and maintenance. Propofol is a newer agent that shows promise as an intravenous anesthetic.

E. Prophylactic atropine is not generally necessary, as the dysrhythmia generally disappears when the stimulus is removed. Bradycardia is benign in most cases and is not accompanied by hypotension. In addition, the reflex seems to fatigue as the procedure progresses. The depth of anesthesia and adequacy of ventilation should be evaluated. The use of atropine is controversial, but 0.01 to 0.02 mg/kg often enables the operation to proceed without delay if bradycardia persists.

F. Postoperative vomiting is common following ophthalmologic surgery, occurring in up to 85% of patients. No method available can completely eliminate this problem. Intraoperative intravenous droperidol, 0.05 to 0.075 mg/kg, has been successful in decreasing vomiting. Other agents have also been used with varying degrees of success. Adequate intravenous rehydration and pain relief also may decrease the incidence of vomiting. Forcing oral fluids prior to discharge from the hospital has been implicated as a cause of vomiting. Postoperative vomiting usually is not severe enough to require hospitalization and is tolerated in the home environment.

G. Analgesics do not necessarily prolong the time to discharge from the hospital. Drugs stronger than acetaminophen may be necessary in the immediate postoperative period in the recovery room. Intravenous nalbuphine, 0.1 mg/kg, has been successful. Intravenous fentanyl, 0.5 to 1.0 μg/kg, may also be used, particularly in the older child and adolescent.

H. Ketamine, given intravenously, 0.5 to 1 mg/kg, or intramuscularly, 4 to 5 mg/kg, maintains ocular muscle tone, allowing the surgeon to hear muscle potential and see immediate results of the injection. Tracheal intubation is generally not required.

I. Many patients are former premature infants and may have chronic lung disease. Intravenous narcotics or inhalation agents can be safely used. Temporary postoperative mechanical ventilator support may be necessary. Infants whose postconceptual age is less than 44 weeks should be monitored for apnea or bradycardia for at least 18 hours postoperatively.

J. Both succinylcholine and tracheal intubation raise intraocular pressure (IOP). Intravenous and volatile agents, with the exception of ketamine, either decrease or have little effect on IOP. Ocular pressure measurements should be performed after induction, before tracheal intubation. A deep plane of anesthesia minimizes elevations in IOP. The use of muscle relaxants prevents coughing during the procedure. Emergence and extubation should be as quiet as possible. The use of intravenous lidocaine, 1.5 to 2.0 mg/kg, prior to extubation may help to decrease the incidence of coughing and laryngospasm after extubation.

K. An open globe often results from traumatic injury. Patients are often at increased risk of pulmonary aspiration. Induction must avoid coughing, straining, or large elevations in blood pressure, and intubation should be rapid. A smooth, rapid induction and intubation can normally be obtained using thiopental, intravenous and/or topical lidocaine, narcotics, and nondepolarizing muscle relaxants, accompanied by a volatile agent. A peripheral nerve stimulator aids in obtaining a satisfactory level of muscle relaxation. Succinylcholine elevates IOP and is generally avoided. Extubation should be as quiet as possible, but the presence of a full stomach may necessitate extubation after airway protective mechanisms have returned.

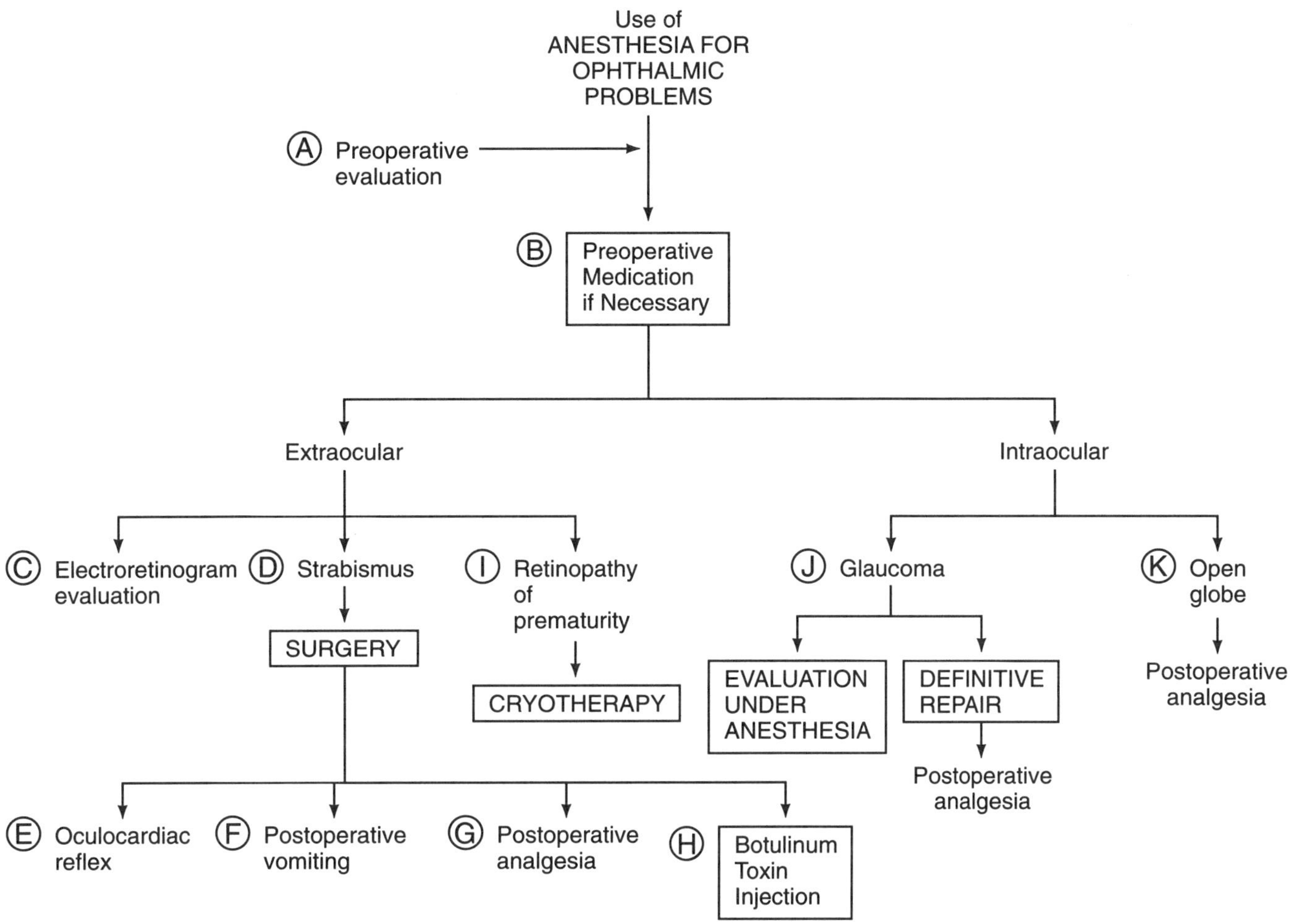

References

Abramawitz MD, Oh TH, Epstein BS, et al. The antiemetic effect of droperidol following outpatient strabismus surgery in children. Anesthesiology 1983; 59:579.

Chi OZ, Ryterband S. Visual evoked potentials during thiopentone fentanyl–nitrous oxide anaesthesia in humans. Can J Anaesthesiol 1989; 36:637.

Duncalf D. Anesthesia and intraocular pressure. Bull NY Acad Med 1975; 51:374.

Magora F, Collins V. The influence of general anesthetic agents on intraocular pressure in man. Arch Ophthalmol 1961; 66:806.

Pandey K, Bandola RP, Kumar S. Time course of intraocular hypertension produced by suxamethonium. Br J Anaesthesiol 1972; 44:191.

Watcha MF, Simeon RM, White P, Stevens JL. Effect of propofol on the incidence of postoperative vomiting after strabismus surgery in pediatric outpatients. Anesthesiology 1991; 75:204.

EVALUATION UNDER ANESTHESIA

Gerhard W. Cibis, M.D.

A. The need for evaluation under anesthesia (EUA) is among the most misunderstood aspects of pediatric ophthalmology practice by other health care providers and third-party payers. Usually parents are aware of their child's lack of cooperation for needed testing. Good pediatric ophthalmology care requires that the EUA not be avoided because of a fear of the anesthesia (see p 308). When a child is at significant risk for an ocular disease, if the proper examination cannot be carried out in the office, an EUA should be done. We are able to hold down, if necessary, and adequately examine most children. However, certain ocular evaluations cannot be adequately performed with a struggling child. When these are imperative to good care, an EUA is needed.

B. Conscious sedation consists of chloral hydrate. The patient is asleep but arousable. With this sedation, children are too easily aroused to do fundus photography or other manipulations such as indirect retinoscopy or gonioscopy. Conscious sedation also works well for electroretinography (ERG) and radiologic studies such as CT and MRI. The dose of chloral hydrate used is 40 to 100 mg/kg body weight. The lowest dose is administered orally. After a wait of 20 minutes, if sedation is inadequate, doses are increased in 20 mg/kg increments up to the maximum. Fox et al. used chloral hydrate in 302 patients without complications.

C. Postsurgical aphakia, retinoblastoma cases, certain hereditary retinal detachment conditions such as juvenile retinoschisis, Walker-Warburg syndrome, Marfan syndrome, and high myopia need examination of the retinal periphery including scleral indentation. The number of such examinations and their timing vary with the exact diagnosis.

D. Patients at risk for congenital, infantile, and juvenile glaucoma need careful intraocular tension measurements before and after surgical and medical intervention. When these measurements cannot be reliably obtained in the office, an EUA is indicated. Gonioscopy needs to be done to ascertain congenital chamber angle abnormalities. This cannot be done in the office with a struggling child. An EUA is imperative (see pp 312, 314, 316).

The number of examinations varies with the degree of pressure control. We do an EUA 6 weeks after glaucoma surgery and then twice every 3 months, then twice every 6 months, then yearly if pressures are well controlled, and more often if not.

E. Unexplained vision loss may require careful direct fundus examination, which may not be possible simply by holding down an uncooperative older child. Other tests such as visual evoked response and ERG and photography may be needed which require more cooperation. Infants can generally be bundled up and given chloral hydrate sedation. Older children may require an EUA.

F. A careful slit-lamp examination may be needed and is not possible in the office. Metabolic disorders with subtle corneal clouding may not be diagnosable simply by direct inspection. Conjunctival biopsy may be needed (see p 302). Corneal ulcers and infection may need scraping and careful observation.

G. I personally perform EUAs on surgically aphakic children once a year until proper retinal examinations can be done in the office. This is not the choice for all practitioners.

Reference

Fox BES, O'Brien CO, Kangas KJ, et al. Use of high dose chloral hydrate for ophthalmic exams in children. A retrospective review. J Pediatr Ophthalmol Strabismus 1990; 27:242.

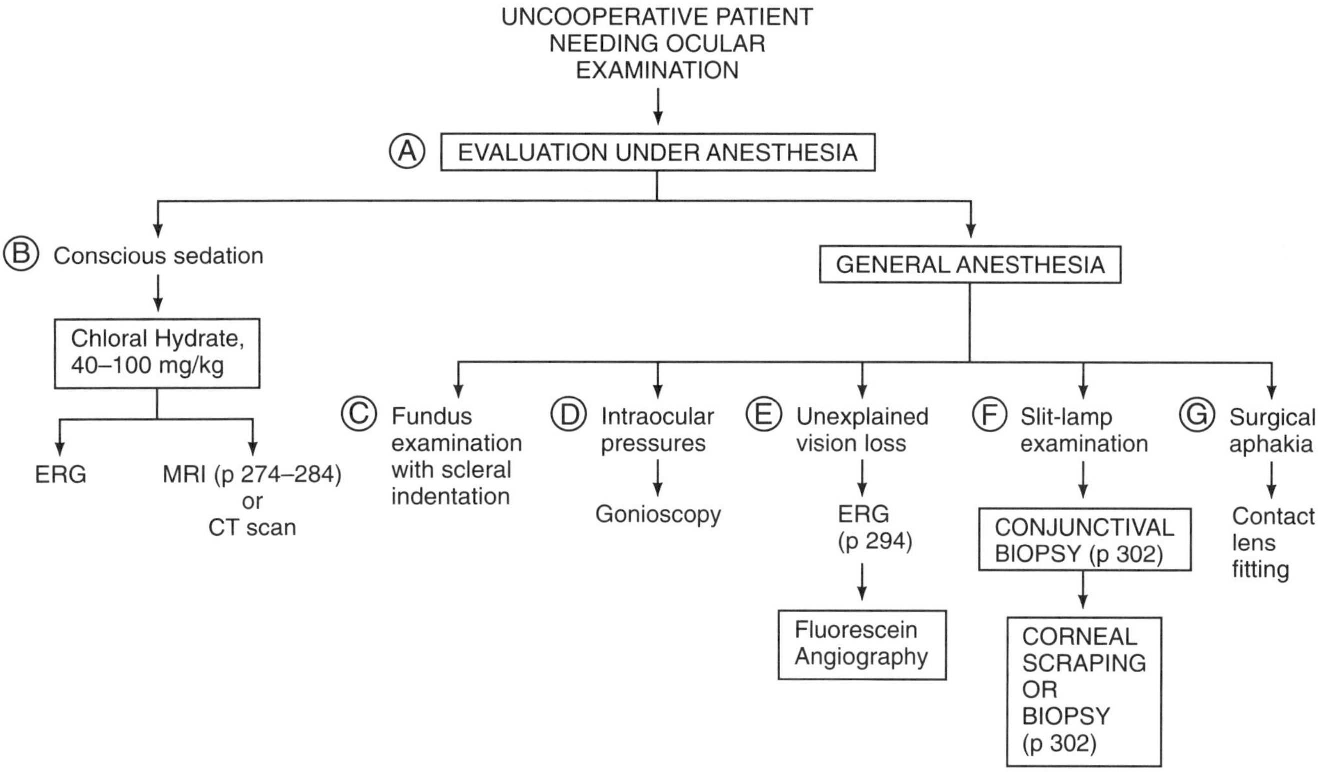
UNCOOPERATIVE PATIENT NEEDING OCULAR EXAMINATION
(A) EVALUATION UNDER ANESTHESIA
(B) Conscious sedation
Chloral Hydrate, 40–100 mg/kg
ERG
MRI (p 274–284) or CT scan
GENERAL ANESTHESIA
(C) Fundus examination with scleral indentation
(D) Intraocular pressures
Gonioscopy
(E) Unexplained vision loss
ERG (p 294)
Fluorescein Angiography
(F) Slit-lamp examination
CONJUNCTIVAL BIOPSY (p 302)
CORNEAL SCRAPING OR BIOPSY (p 302)
(G) Surgical aphakia
Contact lens fitting

INFANTILE GLAUCOMA

Gerhard W. Cibis, M.D.

A. Infantile glaucoma is a general term often used interchangeably with developmental glaucoma, primary congenital glaucoma, and glaucoma of any cause at an early age. Forty-five percent of patients have associated developmental defects, usually anterior segment dysgenesis (see p 140). A history of a glaucoma-associated syndrome such as Sturge-Weber, Rieger, or Lowe's syndrome is important in that glaucoma needs to be ruled out in such patients. This type of glaucoma is called developmental. Primary congenital glaucoma displays a developmental abnormality of the anterior chamber, but it is not consistently associated with systemic or other ocular anomalies. The condition is believed to have a genetic basis. Secondary glaucoma occurs with retrolental fibroplasia, retinoblastoma, juvenile xanthogranuloma, keratouveitis, intraocular surgery, and trauma. Characteristic clinical findings may include photophobia, buphthalmos, epiphora, corneal clouding, and blepharospasm. At other times, glaucoma needs to be suspected simply on the basis of associated systemic or ocular abnormalities.

B. Examination in the office may rule out glaucoma without resorting to anesthesia. If there is no buphthalmos or glaucoma-associated syndrome, it may be avoided by proving that pressures are normal. Applanation tensions can be performed in an awake infant kept hungry and fed at the time of the test. Infant intraocular pressures are lower than those of adults, around 10 mm Hg. Anesthesia lowers the pressure variably, depending on stage of anesthesia and time anesthetized. One should measure tensions as soon as the child is intubated for most consistent results. If the condition is unilateral, comparison of right to left eye is helpful. Both pressures may be below 20, but the difference is significant.

C. Photophobia and epiphora can occur before buphthalmos or clinically apparent clouding. Photophobia is a common nonspecific finding in children with many different disorders (see p 86).

D. The neonatal cornea averages 10 to 10.5 mm and grows by 0.5 to 1 mm in the first year. Vertical and horizontal diameters differ, and both should be measured. Haab's striae with borderline buphthalmos establish the diagnosis if forceps injury has been ruled out. Megalocornea is a rare condition in which both corneas exceed 13 mm in horizontal diameter with no other associated anomaly.

E. By itself, epiphora is usually due to causes other than glaucoma.

F. The microscope, preferably with slit attachment, is needed to evaluate the cloudy cornea and determine the level of the clouding. Epithelial edema comes first, and the stroma is involved only in long-standing pressure elevation.

G. True epithelial edema has bullae and clears with pressure, glycerine, scraping off the epithelium, or lowering intraocular pressure by medication. This helps to differentiate it from other types of epithelial clouding. Short-term use of Timoptic or Diamox is appropriate to clear the corneal clouding for diagnostic purposes, to control pressure until surgery can be arranged, or to be able to perform goniotomy. Long-term medical therapy alone is not. Surgery is the treatment of choice for infantile glaucoma. Medications may be used following surgery. Pupillary constricting medications are ineffective in congenital glaucoma because of the insertion of the ciliary muscle onto the trabeculum rather than the scleral spur.

H. Cupping and axial length are reversible in congenital glaucoma and help to follow pressure regulation. These measurements should be made on first and follow-up examinations.

I. The chamber angle can be normal in developmental glaucoma, for example with Sturge-Weber or rubella syndrome. In congenital glaucoma there are typical changes of high iris insertion on the trabecular meshwork, a thickened meshwork (Barkan's membrane), and iris strands, or the angle may be normal. If other signs such as buphthalmos and/or pressure elevation exist, surgery is indicated even with a normal-appearing angle. Conversely, a glaucomatous chamber angle alone without pressure rise is no reason to do glaucoma surgery: 40% of the Lowe's syndrome patients do not manifest glaucoma until 6 years of age, although all Lowe's syndrome patients have anomalous chamber angles.

J. If pressure elevation is not dramatic enough and other findings are borderline, simply repeat the evaluation under anesthesia (EUA) 1 to 3 months later depending on how likely or unlikely you think glaucoma to be, and remeasure pressure, cupping, and axial length. With relatively low pressure elevation or right-left eye difference, when one eye is clearly normal, and these parameters change, surgery is indicated. In glaucoma-associated cases with an anomalous chamber angle, repeat the EUA in 6 months or 1 year, then yearly until pressures can be taken in the office. See the patient clinically in the interval to look for signs of change that indicate glaucoma; if they are present, do an EUA earlier. Use the same parameters for post-surgery status checks, usually 1 month after surgery and then at 3-month intervals and longer if pressure and other findings are stable.

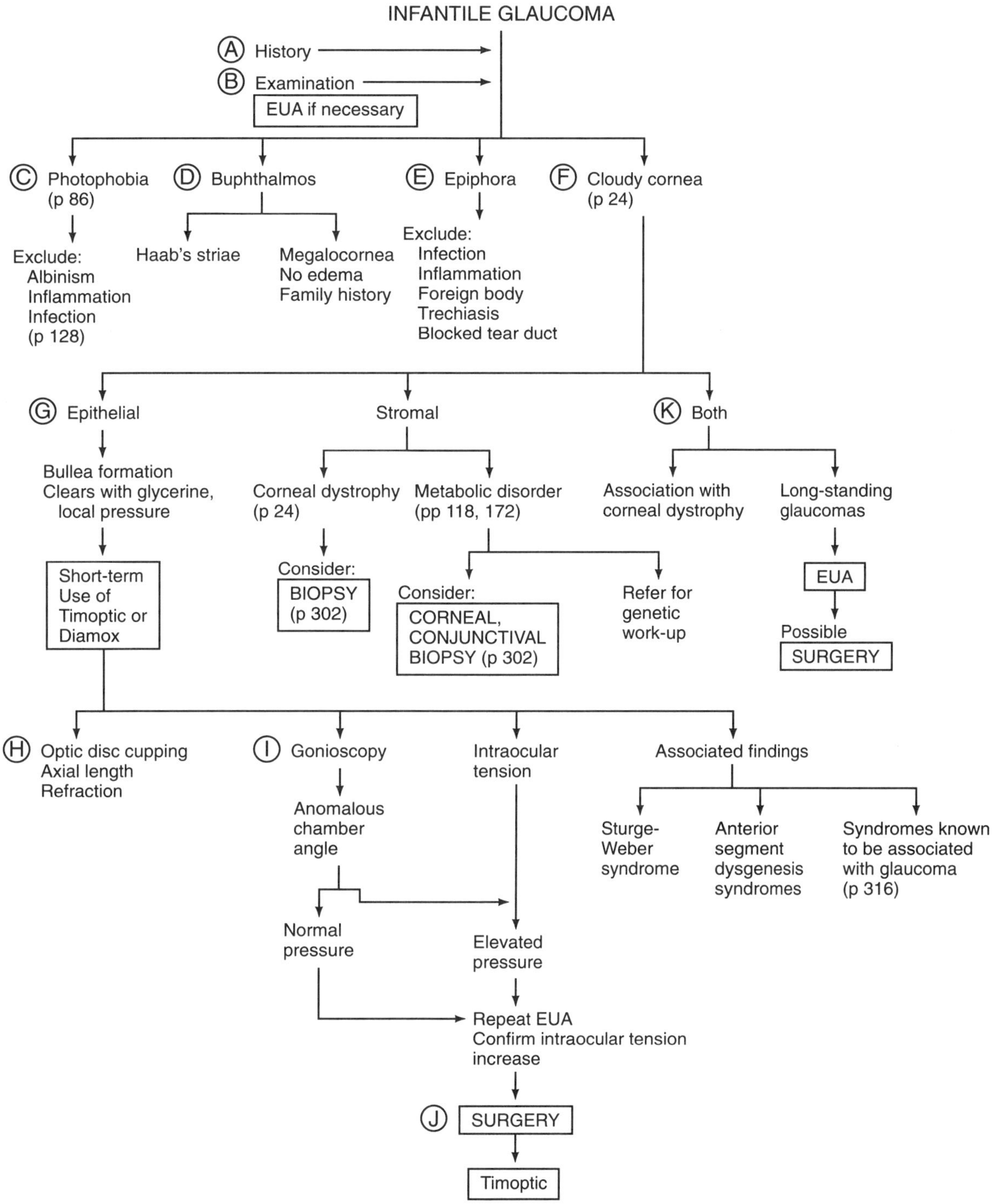

K. Corneal dystrophies (see p 20) such as congenital hereditary endothelial dystrophy (CHED) can be associated with congenital glaucoma. CHED can have epithelial edema on the basis of poor or no endothelium with normal pressure. Lack of buphthalmos differentiates them, but both can be present in the same eye.

References

Cibis GW. Congenital glaucoma. J Am Opt Assoc 1987; 58:728.

Cibis GW, Tripathi RC. The differential diagnosis of Descemet's tears (Haab's striae) and posterior polymorphous dystrophy bands. Ophthalmology 1982; 89:613.

Dickens CJ, Hoskins HD. Diagnosis and treatment of congenital glaucoma. In: Ritch R, Shields MB, Krupin T, eds. The glaucomas. St. Louis: CV Mosby, 1989:773.

Hoyt C, Lambert S. Childhood glaucoma. In: Taylor D, ed. Pediatric ophthalmology. Boston: Blackwell Scientific, 1990:319.

Waring GO, Rodriqueza MM, Laiabson PR. Anterior chamber cleavage syndrome: A stepladder classification. Surv Ophthalmol 1975; 20:3.

JUVENILE-ONSET GLAUCOMA INCLUDING APHAKIA

John R. Samples, M.D.

A. When glaucoma becomes apparent in later childhood or early adulthood, it is often termed juvenile glaucoma. The eye stops lengthening in response to elevated intraocular pressure (IOP) at 3 years of age, so that age is often taken as the division between infantile and juvenile glaucoma. Some glaucomatologists apply the term *juvenile glaucoma* to all open-angle glaucomas occurring in young adulthood.

B. Juvenile-onset glaucoma indicates a dysfunctional trabecular meshwork. This may be on a developmental embryologic basis, as in late-onset glaucoma in Lowe's syndrome, or on the basis of the trabecular meshwork becoming abnormal with time. Examples are the senile meshwork changes reported in some cases of Sturge-Weber syndrome (p 138) and the accumulation of mucopolysaccharides in the meshwork of patients with mucopolysaccharidoses.

C. Secondary angle closure is also a cause of juvenile glaucoma. Post-inflammatory synechiae occur with cataract surgery or uveitis. Late-onset open-angle glaucoma occurs in syndromes associated with glaucoma, such as Sturge-Weber syndrome.

D. Aphakic glaucomas include both open-angle aphakic glaucoma and angle-closure glaucoma secondary to synechiae and are probably underappreciated. *Monitoring of IOP and the appearance of the optic nerve at yearly intervals in all pediatric patients who have undergone cataract extraction is advisable.*

E. IOPs may be elevated. In children over the age of 3 years, it is often possible to measure the IOP with a hand-held applanation tonometer. If co-operation is lacking, an examination under general anesthesia (EUA) or with chloral hydrate may be undertaken.

F. Time and patience help many children successfully complete visual field testing. It may help to test only one eye at a time and to give frequent breaks and substantial encouragement. Some children perform well on perimetry examinations using the Humphrey test. New, fast perimetry strategies like the Humphrey fastpack may be especially useful.

G. Diagnosis of juvenile glaucoma is often based on the appearance of the optic nerve. Children often tolerate increased IOP better than adults without developing cupping. Observation at frequent intervals may help to better establish the diagnosis. Frequency of observation must be based on risk factors and physical findings.

H. Juvenile open-angle glaucomas may be treated with medications, depending upon the age of the patient and side effects of the antiglaucoma agents selected. Beta blockers may be used with good results. However, it is important to monitor carefully for toxicity because the literature indicates that very high blood levels may be achieved. Parents should use punctal occlusion to limit the systemic absorption of these medications. The pediatrician should be notified that a beta blocker is being used, and parents should be cautioned to observe the child for unexplained cough or decreased exercise tolerance. Beta blockers should not be used in patients with asthma. A cardioselective beta blocker like betaxolol may offer some advantages in pediatric use.

Miotics like pilocarpine and carbachol are poorly tolerated. However, such medication is traditionally used after goniotomy and may be of value in lowering the pressure. Local side effects may include eye irritation and brow ache. Epinephrine-containing drugs are generally not used because of their limited potency. Carbonic anhydrase inhibitors may successfully lower IOP. Parents need to be informed about the possible systemic side effects, including kidney stones and potentially life-threatening bone marrow aplasia. These drugs should not be used if there is a history of sulfa allergy. A complete blood count prior to their use, at 2 months after they are initiated, and again at 6 months is advised. Such blood tests seem logical in children in whom obtaining an accurate history is more difficult. Topical carbonic anhydrase inhibitors may be very useful in treating pediatric patients. All antiglaucoma medications have significant side effects, and the decision to treat needs to be weighed carefully against that possibility.

I. Decisions regarding surgical treatment must depend in part on the visual potential of the eye, how well the patient has tolerated medication, and an assessment of postoperative compliance.

J. Laser trabeculoplasty has no place in the management of pediatric aphakic glaucoma. Pupillary block may be effectively treated with laser iridotomy. YAG laser goniotomy has been reported to be successful.

K. Cyclocryotherapy has been a traditional treatment for pediatric aphakic glaucoma. It carries a significant risk of phthisis and is painful. Laser cyclophotocoagulation is less painful and carries less risk of phthisis but may require more repeat treatments. The inflammatory response induced by laser cyclodestructive procedures generally seems to be less than that seen with cyclocryotherapy.

L. Traditional filtering surgery has not been successful in pediatric patients. However, this is changing with reports on the adjunctive use of 5-fluorouracil and mitomycin-C. These drugs are not approved for use in pediatric patients, and it is especially important that full consent be obtained prior to their use.

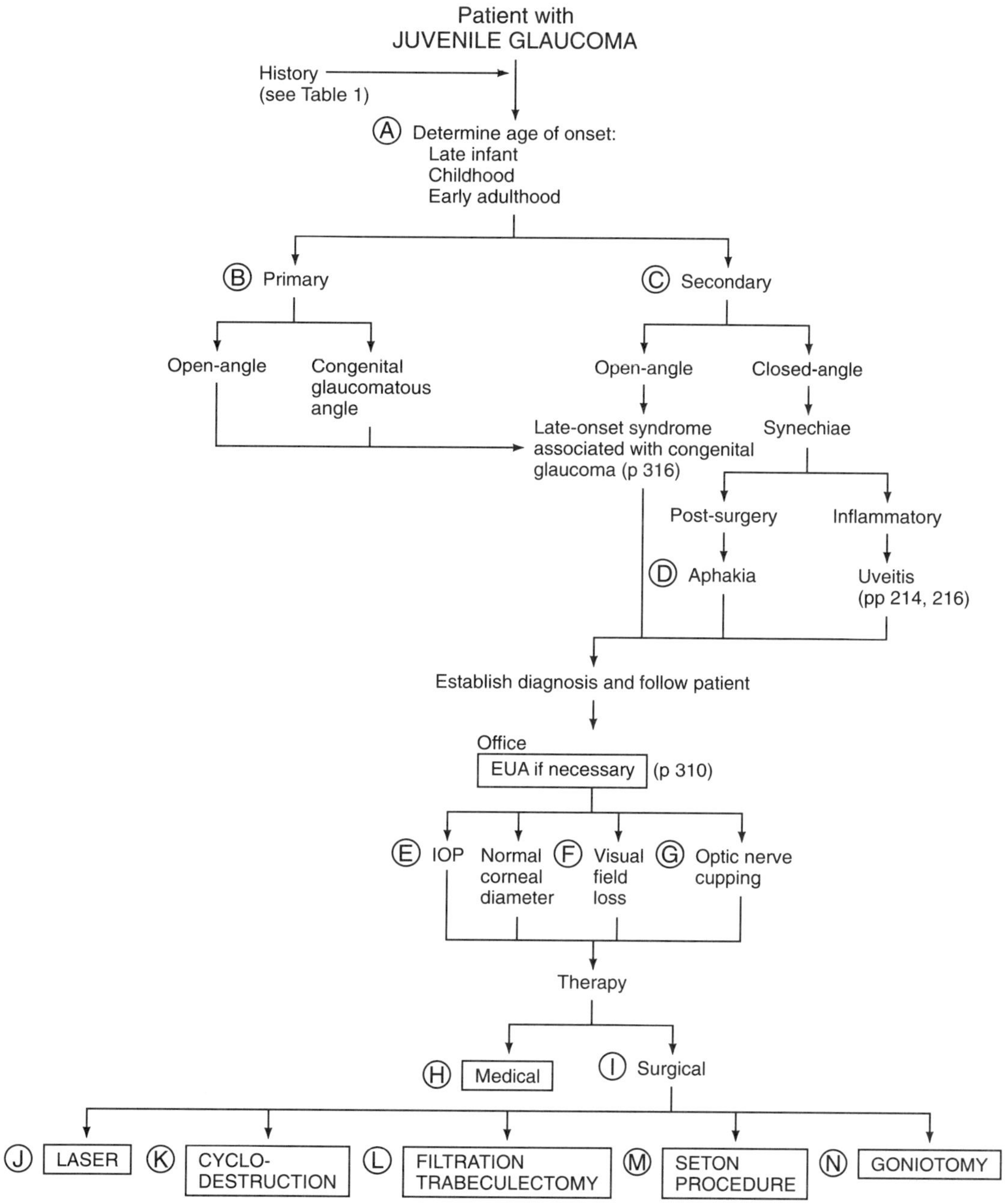

M. Seton procedures can be very effective but are fraught with complications. An ophthalmologist electing to perform these procedures should either have significant experience with them in adults before employing them in children or have extensive pediatric glaucoma surgical experience.

N. Goniotomy ab interno is done with a knife extended across the chamber to the opposite angle to incise it for 2 to 4 clock hours. Goniotomy ab externo (trabeculotomy) introduces a probe into Schlemm's canal from the scleral site. Usually a scleral flap is made as with a trabeculectomy. If the canal cannot be found, as commonly happens in congenital glaucoma from anatomic malformation, conversion to a trabeculectomy can readily be done intraoperatively with this approach.

TABLE 1 Glaucoma Risk Factors

Family history of glaucoma
Diabetes
Race
Myopia
Family history of glaucoma-associated syndrome
Steroid use

References

Cibis GW. Congenital glaucoma. J Am Opt Assoc 1987; 58:728.

Kwitko ML. Glaucomas in infants and children. New York: Appleton-Century-Crofts, 1973:185.

CONDITIONS ASSOCIATED WITH CHILDHOOD GLAUCOMA

Gerhard W. Cibis, M.D.

A. The history or suspicion of a congenital syndrome should alert one to the possibility of glaucoma. Appropriate examination and supervision of such patients to look for development of glaucoma are critical. After the age of 3 years, the globe fails to enlarge with increased intraocular pressure, and buphthalmos is therefore not a reliable sign in older children who have conditions making them susceptible to glaucoma. Careful examination of the cornea for clouding, intraocular tension measurement, and optic disc observation for signs of glaucomatous damage are important.

B. Inflammation from whatever cause can result in synechiae formation or pupillary block glaucoma. With retinopathy of prematurity (ROP) and persistent primary hyperplastic vitreous (PPHV), the retrolental mass pushes the iris lens diaphragm forward, occluding the chamber angle. For PPHV, prophylactic peripheral iridectomy is advocated. For ROP, lensectomy may make enough room to avoid angle occlusion. In both cases vision is usually poor and surgery is done to avoid pain and enucleation.

Glaucoma with juvenile xanthogranulomatosis is caused by tumor cells occluding the chamber angle. Spontaneous hyphema also occurs. Radiation dissolves the lesion and can save the eye. A similar mechanism can account for examples of glaucoma with retinoblastoma in which tumor cells block the chamber angle and rubeosis of the iris occurs. The tumor can mechanically narrow the chamber angle as well. Intraocular surgery is contraindicated. With Coats' disease an exudative retinal detachment and anterior chamber inflammation and infiltration with cholesterol crystals occur. Autoimmune disorders leading to uveitis are usually associated with low intraocular pressure. Lens iris synechiae can result in pupillary block glaucoma. Peripheral synechiae cause angle-closure glaucoma. Proper anti-inflammatory medications such as steroids can induce glaucoma in genetically susceptible individuals.

C. Pigmentary glaucoma is usually seen in young myopic males. As in the adult version, Krukenberg spindle is present. Pigment clogs the chamber angle and is visible on gonioscopy. There is iris transillumination.

D. Surgical and nonintentional trauma can induce glaucoma. With hyphema the blood can clog the chamber angle. Treatment is medical and surgical if pressure cannot be controlled conservatively. Surgically induced glaucoma, usually in aphakia, results from damage to the chamber angle with synechiae formation. Chronic inflammation also plays a role. Again, because of lack of enlargement of the globe from elevated pressures after age 3, the slow development of the pressure rise, and the difficulty of taking pressures in children, such cases are often missed or diagnosis is inordinately delayed. Regular monitoring of pressures and optic nerves in post-cataract cases is crucial. Pupillary block from vitreous incarceration in the pupil is another mechanism for aphakic glaucoma. Several mechanisms may occur simultaneously and need to be considered for proper therapy.

E. Genetic conditions with known association to glaucoma are listed. Most of these have anomalous chamber angles. Some such as Marfan's syndrome can have glaucoma from several mechanisms. Not all patients with any syndrome develop glaucoma. Only about half of Lowe's syndrome cases develop it, but all have cataracts. With aniridia the iris stump closes off the chamber angle. Glaucoma occurs usually between 5 and 10 years of age. Some advocate prophylactic iridectomies. Filtering surgery in Sturge-Weber and Klippel-Trenaunay syndromes can be complicated by expulsive hemorrhage (p 138).

F. Two mechanisms exist in subluxated lenses: angle closure from the lens pushing the iris forward or from actual displacement of the lens into the anterior chamber. The latter mechanism is more common with microspherophakia, as occurs in the Weill-Marchesani and Conradi syndromes.

References

Cibis GW. Congenital glaucoma. J Am Opt Assoc 1987; 58:728.

Cibis GW, Tripathi RC, Tripathi BJ. Glaucoma in Sturge-Weber syndrome. Ophthalmology 1984; 91:1061.

Dickens CJ, Hoskins HD. Epidemiology and pathophysiology of congenital glaucoma. In: Ritch R, Shields MB, Krupin T, eds. The glaucomas. St. Louis: CV Mosby, 1989:761.

Hoyt C, Lambert S. Childhood glaucoma. In: Taylor D, ed. Pediatric ophthalmology. Boston: Blackwell Scientific, 1990:319.

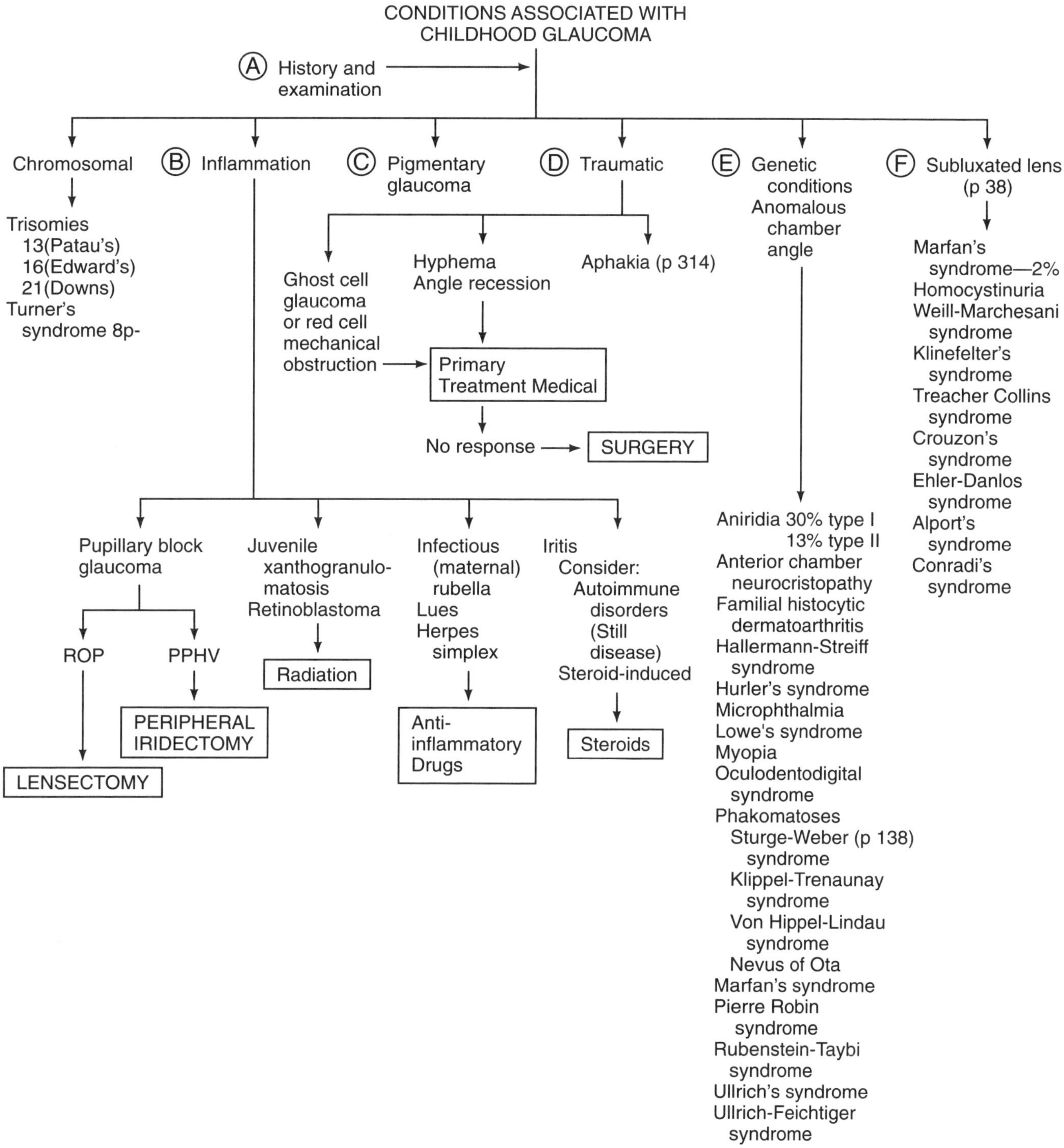
CONDITIONS ASSOCIATED WITH CHILDHOOD GLAUCOMA
(A) History and examination
Chromosomal
Trisomies 13(Patau's) 16(Edward's) 21(Downs)
Turner's syndrome 8p-
(B) Inflammation
Pupillary block glaucoma
ROP
LENSECTOMY
PPHV
PERIPHERAL IRIDECTOMY
Juvenile xanthogranulomatosis
Retinoblastoma
Radiation
Infectious (maternal) rubella
Lues
Herpes simplex
Anti-inflammatory Drugs
Iritis
Consider: Autoimmune disorders (Still disease)
Steroid-induced
Steroids
(C) Pigmentary glaucoma
(D) Traumatic
Ghost cell glaucoma or red cell mechanical obstruction
Hyphema
Angle recession
Aphakia (p 314)
Primary Treatment Medical
No response
SURGERY
(E) Genetic conditions
Anomalous chamber angle
Aniridia 30% type I
13% type II
Anterior chamber neurocristopathy
Familial histocytic dermatoarthritis
Hallermann-Streiff syndrome
Hurler's syndrome
Microphthalmia
Lowe's syndrome
Myopia
Oculodentodigital syndrome
Phakomatoses
Sturge-Weber (p 138) syndrome
Klippel-Trenaunay syndrome
Von Hippel-Lindau syndrome
Nevus of Ota
Marfan's syndrome
Pierre Robin syndrome
Rubenstein-Taybi syndrome
Ullrich's syndrome
Ullrich-Feichtiger syndrome
(F) Subluxated lens (p 38)
Marfan's syndrome—2%
Homocystinuria
Weill-Marchesani syndrome
Klinefelter's syndrome
Treacher Collins syndrome
Crouzon's syndrome
Ehler-Danlos syndrome
Alport's syndrome
Conradi's syndrome

INDEX

t indicates table
f indicates figure

C

F

G

H

R

S

W

X

Y

Z